Lecture Notes in Computer Science 5889

Commenced Publication in 1973
Founding and Former Series Editors:
Gerhard Goos, Juris Hartmanis, and Jan van Leeuwen

Andreas Holzinger   Klaus Miesenberger (Eds.)

HCI and Usability
for e-Inclusion

5th Symposium of the Workgroup
Human-Computer Interaction and Usability Engineering
of the Austrian Computer Society, USAB 2009
Linz, Austria, November 9-10, 2009
Proceedings

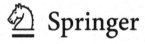 Springer

Volume Editors

Andreas Holzinger
Medical University of Graz (MUG)
Research Unit HCI4MED
Institute for Medical Informatics,
Statistics and Documentation (IMI)
Auenbruggerplatz 2/V, 8036, Graz, Austria
E-mail: a.holzinger@tugraz.at

Klaus Miesenberger
University of Linz
Institut Integriert Studieren
Altenbergerstraße 49, 4040, Linz, Austria
E-mail: klaus.miesenberger@jku.at

Library of Congress Control Number: 2009938712

CR Subject Classification (1998): H.5, D.2, J.3, J.4

LNCS Sublibrary: SL 2 – Programming and Software Engineering

ISSN   0302-9743
ISBN-10   3-642-10307-3 Springer Berlin Heidelberg New York
ISBN-13   978-3-642-10307-0 Springer Berlin Heidelberg New York

springer.com

© Springer-Verlag Berlin Heidelberg 2009
Printed in Germany

Typesetting: Camera-ready by author, data conversion by Scientific Publishing Services, Chennai, India
Printed on acid-free paper   SPIN: 12794980   06/3180   5 4 3 2 1 0

Preface

The Workgroup Human–Computer Interaction & Usability Engineering (Arbeitskreis HCI&UE) of the Austrian Computer Society (Österreichische Computer Gesellschaft, OCG) has been serving as a platform for interdisciplinary exchange, research and development since February 2005. While human–computer interaction (HCI) traditionally brings psychologists and computer scientists together, the inclusion of usability engineering (UE), which is a software engineering discipline and ensures the appropriate implementation of applications, has become indispensable.

Our 2009 topic was therefore Human–Computer Interaction & Usability for e-Inclusion (HCI4e-I), culminating in the 5th annual Usability Symposium USAB 2009 held during November 9–10, 2009 in Linz, Austria (http://usab.icchp.org), organized together with the Workgroup Information Technology for People with Special Needs (OCG Arbeitskreis IT für Menschen mit besonderen Bedürfnissen).

The term e-inclusion, also known as digital inclusion, is used within the European Union to encompass all activities related to the achievement of an inclusive information society.

New information technologies always bring the risk of a digital divide, and consequently e-Inclusion wants to put emphasis on a digital cohesion and on enhancing opportunities with IT into all segments of the European population, including disadvantaged people, e.g., due to lack of education (e-Competences, e-Learning), age (e-Ageing), gender apartheid (equality=e-Quality), disabilities (e-Accessibility), ill health (e-Health) etc. At the European level, e-Inclusion is part of the third pillar of the 2010 policy initiative, managed by the Directorate General for Information Society and Media of the European Commission.

We are convinced that the solution to these challenges can be found at the intersection of the disciplines pedagogy, psychology and computer science (informatics).

The interface of this trinity encompasses thinking, concepts and methods from the humanities, from natural science and from engineering science. Engineering science carries the most responsibility and ethical demands since engineers are the ones who ensure the appropriate development.

The daily actions of the end users must be the central concern, supporting them with newly available and rapidly emerging, ubiquitous and pervasive technologies.

Obviously, an interdisciplinary view produces specific problems. On the one hand government, universities and industry require interdisciplinary work. However, younger researchers especially, being new to their field and not yet firmly anchored in one single discipline, are still in danger of "falling between two seats."

It is certainly easier for researchers to gain depth and acknowledgement in a narrow scientific community by remaining within one single field. Everybody accepts the necessity for interdisciplinary work; however, it is difficult to gain honor.

We are of the firm opinion that innovation and new insights often take place at the junction of two or more disciplines; consequently, this requires a much broader basis of knowledge, openness for other fields and more acceptance.

This is challenging, but also laborious, because working in any interdisciplinary area necessitates the ability to communicate with professionals in other disciplines and most of all a high willingness to accept and incorporate their points of view.

USAB 2009 was again organized in order to promote this closer collaboration between software engineers, psychology researchers and educational professionals.

USAB 2009 received a total of 60 submissions. We followed a careful and rigorous two-level, double-blind review process, assigning each paper to a minimum of three and maximum of six reviewers. On the basis of the reviewers' results, 12 full papers (> 14 pages) and 26 short papers were accepted.

USAB 2009 can be seen as a bridge within the scientific community, between computer science, psychology and education.

Everybody who gathered together to work for this symposium displayed great enthusiasm and dedication.

We cordially thank each and every person who contributed toward making USAB 2009 a big success, for their participation and commitment: the authors, reviewers, sponsors, organizations, supporters, all of the organization team, and all the volunteers, without whose help this bridge would never have been built.

November 2009   Andreas Holzinger
                                                 Klaus Miesenberger

Organization

Programme Chairs

Andreas Holzinger   Medical University Graz & Graz University of Technology, Austria

Klaus Miesenberger   University of Linz, Austria

Programme Committee

(in alphabetical order)

Patricia A. Abbot	Johns Hopkins University, USA
Ray Adams	Middlesex University London, UK
Dominique Archambault	Université Pierre et Marie Curie, France
Sheikh Iqbal Ahamed	Marquette University, USA
Henning Andersen	Risoe National Laboratory, Denmark
Keith Andrews	Graz University of Technology, Austria
Sue Bogner	Institute of Human Error, LLC Bethesda, USA
† Noelle Carbonell	Universite Henri Poincare Nancy, France (died on April 11, 2009)
Tiziana Catarci	Universita di Roma La Sapienza, Italy
Luca Chittaro	University of Udine, Italy
David Crombie	Utrecht School of the Arts, The Netherlands
Matjaz Debevc	University of Maribor, Slovenia
Alan Dix	Lancaster University, UK
Judy Edworthy	University of Plymouth, UK
Peter L. Elkin	Mayo Clinic, Rochester, USA
Jan Engelen	Katholieke Universiteit Leuven, Belgium
Daryle Gardner-Bonneau	Western Michigan University, USA
Andrina Granic	University of Split, Croatia
Eduard Groeller	Vienna University of Technology, Austria
Sissel Guttormsen	University Bern, China
Martin Hitz	Klagenfurt University, Austria
Timo Honkela	Helsinki University of Technology, Finland
Ebba P. Hvannberg	University of Iceland, Reykjavik, Iceland
Julie Jacko	Georgia Institute of Technology, USA
Chris Johnson	University of Glasgow, UK
Anirudha N. Joshi	Indian Institute of Technology, Bombay, India
Georgios Kouroupetroglou	University of Athens, Greece
Denise Leahy	Trinity College Dublin, Ireland
Erik Liljegren	Chalmers Technical University, Sweden
Zhengjie Liu	Dalian Maritime University, China
Silvia Miksch	Donau University Krems, Austria

Lisa Neal   Tufts University School of Medicine Boston, USA
Alexander Nischelwitzer   University of Applied Sciences Graz, Austria
Shogo Nishida   Osaka University, Japan
Hiromu Nishitani   University of Tokushima, Japan
Nuno J Nunes   University of Madeira, PT
Anne-Sophie Nyssen   Université de Liege, Belgium
Erika Orrick   GE Healthcare, Carrollton, USA
Philipe Palanque   Université Toulouse, France
Helen Petrie   University of York, UK
Margit Pohl   Vienna University of Technology, Austria
Robert W. Proctor   Purdue University, USA
Harald Reiterer   University of Konstanz, Germany
Anxo C. Roibas   University of Brighton, UK
Anthony Savidis   ICS FORTH, Heraklion, Greece
Albrecht Schmidt   Fraunhofer IAIS/B-IT, Uni Bonn, Germany
Andrew Sears   UMBC, Baltimore, USA
Ahmed Seffah   EHL Lausanne, Switzerland
Katie A. Siek   University of Colorado at Boulder, USA
Cecília Sik Lanyi   University of Pannonia, Hungary
Daniel Simons   University of Illinois at Urbana Champaign, USA
Christian Stary   University of Linz, Austria
Constantine Stephanidis   ICS FORTH, Heraklion, Greece
Zoran Stjepanovic   University of Maribor, Slovenia
A Min TJOA   Vienna University of Technology, Austria
ManFranceed Tscheligi   University of Salzburg, Austria
Gerhard Weber   Technische Universität Dresden, Germany
Karl-Heinz Weidmann   FHV Dornbirn, Austria
William Wong   Middlesex University, London, UK
Panayiotis Zaphiris   City University London, UK
Jürgen Ziegler   Universität Duisburg Essen, Germany
Ping Zhang   Syracuse University, USA
Jiajie Zhang   University of Texas Health Science Center, USA

Organizing Committee

(in alphabetical order)
Eugen Mühlvenzl   Austrian Computer Society (OCG)
Christine Haas   Austrian Computer Society (OCG)
Andreas Holzinger   Austrian Computer Society (OCG)
Elisabeth Waldbauer   Austrian Computer Society (OCG)

Local Host

(in alphabetical order)
Barbara Arrer   University of Linz
Priska Feichtenschlager   University of Linz
Klaus Miesenberger   University of Linz

Roland Ossmann	University of Linz
Andrea Petz	University of Linz
Christian Schult	University of Linz

Members of the WG HCI&UE of the Austrian Computer Society

(in alphabetical order - status as of September 21, 2009, Total: 197)

Ackerl, Siegfried	Gorz, Karl
Albert, Dietrich	Graf, Sabine
Ahlstroem, David	Graf, Sylvia
Aigner, Wolfgang	Grechenig, Thomas
Andrews, Keith	Granic, Andrina
Auer, Michael	Grill, Thomas
Auinger, Andreas	Goldmann, Thomas
Baillie, Lynne	Groeller, Edi
Baumann, Konrad	Gross, Anne
Bärnthaler, Markus	Haas, Christine
Bechinie, Michael	Haas, Rainer
Behringer, Reinhold	Haberfellner, Tom
Bernert, Christa	Hable, Franz
Biffl, Stefan	Hacker, Maria
Binder, Georg	Hackl, Erich Patrick
Bloice, Marcus	Hailing, Mario
Breiteneder, Christian	Haug, Bernd
Brugger, Martin	Hauser, Helwig
Burgsteiner, Harald	Hellberg, Philip von
Christian, Johannes	Heimgärtner, Rüdiger
Dirnbauer, Kurt	Herget, Martin
Derndorfer, Christoph	Hitz, Martin
Debevc, Matjaz	Hoeller, Martin
Dorfinger, Johannes	Holzinger, Andreas
Ebner, Martin	Hruska, Andreas
Eckhard, Benedikt	Huber, Leonhard
Edelmann, Noelle	Hussain, Zahid
Ehrenstrasser, Lisa	Hyna, Irene
Erharter, Dorothea	Jaquemar, Stefan
Errath, Maximilian	Jarz, Thorsten
Ferro, Bernhard	Kainz, Regina
Figl, Kathrin	Keki, Susanne
Flieder, Karl	Kempter, Guido
Freund, Rudi	Kittl, Christian
Frühwirth, Christian	Kingsbury, Paul
Füricht, Reinhard	Kleinberger, Thomas
Geierhofer, Regina	Koller, Andreas
Geven, Ajan	Kotsis, Gabriele
Glavinic, Vlado	Költringer, Thomas

Kohler, Kirstin
Kreuzthaler, Markus
Kriglstein, Simone
Krieger, Horst
Kriegshaber, Ursula
Kroop, Sylvana
Kohler, Kirstin
Krümmling, Sabine
Kuenz, Andreas
Kment, Thomas
Lanyi, Cecilia
Leeb, Christian
Lenhardt, Stephan
Lugmayer, Arturri
Luneski, Andrej
Loidl, Susanne
Leitner, Gerhard
Leitner, Hubert
Linder, Jörg
Maier, Edith
Maitland, Julie
Makolm, Josef
Mangold, Pascal
Manhartsberger, Martina
Mayr, Stefan
Meisenberger, Matthias
Melcher, Rudolf
Messner, Peter
Miksch, Siliva
Miesenberger, Klaus
Mittenecker, Georg
Motschig-Pitrik, Renate
Musil, Sabine
Müller, Regine
Mutz, Uwe
Nedbal, Dietmar
Nemecek, Sascha
Nischelwitzer, Alexander
Nowak, Greta
Otjacques, Benoît
Oppitz, Marcus
Osterbauer, Christian
Parvu, Andrej
Pellegrini, Tassilo
Peischl, Bernd
Pesendorfer, Florian
Pohl, Margit

Purgathofer, Peter
Rauhala, Marjo
Ramkinson, Arun
Reichl, Peter
Richter, Elisabeth
Richter, Helene
Riener, Andreas
Robier, Hannes
Safran, Christian
Sahanek, Christian
Schaupp, Klaus
Scheugl, Max
Schloegl, Martin
Schreier, Günther
Schwaberger, Klaus
Schwantzer, Gerold
Searle, Gig W.
Sefelin, Reinhard
Seibert-Giller, Verena
Seyff, Norbert
Simonic, Klaus-Martin
Slany, Wolfgang
Sorantin, Erich
Sorantin, Felix
Spangl, Jürgen
Sproger, Bernd
Stanglmayer, Klaus
Stary, Christian
Stenitzer, Michael
Stickel, Christian
Stjepanovic, Zoran
Stiebellehner, Johann
Thümer, Herbert
Thurnher, Bettina
Tjoa, A Min
Tscheligi, Manfred
Urlesberger, Berndt
Vecsei, Thomas
Vogler, Robert
Waclick, Olivia
Wagner, Christian
Wagner, Claudia
Wahlmüller, Christine
Wally, Bernhard
Wassertheurer, Sigi
Weidmann, Karl-Heinz
Weippl, Edgar

Werthner, Hannes
Wimmer, Erhard
Windlinger, Lukas
Wöber, Willi
Wöber, Willi
Wolkerstorfer, Peter
Wotawa, Franz

Wohlkinger, Bernd
Wolkersdorfer, Peter
Zagler, Wolfgang
Zellhofer, Norbert
Ziefle, Martina
Zorn-Pauli, Gabriele

Sponsors

We are grateful to the companies, institutions and organizations for their support in our aims to bridge science and industry. Their logos are displayed at: http://usab.icchp.org/

Table of Contents

Usability Testing, Evaluation, Measurement: Education, Learning and e-Inclusion

Special Session: Design for Adaptive Content Processing

Heuristics and Theory Based Research: Grounded Theory, Activity Theory and Situated Action

Special Session: Smart Home, Health and Ambient Assisted Living

User Centred Design and Usability Practice: Showcases and Surveys

Applications and Analyses: Interaction, Assistive Technologies and Virtual Environments

Analyses and Investigations: Communication, Interfaces and Haptic Technology

Closing: New Technologies and Challenges for People with Disabilities

The Changing Face of Human-Computer Interaction in the Age of Ubiquitous Computing

Yvonne Rogers

Pervasive Interaction Lab,
Open University, Milton Keynes,
MK7 6AA, UK
y.rogers@open.ac.uk

Abstract. HCI is reinventing itself. No longer only about being user-centered, it has set its sights on pastures new, embracing a much broader and far-reaching set of interests. From emotional, eco-friendly, embodied experiences to context, constructivism and culture, HCI research is changing apace: from what it looks at, the lenses it uses and what it has to offer. Part of this is as a reaction to what is happening in the world; ubiquitous technologies are proliferating and transforming how we live our lives. We are becoming more connected and more dependent on technology. The home, the crèche, outdoors, public places and even the human body are now being experimented with as potential places to embed computational devices, even to the extent of invading previously private and taboo aspects of our lives. In this paper, I examine the diversity of lifestyle and technological transformations in our midst and outline some 'difficult' questions these raise together with alternative directions for HCI research and practice.

Keywords: Human–Computer Interaction, Ubiquitous Computing, Pervasive Technology, Methods, Human Values, Research Agenda, Future Technologies.

1 Introduction

Our world is becoming suffused with technologies that have the potential to profoundly change how we live. Computers now intrude on our lives as well as disappear into the world around us; they monitor as well as guide us; and they coerce as well as aid us. They are increasingly becoming part of our environments, in public spaces such as airports, garages, and shopping malls as well as in the private spaces of our homes and offices. As part of this transformation, our minds are extending more into the world. It is commonplace for people to use online calendars to remind them to send a birthday card to a friend and Google information on their mobile during ongoing conversations at dinner parties. People who own an iPhone are noticing how it is taking over more and more brain functions, increasingly replacing and augmenting parts of their memory, such as storing addresses and numbers that once would have required cognitive effort to recall [1]. Car Sat-Nav (GPS) systems have also replaced map reading; drivers can now follow simple instructions reducing the cognitive effort that was needed to work out the best route.

A. Holzinger and K. Miesenberger (Eds.): USAB 2009, LNCS 5889, pp. 1–19, 2009.
© Springer-Verlag Berlin Heidelberg 2009

At the same time affordable computing devices, especially mobile phones, have become more accessible across the globe. More people than ever are using a computing device of one form or other, be they a retiree in Austria, a schoolchild in Africa or a farmer in Ecuador. The way children learn is also changing as more and more technologies are assimilated into their lives [2]. For example, how it happens (e.g., taking part in a discussion with people from all over the world on Second Life) and when it happens (e.g. listening to a podcast about pollution while cycling home) is diversifying. The number of elderly people is increasing as a proportion of the total population. Those growing old in the next ten years will have become accustomed to using computers and mobile phones in their work and leisure. Hence, the need to design computer applications for old people who have not used email or the Web will no longer be a major concern but designing social network sites, creative tools, etc., for healthy, active seventy year olds will.

Technological developments, therefore, are not only altering the way we grow up and grow old, but pervading almost every aspect of our lives, from shopping to medicine, increasing our reliance on them. We are spending more time, and devoting more effort to being in touch with each other than ever before. Our unbridled desire to keep in touch is equaled by our desire to capture more information about our lives and our doings than ever before. What it means to record, why we record and what we do with the collected materials is also changing. This is happening not just at a personal level, but also at the level of government, institutions and agencies.

What do all these changes mean for the field of Human-Computer Interaction and those who research 'user experiences' and practice 'UX design'? In an effort to keep abreast, HCI research is also changing apace: from what it looks at, the lenses it uses and what it has to offer. No longer only about being user-centered, it has set its sights on pastures new, embracing a much broader and far-reaching set of interests. From emotional, eco-friendly, embodied experiences to context, constructivism and culture. Its mission, purpose, goals and methodologies, that were well established in the 80s, have all greatly expanded to the point that "HCI is now effectively a boundless domain" [3] and is "bursting at the seams" [4]. Everything is in a state of flux: the theory driving the research is changing, a flurry of new concepts are emerging, the domains and type of users being studied are diversifying, many of the ways of doing design are new and much of what is being designed is significantly different. What was originally a confined problem space with a clear focus that adopted a small set of methods to tackle it – that of designing computer systems to make them more easy and efficient to use by a single user – is now turning into a more diffuse problem space with a less clear purpose as to what to study, what to design for and which methods to use.

Much is to be gained from this rapid expansion. A danger, however, is that the field may spiral out of control [5] and lose its identity [6]. The trivial and the serious may sit side-by-side and where everything and anything is potentially a topic for HCI. While 'living without parental controls' [7] can be liberating and inevitable in a rapidly transforming society, the questions HCI researchers ask, the purpose of their endeavors and the motivation behind them need continued scrutiny, debate and reflection, if their outputs are to continue to be of relevance and value to society. Part of this will entail setting new agendas; determining what to throw out and what new topics and concerns to focus on. Even its very core – prescribing usability, i.e., how to design 'easy-to-use' tools – needs rethinking since *using* technology in its various manifestations, is second nature to most people and hence unproblematic. The classic interface horror stories, such as the flashing VCR, are being superseded by more pressing matters that face society in the 21st century, such as how pervasive technologies are intruding and extending our physical bodies, cognitive minds and social lives. These are the concerns that the HCI community needs to wrestle with; explicating what it means to be human in an age of ubiquitous computing [8].

In this paper, I explore some new directions for HCI research and practice. I consider how the HCI community of researchers, practitioners and designers can play a new role in shaping society's evolving relationships with computer technologies. I argue that a quite different mindset is needed than the 'easy-to-use' and 'comfortable living' philosophies that have motivated much HCI and ubiquitous computing research. A new research agenda is proposed which sets out how to augment everyday activities using the portability, pervasiveness and computational power of ubiquitous infrastructures and mobile devices [8, 9]. Examples from some of my current research projects are presented to illustrate this alternative approach; one that is based more on exploring human values than simply offering prescriptive advice. Finally, I outline an overarching framework for guiding HCI that contrasts past and present concerns.

2 New Directions for Research

Several researchers have begun to reflect on the perspectives, paradigms and scope of the field of HCI. One trend has been to characterize the developments in HCI in terms of particular epochs or movements. For example, it has been argued that HCI research is entering a third paradigm that is much broader in its remit than the information processing approach of the 80-90s (described as the second paradigm) and the Human Factors work (labeled as the first paradigm) of the 70-80s [10]. Notions of context of use, the social situation of interaction, seamfulness and emotion are outlined as key research concerns, derived largely from sociology, design and the arts. They also propose that researchers seek multiple interpretations to obtain a "more complete overall understanding of the nature of interaction" of the phenomena being observed and analyzed. Similarly, a set of 'third wave challenges' has been outlined for HCI [11] but which suggests that the second wave (akin to the second paradigm) should not be abandoned but studied alongside them using a range of methods and conceptual approaches.

In a more far-reaching and forward-looking report, Being Human, Abigail Sellen, Tom Rodden, Richard Harper and myself [8] summarize the many changes afoot and suggest a new frame for understanding society's relationship with technology. We propose that HCI needs to put human values centre stage, considering both positive and negative aspects of the diversity of new technologically-mediated experiences. In terms of positive experiences, we explore how people use technology to pursue healthier and more enjoyable lifestyles, expand their creative skills with digital tools, and instantly gain access to information never before available. In terms of negative concerns, we explore how governments have become more reliant on computers to control and constrain society, criminals have become more cunning in deceiving people via digital means, and people worry more about what information is stored about them and who has access to it. We conclude by proposing that HCI researchers should be exploring this wider spectrum of user experiences, and in so doing, providing more in-depth explanations, accounts and implications that can inform the design, use and acceptance of future technologies, at personal, social and cultural levels. These outputs should also be of a form that can impact on government policy, in ways that move beyond simply providing guidelines for work practices or interface design.

In so doing, HCI will have to address a set of demanding, all-encompassing and socially awkward questions. To start the process, Being Human proposes five main transformations that are happening in society followed by a series of questions that need to be addressed for each. The changes are:

- the end of interface stability
- the growth of techno-dependency
- the growth of hyper-connectivity
- the end of the ephemeral
- the growth of creative engagement

2.1 The End of Interface Stability

The "interface" with computers is changing to such an extent that it is no longer as clear as when people interacted with PCs. At one end, situated displays and sensors are becoming embedded in buildings, airports and other public spaces, tracking our movements and displaying relevant information in these spaces, such as advertisements of products that are assumed to match our interests. At the other, our interactions with technology are becoming more personal and intimate. For example, we now carry in our pockets and our handbags multiple points of contact to a computational infrastructure. With the shift to medical monitoring and embedded devices this is likely to get closer still. Indeed, it may be difficult to define the boundary at all when devices are embedded within us.

The transformation in interface boundaries relative to our own bodies raises many new questions about how we might interact with new technologies. As the boundary moves closer to us, so the focus of the interaction needs to be better understood by the individual and how it will impact their own personal experience. As these devices become part of us, it raises issues about what defines an individual, and whether embedded devices are part of that definition. However, the issues are more complicated than this. Personal, intimate devices can be networked and therefore can interact with other people and other devices within the wider environment. We need to consider the spectrum of interfaces, ranging from private and personal interaction at one end to public and aggregated interaction at the other. At any one moment in time it means we can be simultaneously interacting with multiple boundaries, some under our control and some not. This causes shifts in what we will perceive as personal space, and what is shared.

2.2 The Growth of Techno-Dependency

The current generation of teenagers has grown up with the Web at their fingertips, instant availability through mobile phones, access to vast archives of their personal music and photographs, and video and TV on demand. They also take for granted older technologies such as calculators, word processors, and email. But what happens when the Internet or a mobile network provider goes offline? People become suddenly aware of their dependence, or even addiction, to email and the Web.

Techno-dependency raises a number of fundamental questions to do with what it means to be human. A controversial concern is the extent to which we will become increasingly dependent on computing technologies acting on our behalf, constantly reminding and telling us what to do. While it might make our lives easier it might come at a cost; for example, we might lose our mental ability to remember. But will this matter, if technology is always at hand [cf 1]?

Another topic that warrants systematic research is whether our ability to pay attention and focus is being affected by the multiple channels of digital information that can now be accessed simultaneously on a PC. Could it be that people who spend lots of time in front of a computer monitoring multiple sources of information are worse at switching between tasks and less able to focus exclusively on a single source? Recent findings suggest that it might be the case and that individuals who partake most in channel-hopping may also suffer the most. A recent study has found that participants who are 'heavy media multi-taskers' were worse at task switching than those classified as 'light media multi-taskers' because they were more susceptible to interference from irrelevant environmental stimuli and irrelevant representations in memory [12]. Hence, far from being able to deftly switch between multiple IM sessions, check up something on Wikipedia, play patience and an online game of chess, while apparently writing an essay, heavy media users are likely to be more easily distracted by the multiple streams of information and ongoing activities than those who are focused more on writing their essay and who may only allow themselves to check their email once every hour. Moreover, heavy users may actually be deceiving themselves: assuming they can benefit from multi-surfing and multi-tasking but which may prove to be more detrimental to them.

2.3 The Growth of Hyper-Connectivity

There has been an explosive growth in connectivity to individuals and society at large. People now connect 24/7 with many more people than ever before, be it friends, family, colleagues or strangers. Teenagers used to brag about how many friends they had online, but now take it for granted that everyone has several hundred 'friends' on Facebook. The boundaries between being at work, at home or out socializing are dissolving. It is accepted for people to be emailing or texting their colleagues in the early hours while playing a game of poker with people they have never even met.

Traditional, socially accepted conventions and etiquette governing how we communicate, when we communicate, and whom we communicate with are rapidly disappearing, with new ones replacing them. For example, students feel it is perfectly acceptable to email their professors with excuses for late assignments using informal text slang. Professors, however, may feel differently. Spontaneously emerging codes of conduct are also appearing when using communication technologies. These include right and wrong behaviors, such as not looking at others or by abstaining altogether from using Facebook in particular contexts (such as when sitting next to a stranger on the bus). Moreover, in a recent study [13] it was found that those students who update others' status or those who use Facebook during classes can seem to be in conflict with the code of conduct that one would expect outside of the Facebook community and that this breach can suggest a privileged position inside that community (e.g., one's Facebook friends) or a judgment towards the outsiders (e.g., the lecturers).

Such hyper-connectivity and rapidly changing social rules raise a number of fundamental issues for understanding how people manage and cope with the increasing demands of perpetual communication. Are they able to adapt and keep up with the new social trends or is the basic human need to disconnect and spend time on their own, or with close friends and family, being detrimentally invaded?

2.4 The End of the Ephemeral

Another transformation that is taking place is the 'expanding digital footprint'. Increasing amounts of information – that previously was largely transient and ephemeral – are being recorded and stored permanently as digital data. These include verbal conversations, emails, photos, texts, blogs, tweets, online purchases, banking transactions, and video footage taken by CCTV cameras and personal cameras/phones. Furthermore, many of these are tagged and indexed. Photos of people taken at a party, school event or at a restaurant can end up appearing on Flickr with associated names but without the tagged people ever realizing or giving permission.

In addition, an assortment of sensors have been experimented with in our homes, hospitals, public buildings, physical environments and even our bodies to detect trends and anomalies, providing a dizzying array of digital data about our health, movements, changes in the environment and so on. A number of location and tagging technologies have been developed, such as RFID, satellite, GPS and ultrasonics, to enable certain categories of information to be tracked and detected. Smartphone applications are now appearing that enable details about people's whereabouts and itineraries to be tracked online as they travel. Again, such information can be without them ever being aware it is available to the public.

In the last few years, there has been an increase in 'assisted living' projects that aim to help elderly people to remain more independent. In one of the early projects a residential care home was wired throughout with a variety of sensors [14]. These included badges on the patients and the caregivers and switches on the room doors that detected when they were open or closed. Load sensors were also used to measure and monitor weight changes of people while in their beds; the primary aim was to track trends in weight gain or loss over time. But the sensors could also be used to infer how well someone was sleeping. If significant movement was detected during the night this could enable a caregiver to see whether the person was having trouble sleeping (and if there was a huge increase in weight this could be inferred as someone else getting in or on the bed). More recently, researchers at the Fraunhofer Institute in Germany have been placing sensors in the toilet, tap, and carpet so that they can detect even more of an elder's intimate activities and record them electronically. They are even putting sensors in the toothpaste tube to record how frequently they are cleaning their teeth.

Such panopticon developments elicit a knee-jerk reaction of horror in many of us. While the motives behind such projects are altruistic, they can also be naïve, overlooking how vulnerable people's privacy and self-respect may be being violated. HCI researchers could make an important contribution by examining the social implications of recording, tracking and re-representing people's movements, conversations, actions and transactions, and whether a person's right to privacy being breached. For example, they could investigate whether different kinds of people mind their everyday habits, such as sleeping, eating, etc., being videoed and sensed, especially when they are not looking their best.

Case Study: A Futuristic Dieting System

One area where new technologies are being developed is for personal healthcare and wellbeing. While offering many benefits to people they can raise contentious issues pertaining to privacy, security and acceptance. How might HCI researchers begin to address these? Consider the following fictitious scenario developed by [15]:

"A company has developed a new wearable technology intended to help people lose weight called DietMon. The main character is Peter, a businessman in his early forties, who is overweight and would like to slim down. He claims he has been keeping a food diary, which shows that he does not eat that much. He also claims to be doing as much exercise as he can fit in with his busy life. However, nothing seems to be able to stop him gaining weight. So, the doctor invites him to try DietMon, a new technology that will assist him in his endeavor to slim down. He will have to wear glasses (fitted with clear lenses for those who don't normally wear them) that are enhanced with invisible cameras hidden in the frames; the cameras take a picture of every food that Peter looks at for more than three seconds and sends it to a database where the system cross-references it in order to identify the approximate number of calories contained in that food. The system will then send a text message to Peter's mobile phone to let him know. If Peter looks at a menu, the system identifies and sends him back the calorific value of each item in the menu. Peter will also have to have a tiny microchip implanted in his wrist, which will record the physiological changes taking place in his body as he eats (for instance, sugar or alcohol levels in the blood). The system sends the data recorded to his doctor, so that she can check whether he is keeping on track, and back to him, to keep him informed on how he is doing. As Peter approaches his daily calorific allowance, the system will send him an alert to let him know that he should stop eating. If he takes the glasses off or forgets to put them on, the microchip will still keep track of his food intake."

To explore the privacy, security and trust concerns this scenario raises, we have developed a new method, called ContraVision. The scenario is represented as two videos, one portraying it in a positive light and the other in a negative light. The two videos take Peter through a series of situations in which he has to manage his relationship with the technology, with food and with his family and colleagues. These are the same in both videos (e.g., having breakfast, walking past a cake shop, going for a meal) but the reactions and actions of Peter vary in subtly different ways for the positive and negative setting. For example, Fig. 1 is a still from the positive video, depicting Peter in a positive light. He is at a colleague's birthday party demonstrating how the dieting system works. Fig. 2 is a still from the negative video, showing Peter looking guilty as he is tempted to eat the pastry, when his wife opens the kitchen door.

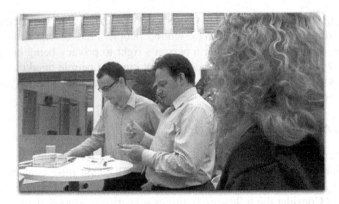

Fig. 1. A still from the positive video. Peter gives his colleagues a demonstration of how the dieting system works. One of his colleagues is wearing Peter's glasses while Peter waits for the text with the calorie count to reach his mobile. (Mancini et al., 2009).

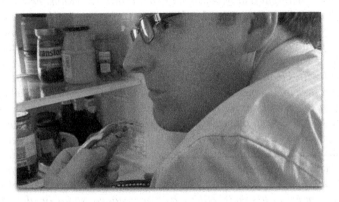

Fig. 2. A still from the negative video. Peter is about to be caught by his wife in the act of stealing a pastry from the fridge. (Mancini et al., 2009).

Participants from varied backgrounds viewed and discussed either the positive or negative video. A wide spectrum of reactions and concerns was elicited and which varied depending on the type of video watched. As might be expected, a number of topics were raised in both, including safety, trust, security, physical intrusion, possible uses and potential misuses of the information recorded and relayed and different forms of privacy breach. The videos also raised concerns that we were not expecting, including how the system would impact on their identity, self awareness, self perception and self representation to others; different levels of openness and deception and stress deriving from the use of deception; levels of control and freedom, and pressure deriving from lack of these; intrusion in and influence on personal and social behavior.

Hence, what might appear as a seemingly benign personal healthcare technology, meant to help people lose weight by giving them up-to-date information about food they are tempted or wish to eat, could end up being a much more pernicious system that not only could invade an individual's privacy, but also their sense of identity and how they interact with others.

2.5 The Growth of Cognitive Engagement

The four transformations described so far have focused primarily on the potential negative concerns of our ever-expanding relationship with technologies. The case study above illustrated how we can begin to explore in-depth the personal, social and cultural aspects of future technologies. However, it should be stressed that there are many opportunities for novel technologies to be designed that can augment and enhance how people learn, live and work in positive ways. Recent commercial examples include embodied physical games, such as the Wii and collaborative learning technologies, such as multi-touch tabletops. Another creative development is the highly succesful smartphone Apps that are designed by and for everyday people. A diverse range of experiences has been created providing people with many shared moments of fun and pleasure. A very popular music example is Shazam (www.shazam.com) that lets the mobile phone user find out which commercially recorded song is currently playing from any loudspeaker (e.g., radio, TV, stereo) that they can then share with their family and friends.

Innovative mixed reality, physical-digital spaces and sensor-rich physical environments have also been developed in Ubicomp research that enable people to engage and use multiple representations in novel ways: in scientific and working practices and in collaborative learning and experimental games. One example, that pioneered a new approach to augmented learning as part of the EQUATOR project, was the Hunting of the Snark game designed for young children [16]. The goal was to provoke their imagination and reflection through novel couplings of physical activities and digital representations. Pairs of children, aged between 6-8, had to discover as much as they could about an imaginary creature, called the Snark – its appearance, its likes and dislikes – by physically interacting with it in various activity spaces. The children had to perform certain kinds of embodied actions in these spaces, such as flying, dancing, walking and feeding. The Snark never appeared in its entirety but only as digital glimpses (animations, sounds and images) in response to the children's physical actions. The Snark responded by crying, laughing or showing appreciation or disgust to what it was fed. Children who played the game were fascinated by the abstract representations of the Snark that surfaced in the activity spaces and tried to work out how their physical actions caused them to appear. After the game, the children often gave lengthy narratives of the Snark's personality and behaviors that were based on their different glimpses when flying, dancing and feeding it.

A question when developing novel ubiquitous applications for creative engagement is how do they compare with those offered by more conventional GUI interfaces – that can be much cheaper and more practical to make? For example, is it not the case that children can be highly creative and imaginative when given simply a cardboard box to play with? If so, why go to such lengths to provide them with new tools? The debate is redolent of whether it is better for children to read a book or watch a 3D Imax movie. One is not necessarily better than the other: the two provide quite different experiences, triggering different forms of imagination, enjoyment and reflection. Likewise, ubiquitous technologies can be developed to both provoke and stimulate, and in doing so promote different kinds of learning and collaboration. Combining physical interaction, through manipulation of objects or tools or through physical body postural movement and location, with new ways of interacting, through ecologies of inter-connected digital technologies offers new opportunities compared with interacting solely with digital representations or solely with the physical world. In turn, this can encourage or even enhance further exploration, discovery, reflection and collaboration.

3 Proactive People Rather Than Comfortable Living

I have argued how human values need to become more central in HCI research, where researchers explore both positive and negative aspects, at personal, social and cultural levels. In addition, I argue that we need to design new technologies to encourage people to be proactive in their lives, performing ever greater feats, extending their ability to learn, make decisions, reason, create, solve complex problems and generate innovative ideas [9]. Such a view, however, is in sharp contrast with the prevailing vision of 'calm computing' that has influenced much of the research in ubiquitous computing, that was originally proposed by Mark Weiser in the early 90s. I argue why it is timely to move on and consider how ubiquitous computing can engage people.

Weiser's [17] central thesis was that while "computers for personal use have focused on the excitement of interaction...the most potentially interesting, challenging and profound change implied by the ubiquitous computing era is a focus on calm." Given the likelihood that computers will be everywhere, in our environments and even embedded in our bodies, he argued that they better "stay out of the way" and not overburden us in our everyday lives. His picture of calm technology portrayed a world of serenity, comfort and awareness, where we are kept perpetually informed of what is happening around us, what is going to happen and what has just happened.

In the last 15 years, Weiser has inspired governments, researchers and developers across the globe. Most prominent was the European Community's Disappearing Computer initiative in the late 90s and early 2000s, that funded a large number of research projects to investigate how information technology could be incorporated into everyday objects and settings and to see how this could lead to new ways of supporting people's lives that went above and beyond what was possible using desktop machines. Other ambitious and far-reaching projects included MIT's Oxygen, HP's CoolTown, IBM's BlueEyes, Philips Vision of the Future and attempts by various telecom companies and academia to create the ultimate 'smart home', e.g., Orange-at-Home and Aware Home. A central aspiration running through these early efforts was that the environment, the home, and our possessions would be aware, in order to adapt and respond to our varying comfort needs, individual moods and information requirements. We would only have to walk into a room, make a gesture or speak aloud and the environment would bend to our will and respond or react as deemed appropriate for that point in time.

Considerable research effort has been spent realizing Weiser's vision in terms of the development of infrastructures, devices and applications – to enable people to live calm lives. My beef with this approach is that as advanced and impressive as these endeavors have been in ubiquitous computing research (Ubicomp) they still do not match up to anything like Weiser's world of calm computing. There is an enormous gap between the dream of comfortable, informed and effortless living and the accomplishments of Ubicomp. As pointed out by Greenfield [18] "we simply don't do 'smart' very well yet" because it involves solving very hard artificial intelligence problems that in many ways are more challenging than creating an artificial human.

In contrast, I argue that a more productive direction for ubicomp research is to augment everyday activities using the portability, pervasiveness and computational power of ubiquitous infrastructures and mobile devices [5]. This idea essentially builds on Doug Engelbart's pioneering research program in the 60s for using distributed computer technology to augment the human intellect. By this he meant increasing the capabilities of a person so that they could make more rapid decisions, understand complex situations and find solutions to problems that seemed insoluble without the aid of technology. His ultimate goal was to develop technologies that could help people solve the world's increasingly complex problems. His approach was to show how the computing technology of the day could be designed to manipulate information directly, and which could thereby enable a new way of thinking about how humans work, learn, and live together. Despite his technological successes – notably the invention of hypertext, GUIs and the mouse – Engelbart's [19] research agenda for how computing could improve human life has not had the impact it should have had [20]. For example, Alan Kay and Andries Van Dam have recently lamented today's practitioners' lack of curiosity and awareness of historical context, "we're incredibly wedged…conceptually, technically, emotionally, and psychologically into a tiny and boring form of computing that is not even utilitarian." [quoted in 20].

In revisiting Engelbart's original idea, we can think more generally about how human behavior rather than the human intellect can be augmented with personal, social and cultural technologies, which aim to *actively* extend what people can do. In addition, we can begin to experiment with new technologies that might begin to shed light on elusive philosophical and psychological questions about the mind and human behavior that have taxed researchers for centuries. Hence, augmentation can be both enlightening and empowering. To illustrate how this might be achieved, I present two examples from my ongoing and future research projects, called e-sense and CHOICE.

The e-Sense Project: Extending Minds, Senses and Bodies

The e-sense project is funded by the UK's Arts, Humanities, Research Council (AHRC) as speculative research to investigate the theory of the Extended Mind [1] and explore how our mind and senses can be extended through designing novel technologies. The extended mind views the human cognitive system as a plastic hybrid of biological and non-biological components, including external representations and technologies. This perspective has profound implications for our notion of what it means to be human, pointing to the potential to change thought and action by integrating new technologies and information sources. Our approach has been to create an array of vibro-tactile interfaces and monitor both their use and the user experiences [21, 22]. From this we can gain knowledge about how to build useful sensory augmentation technologies as well as important insights into the extended mind perspective. In our interdisciplinary approach, conceptual philosophical analysis feeds into the design of systems and user studies reciprocally feed back into philosophy.

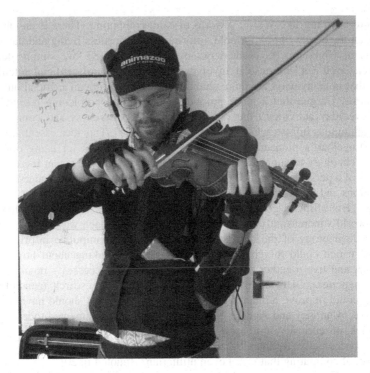

Fig. 3. A prototype of a motion capture and vibro-tactile feedback system for tracking and improving bowing actions when learning to play the violin [from 23]

We have also begun to develop vibro-tactile technologies that increase children's awareness of their body posture when they are learning to play stringed instruments and when singing. Initial studies using motion capture technology to track bowing actions coupled with visual and vibro-tactile feedback have shown how different forms of multi-modal feedback that corresponds to 'corrective' tracking are effective techniques that can improve technique [see Fig. 3]. We are currently developing other engaging and playful tools that can motivate children to practice regularly [23].

The CHOICE Project: Instant Information For In Situ Decision-Making

The CHOICE project is concerned with how new forms of augmented reality can be exploited to enable people to have 'instant information' at their fingertips that help people make more informed choices about values they care about when confronted with multi-dimensional information. Augmented Reality (AR) is becoming available that uses Smartphones and other ubiquitous technologies. For example, Pattie Maes (Media Lab, MIT), in her much talked about 2009 TED presentation, demonstrated how her team's "6th Sense" wearable device, comprising a wearable camera, a mirror and a tiny battery-powered Pico projector could superimpose relevant digital information onto the surfaces in the environment, like people's hands, clothing and food packaging. QR Codes (unique black and white chequered boards) are appearing on consumer products that when photographed, using an enabled mobile phone, will instantly bring up a game, video or informative website.

Our research project is investigating whether instant information provided by mobile AR can make it easy for people to do the right thing in the context of food shopping. We are examining, firstly, whether people can read and act upon such 'instant information' and secondly, whether AR has the desired galvanizing effect; encouraging and empowering people to act upon various social causes (e.g., reducing carbon emissions) or improve their well-being (e.g., changing their diet). Rather than providing more information to enable consumers to compare when making a choice, we propose a better strategy is to design technological interventions that provide just enough information and in the right form. Our solution is to exploit new forms of augmented reality technology to enable 'information-frugal' decision-making, in the context of an intensive activity replete with distractions (i.e., shopping in a supermarket or deciding at the kitchen table what to have for dinner). To this end, we are developing a family of mobile, social and computational devices that will display visualizations of multi-dimensional data at opportune times to see if it can help people make more informed decisions.

Recent research in cognitive psychology has shown how people tend to use simple heuristics when making decisions [24]. A theoretical explanation is that human minds have evolved to act quickly, making 'just good enough' decisions by using fast and frugal heuristics. People typically ignore most of the available information and rely only on a few important cues. In the supermarket, shoppers make snap judgments based on a paucity of information, such as buying brands they recognize, are low-priced, or have attractive packaging [25]. This raises the question of whether people can pay attention to more information, such as nutritional, ethical, and environmental features, regardless of whether it is instant relevant information. Rather than simply providing more information that enable consumers to compare when making a choice, we are determining how to design technological interventions that provide just enough information and in the right form.

4 New Directions for Practice

So far I have explored new directions for HCI research. In this part of the paper, I consider new directions for HCI practice. During the last 10 years, significant strides have been made already in academe and industry, to develop an armory of methodologies and practices. Innovative design methods, unheard of in the 80s, have been imported and adapted from far afield to study and investigate what people do in diverse settings. Ethnography, informant design, cultural probes, experience sampling and scenario-based design are examples of these. New ways of conceptualizing the field are also emerging. For example, many aspects of the user experience (UX) and ways of measuring it have been articulated by practitioners and are now common parlance. The focus is more on what is being done (i.e., designing interactions) and felt (user's experience) rather than the components it is being done to (i.e., the computer, the human). The nature of the user experience and how it unfolds over time is measured by its subjective qualities, such as what interacting with a device feels like to use, e.g., a MP3 player or a pet robot. Concepts such as pleasure, aesthetics, fun and flow, on the one hand, and boredom, annoyance and intrusiveness, on the other, have been used to describe the multifaceted nature of such experiences. The whole life cycle of people's response to technology is also being detailed, from when it first grabs their attention and entices them, through their ongoing relationship with that technology.

New measuring instruments (e.g., eye tracking) are also emerging that can record in fine detail how the body and senses are engaged when interacting with new computing developments – whether it be a new mobile social network service, a blue-toothed enabled GPS system or the latest web advertising. While surveys, user testing and expert reviews persist as staples alongside the classic user-centered design methods, such as storyboarding, scenarios, and low-tech prototyping methods, new technical innovations are turning heads. For example, the current wave of interest in multivariate tools (e.g., AB testing) that enable closer coupling between design and testing of live website components is one such development.

Practitioners are reinventing themselves to keep up with the technological and life style changes in our midst. But is this enough? Can and should they be considering the wider spectrum of human experiences, especially those that focus on positive and negative human values? A difficult challenge is how they can capture and analyze the bigger picture in terms of requirements, design recommendations, principles and implications. Consider the following hypothetical scenario for which a new system has been developed (again for personal healthcare but for which commercial products actually exist):

The number of children diagnosed with Type 2 Diabetes is on the rise, worldwide – a disease that requires constant management and can be very stressful for all concerned. A medical company has developed a new 'well being' monitoring device that periodically sends the latest recording of the child's blood sugar level to subscribing remote cell phones. A goal is to provide reassurance for parents that their child's condition is stable during school time when they are not around to assist. A UX consultancy company has been hired to assess the usability of this service. How might they accomplish this?

An obvious starting point would be to test the legibility and appropriateness of the recordings sent from the monitoring device to the cell phones. Is the form of representation used to convey the readings reassuring to the parents at a glance or do they have problems understanding what they mean, especially when the sugar levels vary from what they expect at that time of day? Are the danger warnings set at the right level? But then there are behavioral measures that need to be considered to determine whether the service is reassuring: How often do the parents use the service on their mobile phones? Do they get more anxious when calling it? What do they think each time they read it? Do they feel the urge to call their child? Should the device also communicate what activities the child is engaged in? And so on.

In conjunction, the UX of the wearer of the monitoring device – in this case the child – would need to be assessed. This raises a whole set of additional questions: Would the child have any control over what and when the recordings were relayed or would it be automated? Should the device signal to the child whenever a parent has called in to get a reading? What happens if the parents don't call in for sometime?

Will the child worry? Will the child become more dependent on them? How often does the child look at the readings? Do they get more or less anxious knowing their parents are looking out for them? Will they think their parents are checking up on them and they would rather they didn't? And so on.

This scenario is representative of many others on the brink. The monitoring of others, the capture of, access to and management of people's personal information, however benign in its intentions, is likely to pervade all aspects of our personal lives. It is no longer enough that practitioners think about how best to design and evaluate applications or services for users, they need also to think about how the technologies will be used by and affect networks of users, such as families, communities and different social groups. A challenge facing practitioners, therefore, is to consider how the more elusive ethical, personal and wider societal concerns can be folded into the UX mix

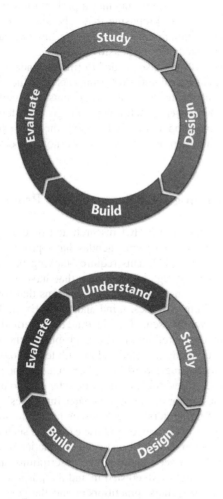

Fig. 4. *Top:* The conventional user-centered research and design model. *Bottom:* The extended five-stage research and design model encompassing a new stage of conceptual analysis or "understanding " of human values (from Harper et al., 2008).

such that they can be sensibly addressed when designing new technologies and services. How realistic and feasible is it? Many of the concerns may not be amenable to their repertoire of methods, usability metrics and design solutions. Moreover, the thorny ones are unlikely to be fixed in the way in which products (sic) have been improved through suggested changes. There is also likely to be several conflicting issues and complex webs of issues.

Taking into account human values, therefore, will be a very different undertaking compared with seeking to attain the design goals of efficiency, effectiveness and utility. Design trade-offs need to be considered not in terms of time and errors, but in terms of the weighing up of the various moral, personal and social impacts on the various parties who will be affected by the proposed technology. In the Being Human report we argue for the inclusion of a new stage in the user-design process, coined 'understand' (see Fig. 4). While understanding a problem has traditionally been part of the initial study phase, we are proposing that it be elevated to be a more explicit process, where the various human values at play are thought through and the trade-offs examined in a more systematic and sensitive way.

A new set of thinking tools are also needed to fill the 'understand' phase, ones that can be used to articulate and resolve the differing sets of values and questions arising from them. Philosophical debate, thought experiments and scenarios are promising candidates for starters. However, practitioners can go one step further: developing accessible frameworks and models that will enable them to explore through a new form of argumentation, and map out the interplay of moral, social and personal issues with their clients.

5 Conclusions: Framing HCI Research and Practice

I have suggested new directions for HCI research and practice that cover a broader spectrum of concerns than other recent agendas have promoted, such as the third paradigm [10] and third wave [11]. This requires moving beyond 'felt experiences' and 'enjoyable/comfortable living' philosophies that have permeated much recent research to encompassing a range of 'difficult' questions that focus on human values and augmentation of the human senses, mind and body. Examples from some of my current research projects were presented to illustrate this alternative approach.

A motivation was to begin rethinking the contribution the HCI community can make to understanding our changing relationship with technology. When asked what I do for a living I find it increasingly hard to explain in a sentence, in the way I used to be able to 10 years ago, i.e., 'designing computers to be easy to use'. Instead, I fumble with phrases, such as 'designing engaging computer interfaces', 'what it means to be human in a world full of computers', and 'I research mobile and sensor-based technologies that can track your every move' and use examples such as the iPhone and the Surface by way of illustration. Maybe I just need to practice a new elevator talk but, seriously, we are in need of a set of new terms, descriptions, and other abstractions that articulate the concerns we are interested in and the purpose behind what we do – and which, importantly, researchers, practitioners and the general public understand and feel comfortable using. We need to begin to engage in more dialogues, identifying areas of conceptual richness and problem articulation.

Table 1 presents my attempt at framing the burgeoning scope of HCI in the age of ubiquitous computing. It contrasts past concerns with future ones along four dimensions. Firstly, in terms of a frame of reference, it suggests that HCI's focus on users should be replaced with context. This shift reflects the broadening of issues, covering personal, social and cultural aspects of technology use and augmentation. Secondly, it notes how the methods, theory and perspective of HCI have in the past followed either the scientific approach (e.g., conducting experiments based on cognitive theory and doing user testing) or interaction design (e.g., prototyping, user studies, ethnography) should be replaced with multiple methods (including experiments and ethnography) that previously might have been considered incommensurate, but which can be mixed and even mashed in order to probe and analyze the wider and sometimes elusive set of concerns. Thirdly, it suggests that the current way of working together inspired by interdisciplinarity should make way for more transdisciplinarity. The 'trans' refers to integrative knowledge based on the convergence of concepts and methods from different research areas, including computing, philosophy, embodied psychology, art and design, ethics and engineering. It involves moving between the big picture and the details of a research question, using a combination of strategies, design methods and theories. For example, this might involved the application of philosophical theory to technological innovation, where conceptual philosophical analysis is fed into the design process and the experiences of being engaged in user studies are fed back into the philosophical analyses. Fourthly, whereas in the past, outputs from HCI research and practice have been either accounts or rich descriptions from ethnographic research; models of the user or the user experience; and conceptual or evaluative tools for analysis, future outputs should provide insights into how to develop engaging user experiences and human augmentation that, importantly, explore the whole gamut of human values that are impinged upon.

Table 1. Framing past and future concerns for HCI

Concern	Past	Future
Frame of reference	• users	• context
Method, theory and perspective	• scientific approach • interaction design	• multiple • mixing and mashing
Working together	• interdisciplinarity	• transdisciplinarity
Outputs	• ethnographies • models and tools for analysis • design guidance	• insights • creating new ways of experiencing • value-based analyses

Acknowledgements

The projects mentioned in the paper have has been partly funded by the EPSRC (PRiMMA) and the AHRC (e-sense). Thanks to Abigail Sellen, Tom Rodden and Richard Harper who co-authored 'Being Human: HCI in the Year 2020' with me.

References

1. Clark, A.: Supersizing the Mind. Oxford University Press, Oxford (2008)
2. Rogers, Y., Price, S.: How mobile technologies are changing the way children learn. In: Druin, A. (ed.) Mobile Technology For Children, pp. 3–22. Elsevier, Burlington (2009)
3. Barnard, P.J., May, J., Duke, D.J., Duce, D.A.: Systems interactions and macrotheory. Transactions On Computer Human Interaction 7, 222–262 (2000)
4. Rogers, Y.: New theoretical approaches for human-computer interaction. Annual Review of Information, Science and Technology 38, 87–143 (2004)
5. Rogers, Y.: Is HCI in danger of spiraling out of control? Interactions 64, 8–9 (2005)
6. Grudin, J.: Is HCI homeless? In search of inter-disciplinary status. Interactions 13(1), 54–59 (2006)
7. Grudin, J.: Living without parental controls: the future of HCI. Interactions 14(2), 48–52 (2007)
8. Harper, R., Rodden, T., Rogers, Y., Sellen, A.: Being human: HCI in the year 2020. Microsoft (2008)
9. Rogers, Y.: Moving on from Weiser's vision of calm computing: engaging Ubicomp experiences. In: Dourish, P., Friday, A. (eds.) UbiComp 2006. LNCS, vol. 4206, pp. 404–421. Springer, Heidelberg (2006)
10. Harrison, S., Tatar, D., Sengers, P.: The three paradigms of HCI. In: CHI 2007. ACM, New York (2007)
11. Bødker, S.: When second wave HCI meets third wave challenges. In: Mørch, A., Morgan, K., Bratteteig, T., Ghosh, G., Svanaes, D. (eds.) Proceedings of the 4th Nordic Conference on Human-Computer Interaction: Changing Roles, pp. 1–8. ACM, New York (2006)
12. Ophir, E., Nass, C., Wagner, A.: Cognitive control in media multitaskers. PNAS Early Edition online, http://www.pnas.org/cgi/10.1073/pnas.0903520106
13. Mancini, C., Thomas, K., Rogers, Y., Price, B.A., Jedrzejczyk, L., Bandara, A., Joinson, A.N., Nuseibeh, B.: From spaces to places: emerging contexts in mobile privacy. In: Ubicomp Proceedings. LNCS, pp. 1–10. Springer, Heidelberg (2009)
14. Beckwith, R., Lederer, S.: Designing for one's dotage: UbiComp and residential care facilities. In: Conference on the Networked Home and the Home of the Future, HOIT (2003), http://www.crito.uci.edu/noah/HOIT
15. Mancini, C., Rogers, Y., Bandara, A., Coe, T., Jedrzejczyk, L., Joinson, A.N., Price, B.A., Thomas, K., Nuseibeh, B.: ContraVision: Widening the spectrum of users' reactions and concerns to personal technology. Submitted to CHI 2010. ACM, New York (2010)
16. Rogers, Y., Muller, H.: A framework for designing sensor-based interactions to promote exploration and reflection. International Journal of Human Computer Studies 64(1), 1–15 (2006)
17. Weiser, M.: The computer for the 21st century. Scientific American 265(3), 94–104 (1991)
18. Greenfield, A.: Everyware: The Dawning Age of Ubiquitous Computing. New Riders, Berkeley (2006)

19. Engelbart, D.C.: Augmenting human intellect: a conceptual framework. SRI Report, AFOSR-3233 (1962)
20. Frenkel, K.A.: A difficult, unforgettable idea. CACM 52(3), 21 (2009)
21. Bird, J., Holland, S., Marshall, P., Rogers, Y., Clark, A.: Feel the Force: using tactile technologies to investigate the extended mind. In: Proceedings of Devices that Alter Perception (DAP 2008), pp. 1–4 (2008)
22. Bird, J., Marshall, P., Rogers, Y.: Low-Fi Skin Vision: A case study in rapid prototyping a sensory substitution system. In: Proceedings of the 23rd Conference on Human Computer Interaction 2009, Cambridge, UK (2009)
23. Van der Linden, J., Schoonderwaldt, E., Bird, J.: Towards a real-time system for teaching novices correct violin bowing technique. In: Proceedings of the International Workshop on Haptic Audio-Visual Environments and Games, HAVE, IEEE Instrumentation and Measurements, to be held November 2009, Italy (2009)
24. Gigerenzer, G., Todd, P.M., et al.: Simple Heuristics That Make Us Smart. Oxford University Press, New York (1999)
25. Todd, P.: How much information do we need? European Journal of Operational Research 177, 1317–1332 (2007)

Different Perspectives on Technology Acceptance: The Role of Technology Type and Age

Katrin Arning and Martina Ziefle

Human Technology Centre (HumTec), RWTH Aachen University
Theaterplatz 14, 52062 Aachen, Germany
{arning,ziefle}@humtec.rwth-aachen.de

Abstract. Although eHealth technologies offer an enormous potential to improve healthcare, the knowledge about key determinants of acceptance for eHealth technology is restricted. While the underlying technology of eHealth technologies and Information and Communication technology (ICT) is quite similar, utilization contexts and using motives are quite different. In order to explore the role of technology type on acceptance, we contrasted central application characteristics of both technology types using the scenario technique. A questionnaire was administered (n = 104) measuring individual variables (age, gender) and attitudes regarding an eHealth application (blood sugar meter) in contrast to an ICT device (Personal Digital Assistant, PDA). Older users basically approved the utilization of health-related technologies and perceived lower usability barriers. In addition, we identified main utilization motives of eHealth technology and technology-specific acceptance patterns, especially regarding issues of data safety in the eHealth context. Effects of age and gender in acceptance ratings suggest a differential perspective on eHealth acceptance. Finally, practical interventions were derived in order to support eHealth device design and to promote acceptance of eHealth technology.

Keywords: technology, eHealth, ICT, acceptance, user diversity, age, gender, usability.

1 Introduction

European health care systems will have to face enormous challenges in the coming years, which are caused by fundamental demographic changes, decreasing financial budgets for health care and innovative technological developments.

Demographic changes. Life expectancy in Western Europe has increased consistently since the 1950s by around 2.5 years per decade, and it is expected to continue to increase. At the same time, within the EU, a decrease in population is predicted due to migration patterns and low fertility rates [1]. A combination of these factors, as well as the ageing of the 'baby boomer' generation, will lead to dramatic changes in the demographic structure of Europe in the next fifty years. According to national census data every third inhabitant in Germany in 2050 will be 60 years or older, almost 50% of the population will be older than 50 years [2]. The proportion of people aged 80 years or

A. Holzinger and K. Miesenberger (Eds.): USAB 2009, LNCS 5889, pp. 20–41, 2009.

older will outnumber the proportion of newborns. Considering the life expectancy of each generation, the societies' aging process is already predetermined. Increasing birth rates or immigration might have a moderating role; however the process of demographic change is irreversible and will fundamentally change our society [1]. Therefore, one of the central challenges of political and health care systems in the 21st century is to master the demands of an aging society.

Decreasing financial budgets for healthcare. The growing number of older adults increases demands on the public health care system and on medical and social services. Chronic diseases, which affect older adults disproportionately, contribute to disabilities, diminish quality of life, and increase health- and long-term-care costs. The health-care cost per capita for persons aged >65 years in developed countries is three to five times higher than the cost for persons aged <65 years, and the rapid growth in the number of older persons, coupled with continuing advances in medical technology, is expected to create upward pressure on health- and long-term-care spending [3]. Due to changing family structures (smaller families living decentralized due to divorces, job-related mobility, etc.) informal health care services provided by relatives, who care for their older family members, are also predicted to decrease. Therefore, a growing number of frail older people will need long term care provided by official health care systems and the demand for long-term care is predicted to triple by 2051 [4].

Innovative technical developments. On the other side, the ongoing technological change and innovations in information and communication technology (ICT) will provide promising possibilities to face the growing pressure on health care systems, i.e. to improve patients' medical care and reduce the financial pressure on health care systems. Technical innovations will offer novel and/or improved medical diagnosis, therapy, treatment and rehabilitation possibilities. Besides progress in biomedical sciences or genetics, especially *eHealth technologies and applications* offer an enormous potential to reduce the pressure on health care systems, because they deliver significant improvements in access to and quality of care for users/patients and the efficiency and productivity of the health sector [5, 6].

1.1 eHealth Technologies

eHealth technologies cover the interaction between patients and health-service providers, institution-to-institution transmission of data, or peer-to-peer communication between patients or health professionals. eHealth technologies also include health information networks, electronic health records, telemedicine services, and personal wearable and portable communicable systems in the small screen sector (e.g. wristwatches, PDA) for continuously monitoring patients' health conditions and providing health-related information [5, 7-9].

Health-related technologies promise to deliver significant improvements in access to care, quality of care, and the efficiency and productivity of the health sector. Both, patients and healthy users can benefit enormously from eHealth technologies by increasing their mobility. eHealth technologies support their users in managing their own diseases, risks – including work-related diseases – and lifestyles. An effective integration of eHealth applications could also improve users' quality of life by enabling safer independent living and increased social inclusion. For example, eHealth could help older and disabled people to remain in their own homes for longer by providing them and their caregivers with increased safety and reassurance, reducing social isolation, and supporting treatment, rehabilitation and intermediate care. Summarizing so far, eHealth technologies and applications can help to shorten or to completely avoid the stay of patients in hospitals or rehabilitation centres, to enhance patient safety and therapeutic success at home after discharge from hospital and to maintain a prolonged independent lifestyle. Moreover, eHealth applications also have the potential to provide flexible forms of support that meet the individual needs of other stakeholders such as care-providers and therapists.

However, in order to fully exploit the potential of eHealth applications, not only aspects of technical feasibility but also of acceptance and usability issues of eHealth applications have to be considered. Improved health care services - especially in the home-care and rehabilitation sector - substantially depend on the ability and the acceptance of recipients to use eHealth applications. However, the knowledge about the antecedents of eHealth acceptance and utilization behaviour on the user side is restricted. Therefore it is necessary to explore and analyze user acceptance of eHealth technologies.

1.2 Technology Acceptance

The issue of technology acceptance has been researched from multiple perspectives, e.g. information theory, diffusion of information or social psychology. It can be described as the approval, favourable reception and ongoing use of newly introduced devices and systems. The majority of theoretical models of technology acceptance refers to the acceptance of information and communication technologies (ICT) in a job-related context [10].

The most influential approach of ICT acceptance and utilization is the Technology-Acceptance-Model (TAM)[10]. Based on the theoretical assumptions of the Theory of Reasoned Action [11] the TAM offers a link between technology acceptance and actual utilization behaviour. According to the assumptions of the Theory of Reasoned Action, an individuals' behaviour is determined by the intention to show certain behaviours. This intention is a function of one's own attitude toward the behaviour and individual norms. According to the TAM, a users' decision to use a new technology is determined by the behavioural intention to use the technical system. This behavioural intention is in turn determined by the perceived ease of use of the technical system and its perceived usefulness. The ease of use describes "the degree to which a person believes that using a particular system would be free from effort", the perceived ease of use is "the degree to which a person believes that using a particular system would enhance his or her job performance" [10]. Empirical studies proved that the perceived ease of use and usefulness were the main predictors of technology acceptance and actual system usage [12-14]. However, one of the main criticisms of the TAM was that external factors such as the influence of individual user variables on technology acceptance were almost completely disregarded. In the extended version of the TAM [15] a number of external variables was added, which were assumed to influence the behavioural intention to use a system, e.g. social and cognitive processes (subjective norm, system image and relevance, quality of output). The latest version of the TAM

– the UTAUT model (Unified Theory of Acceptance and Usage of Technology) [16] – assumes four key constructs (performance expectancy, effort expectancy, social influence, and facilitating conditions), which are direct determinants of technology usage intention and behaviour. Individual user variables such as gender, age, experience, and voluntariness of use are assumed to mediate the impact of the four key constructs on usage intention and behaviour.

Another characteristic of existing models of technology acceptance such as the TAM and its successors is that they almost exclusively focus on acceptance patterns of information- and communication technologies, predominantly in a job-related context. A transfer of their assumptions on eHealth technology acceptance is highly disputable though this has not been analyzed yet. Up to now, only a few studies investigated the special nature of eHealth technology acceptance [17-22]. However, we assume that the acceptance of eHealth technology distinctly differs from acceptance-patterns of ICT for several reasons: First, the *utilization context* of eHealth technologies will be different from ICT usage as eHealth devices will not be used voluntarily, but for medical reasons. Moreover, although eHealth applications might improve patient safety and reassurance, they refer to "taboo-related" areas, which are strongly associated with disease and illness. Second, utilization *motives* will be different, because using an eHealth device, e.g. to keep informed about one's own health status is not comparable to e.g. mobile phone usage to communicate with friends. In recent studies it was found that participants – in case of using an eHealth device- reported to fear to be continuously controlled- while this was not ascribed to a device in the ICT context, as e.g. a mobile phone [17-22]. Third, a higher *heterogeneity* in user groups and an even stronger impact of individual factors on acceptance is expected for eHealth technologies, as users/patients might be far older than "typical ICT-users" and they might additionally suffer from multiple physical and psychological restraints in comparison to healthy user groups. In the following section, the factors contributing to a higher heterogeneity in user groups will be described in more detail.

1.3 The Impact of User Variables on Technology Acceptance

In the last decades, the "human factor" or the user perspective has received more attention in research and the development of technical solutions [23-28]. However, the integration of user characteristics in the design process and in the explanation of technology acceptance still has been mainly restricted to information- and communication technologies like computers, mobile phones, Internet, etc. ICT have proliferated into most professional and private areas and they are voluntarily used even in older age groups. ICT are predominantly perceived in a positive way because they facilitate communication, information access and many activities of daily living [19, 29].

However, from ICT-research it is also known that technology perception, acceptance and utilization behaviour varies considerably among users. ICT acceptance is affected by individual differences such as demographic variables, experience, cognitive abilities, cultural factors und personality factors [30-35]. Research concordantly showed that older adults express lower levels of technology acceptance and that they more hesitantly adopt new technologies [19, 36]. Moreover, especially older users with restricted levels of technical experience or computer knowledge and age-related declines cognitive abilities (spatial and memory abilities) face greater difficulties in acquiring ICT skills and successfully interacting with ICT devices and perceive higher usability and acceptance [26, 33, 34, 37]. Apart from that restricted self-confidence to use technical devices also exerted negative effects on technology acceptance [38]. As potential users of eHealth applications might suffer from multiple physical und psychological restraints (e.g. restricted mobility, medicament-induced side-effects, pain, dementia, cognitive deficits, etc.), an even stronger (negative) impact of individual factors on eHealth technology acceptance is expected than in healthy user groups.

Beyond the above-mentioned individual variables, which generally reduce technology acceptance, we identified factors in previous studies, which promote technology acceptance – especially in older users [21, 22, 26, 28, 29]. Older users basically are highly interested in the technological progress and new technical developments, but they are much more critical regarding usability issues [19, 39]. Seniors are more likely to accept technologies (ICT), when the usefulness or benefits of system usage are made transparent, and when comprehensive instructional support (tutor, manuals, help system) is provided [19, 39].

However, as not only the characteristics of potential users, but also the usage context (medical reasons, mandatory usage) and usage motives (health-related reasons) of eHealth technologies distinctly differ from those of ICT, we doubt that existing knowledge about the user perspective in ICT can be one-to-one transferred to eHealth technologies, but that further research is necessary to explore the complex picture of acceptance factors and their interdependency. In the following section the research aims of the present study are described.

1.4 Research Aims

The current study aimed for an investigation of the complex nature of eHealth acceptance and its comparability to ICT acceptance patterns. A user/patient-centred approach was pursued, which considered the characteristics of a highly heterogeneous user group in a health-related utilization context.

First, general issues of eHealth acceptance were investigated, in order to gain insight into central determinants of eHealth acceptance.

Second, a comparative analysis of ICT- and eHealth acceptance patterns was conducted. As we assumed that the utilization context and utilization motives of eHealth technologies would be different from ICT, we contrasted central application characteristics of both technology types using the scenario technique.

Third, the exploration of factors contributing to eHealth acceptance and knowledge about context-specificity of technology acceptance will provide valuable insights into information needs, usability demands usage contexts and mental models of potential users, which can support designers of eHealth devices and applications in developing "acceptable" products.

2 Methodology

In the following section, more detailed information about the questionnaire, the scenario technique and the study sample will be provided.

2.1 The Questionnaire

In order to examine a large number of participants and to consider the diversity within the older age group, the questionnaire-method was chosen. The questionnaire was designed to obtain information about (1) demographic data (age, sex, education), (2) health-related variables (health status), (3) equipment with ICT and eHealth technologies, and (4) attitude towards eHealth technology (general attitude, confidence and intention to use eHealth, conditions and advantages of eHealth usage, utilization scenarios).

Before administering the questionnaire it was revised by a sample of older adults (n = 10) and by a usability expert with respect to issues of comprehensibility and wording of items. The final version of the questionnaire comprised closed multiple-choice and open-ended questions. Multiple-choice items had to be answered on a six-point Likert scale ranging from 1 (do not agree at all) to 6 (fully agree). Mean values < 3.5 were regarded as disapproving answers, values > 3.5 as affirmative answers. Additional space for comments was available in order to provide deeper insight into attitudes and needs towards eHealth technologies. The total time to fill in the questionnaire took approximately 30 minutes.

Scenario Technique

In order to examine the context-specificity of technology acceptance (ICT vs. eHealth) we used the scenario technique. Two utilization scenarios were presented, in which participants were asked to assess functionalities, characteristics and utilization barriers of a PDA (ICT scenario) and a blood sugar meter (eHealth scenario). As exactly the same functionalities, characteristics and utilization barriers were presented in both scenarios (Figure 1), differences in ratings can be attributed to the different technology type (ICT vs. eHealth).

The instruction in the ICT scenario was: "Imagine, your boss would ask you to use a PDA (a pocket computer with a digital diary, a digital to-do-list and a digital address book) at work for the next 14 days. Please indicate if you would approve the following functions and characteristics of a PDA."

In the eHealth scenario, the instruction was: "Imagine, you suffer from diabetes and your doctor would ask you to use a Blood Sugar Meter (a pocket computer which stores your blood sugar values) for the next 14 days. Please indicate, if you would approve the following functions and characteristics of a Blood Sugar Meter.

Both instructions contained a picture of a PDA or a Blood Sugar Meter, respectively, in order to facilitate the recognition of both technical devices and to enhance the comprehensibility of the instruction.

2.2 The Sample

The data of 104 respondents, 52 university students (m = 25.4 years, s = 4.2, 55.6% female and 52 older adults (m = 55.8, s = 8.4, 48% female) was analyzed. Both age groups did not differ in their educational background. Regarding the recruitment of participants a benchmark procedure was pursued: "younger and comparably healthy older adults" were questioned, which were still active part of the work force. This selection of the "best user case" was based on the assumption that this sample might resemble the group of "future seniors". Respondents of the older age group came from

Contrast of technology scenarios		
Technology type	ICT	eHealth
Technical Device	Personal Digital Assistant (PDA)	Blood Sugar Meter (BSM)
Device example used in the instruction	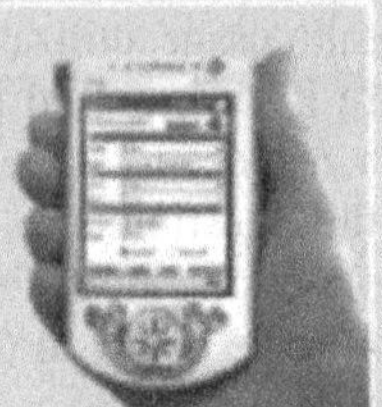	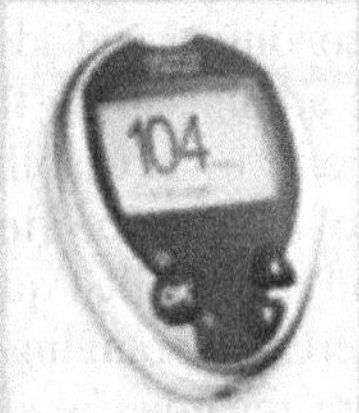
Characteristics and functions of the device	Automatic data storage Automatic data transfer Warning signal for misentries Reminder signal for appointments Password protection Data security Data diagram Handy size	
Utilization barriers	Exposure of personal data Monitoring by technology Technology dependency Restrained usability Feeling controlled by technology Technology too close to own body Visibility of the device for others Abundance of technology Unwilling to adapt to techn. innovations Impersonality of technology Fear of radiation Feeling embarrassed to use technology	

Fig. 1. Contrasting of technology scenarios (ICT vs. eHealth)

different professional fields (engineers, administrative officers, secretaries, teachers, nurses, architects, physiotherapists, physicians, craftsmen). In the younger group, students of engineering and humanity sciences took part.

3 Results

The results are presented according to the structure of the questionnaire, i.e. first, health-related variables and respondents' equipment with ICT and eHealth technologies are presented, followed by the results regarding attitudes towards eHealth technologies and the comparative analysis of technology-specific acceptance patterns. Moreover, in each section the effects of age and gender are reported. Data was statistically analyzed by t-Tests and ANOVAs. The level of significance was set at $\alpha = 0.05$, but, due to the higher variance in the older sample significance levels of $\alpha = 0.1$ are also reported.

3.1 Health-Related Variables

Health status ratings showed that a rather healthy sample was under study ($m = 4.1$ out of 6 points, $s = 0.9$). According to that finding, the sample was suited to fit in our "best case study sample"- approach (see section 2.2). Older adults reported a generally lower health status than younger adults ($m_{young} = 4.5$, $m_{old} = 3.6$; $F(1,44) = 4.7$, $p < 0.05$). Regarding further health-related variables, such as the number of absence days from work due to sick leave, the number of doctors' appointments or preventive medical check-ups, no age differences were found. Male and female participants did not differ in their self-reported health status. An interaction of age and gender was also not found.

3.2 ICT and eHealth Equipment

Participants were comparably well equipped with ICT (Table 1) such as computers, mobile phones, and digital cameras. However, although the older sample was comparably technology-prone and also well-equipped with personal computers, DVD players, navigation systems and PDA, older adults did significantly less possess mobile phones, video recorders, digital cameras, laptops and computer game consoles.

Table 1. Technical equipment with ICT and eHealth devices for both age groups (in %)

ICT	Young adults	Older adults	p
Mobile phone	98.3	88.0	p < 0.05
Computer	82.9	75.6	n.s.
Video recorder	25.8	65.3	p < 0.01
DVD player	60.0	65.5	n.s.
Digital camera	77.5	53.8	p < 0.05
Navigation system	25.8	35.4	n.s.
Laptop	81.7	27.9	p < 0.01
PDA	7.5	9.6	n.s.
Game console	20.8	2.1	p < 0.05
eHealth	**Young adults**	**Older adults**	**p**
Blood pressure meter	14.8	56.0	p < 0.01
Pulse watch	13.0	20.0	n.s.
Hearing aid	1.9	6.0	n.s.
Blood sugar meter	3.7	12.0	n.s.
In-house emergency call	1.9	2.0	n.s.

Compared to ICT, eHealth devices were considerably less frequent in the total sample. The most frequently owned eHealth device was the blood sugar meter, followed by the pulse watch (for heart rate monitoring during sports). The blood pressure meter was more frequently used in the older group (F(1,100) = 4.4; p < 0.01), presumably due to a higher prevalence of cardiovascular diseases in the older group (16% vs. 3% in the younger group). No effects of gender or interactions of age and gender were revealed.

3.3 Attitude towards eHealth Technology

In the following sections, participants' general attitude and confidence to use eHealth technologies and their intention to use eHealth devices are reported. In addition, the necessary conditions which should be fulfilled for eHealth device usage as well as the perceived advantages or motives of eHealth technology utilization are described.

General Attitude and Confidence to Use eHealth Technologies
In order to assess the general attitude and utilization confidence towards eHealth technology, participants were asked to rate their confidence to use eHealth devices, the perceived usefulness of eHealth devices for themselves and for others and the relative advantage of eHealth devices in relation to conventional medical treatments for themselves and for others.

In Figure 2 and Table 2 it can be seen that the general confidence to use eHealth devices, the usefulness of eHealth for oneself and others and the relative advantage of eHealth for oneself and others were rated positively in the total sample (as indicated by mean values > 3.5).

Interestingly, the usefulness of eHealth technology (t(101) = -7.4; p < 0.01) and the relative advantage in relation to conventional medical treatments was perceived to be significantly higher for others than for oneself (t(100) = -6.0; p < 0.01).

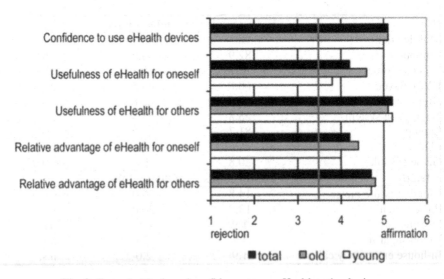

Fig. 2. General attitude and confidence to use eHealth technologies

Older adults reported a significantly more positive attitude towards eHealth technologies (F(1,96) = 17.6; p < 0.01) than the younger group, especially regarding the usefulness of eHealth for themselves. Effects of gender or interactions between age and gender were not found.

Table 2. Mean values of general attitudes and confidence ratings to use eHealth technologies (max. = 6)

	Total	Young adults	Older adults	p
Confidence to use eHealth devices	5.1	5.0	5.1	n.s.
Usefulness of eHealth devices for oneself	4.2	3.8	4.6	p < 0.01
Usefulness of eHealth devices for others	5.2	5.1	5.2	n.s.
Relative advantage of eHealth devices for oneself	4.2	4.0	4.4	n.s.
Relative advantage of eHealth devices for others	4.7	4.7	4.8	n.s.

Intention to use eHealth Devices
Participants were also asked to rate their intention to use specific eHealth devices. As depicted in Figure 3 ("total" bars in black), participants reported a positive intention towards the use of established eHealth devices, such as blood pressure meters, pulse watches, blood sugar meters, in-house emergency calls, and hearing aids. Regarding future eHealth technologies, such as computer rehabilitation exercisers, thirst sensors,

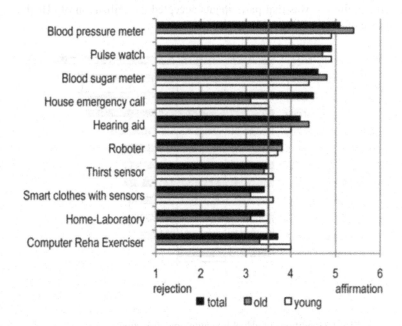

Fig. 3. Intention to use specific eHealth devices

domestic robots, smart clothes with sensors or home laboratories, participants reported an indifferent of even negative attitude (as indicated by mean values < 3.5).

Effects of age, gender, and interactions. Moreover, significant effects of age ($F(10,85) = 2.1$; $p < 0.05$) and gender ($F(10,85) = 1.8$; $p < 0.1$) as well as interactions between age and gender ($F(10,85) = 1.7$; $p < 0.1$) regarding the intention to use specific eHealth devices were detected.

Older adults reported a more positive intention to use blood pressure meters ($F(1,94) = 5.7$; $p < 0.05$), in-house emergency call ($F(1,94) = 3.9$; $p < 0.05$), and blood sugar meters ($F(1,94) = 3.1$; $p < 0.1$) than younger adults. Contrary to that, younger respondents were more positive about using electronic physiotherapists in future ($F(1,94) = 4.5$; $p < 0.05$) in comparison to older participants.

Gender effects were only found for the usage of blood pressure meters, which were more strongly approved by women ($m_{female} = 4.9$, $m_{old} = 4.2$; $F(1,94) = 7.5$; $p < 0.01$).

The interaction between age and gender ($F(1,94) = 3.9$; $p < 0.05$) indicated that the usage of household robots is favoured more strongly by older women and younger men ($m_{young\ female} = 3.3$, $m_{young\ men} = 4.3$, $m_{old\ female} = 4.1$, $m_{old\ men} = 3.6$). Regarding the usage of smart clothes with sensors, especially young men reported a highly positive usage intention, whereas older respondents even rejected the usage of smart clothes with sensors ($m_{young\ female} = 3.1$, $m_{young\ men} = 4.2$, $m_{old\ female} = 3.4$, $m_{old\ men} = 2.8$; $F(1,94) = 3.9$; $p < 0.05$).

Conditions of eHealth Technology Utilization
In a next step participants were queried about necessary conditions, which – to their view – should be fulfilled for an effective, efficient and satisfying interaction with eHealth technology ("I would use eHealth technologies if…"). Most interesting – and the highest rated condition – was that participants accepted the utilization of eHealth devices *only* in case of severe illness (Figure 4).

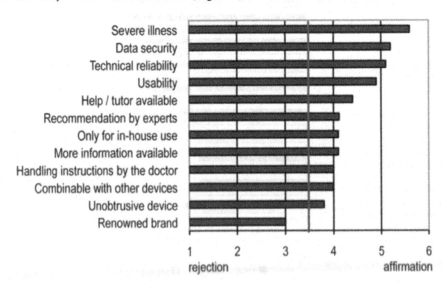

Fig. 4. Conditions of eHealth technology utilization

Further important conditions – apart from a poor personal health status – were technical reliability and data security of eHealth technology, followed by usability aspects and informative help functions. The only aspects or utilization conditions, which were rated as unimportant and negligible, were the devices' brand and the combinability with other devices (e.g. mobile phones). Age differences were also found: In contrast to the younger adult group, older adults significantly more strongly approved the availability of informative help functions (m_{young} = 3.9, m_{old} = 4.7; $F(1,68)$ = 5.5; $p < 0.05$) and data security aspects (m_{young} = 4.9, m_{old} = 5.4; $F(1,68)$ = 3.1; $p < 0.1$). Further effects of age, gender or interactions were not found.

Advantages and Motives of eHealth Technology Utilization
Moreover, participants were asked about perceived advantages and usage motives of eHealth technology utilization. In general, participants approved utilization advantages offered by eHealth technologies (Figure 5, next page).

The highest perceived advantages or utilization motives of eHealth were warning functions in case of emergencies, higher mobility for patients, fast data access, the possibility of a prolonged independent lifestyle and certainty or information about one's own health status. A higher quality of life, a reminding function and a more health-conscious lifestyle as "side-effects" of eHealth usage were also approved. The relief of health system budgets and general attributes of technology ("exciting", "indispensable") were also approved, but to a lower extent. Main effects of age and gender or interactions were not found.

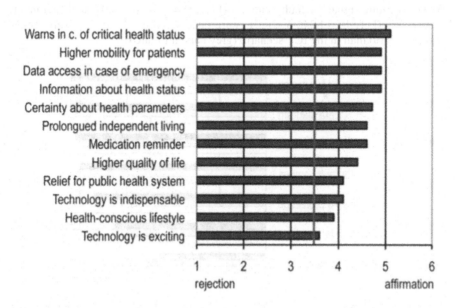

Fig. 5. Perceived advantages and motives of eHealth technology utilization

3.4 Comparison of ICT- and eHealth Technology Acceptance

In the following sections, the results of the technology scenario comparison between job-related ICT usage (using a PDA utilization scenario) and health-related eHealth technology usage (using a Blood Pressure Meter scenario) are reported. First, key characteristics of ICT and eHealth devices are contrasted, and second, perceived utilization barriers for both technology types are detailed.

Comparison of Characteristics and Functions

In two scenarios, in which the utilization of a PDA and a blood sugar meter were described, participants were asked to give ratings about characteristics and functionalities of both technology types.

In general ("total"/black bars in Table 3 and Figure 6), participants approved the given characteristics and functions of a PDA and a blood sugar meter (except "automatic data transfer"). The most important characteristic for participants was the size of the device, followed by a data diagram function for appointments (PDA) or the blood sugar level (BSM), a reminder signal for appointments, a warning signal for faulty entries, password protection and automatic data storage. The only rejection of a technical function (in total) referred to the automatic data transfer function.

However, the ratings regarding characteristics and functions of technical devices differed significantly depending on the specific technology type.

Effects of technology type. Considerable differences in ratings were found for both technology types. The technical functions "automatic data storage" (F(1,98) = 31.4; p < 0.01), "warning signal for faulty entries" (F(1,98) = 12.7; p < 0.01) and "automatic data transfer" (F(1,98) = 80.0; p < 0.01) were rated significantly more positive in the eHealth scenario than in the ICT scenario (grey bars in Figure 6).

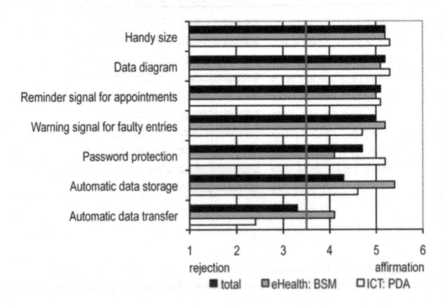

Fig. 6. Characteristics and functions of eHealth (Blood Sugar Meter) and ICT (PDA) devices

In the ICT scenario (white bars in Figure 6), the function "password protection of personal data" was significantly more approved ($F(1,98) = 41.4$; $p < 0.01$), whereas the function "automatic data transfer" was distinctly rejected. For the technical characteristics, "handy size", "data diagram" and "reminder signal for appointments" no statistical differences between the two technology types were found.

Table 3. Mean ratings for characteristics and functions of a PDA and a Blood Sugar Meter (BSM) (max. = 6)

	total	ICT: PDA	eHealth: BSM	p
Automatic data transfer	3.3	2.4	4.1	p < 0.01
Password protection	4.7	5.2	4.1	p < 0.01
Reminder signal for appointments	5.1	5.1	5.0	n.s.
Warning signal for faulty entries	5.0	4.7	5.2	p < 0.01
Data diagram	5.2	5.3	5.1	n.s.
Automatic data storage	4.3	4.6	5.4	p < 0.01
Handy size	5.2	5.3	5.2	n.s.

Effects of age, gender, and interactions. Participants' ratings regarding specific functionalities and characteristics of both technology types were also influenced by main and interacting effects of age and gender.

A handy size of technical devices was significantly more important for younger participants than for older respondents ($m_{young}= 5.4$, $m_{old}= 5.0$; $F(1,98) = 6.7$; $p < 0.05$). For older adults, automatic data storage was more important than for younger adults ($m_{young}= 4.8$, $m_{old}= 5.2$; $F(1,98) = 3.0$; $p < 0.1$), as well as password protection ($m_{young}= 4.4$, $m_{old}= 4.9$; $F(1,98) = 5.7$; $p < 0.05$).

Women approved automatic data storage more strongly than men ($m_{female}= 5.1$, $m_{male}= 4.8$; $F(1,98) = 4.1$; $p < 0.05$). Moreover, automatic data storage is considerably more important for older adults in the eHealth than in the ICT scenario ($m_{ICT\ young}= 4.9$, $m_{eHealth\ young}= 5.3$, $m_{ICT\ old}= 4.2$, $m_{eHealth\ old}= 5.4$), taken from the interaction between age and technology type ($F(1,98) = 5.7$; $p < 0.05$). Password protection is distinctly less important for younger adults in the eHealth than in the ICT scenario, whereas older adults' highly approve a password protection in both technology contexts ($m_{ICT\ young}= 5.2$, $m_{eHealth\ young} = 3.6$, $m_{ICT\ old} = 5.2$, $m_{eHealth\ old}= 4.6$, ($F(1,98) = 8.5$; $p < 0.05$.

Comparison of Utilization Barriers

Participants were also asked to rate utilization barriers in the ICT- and in the eHealth scenario (Table 4).

In general ("total", Table 4), participants disapproved the utilization barriers (mean values < 3.5, "total"/black bars in Figure 7). This suggests a positive utilization motivation of technical devices in general. The only approving rating referred to the barrier "exposure of personal data". Further aspects such as feeling monitored by, controlled by and being dependent from technology, or the fear of health risks (radiation) were not perceived as utilization barriers.

Table 4. Mean values for utilization barrier ratings (max. = 6). Low ratings indicate positive attitude (small barriers).

	total	ICT: PDA	eHealth: BSM	p
Exposure of personal data	4.0	4.1	4.0	n.s.
Monitoring by technology	3.3	3.4	3.1	p < 0.1
Technology dependency	3.2	3.4	3.0	p < 0.05
Restrained usability	3.0	2.9	3.1	p < 0.1
Feeling controlled by technology	3.0	3.4	3.1	p < 0.1
Technology too close to own body	2.6	2.6	2.6	n.s.
Visibility of the device for others	2.4	2.3	2.5	p < 0.05
Abundance of technology	2.8	2.9	2.6	p < 0.05
Rejection of technical innovations	2.9	3.0	2.7	p < 0.05
Impersonality of technology	2.6	2.7	2.5	p < 0.1
Fear of radiation	2.4	2.3	2.4	n.s.
Feeling embarrassed to use technology	2.2	2.0	2.3	p < 0.01

Effects of technology type. In conformity with the findings regarding specific characteristics and functions of technical devices, utilization barriers differed according to the contrasted technology type (ICT vs. eHealth).

Utilization barriers such as the feeling of being monitored ($F(1,99) = 3.3$; $p < 0.1$), and controlled ($F(1,99) = 3.3$; $p < 0.1$) by technology or the impression of being dependent ($F(1,99) = 6.4$; $p < 0.05$) from technology, getting inundated by technology ($F(1,99) = 5.5$; $p < 0.05$), the global rejection of technical innovations ($F(1,99) = 5.1$; $p < 0.05$), the perception of "impersonal" technology ($F(1,98) = 2.8$; $p < 0.1$) or the feeling of being embarrassed to use these technical devices ($F(1,99) = 12.9$; $p < 0.01$) were significantly less pronounced in the eHealth context (grey bars in Figure 7) than in the ICT context (white bars in Figure 7). Thus, the technology type is distinctly affecting usage motives and utilization barriers, and a significantly more positive attitude towards eHealth technologies is present compared to ICT.

Effects of age and gender. Utilization barriers were significantly influenced by main effects of age and gender. No interacting effects were revealed.

Older adults were found to be generally more reluctant and gave consistently higher ratings to each of the single usability barriers ($F(18,36) = 1.8$; $p < 0.1$, Table 5 and Figure 8, next page). In comparison to the younger group, older adults significantly more strongly rejected the exposure of personal data ($F(1,100) = 6.4$; $p < 0.05$), feared to be hampered by restricted usability issues ($F(1,100) = 25.4$; $p < 0.01$), felt monitored by ($F(1,100) = 12.7$; $p < 0.01$), controlled by ($F(1,100) = 12.6$; $p < 0.01$) and dependent from technology ($F(1,100) = 10.1$; $p < 0.05$), refused to "wear" technologies too close to the body ($F(1,100) = 17.1$; $p < 0.01$), complained about the abundance ($F(1,100) = 6.9$; $p < 0.05$) and impersonality of technology ($F(1,100) = 14.0$; $p < 0.01$) and reported a greater fear of radiation ($F(1,100) = 15.8$; $p < 0.01$).

Gender effects were also present: Women significantly more strongly refused to wear technology close to body ($m_{female} = 2.3$, $m_{male} = 2.8$; $F(1,100) = 6.3$; $p < 0.05$).

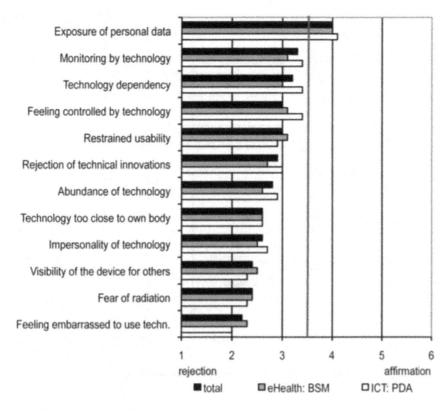

Fig. 7. Barriers to use ICT and eHealth technology. Low ratings indicate positive attitude (small barriers).

Table 5. Age differences in usability barrier ratings (max. = 6)

	Young adults	Older adults	P
Exposure of personal data	3.6	4.4	p < 0.05
Monitoring by technology	2.8	3.8	p < 0.01
Technology dependency	2.8	3.6	p < 0.05
Restrained usability	2.4	3.7	p < 0.01
Feeling controlled by technology	2.8	3.7	p < 0.01
Technology too close to own body	2.1	3.0	p < 0.01
Visibility of the device for others	2.2	2.6	p < 0.1
Abundance of technology	2.4	3.1	p < 0.05
Rejection of technical innovations	2.3	3.5	p < 0.01
Impersonality of technology	2.2	3.0	p < 0.01
Fear of radiation	1.9	2.7	p < 0.01
Feeling embarrassed to use technology	2.0	2.3	p < 0.05

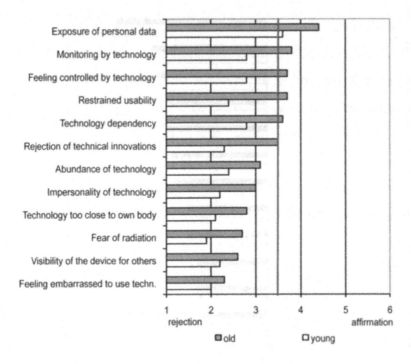

Fig. 8. Age differences in usability barrier ratings

4 Discussion

The present study aimed at an investigation of eHealth acceptance and focused on potential factors, which contribute to persons' attitude towards medical technology as well as on the determinants, which form eHealth technology acceptance. In order to learn more about the impact of technology type and usage context on acceptance outcomes, we compared a scenario, in which either a PDA or a blood sugar meter device was used. Also, the impact of user diversity, i.e. influences of age and gender on acceptance ratings was considered.

4.1 Acceptance of eHealth Technologies

Summarizing so far, participants reported a generally positive attitude towards eHealth technologies. They recognized potential advantages and reported a high motivation to use eHealth technologies. The biggest perceived advantages referred to timely information and, by this, certainty about one's own health status. Also, the possibility to maintain personal independency and mobility and the avoidance of institutionalized care were positive drivers of acceptance. These perceived main advantages refer to vital personal motives, i.e. an unscathed and independent living. Therefore we assume that eHealth technologies have a great potential to become accepted and to improve living conditions of users/patients, if these central motives – information about the health status and maintaining of personal independency and mobility – are adequately considered in technical development and made transparent in an communication or marketing strategy.

Further important aspects, which were identified to contribute to eHealth acceptance, refer to issues of technical reliability and data security as well as usability aspects. Persons who "confide their well-being to technical devices" (a frequent comment of our participants about how they felt about eHealth utilization) expect highest standards regarding technical reliability, system safety and data security. According to that, high quality standards for eHealth technologies have to be defined in order to convey trust regarding the reliability of eHealth technologies. Apart from technical standards, usability standards should also be considered, because users' acceptance will be lost, if restricted usability hampers a successful interaction with eHealth devices.

Another important factor, which influenced acceptance patterns, was the perceived personal closeness or distance to the eHealth topic. The usefulness of eHealth technology was perceived to be higher for others than for one self. Moreover, the majority of participants stated that they would not consider the usage of eHealth or medical technology until they are urged to and poor health conditions require them to do so. On the other side, it is promising that older adults, who usually have a more pragmatic or even rejecting attitude towards technology [29], assessed eHealth technologies more positively than younger adults. We assume that with increasing age adults tend to basically acknowledge the benefits of eHealth applications, but that they also feel intimidated by these new health-technologies, as they cannot appraise the consequences of using these devices for their living context. Further research is necessary to investigate the effect of perceived "closeness / distance" on eHealth acceptance and measures, which will help to reduce the "fear of context" regarding health-related technologies (e.g. demonstrations of eHealth devices on exhibitions, "sightseeing tours" in smart houses, etc.)

Interestingly, a positive perception of eHealth technologies was related to their diffusion rate: established eHealth devices (e.g. blood pressure meter, blood sugar meter) were evaluated more positively than "future" technologies (e.g. smart clothes with sensors), which have not permeated onto broader parts of our society yet. Future studies will have to investigate, if acceptance of future eHealth technologies is influenced by their diffusion rate or "popularity", or if users generally reject the functionalities and characteristics provided by these technologies due to their stigmatizing nature [29].

4.2 Technology-Specificity of Acceptance Patterns

The comparative analysis between ICT and eHealth technology convincingly proved a technology-specificity of technology acceptance. In general, utilization barriers were perceived to be lower in the eHealth scenario than in the ICT scenario. However, it would be misleading to conclude that eHealth acceptance by potential users is easier to obtain than it is in the ICT sector. The evaluation of functions and characteristics of ICT and eHealth technology shows that users in fact differentiate between specific utilization contexts and therefore emphasize different aspects of technology interaction. Issues of data safety (password protection, data storage, safe data transmission) are perceived as much more important and are more willingly accepted in the eHealth context than in ICT context. Moreover, the willingness to exchange or share these data to persons that are perceived as competent (therapists or doctors) is higher for eHealth technology. These results indicate that potential users of eHealth applications demand higher technical reliability and data security on the one hand, and are willing to accept a higher monitoring and surveillance by technology on the other hand.

4.3   User-Specificity of Technology Acceptance Patterns

Also, effects of user diversity were identified to affect acceptance judgements. Age and gender differences suggest that potential users of eHealth technologies differ in their technology acceptance patterns, which requires a more differential perspective on eHealth acceptance. Older adults represent one specific user group, which should be considered in eHealth acceptance research [29]. They perceived higher utilization barriers and reported higher concerns about data safety issues. Gender differences in eHealth acceptance also require special attention: especially older female users reported problems to wear technology too close to the own body. These results confirm outcomes from recent studies of our workgroup [29]. Especially for older and female users of eHealth technology these aspects should be adequately addressed in design and communication (e.g. in training courses). This is of especial importance as - due to higher mortality rates in men [29] - predominately older women are the main end user group of future eHealth technologies [29].

4.4   Limitations of the Study and Future Research

Besides individual variables such as age and gender we assume that further health-related constructs (coping, compliance) have to be considered in a global theoretical model of eHealth acceptance and utilization behaviour. Individuals' coping strategies refer to specific psychological and behavioural efforts that people employ to master, tolerate, reduce, or minimize stressful events. They can be categorized in problem-solving vs. emotion-focused, active or avoidant strategies and were found to affect physical and psychological health outcomes [29]. The construct of compliance has been adopted to describe the degree to which patients follow their provider's recommendations. Modern definitions of compliance emphasize a proactive patient involvement instead of a patient-provider hierarchy [29].

Moreover, current approaches of technology acceptance describe a static perspective on technology acceptance, whereas the acceptance of eHealth applications might have dynamic components, which are influenced by disease-related changes in health state, coping strategies and compliance behaviour. Therefore we suggest the integration of health-related constructs such as compliance and coping-style and dynamic components of acceptance patterns in the theoretical explanation and modelling of eHealth acceptance and utilization behaviour. Moreover, we aim for a longitudinal research approach in order to investigate the process of "acceptance development" and changes in eHealth technology acceptance.

A further note refers to the sample of this study. A comparably young (20-70 years) and healthy sample, which was well equipped with technology (ICT), was under study. Older adults in this sample represent the aging "baby boomer generation", which will become the main target group of future eHealth technologies. Their attitudes and demands have thus to be considered by eHealth technology researchers and developers. However, apart from the main target group of "baby boomers", future acceptance studies should also integrate older (> 70 years) and less healthy user groups, in order to provide a more complete picture of eHealth acceptance.

Finally, an interdisciplinary, user-centred approach is needed, which explores and weighs the contributing factors of eHealth acceptance, considers the demands of a highly heterogeneous user group and the dynamic character of ageing and diseases in a novel, health-related utilization context, identifies barriers and derives practical interventions in order to promote eHealth acceptance.

Acknowledgements

The authors would like to thank Luisa Bremen, Ana Petrova, and Thomas Reitmayer for research support.

This study was supported by the excellence initiative of the German federal and state government.

References

1. Giannakouris, K.: Ageing characterises the demographic perspectives of the European societies. Eurostat 72 (2008)
2. Pötzsch, O., Sommer, B.: Bevölkerung Deutschlands bis 2050 - Ergebnisse der 10. koordinierten Bevölkerungsvorausberechnung. Wiesbaden: Pressestelle Statistisches Bundesamt (2003)
3. Jacobzone, S., Oxley, H.: Ageing and Health Care Costs. Internationale Politik und Gesellschaft Online (International Politics and Society) 1 (2002)
4. Wittenberg, R., Comas-Herrera, A., Pickard, L., Hancock, R.: Future Demand for Long-Term Care in England. PSSRU Research Summary (2006)
5. Demiris, G.: e-health: Current Status and Future Trends in the EU and the US. IOS Press, The Netherlands (2004)
6. Tan, J.K.H.: Healthcare information systems & informatics: research and practices, Hershey (2008)
7. Jähn, K., Nagel, E.: e-Health. Springer, Berlin (2004)
8. Leonhardt, S.: Personal Healthcare Devices. In: Mekherjee, S., et al. (eds.) Malware: Hardware Technology Drivers of Ambient Intelligence, pp. 349–370. Springer, Dordrecht (2005)
9. Holzinger, A., Schaupp, K., Eder-Halbedl, W.: An Investigation on Acceptance of Ubiquitous Devices for the Elderly in a Geriatric Hospital Environment: Using the Example of Person Tracking. In: Proceedings of the 11th international conference on Computers Helping People with Special Needs. Springer, Linz (2008)
10. Davis, F.D.: Perceived Usefulness, Perceived Ease of Use, and User Acceptance of Information Technology. MIS Quarterly 13, 319–337 (1989)
11. Ajzen, I., Fishbein, M.: Understanding Attitudes and Predicting Social Behavior. Prentice-Hall, Englewood Cliffs (1980)
12. Venkatesh, V., Davis, F.D.: A Model of the Antecedents of Perceived Ease of Use: Development and Test. Decision Sciences 27, 451–481 (1996)

13. Schwarz, A., Chin, W.: Looking Forward: Toward an Understanding of the Nature and Definition of IT Acceptance. Journal of the Association for Information Systems 8, 232–243 (2007)
14. Arning, K., Ziefle, M.: Understanding age differences in PDA acceptance and performance. Computers in Human Behavior 23, 2904–2927 (2007)
15. Venkatesh, V., Davis, F.D.: A Theoretical Extension of the Technology Acceptance Model: Four Longitudinal Field Studies. Management Science 46, 186–204 (2000)
16. Venkatesh, V., Morris, M.G., Davis, G.B., Davis, F.D.: User acceptance of information technology: Toward a unified view. MIS Quarterly 27, 3 (2003)
17. Wilson, E.V., Lankton, N.K.: Modeling patients' acceptance of provider-delivered e-health. Journal of the American Medical Informatics Association 11, 241–248 (2004)
18. Stronge, A.J., Rogers, W.A., Fisk, A.D.J.: Human factors considerations in implementing telemedicine systems to accommodate older adults. Telemed Telecare 13, 1–3 (2007)
19. Jakobs, E.-M., Lehnen, K., Walter, M., Vogt, O., Ziefle, M.: Alter und Technik. Eine Studie zur altersbezogenen Wahrnehmung und Gestaltung von Technik. Edition Wissenschaft, Aprimus (2008)
20. Wirtz, S., Jakobs, E.-M., Ziefle, M.: Age-specific issues of software interfaces. In: 9th International Conference on Work With Computer Systems (WWCS), Beijing, China (2009)
21. Gaul, S., Ziefle, M.: Smart home technologies: insights into generation-specific acceptance motives. In: USAB, Linz, Austria (submitted)
22. Ziefle, M.: Age perspectives on the usefulness on e-health applications. In: International Conference on Health Care Systems, Ergonomics, and Patient Safety (HEPS), Straßbourg, France (2008)
23. Rogers, W., Cabrera, E.F., Walker, N., Gilbert, D.K., Fisk, A.D.: A survey of automatic teller machine usage across the adult lifespan. Human Factors 38, 156–186 (1996)
24. Marcellini, F., Mollenkopf, H., Spazzafumo, L., Ruoppila, I.: Acceptance and Use of Technological Solutions by the Elderly in the Outdoor Environment: Findings from a European Survey. Zeitschrift für Gerontologie und Geriatrie 33, 169–177 (2000)
25. Bay, S., Ziefle, M.: Design for all: User characteristics to be considered for the design of phones with hierarchical menu structures. In: Luczak, H., Zink, K.J. (eds.) Human factors in organizational design and management, pp. 503–508. IEA Press, Santa Monica (2003)
26. Ziefle, M., Bay, S.: Transgenerational Designs in Mobile Technology. In: Lumsden, J. (ed.) Handbook of Research on User Interface Design and Evaluation for Mobile Technology, pp. 122–140. IGI Global (2008)
27. Ziefle, M., Bay, S.: How older adults meet complexity: Aging effects on the usability of different mobile phones. Behaviour and Information Technology 24, 375–389 (2005)
28. Arning, K., Ziefle, M.: Barriers of Information Access in Small Screen Device Applications: The Relevance of User Characteristics for a Transgenerational Design. In: Stephanidis, C., Pieper, M. (eds.) ERCIM Ws UI4ALL 2006. LNCS, vol. 4397, pp. 117–136. Springer, Heidelberg (2007)
29. Arning, K., Ziefle, M.: What older user expect from mobile devices: An empirical survey. In: Pikaar, R.N., Konigsveld, E.A., Settels, P.J. (eds.) Proceedings of the 16th World Congress on Ergonomics (IEA). Elsevier, Amsterdam (2006)
30. Czaja, S.J., Sharit, J.: Age Differences in Attitudes Toward Computers. Journal of Gerontology 5, 329–340 (1998)
31. Ellis, D.R., Allaire, J.C.: Modelling computer interest in older adults: The role of age, education, computer knowledge and computer anxiety. Human Factors 41, 345–364 (1999)
32. Freudenthal, D.: Age differences in the performance of information retrieval tasks. Behaviour and Information Technology 20, 9–22 (2001)

33. Arning, K., Ziefle, M.: Effects of cognitive and personal factors on PDA menu navigation performance. Behavior and Information Technology (in press)
34. Arning, K., Ziefle, M.: Understanding age differences in PDA acceptance and performance. Computers in Human Behavior 23, 2904–2927 (2007)
35. Holzinger, A., Searle, G., Nischelwitzer, A.: On some Aspects of Improving Mobile Applications for the Elderly. In: Stephanidis, C. (ed.), pp. 923–932. Springer, Heidelberg (2007)
36. Melenhorst, A.S., Rogers, W.A., Caylor, E.C.: The use of communication technologies by older adults: Exploring the benefits from an users perspective. In: Proc. of the Human Factors and Ergonomics Society 45th Annual Meeting (2001)
37. Kelley, C., Charness, N.: Issues in training older adults to use computers. Behaviour and Information Technology 14, 107–120 (1995)
38. Levine, T., Donitsa-Schmidt, S.: Computer use, confidence, attitudes and knowledge: a causal analysis. Computers in Human Behavior 1, 125–146 (1998)
39. Arning, K., Ziefle, M.: Ask and you will receive: Training older adults to use a PDA in an active learning environment. International Journal of Mobile Human-Computer Interaction (in press)

A Mixed-Method Approach on Digital Educational Games for K12: Gender, Attitudes and Performance

Effie Lai-Chong Law[1], Tim Gamble[1], Daniel Schwarz[2],
Michael D. Kickmeier-Rust[3], and Andreas Holzinger[4]

[1] University of Leicester, LE1 7RH, Leicester, UK
Department of Computer Science
elaw@mcs.le.ac.uk,
gamble@mcs.le.ac.uk
[2] TAKOMAT GmbH, Neptunplatz 6b,
50823 Köln, Germany
dan@takomat.com
[3] Graz University, A-8010 Graz, Austria
Department of Psychology, Cognitive Science Section
michael.kickmeier@uni-graz.at
[4] Medical University Graz, A-8036 Graz, Austria
Institute for Medical Informatics, Statistics & Documentation (IMI)
Research Unit HCI4MED
andreas.holzinger@medunigraz.at

Abstract. Research on the influence of gender on attitudes towards and performance in digital educational games (DEGs) has quite a long history. Generally, males tend to play such games more engagingly than females, consequently attitude and performance of males using DEGs should be presumably higher than that of females. This paper reports an investigation of a DEG, which was developed to enhance the acquisition of geographical knowledge, carried out on British, German and Austrian K12 students aged between 11 and 14. Methods include a survey on initial design concepts, user tests on the system and two single-gender focus groups. Gender and cultural differences in gameplay habit, game type preferences and game character perceptions were observed. The results showed that both genders similarly improved their geographical knowledge, although boys tended to have a higher level of positive user experience than the girls. The qualitative data from the focus groups illustrated some interesting gender differences in perceiving various aspects of the game.

Keywords: User experience, UX, gender differences, digital educational game, DEG, performance, attitude.

1 Introduction

Digital games are omnipresent within the life of the current generation of K12 students. According to a 2008 survey by the Pew Research Center (Washington, DC), 97% of children between 12 and 17 years regularly play computer, Web, portable, or

A. Holzinger and K. Miesenberger (Eds.): USAB 2009, LNCS 5889, pp. 42–54, 2009.
© Springer-Verlag Berlin Heidelberg 2009

console games [1]. Obviously, Digital Educational Games (DEGs) can offer exciting and dynamic environments with which to engage players in meaningful and motivating learning activities and to inspire them to explore a variety of topics and tasks [2], [3], [4], [5], [6].

Play is definitely one of the most important psycho-pedagogical concepts, consequently games, used in an appropriate setting, can be used as splendid educational tools. Nonetheless, some previous research suggests that children in general tend to find such educational games quite uninteresting, and that huge gender differences do exist, implying that boys have a more negative attitude towards so-called edutainment games than girls [7].

Whilst some recent research has indicated that the gender gap is beginning to close (cf. gender similarities hypothesis [8]), whether such a gap-narrowing can be generalized to the domain of computer games remains completely unclear. In fact, the number of girls playing computer games has been increasing tremendously. However, it is still perceived as a masculine activity, and therefore more boys than girls prefer and are willing to spend time on it. Some questions remain relevant: "How much of this is pressure from outside?" and "How many non-academic families see it as acceptable for boys to spend 3 hours in front of a computer, while girls are expected "not to waste their time?" The disparity in gender-specific gameplay pattern is attributable to the stereotypical presentation within games, a general lack of female characters in games, high competitiveness, and limited social interaction [9], [10], [11], [12]. Even children in elementary schools perceive that software is gendered by design. The implication is more than just the attitude towards games; more serious impacts are girls' low confidence in working with computers and avoidance from technology-related fields [13], adversely affecting their employability.

Specifically, Kinzie & Joseph (2008) [7] identified some interesting gender issues in game character preferences, for instance, the children in their study preferred characters to be of their same gender and ethnicity. Presumably, culture with its values, beliefs and norms plays an important role in shaping children's perceptions of game characters. With the above review, we are motivated to study gender differences in the context of a DEG under development. The prototype topic is based on geography. In the first phase, an initial game design concept was developed prior to any implementation. In brevity, the game story was about an alien kidnapping a boy and their flying round the world to collect relevant geographical information. A survey was designed to evaluate the acceptance of the target groups towards the game design, to verify if there are any gender and cultural differences in perceiving the game characters, and to elicit feedback on improving the game concept - a practical means to gather user requirements. In the second phase, an executable prototype was produced.

User tests primarily in the form of observations and questionnaires were implemented to gauge the learning efficacy of the game, user acceptance towards it and different aspects of user experience.

To further explore the issue of gender differences, two focus groups with representative school children were additionally conducted. Results from these three empirical studies (designated as Study 1, 2 and 3, respectively) relevant to gender issues are presented subsequently.

2 Related Work

Research questions addressing the influence of gender on attitudes towards computer games in general and on performance resulting from playing DEGs in particular are not new (e.g. [14]). Previous research on multimedia learning revealed that the mode of presenting learning content significantly affects learning processes, hence the learning performance and is highly related factors including attention, motivation and attitude [15], [16], [17], [18]. However, answers to these questions keep on changing, given the highly dynamic landscape of gaming technologies. Besides, the computer game industry tactically lures more females to become frequent players. Broadly speaking, there exist two major types of factors – personal and technical - contributing to gender differences in computer gameplay patterns.

On the personal level, traits [19], motivation ([6], [12], [20], [21]) and self-concept pertinent to IT competence [22] are salient variables that interact intricately with game design features. Specifically, two genders are observed to differ in achievement needs, with males generally demonstrating a higher level of desire to compete and beat their opponents than females [12], who seem disadvantaged and less effective in competitive settings such as computer games. An apparently weaker competition orientation of females undermines their engagement in computer gameplay. Apparently – because it has not yet been established (to our satisfaction) that this is not inherent in the upbringing, i.e. environmental rather than genetic. We know a number of people – both genders – where this tendency is reversed.

Similarly, males are found to be keener sensation seekers than females as they tend to take risks (e.g. extreme sports) in pursuit of intense feelings and emotional arousal. The notion of sensation seeking has been widely adopted by Zuckerman [23] and other scholars to explicate a range of social phenomena including various types of addictive behaviors. For example, arousal is an interesting, but not fully researched, psychological construct underlying sensation seeking as well as gameplay ([24], [25] [26]). Interestingly, arousal is said to be normally at a higher level in males than females [27]. These observations partly explain gender differences in gametype preferences and their different motivations to play. Males prefer games with confrontational and violent contents entailing fast responses and yearn to gain high scores, sense of control and other personal esteems. In contrast, females appreciate storylines and personalities of game characters to be explored at a relaxing pace and value building relationships with game characters or co-players [10].

Intertwining with competition and sensation seeking orientation is the issue of self concept. Despite insignificant gender difference in online abilities as indicated by some objective measures, females subjectively perceived such abilities to be much inferior to males [22].

Evidence on the trainability of cognitive-perceptual skills, which have traditionally been assumed to be innately stronger in males, seems not yet able to dispel the misconception in females.

In summing up the aforementioned arguments, presumably males tend to play games more engagingly than females; the former are then expected to show significantly higher learning gain from DEGs than the latter. However, recent empirical evidence indicates that no such gender difference can be detected [2]. Indeed, with the increasing awareness of gender differences and their underpinning factors, today's

DEGs are so designed as to eliminate potential biases against any gender by incorporating a range of features and activities [28]. Our project 80Days adopts a gender-sensitive approach by adapting the game to gender-based differences to optimize the learning process. Note, however, the elaboration of the adaptivity mechanism concerned falls outside the scope of this paper.

3 Method and Procedure

3.1 Study 1– A Survey on Initial Design Concepts

Design of the Questionnaire. The questionnaire consists of two major parts. Part A contains five close-end questions on the respondent's gender, age, gameplay habit, gametype preference, and affinity for geography. Specifically, four gametypes – learning, action, strategic and sport – are provided as options to reduce the possible confusion in children; the other taxonomies are deemed rather complex (e.g. [29]). Part B addresses different aspects of the game.

First a synopsis of the game story is presented. Then two close-end questions on the perceived interestingness of stories about aliens/UFO in general and of the game story in particular. An open-end question on describing improvement suggestions is presented. A set of four questions on understanding how respondents identify themselves with the story's main play characters are given. Another set of three questions on the preference of non-play character is posed. The last question is to assess the respondent's intention to play the game in the future.

Participants. Two samples from Germany and England were involved in the survey. They were school children aged between 11 and 14, the target group of the game. In Germany, the survey was conducted in the context of computer games fair.

In England, the survey was administered in the classrooms of the five participating schools. Due to organizational constraints, the survey could only be conducted by the school teachers, who were asked to read aloud a script with similar wordings used in the German event. This step was taken to maximize the comparability of the data collected from the two settings.

Table 1. Demographic data of the survey respondents in the two countries

Country	Number/Age	Girls	Boys	Sub-total
German	Number	78	61	139
	Mean Age (SD)	12.6 (1.1)	12.8 (1.1)	12.7 (1.1)
British	Number	59	83	142
	Mean Age (SD)	12.5 (0.9)	12.7(0.9)	12.6 (0.9)
	Sub-total	137	144	281

3.2 Study 2 – User Tests of the Executable Prototype

Design of the User Test Session: It was conducted in groups of various sizes, ranging from 4 to 14, in the rooms within the respective school premises. Each participant was allocated to one computer where the game was installed and played it on an individual basis.

One or two researchers were present in the rooms all the time to provide help and observe the participants' performance and behaviours. The arrangement of the test session is summarized in Table 2. The instruments listed therein have been developed by the project's research team.

Participants: Two and four secondary schools in England and Austria were involved. Due to some technical problems, some of the participants could not complete the four missions. To compare validly the scores earned in Pre-test ALQ and those in Post-test ALQ, which were based on the contents of the four missions, our data analysis focused on the cases that successfully attempted all the missions.

Besides, considering the differences in the test setting (e.g. larger group size in Austria) and curricular design, data of the British and Austrian samples are not merged whereas data from different schools in the same country are collapsed into one sample.

Table 2. Overview of the arrangement of a user test session

Activity	Objective and Instrument
Introduction	Describe the aim of the evaluation tests and instruct how to operate the laptops and headsets
Fill in the Background Questionnaire	Items: Identifier (ID), gender, age, gameplay frequencies, gametype preference, affinity for geography, subject grades, early involvement, and expectation
Fill in Pre-test Assessment of Learning (ALQ)	16 domain-specific questions, open and close-ended, are based on the content of the game.
View Tutorial	6 open- and close-ended questions about the usefulness and usability of the tutorial material and presentation
Total Pre-Gameplay time: ~ 30 minutes	
Play each of the four micro-missions and fill in "After Mission Questionnaire" (AMQ) right away	Questions of AMQ are adapted to the content of the respective micro-mission. Research on user experience evaluation [28] suggests that data be collected as close to the interactive event as possible. Otherwise, the validity of the data may be compromised.
Total Gameplay time: ~52 minutes	
Fill in the Post-test Assessment of Learning (ALQ)	The same questionnaire used for Pre-test. The rationale is to assess whether the children's knowledge of the geographical concepts covered in the game can be enhanced after playing it.
Usability and User Experience Evaluation of the Game Features	It consists of six sections with each of them focusing on different aspects of the game. The first section "General Game Experience" was adapted from [26].
Debriefing	Summarize the activities of the test session and thank the participants
Total Post-Gameplay time: ~33 minutes	

In this paper, considering the length limit, we just report the findings on the British sample. Thirty-six children from the two British schools, of which the academic performances and infrastructure were comparable, could play through the four missions; the average age was 13 years old; 16 of girls and 20 are boys.

3.3 Study 3 – Focus Groups

Procedure: Prior to taking part in focus groups, participants were asked to play through the whole game without being required to fill in any questionnaire except the one for background data. Subsequently, focus groups were conducted as follows:

- Introduction: Participants were explained the purpose of the focus group
- Game recall exercise: Each participant was given a stack of Post-it notes and asked to write down whatever they could remember about the game.
- Sharing game recollections: Participants were presented three A3 sized sheets, one for each: "Positive" (green), "Neutral" (yellow) and "Negative" (red). They were asked to stick their notes to the respective sheets based on their own judgment how to categorise their notes.
- Guided discussions on different aspects:
  - o Gameplay, e.g. *"In the whole game, which game character do you think you are supposed to be and which one would you like to be?"* (NB: the rationale is to understand if there is any mental gap in role adoption)
  - o Game characters and game story, e.g. *"How would you change the alien so that you will like him better?"*
  - o Learning part, e.g. *"How would you compare learning geography through the game with through normal classroom teaching?"*
  - o Geographical content, e.g. *"If you could add any aspect of Geography to the 80Days game, what would it be and how would you do it?"*
- Debriefing

Participants: Two single-gender groups, five boys and five girls, from a British secondary school (different from that in Study 2) were involved. Their participations were voluntary. The average age was 13.4 for the female group and 14.0 for the male one. All the participants, except one girl who had never played computer games before, were frequent gamers.

4 Results and Discussion

4.1 Study 1 – Survey

Results show that half of the British boys (52%) play games everyday and half of the German boys (51%) play games more than twice per week. Interestingly, 14% and 12% of the British and German girls report that they have never played games, whereas all of the British boys have played games. 45% of the German girls play games less than once per week whilst 44% of their British girls play more than twice per week. These figures seem to suggest that (i) Boys tend to play games more frequently than girls, irrespective of the country of residence; (ii) the British children tend to play games more frequently than their German counterparts. To investigate whether these observations are statistically significant, we performed the linear categorical regression analysis. The value of $R^2 =$ .25 indicates that the two predictor variables *gender* and *country* can explain only 25% of the variations of the gameplay frequencies. Results show the significant effect of the predictor *gender* (beta = .49, t = 9.32, $p<.001$)) and the non-significant effect of the covariate *country* (beta = -.017, t =-.136, $p>0.05$). Boys tend to play games more frequently than girls, and the country of residence does not have a strong effect on the children's gameplay frequency.

Cramer's V was used to evaluate whether *gender* was associated with *gametype preferences*. The most preferable gametype for both the British girls (51.7%) and boys (49.5%) are Action, followed by Strategic and Sport. The least preferable gametype is Learning with only 3.2% and 2.2% for the girls and boys, respectively. The value of the Pearson chi-square equals 0.581 ($p =$. 901), indicating that *gender* and *gametype preference* for the British sample are **not** significantly related. In contrast, the German sample demonstrates a slightly different pattern from their British counterparts.

The most preferable gametype for the German girls is Strategic (40.7%), followed by Action and then Sport; the most preferable gametype for the German boys is Action (54.3%), followed by Strategic and then Sport. The least preferable gametype is Learning with 13.2% and 3.2% for the girls and boys, respectively. The value of the Pearson chi-square equals 13.972 (p = .003), indicating that *gender* and *gametype preference* for the German sample are significantly related.

With the aim of evaluating to what extent the respondents tended to associate the Boy's (the main play character) attributes with their own, they were asked to rate first the Boy and then themselves, using a 7-point scale, with respect to six pairs of contrasting adjectives adapted from the instrument Speech Evaluation Instrument [4] consisting of three subscales – superiority, attractiveness and dynamism, against which the entity of interest is evaluated:

- *Superiority*: Intelligent vs. Unintelligent; Uneducated vs. Educated;
- *Attractiveness*: Friendly vs. Unfriendly; Cold vs. Warm;
- *Dynamism*: Peaceable vs. Aggressive; Talkative vs. Shy

The exercises resulted in a set of so-called "Boy-based ratings" and another set of "Me-based ratings". We computed the correlations among them independently for the German and British samples.

A number of statistically significant correlations are found. Nonetheless, based on our research interest, we explore whether there are gender differences in perceiving the relationships between the Boy's attributes, between the Me attributes, and between these two sets. Interestingly, results consistently show that the German female respondents tended to perceive the attribute interrelations, be they applied to the Boy or themselves, in a more complicated manner than did their male counterparts. Presumably, the German male respondents may associate their own attributes with the Boy's (same gender) more strongly than the female respondents (opposite gender) do; however, the empirical results indicate otherwise. In contrast, the British respondents' perceptions, irrespective of gender, are less complicated than those of their German counterparts.

Interestingly, the British male respondents tend to perceive the associations in a more complex way than their female ones – a reverse of the trend demonstrated by the German sample. Fig. 1 and Fig. 2 illustrate the results of how the respondents perceive the associations between the game main play character ("Boy") and themselves ("Me").

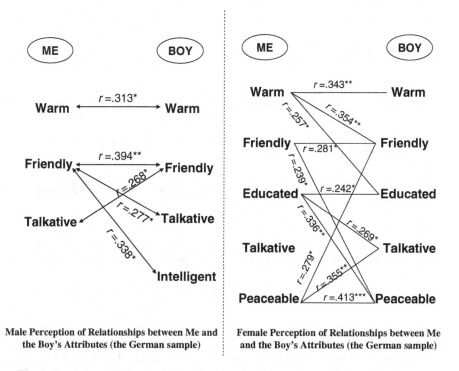

Male Perception of Relationships between Me and the Boy's Attributes (the German sample)

Female Perception of Relationships between Me and the Boy's Attributes (the German sample)

Fig. 1. Gender-specific perceptions of the play character and oneself (German sample)

Contrasts are observed across gender and culture. We also aim to find out whether those who perceived a stronger "Boy-Me" association might have a higher tendency to play the game in the future (i.e. the last question of the survey) by summing the absolute differences in ratings over the six pairs of adjectives.

While there is a moderately significant correlation for the British sample (r =-.24, N = 199, $p<.05$), it is not significant for the German sample.

4.2 Study 2: User Tests of the Executable Game Prototype

Our basic assumption is that by completing the four Missions of the game the participating children can gain better understanding of the geographical contents addressed therein. The improvement can be measured in terms of the significant difference in their performance between the Pre-Assessment and Post-Assessment of Learning Questionnaire (Pre-ALQ vs. Post-ALQ). The British participants demonstrated statistically significant learning gains (Pre-ALQ: mean = 20.8; Post-ALQ: 27.4; $t = 5.25$, $df = 35$, $p<.001$). When breaking down the data by gender, some interesting observations are obtained. In both Pre-ALQ and Post-ALQ, the boys performed significantly better

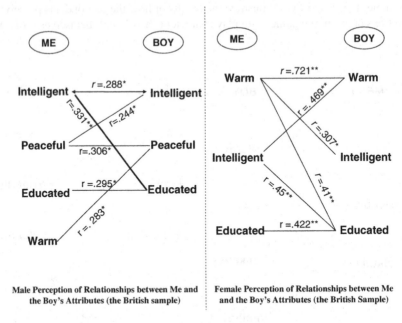

Male Perception of Relationships between Me and
the Boy's Attributes (the British sample)

Female Perception of Relationships between Me
and the Boy's Attributes (the British Sample)

Fig. 2. Gender-specific perceptions of the play character and oneself (British sample)

than the girls (p <.05). The girls gained on average 5.1 points with the range of difference being -6 to 14 whereas the boys gained on average 7.8 points with the range of
difference being -9 to 23 (Note that some children lost rather than gained points after
the gameplay; we speculate that either they made guesses in Pre-ALQ or got confused
about certain concepts during the gameplay).

However, the boys did *not* improve to a significantly larger extent than did the girls.
In other words, both genders benefited from the gameplay in terms of knowledge gain,
but it did not privilege the boys or frequent gamers (i.e. gameplay frequency is a non-
significant covariate). Existing literature suggests that evaluation of children's game
experience should address seven dimensions, including *challenge, competence, flow,
immersion, negative affect, positive affect and tension* ([30]). Accordingly, 14 statements are adapted for evaluating our game, two for each dimension (Table 3). The
participants are asked to rate each of them with a 5-point Likert scale with the right-
most and leftmost anchors being 'not true at all' and 'very true', respectively.

Results indicate that significant gender differences can only be found in two dimensions, namely *Competence* (S7) and *Flow* (S8, S14). The girls rated themselves
lower in Competence than did the boys (Mg = 2.3, Mb=1.4; t = 2.4, p<.05; NB: the
higher the rating in S7, the lower the perceived competence is).

This seems to be a much investigated and frequently documented phenomenon –
particularly in human resources, one is even advised to add 10% to a female assessment of herself and to deduct 10% from a male assessment. In contrast, the boys rated

significantly higher than did the girls in S8 ($Mg = 3.1$, $Mb=4.0$, $t = 2.4$, $p<.05$) and S14 ($Mg = 3.1$, $Mb= 4.0$, $t = 2.5$, $p<.05$).

Table 3. Seven dimensions of general game experience

S1.	Playing this game was useful for me to learn geography	(Challenge)
S2.	This game was interesting for me	(Positive Affect)
S3.	I put a lot of effort in playing the game	(Challenge)
S4.	Playing this game was a waste of my time	(Negative Affect)
S5.	I felt frustrated when playing the game	(Negative Affect)
S6.	I felt proud when I finished the game	(Competence)
S7.	The game was too difficult for me	(Competence)
S8.	I could concentrate easily on the game activities	(Flow)
S9.	I had the feeling of controlling the game	(Positive Affect)
S10.	I was completely absorbed by the game	(Immersion)
S11.	I felt exhausted after playing the game	(Tension)
S12.	I had the feeling that I had returned from a journey	(Immersion)
S13.	I felt time pressure	(Tension)
S14.	I was fast at reaching the target of the goal	(Flow)

As the feeling of flow [31] is imperative for engaging in gameplay, it can be inferred that the boys had stronger positive experience through playing the game than did the girls.

4.3 Study 3 – Focus Groups

The focus groups were audio-taped and transcribed in verbatim. Some interesting gender-specific findings are obtained. In game recollections, only two boys named a negative feature: the character Aunt (i.e. a static 3D female figure presenting geographical information via a text window) and controls of the Spaceship. In contrast, each of the five girls named at least two negative features, including the Aunt and the Spaceship. This observed differences suggest that the boys had a higher acceptance towards the game than did the girls. In guided discussions, all the five boys and only one girl considered flying UFO the most positive aspect. Three girls appreciated the graphics the most and criticized that there was too much talking in the game. With regard to the role adoption, it seemed that both genders had difficulty in recognizing that they were supposed to play the role of the abducted Boy. One girl, who was able to do so, uttered: "You were the boy. You were looking through his eyes" whereas another stated surprisingly: "I never even knew we were playing with him. I didn't even know we were that person." Concerning the learning part, both groups mentioned the importance of getting explanation. Some girls remarked: "The teacher gives you more of an explanation … you can ask them (the teacher) if you're stuck". Similarly, a boy mentioned "In the classroom you've got an explanation… but in the game it just tells you you've got to go here and name the countries, like it doesn't give you an explanation." Interestingly, some boys suggested lengthening the missions but some girls suggested shortening them. Quite unexpectedly, none of the girls proposed including a female game character (instead of or in addition to the Boy) whereas one boy recommended providing a choice of a male or female play character.

5 Concluding Remarks

Previous research suggests that children, especially boys, tend to find learning games boring. It is corroborated by our findings of Study 1 that, among the four gametypes, the learning game is least preferable and that girls are more positive towards it than boys. Existing research also suggests that children tend to prefer game characters that are in some way "like me". Cultural preferences for normative personal qualities may influence children's preferences for the characters they play. While there are some very interesting gender and cultural differences in interpreting the main play character's qualities and in associating those qualities to theirs, such associations do not affect their intention to play the game. The setting, where the survey was conducted, could have impact on the children's perception and acceptance of the game: the relaxing atmosphere in the game fair with the exhibitors as opposed to the more structured classroom environment with the teacher. Results of Study 2 suggest that both genders could benefit to a similar extent from playing the game in terms of domain-specific knowledge gain. Interestingly, the female participants found the game more difficult to play than did the boys. In other words, the girls' perceived competence in gameplay was significantly lower than the boys'. This observation is consistent with the earlier research. In the same vein, the boys had experienced a significantly higher level of flow feelings, which are important for engaging in and enjoying a game. Findings of the two single-sex focus groups also suggest gender-specific likes and dislikes towards different aspects of the game. Surprisingly, the girls tended to be more critical. Currently, we are exploring psychosocial theories to explicate the phenomena observed and their implications on future work.

References

1. Hoffmann, L.: Learning through games. Communications of the ACM 52(8), 21–22 (2009)
2. Papastergiou, M.: Digital Game-Based Learning in high school Computer Science education: Impact on educational effectiveness and student motivation. Computers & Education 52(1), 1–12 (2009)
3. Law, E.L.-C., Kickmeier-Rust, M.D., Albert, D., Holzinger, A.: Challenges in the Development and Evaluation of Immersive Digital Educational Games. In: Holzinger, A. (ed.) HCI and Usability for Education and Work, 4th Symposium of the Workgroup Human-Computer Interaction and Usability Engineering of the Austrian Computer Society, pp. 19–30. Springer, Heidelberg (2008)
4. Robertson, J., Howells, C.: Computer game design: Opportunities for successful learning. Computers & Education 50(2), 559–578 (2008)
5. Kickmeier-Rust, M.D., Peirce, N., Conlan, O., Schwarz, D., Verpoorten, D., Albert, D.: Immersive Digital Games: The Interfaces for Next-Generation E-Learning? In: Stephanidis, C. (ed.) HCI 2007. LNCS, vol. 4556, pp. 647–656. Springer, Heidelberg (2007)

6. Holzinger, A., Pichler, A., Maurer, H.: Multi Media e-Learning Software TRIANGLE Case-Study: Experimental Results and Lessons Learned. Journal of Universal Science and Technology of Learning, 61–92 (2006),
http://www.justl.org/justl_0_0/multi_media_
elearning_software/justl_0_0_0061_0092_holzinger.pdf
7. Kinzie, M.B., Joseph, D.R.D.: Gender differences in game activity preferences of middle school children: implications for educational game design. ETR&D-Educational Technology Research and Development 56(5-6), 643–663 (2008)
8. Hyde, J.S.: The gender similarities hypothesis. American Psychologist 60(6), 581–592 (2005)
9. Agosto, D.E.: Design vs. content: A study of adolescent girls' website design preferences. International Journal of Technology and Design Education 14(3), 245–260 (2004)
10. Agosto, D.E.: Girls and Gaming: A summary of the research with implications for practice. Teacher Librarian 31, 8–14 (2004)
11. Gentry, M., Gable, R.K., Rizza, M.G.: Students' perceptions of classroom activities: Are there grade-level and gender differences? Journal of Educational Psychology 94(3), 539–544 (2002)
12. Hartmann, T., Klimmt, C.: Gender and computer games: Exploring females' dislikes. Journal of Computer-Mediated Communication 11(4) (2006)
13. Gartner: Report: Women and men in IT: Breaking through sexual stereotypes, http://www.gartner.com/it/sym/2006_/esc18/esc18_home.jsp (last access: 2009-09-14)
14. Gorriz, C.M., Medina, C.: Engaging girls with computers through software games. Communications of the ACM 43(1), 42–49 (2000)
15. Sanders, A.F.: Elements of Human Performance: Reaction Processes and Attention in Human Skill. Lawrence Erlbaum, New York (1998)
16. Kettenanurak, V., Ramamurthy, K., Haseman, W.: User attitude as a mediator of learning performance improvement in an interactive multimedia environment: an empirical investigation of the degree of interactivity and learning styles. International Journal of Human-Computer Studies 54(4), 541–583 (2001)
17. Holzinger, A., Kickmeier-Rust, M., Albert, D.: Dynamic Media in Computer Science Education; Content Complexity and Learning Performance: Is Less More? Educational Technology & Society 11(1), 279–290 (2008)
18. Holzinger, A., Kickmeier-Rust, M.D., Wassertheurer, S., Hessinger, M.: Learning performance with interactive simulations in medical education: Lessons learned from results of learning complex physiological models with the HAEMOdynamics SIMulator. Computers & Education 52(2), 292–301 (2009)
19. Bonanno, P., Kommers, P.A.M.: Exploring the influence of gender and gaming competence on attitudes towards using instructional games. British Journal of Educational Technology 39(1), 97–109 (2008)
20. Ebner, M., Holzinger, A.: Successful Implementation of User-Centered Game Based Learning in Higher Education – an Example from Civil Engineering. Computers & Education 49(3), 873–890 (2007)
21. Holzinger, A., Pichler, A., Almer, W., Maurer, H.: TRIANGLE: A Multi-Media test-bed for examining incidental learning, motivation and the Tamagotchi-Effect within a Game-Show like Computer Based Learning Module Educational Multimedia, Hypermedia and Telecommunication 2001. Association for the Advancement of Computing in Education, Charlottesville (VA), pp. 766–771 (2001)

22. Hargittai, E., Shafer, S.: Differences in actual and perceived online skills: The role of gender. Social Science Quarterly 87(2), 432–448 (2006)
23. Zuckerman, M.: Sensation seeking: Beyond the optimal level of arousal. Erlbaum, Hillsdale (1979)
24. Brehm, J.W., Self, E.A.: The Intensity of Motivation. Annual Review of Psychology 40, 109–131 (1989)
25. Hanoch, Y., Vitouch, O.: When less is more - Information, emotional arousal and the ecological reframing of the Yerkes-Dodson law. Theory & Psychology 14(4), 427–452 (2004)
26. Stickel, C., Fink, J., Holzinger, A.: Enhancing Universal Access – EEG based Learnability Assessment. In: Stephanidis, C. (ed.) HCI 2007. LNCS, vol. 4556, pp. 813–822. Springer, Heidelberg (2007)
27. Lucas, K., Sherry, J.L.: Sex differences in video game play: A communication-based explanation. Communication Research 31(5), 499–523 (2004)
28. Boyle, E., Conolly, T.: Games for learning: Does gender make a difference? In: Conolly, T., Stansfield, M. (eds.) 2nd European Conference on Games Based Learning, pp. 69–75. Academic Publishing (2008)
29. Apperley, T.H.: Genre and game studies: Toward a critical approach to video game geners. Simluation & Gaming 37(1), 6–23 (2006)
30. Poels, K., IJsselsteijn, W.A., de Kort, Y.A.W., Van Iersel, B.: Digital Games, the Aftermath. Qualitative insights into Post Game Experiences. In: Bernhaupt, R. (ed.) Evaluating User Experiences in Games. Springer, Heidelberg (in press)
31. Hassenzahl, M.: The effect of perceived hedonic quality on product appealingness. International Journal of Human-Computer Interaction 13(4), 481–499 (2001)

Improving Cognitive Abilities and e-Inclusion in Children with Cerebral Palsy

Chiara Martinengo[1] and Francesco Curatelli[2]

[1] University of Genova - Italy, Dept. of Mathematics (DIMA)
martinen@dima.unige.it
[2] University of Genova - Italy, Dept. of Electronics (DIBE)
curatelli@unige.it

Abstract. Besides overcoming the motor barriers for accessing to computers and Internet, ICT tools can provide a very useful, and often necessary, support for the cognitive development of motor-impaired children with cerebral palsy. In fact, software tools for computation and communication allow teachers to put into effect, in a more complete and efficient way, the learning methods and the educational plans studied for the child. In the present article, after a brief analysis of the general objectives to be pursued for favouring the learning for children with cerebral palsy, we take account of some specific difficulties in the logical-linguistic and logical-mathematical fields, and we show how they can be overcome using general ICT tools and specifically implemented software programs.

Keywords: e-inclusion, cognitive development, mathematical learning, motor disability, cerebral palsy, educational software.

1 Introduction

Computers are currently important tools for increasing information or productivity in various fields (education, job, personal communication, etc.). In particular, in the last years their importance has emerged to get the objective of e-inclusion, where this term refers to both narrow objectives of global accessibility to ICT by all citizens, and ampler objectives of better people integration obtainable with ICT [1]. The aim is to make it possible for all citizens the participation to the information society, the improvement of social relationships, the improvement of job possibilities and, in general, the active participation to the cultural patrimony of the society. Such objectives are important for all people, but mainly for the disabled persons; in fact ICT can dramatically increase their integration in the society by providing tools for overcoming the motor, perceptual or cognitive difficulties that make this participation difficult.

Overcoming the motor and perceptual difficulties, through the study and design of suitable interfaces for each specific disability, is obviously the first objective. In fact, this allows many disabled people (mainly adults, for whom the disability has been acquired and the cognitive abilities are normal) to achieve good levels of e-accessibility. However, although necessary, such solutions are often not enough

A. Holzinger and K. Miesenberger (Eds.): USAB 2009, LNCS 5889, pp. 55–68, 2009.

when the disability concerns children. In fact, in disabled children the cognitive development is not yet completed, and it can be made very difficult by disability. For example, this is the case for motor-impaired children with cerebral palsy, whose cognitive development is slowed down or prevented both by the neurological damage suffered and by the fact that their motor disabilities make much more difficult to live the experiences that normally concur to the development of the cognitive abilities in non-disabled children.

Children with cerebral palsy typically suffer from cognitive troubles which are directly imputable to the extension of the lesions in the cerebral areas that are appointed to the high-level cognitive functions (e.g., the language). However, there are also cognitive disorders which are not the direct consequence of a lesion, but are due to the limitations imposed by the motor impairment, especially when it is significant. In fact, the formation of the knowledge in the first years of life is tightly tied to: the exploratory activity, the ability to perform motor actions and objects manipulation in the surrounding world, and the ability to pick up information from the environment by exploring and modifying it through own actions [2,3,4]. Therefore, as the intellectual operations originate from real actions, it is necessary to verify how the limitations of the motor experiences do influence learning, and therefore the mental development of the children; in fact, during the first 18 months of life the mental and the motor activities are hardly dissociable [5]. Nevertheless, on one side the motor problems are not a sure sign of mental retardation, and on the other side the relation between motor functionalities and cognitive activities varies in very remarkable measure during the different phases of the development. In fact, the importance of the direct experience, and therefore of the integrity of the motor functionalities, already decreases starting from the second infancy [6].

Therefore, for motor-impaired children ICT can provide a very useful support, not only to overcome the motor barriers for accessing to computers and Internet, but also for the cognitive development of the children. In fact, after an accurate task analysis has defined for a child the most suitable methods, plans and timelines for learning, the use of ICT computation and communication tools make it easier to put into effect the required learning plans in both the logical-linguistic and logical-mathematical fields [7].

Starting from these motivations, our research has concerned the use of ICT for the cognitive development of motor-impaired children by cerebral palsy and learning difficulties in the frame of mild mental retardation; in this field we have a direct experience because this is the condition of our daughter Margherita. We have followed our daughter, who has just taken the middle school exam, for all her path of studies, cooperating with the scholastic structures and integrating her learning path with specific homework. Our professional formation has allowed us to look for and to find suitable methodological tools as well as to select, and eventually implement, some educational tools to favour the cognitive development of Margherita. Anyway, even if our interest has been particularly focused to cerebral palsy, some ideas contained in this work could be valid in other cases in which disability involves mild cognitive retardation.

2   Learning in the Logical-Linguistic Field

2.1   General Objectives

The basic learnings inherent to the spoken and written language are of fundamental importance for the cognitive development, and therefore for the integration in the society. In fact, on them is founded the acquisition of thought tools that are important, not only for the scholastic job in general, in whatever disciplinary field it be developed, but mainly for the global formation of the person. This produces a better self-awareness and a better awareness of the relation with the external world and with own history. In other words, we can tell that such learnings are essential to acquire a *orientation* [8]. In the field of the psychology of the development age, H.S. Sullivan introduced the concept of *orientation in the life*, which is reached through several subsequent phases [9].

For this reason, already in the first years of school it is important to define objectives of general cognitive type:

a) attainment of the aware control of thought activity, when this is spontaneously manifested by the child, and
b) promotion of the thought activity, when this shows low autonomy;
c) connection between the *thought* and his *representation* (graphical, spoken verbal, written verbal;
d) connection between the *thought* and the *reality*, so that the thought activity become able to take into account the constraints put by the external world, and so to face more and more complex real situations;
e) efficient management of the memory, both to remember past actions and stories and to insert in the memory important elements related to new experiences.

Our experience in this field is both direct, through the scholar path of our daughter, and indirect, through the interaction and the exchange of opinions with other parents and teachers. Therefore, we can reasonably affirm that, during the primary schools and towards disabled children, the above objectives are pursued in a very partial way, mainly concerning points a), b), c) and d). In particular, one of the most serious and frequent lacks is given by the fact that the educational lines adopted by teachers towards disabled children often are limited to pursue the objective of rote learning rather than of building the capabilities to understand and think.

On the basis of our experience, we think that, mainly when the disabled pupil shows low autonomy in the production of thought, it is essential to perform a suitable diagnosis of his/her situation, limits and potentialities, which allow to reach the individualization of the best strategies for overcoming the learning difficulties.

2.2   Difficulties and Solutions for Children with Cerebral Palsy

Going into detail, now we treat the case of children with motor disability due to cerebral palsy and with learning difficulties in a frame of mild mental retardation.

On the basis of our experience we have been able to directly ascertain that in these cases the difficulties in the linguistic field can be subdivided, at a first level of analysis, into two types:

- Operational difficulties; for example those in handwriting, due to motor disability, or in reading, due to problems in visual coordination, or in reading/ writing, due for example to problems in the short- and long-term memories.
- Cognitive difficulties, especially in the semantic understanding of the text and in the autonomous production of text.

Some operational difficulties in the acquisition, in relatively fast times, of handwriting are surely present when the thin movements of the hands are compromised from the motor disability. Such difficulties can be solved, or anyway mitigated, through the use of the computer, obviously in different ways according to the type and level of disability. It is important to notice that the solution to this type of operational difficulty can also have very positive repercussions on the cognitive field. In fact, the autonomy in writing is a primary objective; achieving the possibility to autonomously express in writing his/her own thought is, for the child in general and particularly for the disabled child, a fundamental finishing line for his/her personal growth.

Besides the psychological motivations, such as for example the personal gratification and the increase of self-esteem, which surely are involved in the attainment of an important finishing line, the role of the written language is fundamental in the cognitive growth; in fact, the expression of own thought in writing involves the structuring of the same thought and a return of the thought on the thought itself which actively favours its development. Moreover, the modern educational lines for reading learning are often based on the application of the global method, and therefore they start from the copying of words and simple sentences. Insofar, to give as soon as possible the possibility to write through the use of the computer also make easier reading learning, which is another fundamental element for the development of the thought.

On the basis of our experience, we have been able to verify that a widespread fear, among parents, teachers and specific operators of the sector, is substantially unfounded, i.e., the fear that the early and systematic use of the computer for writing by motor-impaired children be harmful, because it would inhibit the acquisition of the residual ability of handwriting that is made possible by the motor disability of the child. Instead, in our case the early use of the computer since the first year of the primary schools does not have inhibited handwriting, rather it has facilitated its acquisition. In fact, we have verified that handwriting, in the form of copying and in the autonomous production of words or short texts, can be considered by the child a pleasant activity.

Besides, we have ascertained that, going on in the scholar path, the use of the computer from children with cerebral palsy for writing texts (description of situations, answers to questions, imaginative theme) tends to make the written production easier and more effective than the spoken production. In fact, the pupil is more relaxed and can often develop the scholar activity contemporaneously with relaxing passive activities, such as for listening to the music.

2.3   Access to ICT by Children with Cerebral Palsy

Now, we appraise the specific possibilities offered from the computer and communication technologies for the realization of a more effective learning and a real inclusion of the disabled pupil in the information society.

In fact, the computer tools can also play a fundamental role to make gratifying, and at the same time productive from the cognitive point of view, the free time of the child, which otherwise would be much emptier of activities, interests and gratifications than that of the normal coetaneous.

- Writing e-mail messages, the participation to Internet blogs, forums and Facebook facilitate the contact with coetaneous persons of the external world for children that otherwise would be deprived of real and virtual interlocutors.
- Using Internet makes it possible to download drawings, to colour and to modify them with graphics programs on his/her own computer; this stimulates the creativeness of the child. In the last years it is also possible to use on-line video games, to listen unload and transfer music on MP3 readers. The interaction with the computer can stimulate the inventiveness and the reasoning of the child. An illuminating anecdote: one day Margherita transferred some musical files on her own MP3 reader by using a procedure, made possible by Windows XP, which she had discovered autonomously and by functional analogy with other Windows Explorer operations.
- Using Internet search motors allows to access sites containing useful information, such as texts of songs, news, addresses. The possibility to use on-line encyclopaedias, such as Wikipedia, allows to delve into matters of interest for homework or simply for personal curiosity. Moreover, the possibility to access to online electronic documentation replaces, overcoming in efficiency, searching and reading paper books, which typically are not easily accessible (for the difficulty to pick them) and readable (for the difficulty to skim through the pages).

The activities on the computer, used as a stand-alone tool or with the Internet connection, can create a virtuous circle involving: the improvement of the mental coordination and of the cognitive abilities, the improvement of the visual-motor coordination, and the growth of the autonomy and of the self-esteem of the disabled person. This create therefore the favourable conditions so that e-inclusion be not only a theoretical possibility but a real result.

Moreover, ICT allows to reduce the difficulties of access to the computer and to the net in the cases in which the motor disability does not allow to effectively use a normal computer. In fact, in many cases writing of texts by motor-impaired users with cerebral palsy can be made very difficult and slow by the physical limitations. The use of speech recognition interfaces can be useful in some cases, but such solution is not applicable when the disability also concerns the phonatory apparatus. Besides, such solution can be unsuitable for the development of the task in the class by the pupil. In fact, the most diffused solution is to use hardware or software interfaces that allow to: a) increase the speed of text entry, which is measurable in terms of characters per second (CPS) or word per minute (WPM); or to: b) reduce the number of pressed keys, which is measurable in terms of the percentage gain in comparison to the use of hardware or software standard keyboard (KSR). In the first case, the use of special hardware or software alphabetical keyboards, e.g., with greater keys, facilitates the action of the pupil [10] and yields an increase of CPS but not a decrease of KSR, which is unitary. In the second case, the use of software programs for word completion and prediction allows to get KSRs with values going from 30%, with only one suggestion, to more than 50%, with five or more visualized suggestions [11,12]. Consequently, also the text entry time decreases, but less that the improvement of KSR would suggest; this because of the higher cognitive load which is necessary for visual scanning the suggestions [13].

Instead, to reduce KSR without the necessity to use word prediction and its consequent cognitive load, we have adopted a novel pseudo-syllabic, non alphabetical, model, with the definition of a strict and meaningful subset of sequences of letters with high frequencies [14]. The pseudo-syllables are rigorously built by composition of a consonant grapheme $\hat{C}$ and one vowel grapheme $\hat{V}$ (each one constituted by one or more letters or from the empty grapheme) according to the grapheme configurations $\hat{C}\hat{V}$ or $\hat{V}\hat{C}$. So, the keyboard is organized as a 2-dimensional array of keys (orthogonal keyboard); every row is univocally assigned to a vowel grapheme $\hat{V}$ and every column is univocally assigned to a consonant grapheme $\hat{C}$. In this way, a key $\hat{C}\hat{V}$ or $\hat{V}\hat{C}$ is reached fast, with an access to the vowel row and an access to the consonant column. Since the two sets are orthogonal, it is not necessary to perform a complete visual scanning of the keyboard; so, the access is fast and the cognitive load is smaller; the proposed scheme has been applied with success to languages such as Italian and Spanish [14,15]. The obtained KSRs are greater that 34% and 43% when only alphanumeric characters are considered; they are comparable or better than those obtainable by word prediction programs with single suggestion. Anyway the two techniques can be integrated to cumulatively increase the text entry speed. Recently, comparable results have been obtained with English [16].

Currently our research in this field concerns the extension of the pseudo-syllabic model to characterize a greater number of syllabic structures and the study of new models of keyboards.

3   Learning in the Logical-Mathematical Field

3.1   General Objectives

Also the first learnings in the logical-mathematical circle are of fundamental importance for the cognitive development: in fact, they set the bases, not only for the mathematical job of the whole scholastic path, but also and above all for acquiring the ability to analyze, through mental abstract models, reality and to elaborate a suitable feedback to the problematic situations that can be met in the daily life. In particular, the first mathematical learnings set the bases to acquire important finishing lines as:

a) the ability of reasoning which is anchored to the reality;
b) the organization of the thought;
c) more conceptual learnings, such as the meanings of the number and of the basic operations.

However, just during the first learnings, type two major general difficulties arise for the mathematical field.

The first one directly concerns disabled children. Typically, children start the primary school with a series of mathematical modelling experiences that were acquired in family or in the nursery school, and that are almost exclusively based on motor type experiences.

As argued for instance in [17], on the basis of a delved activity of experimentation and research in the nursery school, typically 5 year old children already are rather able facing numerical matters, even if they encounter numbers with more figures. They are able to read and write numbers, they know how to compare them also using complex strategies [18], even if full maturity in the autonomous elaboration of the numerical information grows gradually, together with the mathematical abilities [19].

Instead, in the first years of life the child with motor difficulties is almost totally deprived of that type of experiences; therefore, preschool experiences of mathematical modelling are very poor and absolutely not enough to serve as base for learning the concept of number in its different meanings: ordinal, cardinal, measure, value, and so on. As we have clearly seen in our experience, nothing can be taken for granted, and it is necessary to find specific compensatory strategies to move around the poverty of spatial experiences.

The second difficulty concerns school, teachers and educational lines. In the framework of the first logical-mathematical learnings, the chosen methodological lines, which are often inadequate already for non-disabled children, are almost always entirely unsuitable in case of disability. For instance, an approach that is based exclusively on sets attributes too much importance to the cardinal aspect, and it can constitute an obstacle to the acquisition of the other meanings of numbers [20]. In fact, recent studies on the brain activity have shown that in the various phases of the arithmetic elaboration different cerebral regions are activated. In particular, different regions seem to be specialized in the codification of the manifold meanings of numbers [21]. Therefore the various meanings of numbers cannot be directly deduced the one from the other.

Moreover, the typical didactic path plans, already during the first scholastic years, the use of the numbers in abstract calculations that are totally separated by the meanings of the numbers. This can lead to wrong interpretations of the cognitive situation of a child with disability; as we have seen in our experience, the fact that in the first scholastic years the child knows how to perform simple calculations with the numbers does not at all mean that he/she has understood the different meanings of numbers and operations. We believe that the choice of the more appropriate methodological lines always has to follow a careful and precise diagnosis of the cognitive condition, difficulties and potentialities of the child, and it should be targeted to the individualization of strategies to overcome the difficulties. Unfortunately, such analysis is done only often the relevant offices in a clinical-physician framework (for example the neuropsychiatrist of the advisory bureau or the centre that has in load the child), and the indications that could follow from such analysis remain sometimes disregarded in the real scholar experience.

As is the case for the linguistic field, also for the mathematical field the difficulties can be operational or cognitive; as regards the latter we can cite, as example, the difficulties in acquiring the various meanings of the numbers and of the four basic operations. These being specific matters, this is not the proper place for a detailed analysis of the difficulties that can be found in the logical-mathematical field, analysis that will be done in [22,23]. Instead, in the following paragraph we will consider an example that is, in our opinion very meaningful, of a situation of cognitive difficulty which can receive a valid aid by the use of a suitable program software. Anyway, it is essential that the use of computer tools be inserted within the framework of an approach to the different meanings of the numbers and of the elementary operations; this approach must be closely related to *fields of experience* that be meaningful of the concrete reality in which the child acts [24,25,26,27]. In fact, the use of suitable and real fields of experience favours the recognition of the sense of the problematic situation and allows to build a resolving strategy; this is done by recalling schemes of behaviour that are usual, with a positive reflex for the cognitive development. Here it is also valid what has already been observed, i.e., that the use of the software programs does not have to become a rote exercise, but it must be loaded with meanings. This is possible only if the activities that require the use of the software are preceded, for the time that is judged necessary in every specific case, and accompanied by real activity in the chosen field of experience. In such way, the exercise with the computer recalls concrete and well consolidated contents.

3.2   Difficulties on the Number Line and Theoretical Solutions

One of the most serious difficulties that we have found in our experience have concerned the comparison between two numbers (in particular between relatively large numbers, that is greater than 20, for which the set control is lost) and the connection with the ordinal meaning. In practice it is the difficulty *to see* the numbers inside the number line and to create a mental representation of the number line itself. We have also ascertained how it is difficulty to spontaneously connect and in natural way the concept of *greater than-smaller than* with that of *it follows-it precedes*.

In our experience, we have ascertained that the attempts to acquire a mental representation of the number line through the use of a straight number line drawn on a strip of paper (as those that are normally used at school) have not led up to any meaningful result. The reason for the failure of this approach is the lack of the connection with the temporal dimension; in other words there is not a meaningful experience, in temporal terms, of an ordered sequence to which to associate the sequence of the numbers. This makes meaningless to work on drawn number lines because they are an abstract support, which can be used for performing calculations but these are unrelated to any meaningful context. For example, according to our experience, the uncertainties to mentally determine the subsequent one of a given number or the incapability to mentally determine the previous one of a given number are not due, or minimally, to a memory deficit, but rather to a lack of meaning which to make reference to.

The more natural field of experience to consolidate the ordinal meaning of the numbers is the *calendar* [28]; this framework allows to build the ordinal meaning of the number in tight connection with the ordering of the days, starting from counting numbers, which the child usually already owns, at least for the first numbers. It is opportune, at least for the first activities developed in this field of experience, to use a real calendar, possibly with the succession of the numbers of the days put in vertical. Here are some examples of first activities on the calendar.

Today it is Wednesday, October 14:

1. looks for the day on the calendar
2. what day will it be tomorrow?
3. what day was it yesterday?
4. what is the date on next Sunday?
5. in 4 days, what day will it be?
6. how many days are before October 19?
7. what day was two days ago?

The purpose of these activities is to reach the control of the temporal dimension and the modelling of the flow of the time with the sequence of the numbers. It is therefore fundamental that the vertical strip of the days of the month does not reduce to a succession of abstract numbers but be, as much as possible, full of meanings. Any exercise on the timeline does not have to become an exercise that be an end in itself. The time must be a time of life and events, a time of expectations and memoirs; otherwise, it is not *time* but a new formal abstraction. This can happen by annotating the meaningful events of the life of the child, both the periodic ones, such as going to swimming pool or to the physiotherapist, the birthdays of relatives or schoolmates, and the extemporaneous ones, such as a trip, a visit to grandparents, etc. In this way, the number on the calendar comes to correspond to a meaningful event, which is situated in well precise way in the time, and the search of the number, even if done (at least initially) by counting the days starting from the beginning of the month, is not a simple rote counting as an end in itself, but it is connected to a concrete fact. For example, the child is much more motivated if is asked to look for the date of the day in which he/she will go to the cinema to see a movie that he likes, and to count how many days miss to that date.

In this way, also the classical activities for the development of concepts such as *first, later, while* assume meaning not as abstract categories, but as cultural acquisitions, rich in emotional and affective resonances. Moreover, there is a dialectical relation, of mutual consolidation, between the acquisition of the cultural tools that allow to orient in the temporal dimension, and the acquisition of the psychological dimension of the time, which is based on the concrete experiences of the changes in his/her own life and in the life of the society. The interiorization of the timeline and of the paths on it also allows to acquire some important meanings of the operations. For example, exercise 5 needs an addition, to determine the requested day, whose meaning overcomes the purely set meaning. In fact, to calculate the new date, it is necessary to add the number (ordinal) that represents today's date and the number 4 (cardinal) that represents the number of the days. Instead, exercise 6 is solved in natural way with an addition of completion, which then introduces to one of the meanings of the subtraction.

All these activities can require quite long times, but our experience has shown us that it is necessary not to be in a hurry, neither to lose heart themselves if sometimes it seems that the performed work has been useless and it is necessary to restart afresh. For the reasons that we have previously exposed, the construction of the mental representation of the number line and of the possibility to move on there above is a fundamental step of the cognitive development, so that the time devoted is certainly well.spent. In our experience, we have witnessed during the years to the slow but real consolidation in Margherita of the mental representation of the number line and of the awareness of what is the meaning in moving on it.

In a subsequent phase, time modelling can be extended to the months of the year, and then to the sequence of the years which becomes historical time. We have ascertained that it is very difficult for motor-impaired children to acquire the awareness of historical periods that are quite far away in the time, but this awareness can be reached if specific references to facts and concrete people are used.

In parallel, the modelling of the time can be done with the hours of the day, through the scanning of the time of the day, in hours, minutes, seconds. Here many problems that are useful in the daily life arises, such as: reading the time, to calculate in how much time a certain event will happen, or after how much time a certain event has happened, etc. It is preferable, at the beginning, to use a real clock, which be easily handlable, through which be possible to have a concrete experience of measuring particular time slices, such as one minute, ten minutes, an hour. It has been very meaningful for our daughter to realize how long is an hour by waiting that the minute hand come back again in the position of departure, after having made the whole turn. The objective of all these activities is the control of the daily time, which is a necessary requisite to be able to interact in autonomous and conscious way with the events of the life and power, and to use the interaction and relation potentialities that are made at disposal by ICT.

3.3   An Educational Tool for the Number Line

Many educational tools have been proposed, which use the number line to increase the basic arithmetical skills of students. However, although quite useful in general, the available tools typically do not seem well suited to implement the learning strategies explained above. In particular, they lack an adequate link with real meanings about the numbers put on the line, and they do not allow to use the number line hierarchically, i.e. making it possible to display and surf different lines with different resolutions. Other typical problems, common to most mathematical educational programs, are the excessive emphasis placed on the recreational aspect of the tool (so often distracting the pupils from the real target of the actions), and the limited possibility the teacher or the pupil have to modify the proposed exercises.

To overcome the above limitations, and provide a useful educational tool for the activities on number line, ordinal aspect of numbers and meanings of operations, we have implemented the prototype of a hierarchical timeline software program.

In fact, starting from the default page which displays the days, the temporal resolution can be increased, going into the page of the hours and then of the minutes (by pressing the keyboard key F12), or decreased, going into the page of the months and then of the years (by pressing the keyboard key F11). The navigation inside each page is done by using the keys F1 and F2, or through the arrows. The use of the keyboard keys typically makes it possible the use of the tool also by severely motor-impaired children, who could not use the mouse.

In the hours and minutes pages, time can be displayed also with an analogical or a digital clock to improve the skill in watch reading. The exercise to be performed can be set by either the teacher or the pupil, produced in random way by the program, or loaded from an external file. In the user modality the presence of incoherent data is signalled through an error message; instead, in the random modality the data are already provided respecting some constraints that allow the execution of the problem.

In comparison to a *papery* application of the method described in the previous paragraph, the use of the tool has allowed Margherita to have a much greater operational autonomy. In fact, the possibility to quickly and easily move, both inside the current page and changing the temporal resolution, has allowed a more dynamic and autonomous management of the exercises.

4 Design Guidelines

From the considerations stated in the previous sections, we can argue that with children affected by cerebral palsy the overall objective should be that of building, through exercises and experiences that be connected to real meanings, their capabilities to understand and think; this both in applying educational lines and in using educational tools to support them. However, in too many cases the features of the available educational tools are more suited for rote learning, with the repetition of specific actions triggered by the recognition of specific situations. The result is that, in presence of even minimal changes of the environment conditions, the disabled pupil is not able to manage the new situation because the mechanical execution of exercises that are not linked to real meanings did not aid the pupil to build a better inner capability to understand and react with the environment.

The experience acquired in our work can be consolidated into some basic design principles and guidelines for educational tools that be targetted to children with cerebral palsy:

1. In any suitable educational tool for motor-impaired children, the actions needed to write texts should as much as possible minimize the need of movements that are impossible or very difficult for motor-impaired users. So, whenever possible the tool should use keyboard keys to select actions and move along objects (as it is the case for the timeline). On the other hand, it is anyway convenient to maintain the possibility to use the mouse; this to make easier the work for children with moderate motor-impairment.

2. For tools requiring significant text inputs, it should be added a virtual or hardware multi-letter keyboard which allows the user to input syllabic or pseudo-syllabic texts. In this way the overall typing speed can be significantly increased; moreover this approach can be possible enhanced with completion menus and word prediction to get even higher speed improvements. This is very important because, as we have seen before, a major objective is that the pupil achieves a real autonomy in writing; although it is not possible to formalize specific tool characteristics for directly aiding the cognitive mechanisms of the thought production, this is not the case for the actions that are required to input texts.

3. The mathematical educational tools should not put excessive emphasis on recreational aspects, i.e., they should not be mainly perceived as games; this is important in order not to distract the pupil from the real target of the exercise. Instead, the tools should be as much as possible open, giving the teacher and the pupil the possibility to modify the proposed exercises.

4. Concerning tools for learning the basic arithmetic operations, timeline should be considered the privileged real environment to implement the number line. The timeline should be organized hierarchically, with the possibility to expand and reduce the time resolution (different pages for minutes, hours, days, months, years, ...). Moreover, it should be possible for the pupil to mark the timeline with meaningful events; for example milestone events of the pupil's life can be marked on the years and months pages, while daily actions of the pupil can be marked on the days and minutes pages.

5   Conclusions

In this paper we have seen how, for children with motor disability due to cerebral palsy, the opportunities provided by ICT spread to the possibility to provide a necessary support to the cognitive development the children. In fact, after having individualized the modalities, the contents and the times of learning, the ICT tools allow to put in act, in a more efficient and complete way, the required learnings, both in the logical-linguistic field and in the logical-mathematical field. On the basis of our direct experience with our daughter Margherita, we can conclude that in the logical-linguistic field the activities that are correlated to the use of ICT tools are very useful, not only as leisure and aid to the scholastic learning, but also to improve the motor and visual coordination.

Besides, through the activities on the computer, a virtuous circle can be created which leads to the improvement of the mental coordination, of the cognitive abilities, of the motor and visual coordination, and to the growth of the autonomy and self-esteem of the disabled pupil. On the other hand, we have directly ascertained that the learnings in the mathematical field are much more critical; so, the acquisition of the basic mathematical concepts by the child has to happen with gradualness and verifying the acquisition of the related meanings. ICT tools can be very useful to support the proposed methodology, provided that they have been studied and used in support of real activities in the field of experience chosen, so that the exercise to the computer actually recalls concrete and well consolidated contents. To this aim we have provided some guidelines for designing educational tools that be well suited for the use by children with cerebral palsy.

References

1. UE Ministerial Declaration, Riga (June 2006),
   http://ec.europa.eu/informationsociety/events/ict_riga_2006/doc/declaration_riga.pdf
2. Zanobini, M., Usai, M.C.: Psicologia della Disabilità e dell'Integrazione. Franco Angeli (2005)
3. Benelli, B., D'Odorico, L., Lavorato, M.C., Simion, F.: Formation and Extension of the Concept in a Prelinguistic Child. Italian J. of Psychology 4, 429–448 (1977)
4. Benelli, B., D'Odorico, L., Lavorato, M.C., Simion, F.: Forme di Conoscenza Prelinguistica. Giunti, Firenze (1980)
5. Stella, G., Zanotti, S.: Selective Neuropsychological Problems of Learning in Disability in The Restored infant. In: Proc. 4th EACD Meeting (1993)
6. Stella, G., Biolcati, C.: La Valutazione Neuropsicologica in Bambini con Danno Motorio. In: Bottos, M. (ed.) Paralisi Cerebrale Infantile (2002)
7. Hughes, S.: Another Look at Task Analysis. J. of Learning Disabilities 15(5), 273–275 (1982)
8. Galimberti, U.: Enciclopedia di Psicologia. UTET, Torino (1999)
9. Sullivan, H.S.: The Interpersonal Theory of Psychiatry. Norton & Co., New York (1953)
10. Stone, D., Jarrett, C., Woodroffe, M., Minocha, S.: User Interface Design and Evaluation. Morgan Kaufmann, San Francisco (2005)
11. Zagler, W.L., Beck, C., Seisenbacher, G.: FASTY-Faster and Easier Text Generation for Disabled People. In: Proc. AAATE 2003, Dublin, pp. 964–968 (2003)
12. Wandmacher, T., Antoine, J.Y., Poirier, F.: SIBYLLE: A System for Alternative Communication Adapting to the Context and its User. In: Proc. ASSETS 2007, Tempe, pp. 203–210 (2007)
13. Trnka, K., McCaw, J., Yarrington, D., McCoy, K.F.: User Interaction with Word Prediction: the Effects of Prediction Quality. ACM Trans. on Accessible Computing 1(3), 17:1–34 (2009)
14. Curatelli, F., Martinengo, C.: A Powerful Pseudo-Syllabic Text Entry Paradigm. Int. J. of Human-Computer Studies 64(5), 475–488 (2006)

15. Curatelli, F., Martinengo, C., Mayora-Ibarra, O.: Improving Text Entry Performance for Spanish-Speaking Non-Expert and Impaired Users. In: Proc. CLIHC 2005, Cuernavaca (2005)
16. Curatelli, F., Martinengo, C.: English Orthogonal Keyboard for Efficient Text Entry (2009) (in preparation)
17. AA. VV.: Le Competenze dei Bambini di Prima Elementare: un Approccio all'Aritmetica. In: La matematica e la sua didattica, vol. 1, pp. 47–95 (2004)
18. Teruggi, L.A.: Scritture Numeriche nella Scuola dell'Infanzia. In: Didattica della matematica e rinnovamento curricolare, pp. 119–130 (2001)
19. Girelli, L., Lucangeli, D., Butterworth, B.: Development of Automaticity in Accessing Number Magnitude. J. of Experimental Child Psychology 76(2), 104–122 (2000)
20. Boero, P., Rondini, A.: Bambini, Maestri, Realtà. Rapporto tecnico, vol. 1, Cl. I (1996)
21. Dehaene, S.: The Number Sense: How the Mind Creates Mathematics. Oxford University Press, Oxford (1999)
22. Martinengo, C., Curatelli, F.: On Some Maths Difficulties in Motor-Impaired Children with Cerebral Palsy (2009) (in preparation)
23. Martinengo, C., Curatelli, F.: Moving on the Timeline: Maths Learning Method for Motor-Impaired Children (2009) (in preparation)
24. Scali, E.: Costruzione dei Significati del Numero Naturale in Prima Elementare: il Ruolo dei Campi di Esperienza e la Funzione Mediatrice dell'Insegnante. In: Seminario Nazionale di Ricerca, Pisa (1994)
25. Boero, P.: Semantic Fields Suggested by History: their Function in the Acquisition of Mathematical Concepts. Zentralblatt für Didaktik der Mathematik (20), 128–133 (1989)
26. Boero, P.: The Crucial Role of Semantic Fields in the Development of Problem Solving Skills. In: Mathematical Problem Solving and New Information Technologies, pp. 77–91. Springer, Heidelberg (1992)
27. Boero, P.: Experience Fields as a Tool to Plan Mathematics Teaching from 6 to 11. In: Proc. II It-De Symp. on Didactics of Math., vol. 39, pp. 45–62 (1994)
28. Dapueto, C., Parenti, L.: Contributions and Obstacles of Contexts in the Development of Mathematical Knowledge. Education. Studies in Math. 39(1), 1–21 (1999)

Finding Relevant Items: Attentional Guidance Improves Visual Selection Processes

Sonja Stork[1], Isabella Hild[1], Mathey Wiesbeck[2], Michael F. Zaeh[2], and Anna Schubö[1]

[1] Ludwig Maximilian University Munich, Department Psychology,
Leopoldstraße 13, 80802 Munich, Germany
sonja.stork@lmu.de

[2] Technische Universität München, Institute for Machine Tools and Industrial Management, Boltzmannstraße 15, 85747 Garching, Germany

Abstract. In daily life and at work people are confronted with complex information. Especially elderly or disabled users might be overburdened by the amount of information and distracted by irrelevant items. Due to this, they possibly fail to find and select relevant items in visual search. This could be demotivating for the use of media like the internet or could result in an inability to achieve certain job requirements. A method for supporting performance in visual search tasks is the guidance of attention. The present study compares different methods for attentional guidance. Results show a benefit for peripheral exogenous cues realized as luminance changes in comparison to endogenous central cues. Possible applications for the proposed attentional guidance method are discussed.

Keywords: Information Presentation, Visual Search, Eye Movements, Human Performance, Augmented Reality, Assistive Technology.

1 Introduction

In daily life and in working environments people are confronted with complex information while using media like the internet or various software tools. As dealing with the increasing complexity of information is a challenge for even young and healthy people, especially elderly [1,2] and disabled users need to be supported adequately. Accordingly, there is an increasing need of Assistive Technologies [3]. Nevertheless, following the "Design for All" principle should lead to the development of information technologies and applications which are easily adaptable to the needs of a user besides developing rather specialized tools for certain minorities [4].

One possible solution in this context are multimodal systems [5] because the use of different channels for information presentation enhances the possibility that also disabled people can deal with it. Besides this, also healthy users can be in context conditions where a certain modality is unavailable. Adaptivity [6] and context awareness are therefore key issues for adequate supporting devices. The multimodal account does not rule out the necessity to also support as good as

A. Holzinger and K. Miesenberger (Eds.): USAB 2009, LNCS 5889, pp. 69–80, 2009.

possible within a certain modality, because it might be the only available source of information.

The visual modality is of outstanding relevance, as humans normally gather 70-80% of information via the eyes. Vision is capable of delivering complex information in a short time. The drawback is that sometimes too much visual information is available which makes it difficult to decide which items are relevant. Accordingly, the vision modality can be supported optimally by reducing the amount of information to be processed and guiding selective visual attention.

1.1   Selective Visual Attention and Visual Search

As the human visual system is limited with respect to the number of objects which can be processed simultaneously, selective visual attention has to be directed to areas of interest. Search strategies can help to allocate attention appropriately and efficiently. Bottom-up or stimulus-based mechanisms guide visual attention to objects with certain physical properties, e.g. to salient objects [7]. Those so-called pop-out stimuli enable fast and efficient search, in contrast to more serial and inefficient search where each item has to be scanned one after the other [8]. The difficulty in visual search increases with increasing similarity between target and distractors [9]. In case of overlapping features no target pop-out is possible. Here, search times increase with the number of surrounding distractors.

Many daily life activities include visual search tasks. While searching for apples in the supermarket it might be helpful to look for red or green objects, i.e. prior knowledge can help to direct attention to relevant salient object features. While scanning websites or searching for menu items in software applications such a prior knowledge often is not available, if a user does not know how a certain icon or button looks like. Then every possible item has to be scanned and checked serially. What might be only annoying for young and healthy users could lead to the inaccessibility of certain media or scenarios for elderly and disabled people. Accordingly, investigating cognitive processes and their limitations is one key issue for the development of adaptive support [10,11,12].

1.2   Supporting by Attentional Guidance

Especially for people who have difficulties to apply adequate search strategies and feel rather overburdened by information presentation in complex media attentional guidance can help to select relevant information. There exist different methods for directing attention to specific locations [13]. As described in the beginning salient items are able to capture attention. One method using this bottom-up mechanism is to present salient spatial cues at the position attention should be shifted to. This so-called endogenous, stimulus-driven or peripheral cueing is involuntary in the sense that it leads to automatic and reflexive attention shifts. In contrast, endogenous or central cueing requires a top-down interpretation of a symbolic cue in order to know where the attention has to be shifted to. Any kind of symbol representing the direction or location for the attention shift can serve as endogenous cue. Typically arrows are used. In general, reflexive attention shifts in response to a peripheral salient cue are faster than shifts in response to central cues, which need additional time for the interpretation processes. Attributes like movement, size, orientation, color and transient luminance changes are very effective exogenous cues which enable parallel search [14]. On computer monitors it is easy to present endogenous cues or exogenous cues for items which have to be found on the screen. A possibility to cue relevant item positions also in real world-scenes is the Augmented Reality (AR) technique. Here, the environment is overlaid with additional information at the exact position where it is needed. By using a simple LCD projector it is possible to present also peripheral cues to various contexts [15,16].

1.3 Search Performance and Eye Movements

Typically, visual search performance is measured by the time necessary to find a relevant item among several distractors, i.e. the reaction time for target detection. Another method for the investigation of visual search performance is the tracking of eye movements. Eye fixations can be interpreted as indicator for attention allocation. Eye movement parameters like fixation count and fixation duration provide information on the intensity of information processing of a certain object [17]. Moreover, these eye movement parameters show whether difficulties during the information processing occur [18]. For example, a high fixation count indicates an inefficient visual search [19]. Moreover, eye movement trajectories visualize the search path and can be analyzed in order to investigate search strategies as well as the influence of distracting items. Results from fundamental research have demonstrated that spatial cues can accelerate attention shifts, as well as eye movements and simple reaction times [20].

2   Experiment: Searching Relevant Items

The goal of the present experiment was to evaluate different methods for attentional guidance which are expected to facilitate the visual search of relevant items. Previous results regarding a similar task and setting indicated an advantage of peripheral endogenous cueing, i.e. of highlighting, but differences were not clear cut [16]. Moreover, we were interested in the question up to how many items can be cued efficiently at the same time.

2.1   Methods

Participants. Twentyfour participants (7 female, 17 male, aged between 19 and 42 years, mean age 25.5 years, 22 right-handed) joined the experiment. All had normal or corrected-to-normal vision according to self-report and were naïve as to the purpose of the experiment. Participants received 8 Euro per hour for their participation.

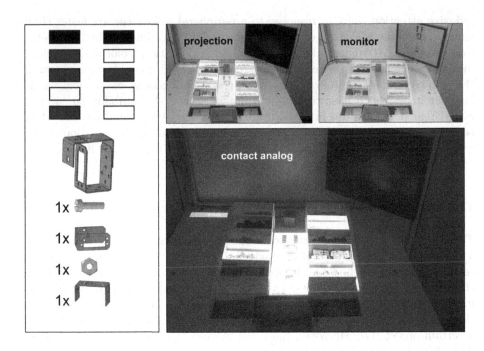

Fig. 1. The item list with goal representation and schematic picture of item locations (left). The three different presentation modes: projection between the item area (top middle), monitor presentation (top right) and contact analog highlighting of item positions (bottom right). The work space was the same in all presentation modes.

Items and Presentation Modes. The task was to search, select and grasp different types of items according to detailed instructions. The items consisted of technical elements (i.e. screws, nuts and metal brackets). Instructions were generated with Powerpoint 2002. Each instruction consisted of a list of items relevant for the current trial (see Fig. 1). The number of relevant different items varied between 1, 2, 4 and 6 per trial. Accordingly, between two and six items were used in the search list and had to be grasped within a trial. Only one exemplar of those items had to be selected and grasped. Above the item list a goal representation consisting of all relevant parts in the item list was presented. This goal representation was used, although the goal state had not to be build, in order to make the memorizing process comparable to previous applied studies in the working context. Items and goal representations were designed by a CAD program (Catia V5R17), a software tool that allows constructing technical 3D models. The pictures were rotated in perspective in order to show as many details as possible.

The instructions were presented via three different presentation modes which differed in respect to the location and content of information presentation. Search information was displayed on the computer monitor or via a projection on the search area. In the monitor and projection condition, a schematic picture of the ten item locations (five left, five right) was depicted on the top, showing the relevant item positions in orange and irrelevant positions in black. The difference between monitor and the projection mode consisted in the location of the information presentation. In the monitor condition, participants had to switch attention between the information presentation that was displayed on a computer screen and the search area over a larger distance than in the projection condition. In the projection mode cues for the relevant item position were closer to the real items than in the monitor condition. Therefore, item positions were supposed to be found more easy and effortlessly. In the contact analog condition all schematic item locations were black. Relevant item locations were directly highlighted by a contact analog projection of white light. This highlighting of items was expected to be helpful for attention allocation resulting in improved search performance. Figure 1 shows the three resulting presentation modes: projection (top middle), monitor (top right) and contact analog (bottom right).

Design. A within-subjects design with repeated measurements was used in the study. Each of the three presentation modes was presented to each participant, the order was balanced. Each presentation condition consisted of 80 search trials, 240 trials in total. The arrangement of item positions was changed after 20 trials (i.e. four times per condition) in order to avoid strong memorizing effects which could eliminate advantages of different presentation modes. The order of item arrangements was randomized. Each number of items (1, 2, 4 and 6 items) was presented in 20 trials per presentation condition in randomized order.

Setup and Apparatus. The setup consisted of a table equipped with a LCD projector (EIKI LC-XB40, 4000 lumen, resolution 1024 x 768 pixel) attached to a plate above. A front-surface mirror was placed in 45° angle orientation in front of the projector enabling the projection of information directly on the search area. Additionally, a computer monitor was placed in front (see Fig. 2).

The search area on the table included five boxes to the left and right as well as a field for instructions (only used in the contact analog and projection condition) and covered 49 x 38 cm. Item boxes were arranged upwards with 12 angles of incline in order to avoid body movements during grasping movements, which would have made the collection of eye movement data more difficult. During the experiment the left eye's gaze position and eye movement duration during the search was recorded via an Eyelink® 1000 system (®2007 SR Research Ldt.; sample rate 500 Hz, pacing interval 1000 Hz, 100% illuminator power) in remote mode. The eye tracker was placed in a hole in the table below the search area. Eye movements of the left eye were registered while using a marker above it. Below the eye tracker a box was placed for collecting the selected and grasped items. The experiment was controlled with MATLAB® R2006b (The MathWorks Inc.) on a Dell Latitude D830 laptop running Microsoft Windows® XP Professional. Eye movement data were recorded by a portable Host PC in DOS mode. The two computers were synchronized for real time data transfer via an Ethernet link by using the Eyelink Toolbox extensions for Matlab [21].

A Polhemus Liberty motion tracking system was utilized for tracking the movement of the right and left hand, but these results are not in the focus of this

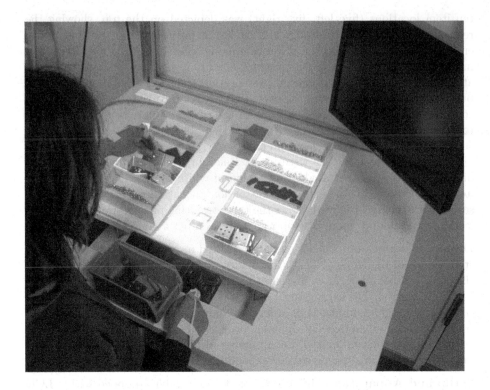

Fig. 2. Experimental setup with the working area, beamer projection, monitor, source of the motion tracker as well as the remote eye tracker. One exemplary participant is selecting and grasping one item with the left hand in order to place it inside the box in front.

paper. A footpedal was positioned below the table in order to make it possible to proceed to the next search step without using the hands. Additionally, the whole session was recorded by a DV camera. The video stream allows for the evaluation of search performance in more detail.

Procedure. Participants sat in front of the table containing the search area. In the beginning participants were instructed during a short training phase in order to familiarize them with the items and setting, but without using the schematic pictures or highlighting. Following this, markers were attached to the right and left index finger. For eye movement recording a marker for remote eye tracking was placed above the left eye. After adjusting the camera position a 5-dot calibration was conducted on the plane of the search area. This calibration was repeated after each presentation condition. Participants were asked to move as little as possible. Then the first condition was introduced, i.e. highlighting or schematic pictures of item position were explained. After pressing the foot pedal a trial started with the presentation of a fixation cross in the center and the instruction to place the index fingers in a starting position left and right of the goal box for the items. Another foot pedal press started the presentation of the search instruction. After all relevant items had been selected and collected to the goal box a food pedal press terminated the trial and started the presentation of the next trial's fixation cross. Participants were instructed to select, pick and place the item as fast as possible, but no explicit time constraint was given. They had to grasp items on the left side with their left hand and items on the right side with their right hand. Moreover, items had to be selected in the depicted order. The whole experiment lasted approximately two hours.

2.2   Data Analysis

For the analysis of completion times the time stamp difference between the initiating and terminating food pedal press was computed for each trial. Accordingly, completion times included search times and times to grasp for all items in a trial. Naturally, the overall completion times in trials with four or six items were longer than completion times for trials with one item, because more elements had to be selected, grasped and collected. In order to estimate the time needed for the selection of one item within a trial overall completion times were divided by the number of relevant items. Thus, the time needed per item could be compared between different item numbers. In the following only completions times per item are reported. For the eye movement analysis the number of fixations per trial (fixation count) was computed with the Eyelink DataViewer software. Overall fixation counts within a trial were also divided by the number of relevant items, resulting in a mean fixation count per item. Means per subject were adjusted by excluding all outlier values below and over two standard deviations. Completion times were entered into a 3 x 4 repeated measurements ANOVA with presentation mode (contact analog, projection, monitor) and item number (1, 2, 4 and 6) as factors. For the statistical analysis of fixation counts the data of the monitor condition had to be excluded, as the eye pupil signal was lost too often during head movements towards the monitor. Accordingly, a 2 x 4 repeated measurements ANOVA was computed with the factors presentation mode (contact analog, projection) and item number (1, 2, 4 and 6).

2.3   Experimental Results and Discussion

In accordance with cueing effects established in cognitive experimental psychology we hypothesized differential effects of peripheral and central cueing on visual search performance.

Figure 3 (left) shows the completion times per item in the contact analog, projection and monitor condition with different item numbers. In general, the completion time per item was reduced if more items had to be selected and grasped, i.e. the completion times for one of four or six items were shorter in comparison to trials with one or two items. Most importantly, the completions times were shorter with contact analog highlighting than in the projection and in the monitor condition. This effect of different presentation modes was significant ($F(2,46) = 12.28$, $p < 0.001$). Post-hoc contrast analysis revealed a significant

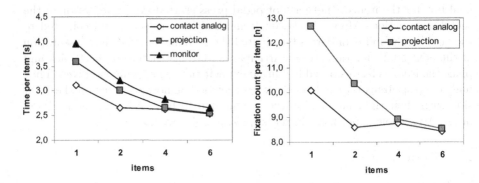

Fig. 3. Completion times per item on the basis of foot pedal presses in the three presentation modes and with different number of items (left). Fixation counts per item on the basis of eye tracker data in the three presentation modes and with different number of items (right).

reduction of completion times with contact analog highlighting in comparison to the projection condition ($F(1,23) = 6.27$, $p < 0.05$) as well as in comparison to the monitor presentation ($F(1,23) = 23.97$, $p < 0.001$). Also, completion times in the projection condition were significantly shorter than in the monitor condition ($F(1,23) = 6.16$, $p < 0.05$).

The variation of item number showed a significant effect on completion times ($F(3,69) = 180.21$, $p < 0.001$). Moreover, a significant interaction between presentation mode and number of items was present ($F(6,138) = 20.65$, $p < 0.001$). Here, a contrast analysis comparing the contact analog and projection condition revealed a significant time reduction with contact analog highlighting between the item numbers 1 to 2 and 2 to 4 but not between 4 to 6 items.

Figure 3 (right) shows the fixation count per item for the contact analog and the projection condition and four different item numbers. In accordance with completion times also the fixation counts were reduced with contact analog presentation in comparison to the projection condition. A significant effect for presentation mode, i.e. contact analog versus projection, was present ($F(1,23) = 12.90$, $p < 0.01$). Also the interaction between presentation mode and number of items was significant ($F(3,69) = 33.00$, $p < 0.001$). Contrast analysis revealed a significant reduction of fixations in the contact analog presentation mode in comparison to the projection condition with 1, 2 and 4 items.

In sum, completions times and fixation counts showed the same pattern of results. The benefit for the contact analog presentation as well as the reduction with more items was present. Both measurements demonstrated the improved performance with peripheral cueing.

Figure 4 shows two exemplary eye movement trajectories of one subject performing the same search task in the contact analog (left) and the projection condition (right). Obviously, in this case contact analog exogenous cueing directed attention more efficiently to the relevant item position. In the projection condition, the schematic picture or endogenous cue was not able to prevent attention

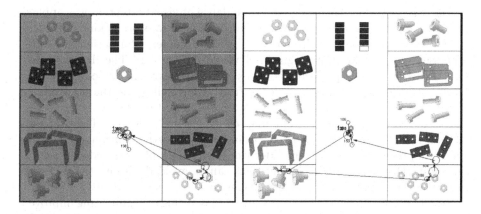

Fig. 4. Two exemplary eye movement trajectories of one subject performing the same search task in the contact analog (left) and the projection condition (right)

allocation and resulting eye movements to a irrelevant item position. Maybe item similarities lead to confusion of item positions.

Complementary to previous results, a significant benefit of the contact analog exogenous spatial cueing was demonstrated. These findings are in accordance to results from cognitive experimental psychology. Importantly, this benefit was only present if the number of items did not exceed 2, that is 20 % of the total item number. Highlighting of more item positions afforded more serial search again.

3   Conclusions and Future Directions

The experiment compared three modes for attentional guidance in order to evaluate facilitation effects for attention shifts to relevant item positions. Exogenous peripheral cueing, i.e. highlighting of item positions, lead to faster completion times and fewer eye fixations in comparison to endogenous symbolic cues presented in the search area or on the monitor. Both the completion times for selecting and grasping relevant items as well as the number of necessary eye fixations showed the same pattern of results, delivering converging evidence for the benefit of contact analog highlighting. In general, the peripheral cue seems to enable a better suppression of irrelevant items. Nevertheless also the projection of schematic item positions enhanced performance in comparison to the monitor presentation. In the present context, symbolic cues seem to be more efficient if they are placed close to the search area. This is plausible, because otherwise attention has to be shifted again between cue and search area. Naturally, this will not be necessary with simple cues like arrows, but maybe the schematic view is already too complex to be memorized at once. Accordingly, especially for elderly and disabled people the peripheral cue is expected to be more helpful, because of the automatic and reflexive mechanism involved.

The demonstrated AR technique for guidance of visual attention was applied to a working scenario but can also be incorporated into other kinds of information systems. Several environments in which complex information has to be processed can benefit from augmented visualizations [22]. The demonstrated solution using a LCD projector is an example for easy and low-cost AR [23]. Moreover, directing attention could be fruitful for facilitating the accessibility of websites as well. Websites typically consist of more than ten items (pictures, icons, etc.) and could benefit from adapted attentional guidance. The proposed method could complement assistive technology supporting learning, education and work processes especially for elderly or disabled people with reduced mental capacities. Distraction by irrelevant items can be avoided without the necessity to reduce the complexity of the overall content.

Results of the present experiment showed that cueing or highlighting improved search performance only if not more than two items were cued. This might be due to the fact that participants had to search for the items in a specific order. Nevertheless, the most obvious effect will be present with the cueing of one specific item. One possibility could be the highlighting of relevant items in dependency of the eye fixation. In our context that means for example that fixation of an item on the item list could lead to respective highlighting of the relevant item position.

Disadvantages of exogenous peripheral cues could be their quickly fading effect and the risk to capture attention while disturbing information processing of other relevant items. Accordingly, cues have to be evaluated and adapted to the content and context of information presentation.

Acknowledgments

The present research was conducted in the project "Adaptive Cognitive Interaction in Production Environments" (ACIPE) within the Excellence Cluster "Cognition for Technical Systems" (CoTeSys) by the German Research Foundation (DFG). The work was funded by grants to M.F.Z and A.S. The authors would like to thank Laura Voss as well as two anonymous reviewers for comments on an earlier version of the manuscript.

References

1. Holzinger, A., Searle, G., Kleinberger, T., Seffah, A., Javahery, H.: Investigating Usability Metrics for the Design and Development of Applications for the Elderly. In: Miesenberger, K., Klaus, J., Zagler, W.L., Karshmer, A.I. (eds.) ICCHP 2008. LNCS, vol. 5105, pp. 98–105. Springer, Heidelberg (2008)
2. Zaeh, M.F., Prasch, M.: Systematic workplace and assembly redesign for aging workforces. Production Engineering - Research and Development 1, 57–64 (2007)
3. Matausch, K., Hengstberger, B., Miesenberger, K.: "Assistec" – A University Course on Assistive Technologies. In: Miesenberger, K., Klaus, J., Zagler, W.L., Karshmer, A.I. (eds.) ICCHP 2006. LNCS, vol. 4061, pp. 361–368. Springer, Heidelberg (2006)

4. Darzentas, J., Miesenberger, K.: Design for All in Information Technology: A Universal Concern. In: Andersen, K.V., Debenham, J., Wagner, R. (eds.) DEXA 2005. LNCS, vol. 3588, pp. 406–420. Springer, Heidelberg (2005)
5. Holzinger, A., Mukasa, K.S., Nischelwitzer, A.K.: Introduction to the special thematic session: Human–computer interaction and usability for elderly. In: Miesenberger, K., Klaus, J., Zagler, W.L., Karshmer, A.I. (eds.) ICCHP 2008. LNCS, vol. 5105, pp. 18–21. Springer, Heidelberg (2008)
6. Sarter, N.: Coping with Complexity Through Adaptive Interface Design. In: Jacko, J.A. (ed.) HCI 2007. LNCS, vol. 4552, pp. 493–498. Springer, Heidelberg (2007)
7. Treisman, A.M., Gelade, G.: A feature-integration theory of attention. Cognitive Psychology 12, 97–136 (1980)
8. Wolfe, J.M.: Visual search. In: Pashler, H. (ed.) Attention, pp. 13–74. Psychology Press, London (1998)
9. Duncan, J., Humphreys, G.W.: Visual search and stimulus similarity. Psychological Review 96, 433–458 (1989)
10. Proctor, R.W., Vu, K.-P.L.: Human information processing: An overview for human-computer interaction. In: Sears, A., Jacko, J. (eds.) The human-computer interaction handbook: Fundamentals, evolving technologies, and emerging applications, 2nd edn., pp. 43–62. CRC Press, Boca Raton (2008)
11. Wickens, C.D., Carswell, C.M.: Information processing. In: Salvendy, G. (ed.) Handbook of human factors and ergonomics, 3rd edn., pp. 111–149. John Wiley, Hoboken (2006)
12. Stork, S., Stößel, C., Müller, H.J., Wiesbeck, M., Zäh, M.F., Schubö, A.: A Neuroergonomic Approach for the Investigation of Cognitive Processes in Interactive Assembly Environments. In: 16th IEEE International Conference on Robot and Human Interactive Communication (ROMAN 2007), pp. 750–755 (2007)
13. Posner, M., Snyder, C., Davidson, B.J.: Attention and detection of signals. Journal of Experimental Psychology: General 109, 160–174 (1980)
14. Wolfe, J.M., Horowitz, T.S.: What attributes guide the deployment of visual attention and how do they do it? Nature Reviews Neuroscience 5, 1–7 (2004)
15. Stößel, C., Wiesbeck, M., Stork, S., Zäh, M.F., Schubö, A.: Towards Optimal Worker Assistance: Investigating Cognitive Processes in Manual Assembly. In: Proc. of the 41st CIRP Conference on Manufacturing Systems, pp. 245–250 (2008)
16. Stork, S., Stößel, C., Schubö, A.: The influence of instruction mode on reaching movements during manual assembly. In: Holzinger, A. (ed.) USAB 2008. LNCS, vol. 5298, pp. 161–172. Springer, Heidelberg (2008)
17. Just, M.A., Carpenter, P.A.: Eye fixations and cognitive processes. Cognitive Psychology 8, 441–480 (1976)
18. Jacob, R.J.K., Karn, K.S.: Eye tracking in Human-Computer Interaction and usability research: Ready to deliver the promises. In: Hyönä, J., Radach, R., Deubel, H. (eds.) The mind's eye: Cognitive and applied aspects of eye movement research, pp. 573–605. Elsevier, Amsterdam (2003)
19. Goldberg, H.J., Kotval, X.P.: Computer interface evaluation using eye movements: Methods and constructs. International Journal of Industrial Ergonomics 24, 631–645 (1999)
20. Crawford, T.J., Müller, H.J.: Spatial and temporal effects of spatial attention on human saccadic eye movements. Vision Research 32, 293–304 (1992)
21. Cornelissen, F.W., Peters, E., Palmer, J.: The Eyelink Toolbox: Eye tracking with MATLAB and the Psychophysics Toolbox. Behavior Research Methods, Instruments and Computers 34, 613–617 (2002)

22. Behringer, R., Christian, J., Holzinger, A., Wilkinson, S.: Some Usability Issues of Augmented and Mixed Reality for e-Health Applications in the Medical Domain. In: Holzinger, A. (ed.) USAB 2007. LNCS, vol. 4799, pp. 255–266. Springer, Heidelberg (2007)
23. Nischelwitzer, A., Lenz, F.-J., Searle, G., Holzinger, A.: Some Aspects of the Development of Low-Cost Augmented Reality Learning Environments as examples for Future Interfaces in Technology Enhanced Learning. In: Stephanidis, C. (ed.) HCI 2007. LNCS, vol. 4556, pp. 728–737. Springer, Heidelberg (2007)

Which Factors Form Older Adults' Acceptance of Mobile Information and Communication Technologies?

Wiktoria Wilkowska and Martina Ziefle

Human Technology Centre, RWTH University
Theaterplatz 14, D-52062 Aachen, Germany
{wilkowska,ziefle}@humtec.rwth-aachen.de

Abstract. Technology acceptance has become a key concept for the successful rollout of technical devices. Though the concept is intensively studied for nearly 20 years now, still, many open questions remain. This especially applies to technology acceptance of older users, which are known to be very sensitive to suboptimal interfaces and show considerable reservations towards the usage of new technology. This study investigates long- und short-term effects on technology acceptance for a personal digital assistant (PDA) in older users. We examined the influence of users' personal factors (computer expertise, technical self-confidence) on acceptance (long-term effects). To assess short-term effects on acceptance, PDA acceptance was measured, after participants were given a PDA tutor training and interacted with a simulated PDA. According to the findings, individual factors largely determine people's acceptance showing that acceptance is mainly influenced by the individuals' learning history with technology. Though, also the tutorial training significantly affected acceptance outcomes, especially in the older group.

Keywords: Technology Acceptance, Perceived Ease of Use, Perceived Usefulness, Age, Computer expertise, Subjective Technical Confidence, Tutorial.

1 Introduction

In contrast to former times, in which the functionality of a technical system as well as aspects of technical feasibility were the main drivers of technical developments, the usability and the need of user-centered interface designs advanced to a key criterion of technological developments in the last decade [e.g., 1, 2, 3, 4, 5, 6]. In several studies published in different research areas (ergonomics, computer science, psychology, economics) it had been convincingly shown that the full benefit of technology decisively depends on usability and ease of use while interacting with technical devices [e.g., 7, 8, 9, 10, 11]. The concentration on the needs and wants of end users is highly opportune facing current societal developments. One development is the profound demographic change with an increasingly aging population. According to population-statistical forecasts, the proportion of people older than 65 years is assumed to rise from 25% to 56% [12]. Another trend is the continuously increasing proliferation of information and communication technology (ICT) in many parts of daily life [13]. Characteristically, the usage of ICT is not longer limited to professional areas. As

A. Holzinger and K. Miesenberger (Eds.): USAB 2009, LNCS 5889, pp. 81–101, 2009.

opposed to the past, when mostly technology prone professionals were the typical end-users of technical products, nowadays broader user groups have access to information technology in various contexts [7, 8, 14, 15, 16] and its effective usage has become an essential requirement in today's working and private life. Apart from business applications, primarily mobile technologies are assumed to specifically support older adults in their daily lives. Referring to this, mobile devices are applicable in different fields, such as for instance medical monitoring, orientation aids, general memory aids or conventional personal data management. Although applications are supposed to be accessible to everyone, a gap between those, who are "computer-literate" and those who are not (predominantly older users) is emerging. Moreover, it should be kept in mind that older users – in comparison to those younger aged – in many cases considerably differ in their needs, abilities and competencies [17, 18, 19, 20, 21]. It is a central claim that these mobile devices are designed to correspond to older users' specificity and diversity [23, 24, 25, 26]. Therefore, mobile devices should be developed in a way that enables (older) people to use them and not only "for technologies sake" [14, 19]; and, what is even more important, that their appropriate quality and constitution tempt the consumer to accept and to use those devices. As long as mobile devices are not easy to use and learn, technical innovations will not have sustained success [19, 21, 27, 28, 29].

1.1 Usability of Technical Devices and Older Users

However, the mobile character of devices still represents higher usability demands. On the one hand, mobile devices are equipped with a specific display technology, which – from the visual ergonomic perspective – has negative effects on information access, especially for older adults [30, 31, 32, 33, 34]. On the other hand, mobile devices are often small-sized with a miniaturized communication window.

The limited screen space is extremely problematic for providing optimised information access. The small window space allows only a few items to be seen at a time, so that the complexity, extension and spatial structure of the menu are not transparent to the user while navigating through it. As a consequence, users are urged to memorize functions' names and their relative location within the menu. Disorientation in handheld devices' menus is a rather frequent problem [35, 36, 37, 38], especially for aged users or those with rather limited computer-related knowledge and experience [7, 16, 24, 26, 38].

In addition, the aging process further aggravates interaction with small screen devices for the older group. Age-related changes in the cognitive system lead to a decline in working-memory capacities, a slowing-down in processing speed and a reduced ability to distinguish relevant from irrelevant information [for an overview, see 17, 18]. As a result, older learners face greater difficulties in extracting relevant information from user manuals or they are overwhelmed with displays with a high information density. A reduced working memory capacity becomes critical when task demands are high, as for example when using novel or complex technical devices. Another profound decline over the life span concerns spatial abilities as well as spatial memory [11, 25, 36, 39, 40]. Older users with reduced spatial abilities experience disorientation and the feeling of "getting lost" while navigating through the menu of software. Thus, regarding performance when using a device, previous studies congruently showed that older users usually have greater difficulties in handling a computer device or in the acquisition of computer skills [40, 41, 42]. However, the knowledge about the influence of age on the acceptance of a technical device and the correlation between usability and acceptance older adults is limited.

1.2 Acceptance of Technical Devices and Older Users

As the utilization of ICT is no longer voluntary and its effective use has become an essential requirement in today's working and private life, the organization of professional and private activities, events and transactions heavily depends on the utilization of technical devices and demands the acceptance and application of ICT from our society. The majority of technology acceptance studies deal with the impact of ICT in the working context and address young and healthy adults as a major user group of information and communication technologies [43, 44, 45, 46, 47, 48]. Comprising the outcomes, it was found that the perceived ease of using a system and the usefulness are the key components of technology acceptance [43, 44, 45, 46, 47, 48, 49]. Recently, user characteristics (economic status, culture, gender, experience and the voluntariness of system usage) had been added to the original model to meet the requirements of understanding technology acceptance in a broader context [41, 46, 49].

It is reasonable to assume that the extent of technology acceptance depends on many more factors, especially in the older group. In this context, the learning history and the experience with technology might be a crucial factor. Technology acceptance – especially when encountering a new technical device – could be impacted by positive or negative experience with the own competence when using previous technical devices and the respective expertise with the usage of technology. It was found [50] that prior experience was associated with ease of use, but did not directly affect the behavioural intention to use the device.

The perceived usefulness of technology was identified to be lower in older adults [19, 29], because they weigh the perceived usefulness against the time to learn how to operate the system. Related to this, balancing procedure is the fear of failure as additional barrier, which is much more pronounced in older than in younger adults. On the other hand, positive experience when handling a new device could completely change acceptance, irrespective of previous learning history, as it could happen – for instance – after older adults receive a suitable tutorial and experience learning success in the subsequent usage of a technical device. The positive effects of appropriate tutors on the performance of novices when using a PDA had been shown in several studies [51, 52, 53, 54, 55], however the studies did not consider yet these effects on acceptance of older novice users.

Concluding, we do not yet fully understand the acceptance patterns of older adults when they deal with new technical devices and how acceptance can be influenced. In this research we would like to contribute to the understanding by examining long-term and short-term effects on older users acceptance of a PDA.

1.3 Question Addressed, Research Model and Hypotheses

We assume that acceptance of PDA usage – operationalized as perceived ease of use (PEU) and perceived usefulness (PU) of the device – is on the one hand influenced by individual factors such as self-confidence when using technology (STC), computer expertise (CE) and age, but on the other hand by the success of interacting with the PDA, which is modulated by the support of a tutorial given prior to interacting with it. The individual factors are considered as long-term effects as they reflect the learning history with technology. In contrast, the influence of the tutorial on performance, and consequently, on acceptance outcomes, can be classified as short-term effects. Beyond the question which of these factors impact acceptance to what extent, we also seek to answer the question, if acceptance is more strongly influenced by long-term, or rather, by short-term effects. A schematic model is illustrated in Figure 1.

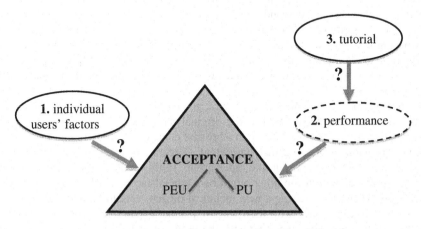

Fig. 1. Research model

According to the proposed model following hypotheses are specified:

H1: Individual factors such as age, computer expertise (CE) and subjective technical confidence (STC) are related to users' acceptance (perceived ease of use and perceived usefulness of PDA). Thereby, younger adults show higher computer-specific knowledge and a higher level of technical self-confidence than older users.

H2: Users with a higher level of CE perceive modern ICT-technologies as easier to use and more useful in comparison to those with lower level of CE.

H3: Users with a higher level of STC perceive modern ICT-technologies as easier to use and more useful in comparison to those with lower level of STC.

H4: Users' performance-effectiveness and -efficiency is related to the acceptance measures.

H5: Tutorial enhances performance on the PDA and affects indirectly users' acceptance. Thereby, older users benefit more from tutorial than younger users.

H6: Perceived ease of use (PEU) and perceived usefulness (PU) are positively related.

2   Research Method

The objective of the study was to revise which factors influence older users' acceptance of widespread mobile ICT-technologies. Based on a former research [7], which focussed exclusively on individual factors taking short-term determinants of acceptance into account, this study widens the acceptance research with an external component, which is an accompanying tutorial. Presumably, supporting novice (especially older) users with detailed instruction about how to realize applications in PDA could encourage their acceptance and therefore their usage of modern ICT-technologies. Since the current study claims to extend the earlier research, efforts were made to keep the method very similar to that used before. In this section the conceptual design and the procedure are described.

2.1 Experimental Variables

In our study we consider four independent and four dependent variables.

Independent Variables. Independent variables can be distinguished in long-term and short-term factors. Long-term variables represent user characteristics age, computer expertise and technical self-confidence, and they are classified as such, because they belong to users' specific learning history in the interaction with technical devices. Short-term effects are characterized as the moderating influence of a positive interaction with the technical device on acceptance.

Long-term factors: The first variable refers to users' age, contrasting younger participants aged between 20 and 29 years and older participants aged between 48 and 68 years. As a matter of fact the variable age acts as an indicator for two different technology generations dividing the sample in a group of users, which grew up with the modern technology, and in another group of users, who acquired their technical abilities over the years.

The second individual variable is directed to the level of computer expertise (CE) participants bring along. In order to find out, to which extent prior computer-specific knowledge would have an impact on acceptance outcomes participants were a priori distinguished in a group with high and a group with lower computer expertise. As older adults usually have lower prior computer knowledge – especially when compared to younger users – the median split procedure was accomplished age-related, forming two expertise groups within each age group according to their computer expertise scores. Thus, both, the older and younger group, held higher and lower computer-experienced subjects.

Additionally, participants' subjective technical confidence (STC), i.e. the degree of confidence to which a person believes in own ability to solve technical problems, was assessed. Similar to CE it was assumed that younger people would generally have a higher level of technical self-confidence in comparison to older users, so that the median splitting in groups of high and low technical self-confidence was conducted age-related as well.

Short-term factors: In order to examine short-term effects on performance, we applied a specific tutor training, which was found to be especially helpful in an earlier study [57]. One part of the sample received the tutor training prior to interacting with the device, while an another part – a control group – did not receive any tutorial help, but had to solve the specified PDA-tasks by their own. The tutorial was specifically developed for support of older adults and had been evaluated as effective in recent studies [55, 57]. Tutor format will be shortly explained in section 2.2.

Dependent Variables. As dependent variables two acceptance measures were surveyed: the perceived ease of use (PEU) and the perceived usefulness (PU) using original items of the Technology Acceptance Model (TAM, [43]; for detailed description see section 2.3). Those variables represented the core of this research and were observed for every manipulation of the independent variables. Additionally, two measurements concerning users' performance (effectiveness, i.e. the number of tasks successfully solved tasks, and efficiency, i.e. the time needed to process the tasks) were taken as the standard for usability [58]. These variables are assumed to reflect the (positive) tutor effect and, according to the specified hypotheses, mediate the tutor effect on acceptance.

2.2   Experimental Procedure

In order to test the research model and to determine the effects of long- and short-term variables on performance, an experimental setting with a simulated PDA was conducted. At the outset participants completed a computer-based questionnaire concerning demographical information (age, gender, educational achievement) and information about the familiarity with common technical devices (usage-length and -frequency of mobile phone and PC, as well as the perceived ease of using them). The fill-out was carried out by using the computer mouse and by choosing adequate answers from the prepared answer-lists. The same method was used later while task solving in PDA-simulation, and guaranteed that all attendees were experienced with the handling of the computer mouse.

Likewise computer-assisted, subjects proceeded a survey regarding technical self-confidence, where they had to tick the correct answers on a six-point scale (from 'strongly agree' to 'strongly disagree'). It was of great importance that STC-levels were assessed prior to using the PDA as the perceived tasks' success or failure could possibly bias STC-ratings. The preliminary data collection finished with a paper & pencil-test with regard to theoretical and practical aspects of computer knowledge and computer expertise, respectively [56].

With a next step participants worked on the simulated PDA and had to manage six prototypic tasks of the electronic organizer. In order to reflect a realistically task context, common applications of the digital diary were chosen (office and data management): three tasks requested entering of given information (e.g., entering of a new contact), and in the other three tasks modifying existing data (e.g., postponing appointment).

All participants were PDA-novices. One part of the sample (n = 40; treatment group) was previously instructed by an audio-visual tutorial (a computerized Microsoft Power-Point® presentation), which showed every single step necessary for successful task solving. Those participants learned two crucial functions needed for smoothly task solution: first, how to input a new entry into the device (button 'new'), and second, how to change corresponding details of an already existing entry (button 'edit'). Another part of the sample (n = 20) – the control group – did not receive tutorial help, but was solely instructed about the character of the imminent tasks. A basic task-information was printed on hardcopy and was present placed always next to participants in all groups (tutor and control), in order to give all participants the possibility to have a look at these instructions during the experiment. For each task there was a time limit of 5 minutes.

After completion of experimental tasks participants were asked to rate perceived ease of use (PEU) and perceived usefulness (PU) of the PDA they were working with. The described experimental procedure is presented schematic in figure 2.

1. Computer-based Questionnaires:
- demographical information
- technical self-confidence (STC)
- technical experience and PEU
  of common ICT (mobile
  phone, personal computer)

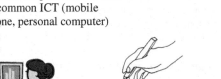

2. Questionnaire to assess **computer expertise** (CE)

3. PDA-simulation: n=40 with prior tutorial; n =20 without prior tutorial

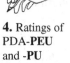

4. Ratings of PDA-**PEU** and -**PU**

Progression of the experiment

Fig. 2. Schematic schedule of experimental procedure

2.3 Materials

Perceived Ease of Use (PEU) and Perceived Usefulness (PU). Users' technology acceptance was assessed by original items from the Technology Acceptance Model [43]. The model integrates two main factors: firstly, the perceived ease of use (PEU) which implies 'the extent to which a person believes that using a particular system would be free of effort', and secondly, the perceived usefulness (PU) which is defined as 'the extent to which a person believes that using a particular system would enhance his or her job performance [43]. The validity and reliability of the items has been proven by several empirical studies [7, 9, 43, 44, 45, 47]. Each of the 12 presented items (6 items for PEU, 6 items for PU) had to be approved or rejected on a five-point Likert-scale ranging from 1 (strongly disagree) to 5 (strongly agree). The maximum to be reached for each acceptance variable was 30 (max. TAM-value = 60 points).

Subjective Technical Confidence (STC). The technical self-confidence was measured by the STC-questionnaire [59]. It determines person's subjective confidence in his or her own ability to solve technical problems. The short version of the test containing eight items (e.g., "Usually, I successfully cope with technical problems", "I really enjoy cracking technical problems") had to be rated on a six-point scale from 1 (strongly disagree) to 6 (strongly agree). The maximum score was 40 points. According to Beier's own studies the reliability of the STC short version reaches satisfactory values (Cronbach's alpha = 0.89). In the present study the reliability of the STC-Scale was even higher (Cronbach's alpha = 0.91).

Computer Expertise (CE). In order to detect participants' level of computer expertise (CE), 18 questions about computer-related knowledge (i.e. theoretical and practical aspects of the computer structure) were placed. The questionnaire [56] had been specifically developed for the difficulty level of older adults (exemplary items are presented in figure 3). Reliability and validity reached satisfying values [56].

A 'search engine' is:
    a) a specific robot for finding defined things autonomously   □
    b) a specific high performance computer for searching the internet   □
    c) a programme to retrieve data on the computer   □
    d) a databank to retrieve information in the internet   □
    e) 'I do not know' ¤   □
Your computer hangs up and you would like to restart it carefully. In order to do that
    a) you press the 'reset' button   □
    b) you press the combination 'Ctrl + Alt + Del'   □
    c) you press the combination 'End + Enter' ¤   □
    d) you turn off the computer and restart it ¤   □
    e) 'I do not know' ¤   □

Fig. 3. Example-items for the computer expertise Questionnaire [56]

A multiple-choice format was chosen for answering the questions. Only one answer could be marked among four alternatives. An additional option "I do not know" was also given. Participants were not given a time limit filling out the questionnaire. The maximum score to be reached was 18.

Experimental Tasks. The experimental tasks referred to frequently used applications of a digital diary, which are standard software and a part of each PDA available on the commercial market. Overall, two task types, 'new entry'- and 'edit'-tasks, should be managed. For the 'new entry'-tasks between 16 and 30 clicks, and for the 'edit'-tasks between 9 and 13 clicks has been necessary to solve the tasks on the shortest way possible. Thus, overall a minimum of 94 clicks needed to be done. In the following, examples of both task types are described:

■ Example for 'new entry'-task: *'You just made an appointment at the coiffeur Salon on Monday, the 2nd March, from 9 am to 11am. Please, enter this appointment into your digital diary and activate a reminder'.*

■ Example for 'edit'-task: *'Last week you made an appointment with your tax adviser on 18th April, from 9 am to 10 am at his office, Stauffenallee, 89. But he just called to ask you, if you could postpone the appointment to the proximate week, the 25th April, same time, same place. Please, change the details of this notice in your PDA'.*

2.4 Participants

A total of sixty adults participated. Thirty young adults (9 males, 21 females) with a mean age of 25.2 years (SD = 2.5; range: 20 – 29 years) and thirty older adults (14 males, 16 females) with a mean age of 60.2 years (SD = 5.6; range: 48 – 68 years) took part. The younger participants were mostly university students of different academic fields (psychology, social science, engineering, communication science). Older users were reached by advertisement in a local newspaper and through their social networks, and covered a broad range of professions and educational levels (e.g. administrative officers, secretaries, teachers, nurses, engineers, physicians). Regarding the recruitment of older participants a benchmark procedure was pursued: "younger and healthy seniors" were aimed. All older adults participating were active parts of the work force, mentally fit and not hampered by stronger age-related sensory and psychomotor limitations. All participants were PDA novices. In order to assure a proper input device usage, participants completed computer-based questionnaires using a computer mouse. There were no great difficulties observed in handling the mouse, confirming participants' reported experience with it.

The technical experience (i.e. usage of mobile phones and computer) disperses in the tested sample. Analyzing holding duration ("For how long have you been working with...") and usage frequency of those technologies ("How often do you work with...") by older and younger adults, we found meaningful differences. In the younger group all participants held mobile phones (MP) as well as personal computers (PC). The mean value for duration of mobile phone holding period was 5.5 years ($SD = 1.6$), and the holding period for personal computer was on average 6.8 years ($SD = 2.5$) in this group. The frequency of usage [rated on a four-point Likert-scale from 1 (= less then once per week) to 4 (= daily)] approaches for both technologies almost the maximum value ($M_{MP} = 3.9$, $SD_{MP} = 0.5$; $M_{PC} = 3.9$, $SD_{PC} = 0.4$) and implies younger users' daily usage of common ICT. In contrast, in the group of older users only 90% ($n = 27$) declared to hold a mobile phone since on average 4.9 years ($SD = 2.5$), and to use it 2-3 times per week ($M = 3$, $SD = 1.1$). Moreover, all of the older participants possessed a PC ($M = 4$, $SD = 3.5$), but 10% of them seemed not to use or only sporadically use it. For the frequency of PC-usage resulted the mean value of 2.6 ($SD = 1.4$), which suggests that older people use their PC on average less than 2-3 times per week. In table 1 the outcomes of T-test for mean differences in the both age groups are presented.

Table 1. T-test for age differences of technical experience and ease of use variables for mobile phone and personal computer

	T	Df	p
Duration for holding a mobile phone	1.1	43.4	> 0.05
Frequency of using a mobile phone	3.6	36.7	< 0.01
Perceived ease of using a mobile phone	-5.3	45.4	< 0.01
Duration for holding a personal computer	3.5	52.4	< 0.01
Frequency of using a personal computer	4.4	30.5	< 0.01
Perceived ease of using a personal computer	-4.1	34.8	< 0.01

Also, the perceived ease of use (PEU) of the investigated devices differed significantly in both age groups. Participants were asked to rate the ease of use for those technologies ("how easy to use is for you ...") on a four-point scale (1 = very easy, 2 = quite easy, 3 = quite difficult, 4 = very difficult). Younger participants rated navigating mobile phone as (very) easy ($M = 1.4$, $SD = 0.5$) and handling personal computer as quite easy (M = 1.9, SD = 0.4). Older participants judged using the small-screen device still as quite easy (M = 2.3, SD = 0.7), but getting along with personal computer was rated on average as quite difficult (M = 2.8, SD = 0.8) in the older group. Those differences in perceiving using common ICT-devices as easy are statistically significant (Table 1) comparing both age groups.

As the analysis for technical experience shows younger people use currently ICT-technologies evidently more frequently and they perceive the usage of these devices as easier in comparison to older users.

3   Results

Results of this study were analyzed by bivariate correlations, multivariate and univariate analyses of variance (M)ANOVA with a level of significance set at 5%. Outcomes within the less restrictive significance level of 10% are referred as marginally significant. The significance of omnibus F-Tests in MANOVA-analyses was taken from Pillai values. Acceptance measures (perceived ease of use and usefulness) were analysed non-parametrically (*Mann-Whitney-U-Test*). In order to integrate the individual factors computer expertise (CE) and subjective technical confidence (STC) as independent variables into the statistical analysis, a median-split method was conducted, respectively. Median values were assessed for the both age groups separately, so that within the particular group the number of participants with parameter values below the group-median (low), and of those who reached values above the group-median (high) was about the same size.

The result section is designed as follows: first, we assess correlative relations and impact of individual factors (age, computer expertise and technical self-confidence) on users' acceptance; second, correlative relationships between performance (supported by tutorial) and PEU and PU are conducted; and third, the influence of tutorial treatment on performance and its effect on acceptance measures are presented.

3.1   Impact of Individual Factors on Acceptance

At first, the analysis of the individual factors on acceptance ease of use and usefulness are of interest. Strictly speaking, ratings should be analysed non-parametrically. However, as we were interested in the interacting effects between independent variables on acceptance, which only can be assessed by (multiple) analysis of variance procedures, we decided to analyse data by the way of MANOVA. In order to be sure that we do not "overestimate" the significance of outcomes, we checked that the main effects yield the same significances in both, parametric and non-parametric testing procedures.

Relationships between Individual Factors and Acceptance. To get a first insight into the data, correlations (Spearman rank analyses) between individual variables and acceptance measures were carried out (table 2). Computer expertise was significantly correlated to both acceptance indicators (PEU: r = .61, p < 0.01; PU: r = .26, p < 0.05): with increasing computer expertise, the perceived ease of use and usefulness of the PDA is rated as higher. Moreover, the factors age and subjective technical confidence were significantly connected to the perceived ease of using the device (age: r = -.50, p < 0.01; STC: r = .44, p < 0.01), but not to the usefulness. Thus, with increasing age and decreasing technical self-confidence, the ease of using the device was rated as lower.

Table 2. Bivariate correlations between computer expertise, technical self-confidence, age and PEU, PU (N = 60). Bold values are significant (* p<0.05; ** p<0.01).

	PEU	PU	Age	Computer expertise	Subjective technical confidence
PEU	1	**.32***	**-.50****	**.61****	**.44****
PU		1	-.13	**.26***	.04
Age			1	**-.59****	**-.43****
Computer expertise				1	**.49****
Subjective technical confidence					1

Now, being aware of these relationships we inspect effects of individual factors on PEU and PU in the next step.

Effects of Age and Computer Expertise on Acceptance. A multiple analysis of variance with the between-factors age and computer expertise on dependent variables PEU and PU revealed highly significant effects of age (F (2,55) = 10.6, $p < 0.01$) and expertise (F (2,55) = 8.8, $p < 0.01$). The interacting effect between these factors though was not statistically relevant (F (2,55) < 1; n.s.). Descriptive analysis shows that the perceived ease of PDA-using was rated higher in the younger adult group (M = 24.4 points; SD = 5.1) in contrast to older users' ratings, which resulted considerably lower with 17.9 (SD = 6.1) out of maximum 30 points (F (1,56) = 21.6, $p < 0.01$). Age, however, did not significantly affect the perceived usefulness (F (1,56) < 1; n.s.): younger users rated the PDA just marginally as more useful (M = 20.2, SD = 5) than older users (M = 18.8, SD = 6.6). The effect of age on acceptance is presented in figure 4 on the left.

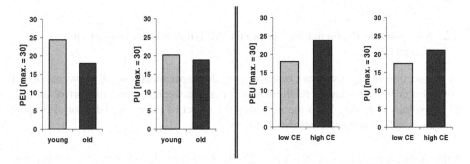

Fig. 4. Effects of age (left) and computer expertise (right) on PEU and PU (N=60)

Moreover, computer expertise revealed to be a major factor on acceptance (figure 4, on the right). Persons with high computer expertise rated the PDA as easier to use than those with lower level of theoretical and practical computer knowledge (F (1,56) = 15.3, $p < 0.01$), and they also judged usefulness of the device as higher (F (1,56) = 5.5, $p < 0.05$). Though, it should be noted that the average ratings for ease of use and usefulness (see table 3) are far from maximum values (20 out of 30 points), showing a basically reluctant acceptance.

Table 3. Means (and SD) for PEU and PU depending on level of computer expertise ($N = 60$)

Level of computer expertise	PEU	PU
Low	18.0 (6.5)	17.5 (6.1)
High	23.7 (5.2)	21.1 (5.2)

Effect of Subjective Technical Confidence on Acceptance. In addiction to computer-related knowledge also technical self-confidence affects users' acceptance judgments. In a MANOVA with factors age and the median-split STC on the dependent measures PEU and PU technical self-confidence showed a marginally significant impact on acceptance (F (2,55) = 2.9, p = 0.06). Persons, which are convinced about own technical abilities (scores above median), perceived ease of PDA-usage as higher than those, who showed rather lower technical self-confidence (scores below median). Interestingly, the latter tend to judge usefulness of the digital organizer even higher than high technically self-confident participants in the sample (for details see table 4). No interacting effect between age and STC (F (2,55) < 1; n.s.) was present.

Table 4. Means (and SD) for PEU and PU depending on level of STC ($N = 60$)

Level of technical self-confidence	PEU	PU
Low	19.9 (6.7)	20.2 (6.4)
High	22.5 (6.0)	18.6 (5.1)

Summarizing the results so far, we can assume that especially age and computer expertise, but also – to a lesser extent – the technical self-confidence affect users' acceptance of the PDA.

3.2 Navigational Performance Supported by Tutor and Its Impact on Acceptance

In this section firstly bivariate correlations of the experimental variables were carried out in order to find relevant relationships between acceptance and supportive as well as individual variables. With the next step the effect of prior applied tutorial on performance and acceptance measures is assessed.

Table 5. Bivariate correlations between PEU, PU and performance (N = 60; **p < 0.01, *p < 0.05)

	PEU	PU	No. of tasks solved	Time on task
PEU	1	.28*	.72**	-.68**
PU		1	.23	-.25
Number of tasks solved			1	-.71**
Time on task				1

Relationships between Performance and Acceptance Measures. Correlation findings for the whole sample ($N = 60$) – as can be seen in table 5 – show that the perceived ease of use is strongly related to performance effectiveness (i.e., number of tasks solved: $r = .72$, $p < 0.01$) and efficiency (i.e., time needed to solve the tasks: $r = -.68$, $p < 0.01$).

Outcomes suggest that users, who solved the experimental tasks faster and more successfully, perceive the PDA as easier to use in comparison to those who performed less effective and less efficiently. Perceived usefulness, in contrast, was not associated with the observed performance parameters (n.s.). These findings partially confirm prior formulated assumption (H4): performance is significantly linked only to PEU; it does not apply to PU. Furthermore, the indicators PEU and PU are related to each other, though not very strong ($r = .28$, $p < 0.05$), confirming H6.

In order to determine if the correlative relationships are equally strong in both age groups, we also execute correlation-analysis separately for the older and the younger users. Moreover, correlative analyses were also carried out separately for the treatment and the control group in order to get more information about the tutor effect (Table 6).

As can be seen in the upper part of table 6, younger users' perceived ease of use is not significantly associated with performance effectiveness (n.s.) but with efficiency in the tutored group ($r = -.62$, $p < 0.01$), indicating that shorter processing time in solving experimental tasks was strongly related to participants' positive opinions about the ease of PDA-use. In the younger group, which was not supported by tutorial (control group), neither effectiveness nor efficiency showed significant coefficients.

Table 6. Bivariate correlations between PEU, PU and performance variables (supported vs. not supported by tutorial) for younger and older users (**p < 0.01, *p < 0.05)

		PEU	PU	No. of tasks solved		Time on task	
				tutor	no tutor	tutor	no tutor
younger users (n=30)	PEU	1	.23	.28	.53	**-.62****	-.08
	PU		1	.19	-.31	-.18	-.34
	Number of tasks solved			1	1	**-.59****	.28
	Time on task					1	1
older users (n=30)	PEU	1	.35	**.62****	.52	-.33	**-.69***
	PU		1	.13	**-.66***	-.12	-.30
	Number of tasks solved			1	1	-.29	-.40
	Time on task					1	1

For the older group (lower part of table 5) we found that persons, who previously received tutorial, rated the ease of use significantly higher the more effective their performance was ($r = .62$, $p < 0.01$); however, the tutor effect was not observed in task efficiency (time on task). In contrast, not tutored users perceived the PDA as more useful the shorter was their processing time ($r = -.69$, $p < 0.05$). In addition, in the older group a significant negative association between effectiveness and perceived usefulness was revealed (r = -.66, p < 0.05) for those adults, who did not receive tutorial, i.e. the higher the number of solved tasks the lower the PU-appreciation.

Effect of Applied Tutorial on Acceptance and Performance. As addressed before, H5 declares an effect of applied tutorial on performance and acceptance. A MANOVA with the factors age (younger vs. older users) and prior tutoring (tutor vs. no tutor) as independent variables, as well performance measures (i.e. effectiveness and efficiency) and acceptance measures (i.e. PEU and PU) as dependent variables was carried out. The outcomes revealed – beyond the effect of age (F (4,53) = 17.5, p < 0.01) – a highly significant positive effect of tutor on performance (F (4,53) = 3.9; p < 0.01).

At first we take a look on the performance (figure 5, right): participants previously instructed by the computerized tutor solved on an average more tasks (M = 2.6, SD = 2.4) than in the control group (M = 2, SD = 2). Similar pattern is obtained for the processing time (in seconds): the tutored group needed less time (M = 943, SD = 383.1) than the control-group (M = 947, SD = 352.7). Thus, participants who were supported by a tutor, worked more effectively and more efficiently than users without such training.

However, the focus of our interest was the effect of tutorial on the acceptance measures (figure 5, left). In the tutored group the perceived ease of use of the PDA was 22.7 (SD = 5.7) points and the perceived usefulness was 20.4 (SD = 6.2) out of maximum 30 points, each. In contrast, in the no-tutor-group the scores for acceptance measures were lower: here, users reached on an average 18 (SD = 6.9) points for perceived ease of use and 17.6 (SD = 4.6) points for perceived usefulness. Thus, users who were instructed by tutor before task solving pronounced considerably higher judgments about the perceived ease of use (single F(1,56) = 10.5, p < 0.01) and they also tended to perceive the electronic organizer as more useful (single F(1,56) = 2.9, p < 0.1) in comparison to those without prior treatment. Thus, the in H5 claimed influence of tutorial on performance and acceptance had been confirmed.

The interaction between the factors age and applied tutorial does not show a significant effect on the dependent variables (F (4,53) = 0.3; n.s.), which shows that the positive effect of the tutor on acceptance was for both age groups equally large.

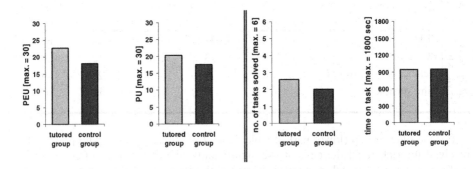

Fig. 5. Effects of tutor on acceptance (left) and performance (right)

Concluding the results in this section, tutorial has a positive effect on performance and, by this, on acceptance of mobile ITC-devices. Especially one aspect of novices' acceptance is strongly related to effectiveness and efficiency of performance: the perceived ease of use. This strong effect, however, fails to appear in regard to another indicator of acceptance, i.e. perceived usefulness.

4   Revision of the Research Model

We started this research with the basic question, to which extent older adults' acceptance of ICT-technologies is influenced by either long-term factors (individual characteristics) or short-term factors (tutor support and performance success). Based on the present research we now can a) furnish the assumed relationships with quantitative data and b) identify the key player on older adults' acceptance.

Long-term Effects. Among the user characteristics, computer expertise is the strongest driver of acceptance. People, who possess a high computer-related knowledge, show higher acceptance of ICT. This was to a lesser extent valid for the young adults ($r = .32$), but asymmetrically stronger for the older group ($r = .54$). The self-confidence when using technology turned out to be also a strong driver on performance ($r = .44$). People with a solid self-confidence in technical matters evaluate the ease of using the devices as significantly higher, but not the usefulness. Though, again, technical self-confidence impacted acceptance more strongly in the older group. The relationships furnished with data are illustrated in Figure 6.

Short-term Effects. Now we look at short-term effects and the question, if a successful performance – mediated by tutor support – comparably influences acceptance outcomes. Overall, high tasks success was positively correlated with acceptance (effectiveness: $r = .68$; efficiency: $r = -.69$). This hints at an important impact of a high usability and a positive experience of participants with the device interaction. If looking at the age groups separately, the tutor specifically supports the efficiency in the young group ($r = -.62$), while in the older group it supports in particular the effectiveness ($r = .62$). Apparently, the tutor is very supportive for both age groups, but the mode of operation is age-related. As the younger users already show a high tasks success, it is the efficiency, which is mainly advantaged. In the older group, which shows naturally a lower processing speed, it is the effectiveness, which is mostly supported.

Concluding we can say, that both, short-term and long-term effects do modulate acceptance outcomes. The success in performance with the device yielded a stronger effect on acceptance compared to the effects, which are carried by user characteristics. However, the positive tutor effect does mainly affect the perceived ease of use and does not impact perceived usefulness likewise. In addition, previous computer experience and expertise as well as – to a lesser extent – technical self-confidence modulate acceptance. It is insightful, that especially the previous computer experience and the familiarity with technology are strong predictors of acceptance in the older group.

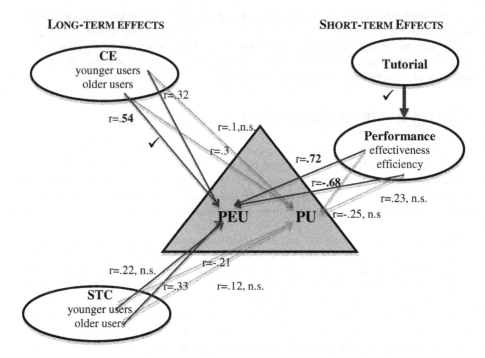

Fig. 6. Revision research model: influence of short- and long-term factors on acceptance (bold: $p < 0.01$). Black lines indicate significant impacts on PEU, grey lines represent insignificant impacts on PU.

5   Discussion and Future Research Duties

The present study was conducted to provide a deeper understanding of factors influencing user's acceptance of popular mobile information and communication technologies, taking a PDA and data management tasks as an example. Two key determinants of technology acceptance [43] were focussed in dependence of age, computer-related knowledge and technical self-confidence. The latter were assumed to be long-term effects. Also, the positive effect of a tutor was investigated, which should impact PDA performance, and by this, the acceptance of its usage (short-term effect).

In the focus of our interest were older users, as the demographic structure in the western world is continuously changing and it is supposable to expect that in the near future the majority of the population – and at the same time the majority of technology users – will be aged. In this regard, there is a need not only for meeting actual demands of the elderly and for appropriate adapting of technical products to this age group, but also, for understanding of basic necessities and customizing the technology market adequate to acceptance requirements.

The results revealed that among the long-term effects, predominately the previous experience and computer expertise were decisive for acceptance outcomes. While this was valid for younger and older users, confirming findings of other studies with mobile technologies [11, 25, 26], this was especially true for the older adults. This finding is very important regarding the impact of future educational efforts and life-long learning concepts. Only older adults' continuous motivation to actively handle technical devices, and to overcome the resentment and fear of failure towards technology may increase computer knowledge in this group on the long run. As has been exemplary found in an evaluative study in terms of computer expertise in older adults [56], an active exploration of technical systems provides those users with appropriate procedural and declarative knowledge components enhancing the perceived ease of using these devices. A successful device interaction on its part reduces computer anxiety and enhances computer-related self-efficacy [7, 8, 40, 41, 60, 61, 62]. However, the need for active participation in the interacting with new technology accepted and approved by older adults is only one side of the story.

The other side is the clear-cut importance of usability demands of technical systems, including the requirement of usable tutorial systems. The positive effect of the tutor on performance, and subsequently, on acceptance also showed that it is of great importance that users of ICT – especially the older ones – are adequately supported. As found, performance increase supported by the tutor enhanced the perceived ease of use, again especially pronounced in the older group. Facing that, any positive interaction with a technical device will shape and modulate the technical self-confidence and will reduce computer anxiety, the significant impact of a high usability of interface designs and age-sensitive tutors come to the fore.

People designing technical interfaces, electronic tutors and digital help systems need to take this sensitive relation between usability and acceptance serious. It should be kept in mind that any devices' technical genius and the promised advantage for users' daily needs can only be recognized and highly valued, if the human properties and cognitive specificities are properly recognized, and highly valued. Thus, whenever the knowledge of both the technical and the human factors are incorporated into current design, the devices may meet the demands of users, designers and manufacturers at the same time.

In the present study, short- and long-term effects could only be detected for one of the key components of technology acceptance [43], the perceived ease of using the PDA. In contrast, no effects on perceived usefulness could be identified, though the perceived ease of use and the perceived usefulness showed a basic correlation in the sample. The lack of the usefulness effect might be due to the specificity of the older group, corroborating earlier findings [19, 29, 34].

Melenhorst et al. [19] for example, explain the reluctance of older adults to weigh technological devices as "useful" by the lack of the perceived advantages, or the benefits. The perceived context-related benefit however is a major motivational factor for using or not using an electronic device. Older adults tend to be present-oriented and, consequently, do not see the need to evaluate technical devices as useful, which will be possibly used in future. The expected gain of the device may be perceived as not worth the trouble (learning cost, frustration and anger about a suboptimal usability [37]). This present-oriented attitude possibly reduces also older adults' preparedness to learn something new and to intensively deal with a new technology. Thus, for older adults, appropriate information about the benefits of technical devices represents an important determinant for using them. Provided the benefits are valued sufficiently high, they may overcome their reluctance and their susceptibility to effects of low usability and interface complexity. Taken this for granted, the usefulness represents the asymmetrically more important facet of technology acceptance for older adults compared to the perceived ease of using the device. Training the skills to handle a new technology should therefore involve information about its specific benefits, from the user's perspective.

On the other hand it is also very plausible that many of the present technical devices do not address a concise and coherent need of older adults beyond augmenting current entertainment and communication practices. In our study, participants did probably not apprehend the basic necessity to use additional device in order to execute day-to-day duties or storage information, and so they perceived the PDA as overall less useful. Future research should therefore include other kinds of device interactions and using contexts (e.g., medical technology), in which technology is basically welcome and needed by the older group.

Acknowledgments. The authors would like to thank all participants, who took part in this study. Many thanks also to Katrin Arning for the research support. This research was supported by the excellence initiative of the German federal and state governments.

References

1. Selwyn, N., Gorad, S., Furlong, J., Madden, L.: Older adults' use of information and communications technology in everyday life. Ageing and Society 23(5), 561–582 (2003)
2. Evans, G., Simkin, M.: What best predicts computer proficiency? Communications of the ACM 32, 1322–1327 (1989)
3. Pruitt, J., Adlin, T.: The Persona Lifecycle: Keeping People in Mind throughout Product Design. Elsevier/Morgan Kaufmann, Amsterdam (2006)
4. Mulder, S., Yaar, Z.: The User Is Always Right: A Practical Guide to Creating and Using Personas for the Web. New Riders Press (2005)
5. Kuniavsky, M.: User profiles. In: Observing the User Experience: A Practitioner's Guide to User Research, pp. 128–157. Morgan Kaufmann, San Francisco (2003)
6. Morrow, D., Miller, L.S., Ridolfo, H., Kokaye, N., Chang, D., Fischer, U., Stine-Morrow, E.: Expertise and aging in a pilot decision-making task. In: Proc. of the Human Factors and Ergonomics Society 48th Annual Meeting, pp. 228–232. Human Factors Society, Santa Monica (2002)
7. Arning, K., Ziefle, M.: Understanding age differences in PDA acceptance and performance. Computers in Human Behavior 23, 2904–2927 (2007)
8. Arning, K., Ziefle, M.: Barriers of information access in small screen device applications: The relevance of user characteristics for a transgenerational design. In: Stephanidis, C., Pieper, M. (eds.) ERCIM Ws UI4ALL 2006. LNCS, vol. 4397, pp. 117–136. Springer, Heidelberg (2007)
9. Adams, D.A., Nelson, R., Todd, P.A.: Perceived usefulness, ease of use, and usage of information technology: A replication. MIS Quarterly 16, 227–247 (1992)
10. Wirtz, S., Jakobs, E.-M., Ziefle, M.: Age-specific issues of software interfaces. In: 9th International Conference on Work With Computer Systems, Beijing, China (2009)
11. Ziefle, M., Bay, S.: Transgenerational Designs in Mobile Technology. In: Lumsden, J. (ed.) Handbook of Research on User Interface Design and Evaluation for Mobile Technology, pp. 122–140. IGI Global (2008)

12. Pötzsch, O., Sommer, B.: Bevölkerung Deutschlands bis 2050 - Ergebnisse der 10. koordinierten Bevölkerungsvorausberechnung. Pressestelle Statistisches Bundesamt, Wiesbaden (2003)
13. Shiffler, G., Smulders, C., Correia, J.M., Hale, K., Hahn, W.M.: Gartner dataquest market databook (2005)
14. Wyeth, P., Austin, D., Szeto, H.: Designing Ambient Computing for use in the mobile healthcare domain. In: Online-Proceedings of the CHI (2001)
15. Leonhardt, S.: Personal Healthcare Devices. In: Mekherjee, S., et al. (eds.) Malware: Hardware Technology Drivers of Ambient Intelligence, pp. 349–370. Springer, Dordrecht (2005)
16. Arning, K., Ziefle, M.: What older user expect from mobile devices: An empirical survey. In: Pikaar, R.N., Konigsveld, E.A., Settels, P.J. (eds.) Proceedings of the 16th World Congress on Ergonomics (IEA). Elsevier, Amsterdam (2006)
17. Fisk, A.D., Rogers, W.A.: Handbook of Human Factors and the Older Adult. Academic Press, San Diego (1999)
18. Craik, F.I.M., Salthouse, T.A.: Handbook of Aging and Cognition. Lawrence Erlbaum, Hillsdale (1992)
19. Melenhorst, A.S., Rogers, W.A., Caylor, E.C.: The use of communication technologies by older adults: Exploring the benefits from an users perspective. In: Proc. of the Human Factors and Ergonomics Society, 45th Annual Meeting (2001)
20. Czaja, S.J., Sharit, J.: Age Differences in Attitudes Toward Computers. Journal of Gerontology 5, 329–340 (1998)
21. Mynatt, E.D., Melenhorst, A.-S., Fisk, A.-D., Rogers, W.A.: Aware technologies for aging in place: understanding user needs and attitudes. IEEE Pervasive Computing 20(3) (2004)
22. Morrell, R.W., Mayhorn, C.B., Bennet, J.: A Survey of World Wide Web Use in Middle-Aged and Older Adults. Human Factors 42(2), 175–182 (2000)
23. Marquie, J.C., Jourdan-Boddaert, L., Huet, N.: Do older adults underestimate their actual computer knowledge? Behaviour and Information Technology 21(4), 273–280 (2002)
24. Arning, K., Ziefle, M.: Effects of cognitive and personal factors on PDA menu navigation performance. Behavior and Information Technology 28(3), 251–269 (2009)
25. Ziefle, M., Schroeder, U.: How young and older users master the use of hyperlinks in small screen devices. In: Proceedings of the SIGCHI Conference on Human Factors in Computing Systems 2007, pp. 307–316. ACM, New York (2007)
26. Ziefle, M.: The influence of user expertise and phone complexity on performance, ease of use and learnability of different mobile phones. Behaviour and Information Technology 21(5), 303–311 (2002)
27. Zimmer, Z., Chappell, N.L.: Receptivity to new technology among older adults. Disability and Rehabilitation 21(5/6), 222–230 (1999)
28. Mynatt, E.D., Rogers, W.A.: Developing technology to support the functional independence of older adults. Ageing International 27(1), 24–41 (2001)
29. Melenhorst, A.-S., Rogers, W.A., Bouwhuis, D.G.: Older adults' motivated choice for technological innovation: Evidence for benefit-driven selectivity. Psychology and Aging 21(1), 190–195 (2006)
30. Oetjen, S., Ziefle, M.: The Effects of LCD's Anisotropy on the Visual Performance of Users of Different Ages. Human Factors 49(4), 619–627 (2007)
31. Oetjen, S., Ziefle, M.: A visual ergonomic evaluation of different screen technologies. Journal of Applied Ergonomics 40, 69–81 (2009)

32. Omori, M., Watanabe, T., Takai, J., Takada, H., Miyao, M.: Visibility and characteristics of the mobile phones for elderly people. Behaviour & Information Technology 21(5), 313–316 (2002)
33. Ziefle, M.: Aging and mobile displays: Challenges and requirements for age-sensitive electronic information designs. In: 9th International Conference on Work With Computer Systems, Beijing, China (2009)
34. Zajicek, M., Hall, S.: Solutions for elderly visually impaired people using the Internet. Human Computer Interaction, 299–307 (2000)
35. Lin, D.-Y.: Age Differences in the Performance of Hypertext Perusal. In: Proceedings of the Human Factors And Ergonomic Society 45th Annual Meeting, pp. 211–215. Human Factors and Ergonomics Society, Santa Monica (2001)
36. Ziefle, M., Bay, S.: How to overcome disorientation in mobile phone menus: A comparison of two different types of navigation aids. Human Computer Interaction 21(4), 393–432 (2006)
37. Ziefle, M., Bay, S.: How older adults meet cognitive complexity: Aging effects on the usability of different cellular phones. Behaviour and Information Technology 24(5), 375–389 (2005)
38. Tuomainen, K., Haapanen, S.: Needs of the active elderly for mobile phones. In: Stephanidis, C. (ed.) Universal Access in HCI: Inclusive design in the information society, pp. 494–498. Lawrence Erlbaum, NJ (2003)
39. Freudenthal, D.: Age differences in the performance of information retrieval tasks. Behaviour and Information Technology 20, 9–22 (2001)
40. Ellis, D.R., Allaire, J.C.: Modelling computer interest in older adults: The role of age, education, computer knowledge and computer anxiety. Human Factors 41, 345–364 (1999)
41. Levine, T., Donitsa-Schmidt, S.: Computer use, confidence, attitudes and knowledge: a causal analysis. Computers in Human Behavior 1, 125–146 (1998)
42. Goodman, J., Gray, P., Khammampad, K., Brewster, S.: Using Landmarks to Support Older People in Navigation. In: Brewster, S., Dunlop, M. (eds.) Mobile Human Computer Interaction, pp. 38–48. Springer, Berlin (2004)
43. Davis, F.D.: Perceived Usefulness, Perceived Ease of Use, and User Acceptance of Information Technology. MIS Quarterly 13, 319–337 (1989)
44. Venkatesh, V., Davis, F.D.: A Model of the Antecedents of Perceived Ease of Use: Development and Test. Decision Sciences 27, 451–481 (1996)
45. Venkatesh, V., Davis, F.D.: A Theoretical Extension of the Technology Acceptance Model: Four Longitudinal Field Studies. Management Science 46, 186–204 (2000)
46. Venkatesh, V., Morris, M.G., Davis, G.B., Davis, F.D.: User acceptance of information technology: Toward a unified view. MIS Quarterly 27 (2003)
47. Schajna, B.: Empirical evaluation of the revised technology acceptance model. Management Science 42, 85–92 (1996)
48. Schwarz, A., Chin, W.: Looking Forward: Toward an Understanding of the Nature and Definition of IT Acceptance. Journal of the Association for Information Systems 8, 232–243 (2007)
49. Arning, K., Ziefle, M.: Different perspectives on technology acceptance: The role of technology type and age. In: USAB 2009, Linz, Austria (submitted, 2009)
50. Argarwal, R., Prasad, J.: Are differences Germane to the acceptance of new Information technologies? Decision Sciences 30, 361–391 (1999)
51. Ziefle, M.: Instruction formats and navigation aids in mobile devices. In: Holzinger, A. (ed.) USAB 2008. LNCS, vol. 5298, pp. 339–358. Springer, Heidelberg (2008)

52. Bay, S., Ziefle, M.: Landmarks or surveys? The impact of different instructions on children's performance in hierarchical menu structures. Computers in Human Behavior 24(3), 1246–1274 (2008)
53. Kirschner, P., Gerjets, P.: Instructional design for effective and enjoyable computer-supported learning. Computers in Human Behavior 22, 1–8 (2006)
54. Sarrafzadeh, A., Alexander, S., Dadgostar, F., Fan, C., Bigdeli, A.: How do you understand that I don't understand? A look at the future of intelligent tutoring systems. Computers in Human Behavior 24, 1342–1363 (2008)
55. Arning, K., Ziefle, M.: Ask and you will receive: Training older adults to use a PDA in an active learning environment. International Journal of Mobile Human-Computer Interaction (2009)
56. Arning, K., Ziefle, M.: Assessing computer experience in older adults: Development and validation of a computer expertise questionnaire for older adults. Behaviour and Information Technology 27, 89–93 (2008)
57. Wilkowska, W., Ziefle, M., Arning, K.: Older adults' navigation performance when using small-screen devices: does a tutor help? In: 9th International Conference on Work With Computer Systems, Beijing, China (2009)
58. EN ISO 9241-11: Ergonomic requirements for office work with visual display terminals. Part 11: Guidance on usability. Beuth, Berlin, Germany (1997)
59. Beier, G.: Locus of control when interacting with technology (Kontrollüberzeugungen im Umgang mit Technik). Report Psychologie 24, 684–693 (1999)
60. Brosnan, M.J.: The impact of computer anxiety and self-efficacy upon performance. Journal of Computer Assisted Learning 14, 223–234 (1998)
61. Busch, T.: Gender differences in self-efficacy and attitudes toward computers. Journal of Educational Computing Research 12, 147–158 (1995)
62. Chua, S., Chen, D., Wong, A.: Computer anxiety and its correlations: a meta analysis. Computers in Human Behavior 15, 609–623 (1999)
63. Holzinger, A., Searle, G., Kleinberger, T., Seffah, A., Javahery, H.: Investigating Usability Metrics for the Design and Development of Applications for the Elderly. In: Miesenberger, K., Klaus, J., Zagler, W.L., Karshmer, A.I. (eds.) ICCHP 2008. LNCS, vol. 5105, pp. 98–105. Springer, Heidelberg (2008)
64. Holzinger, A., Searle, G., Nischelwitzer, A.: On some Aspects of Improving Mobile Applications for the Elderly. In: Stephanidis, C. (ed.) HCI 2007. LNCS, vol. 4554, pp. 923–932. Springer, Heidelberg (2007)

A Usability and Accessibility Design and Evaluation Framework for ICT Services

Özge Subasi[1], Michael Leitner[1], and Manfred Tscheligi[1,2]

[1] CURE, Hauffgasse 3 1110, Vienna, Austria
{subasi,leitner,tscheligi}@cure.at
[2] ICT & S Salzburg, Austria
manfred.tscheligi@sbg.ac.at

Abstract. This paper introduces a step by step framework for practitioners for combining accessibility and usability engineering processes. Following the discussions towards the needs of more user centeredness in the design of accessible solutions, there is a need for such a practical framework. In general, accessibility has been considered as a topic dealing with "hard facts". But lately terms like semantic and procedural accessibility have been introduced. In the following pages we propose a first sketch of a framework, which shows how to merge both usability and accessibility evaluation methods in the same process in order to guarantee a unified solution for both hard and soft facts of accessibility. We argue that by enhancing the user centered design process as the ISO DIS 9241-210 (revised DIN ISO 13407) describes it, accessibility and usability issues may be covered in one process.

Keywords: Universal accessibility, universal usability, older users, process framework.

1 Introduction

Accessibility and usability of ICT applications for an aging population are going to be more and more important. Scholars of both disciplines and interdisciplinary approach have long been indicating a need to combine and even merge these two areas. Still there is no step-by-step methodological framework for practitioners to cover these aspects in projects in a progressing level. But actually lacking of such a frame costs both scholars and industry much time, as the work is to be done almost double and in some cases triple due to lack of concrete organizational structure among different stakeholders and due to a need of evaluating components with different methods for similar purposes. The testing of these issues has been mostly stakeholder based and therefore it was not easy to combine processes (accessibility & usability). Our attempt is to have a broader perspective and to draw a generalist step-by-step framework considering the process from all sides so that each stakeholder can optimize his/her time to concentrate his/her evaluation and evaluate their cooperation possibilities. The introduced framework combines the evaluation of usability and accessibility of products considering all stakeholders and end users in order to improve the quality of end

A. Holzinger and K. Miesenberger (Eds.): USAB 2009, LNCS 5889, pp. 102–110, 2009.

products for the target population. Our approach on the next pages is based on user centered design process. In order to extend and re-describe the framework, we considered several aspects like role of different parties like designers or technical implementers as well as wishes of diverse end-users. During our study, after analyzing the literature from different disciplines we conducted several workshops with different stakeholders and included end-users to most of the stages. To answer the needs of users in our design, we benefited from guidelines, needs and requirements analysis from usability research for older users. Moreover we took the advantages of exchange of knowledge among different parties during iterative development process. We believe that the process we followed is offering a solution for practitioners to make the service both accessible and usable for users. This paper formulizes the theory behind this process in the following pages.

2 Related Work

Next to an aging society, both the increase in need of usage of technology on basic applications like e-government and e-health websites and the "turn of the status of users to active producers of web contents" [16] make it necessity to have a standard framework for designing of accessible and usable web applications. Next to well known and applied guidelines of to WACAG 2.0 principles [25] for accessibility, several guidelines for designing usable websites for older people (a detailed summary available in [14]) are widely applied in the area to deal with these problems. Next to existing heuristics and guidelines for older users, within each new usability study with end-users, many issues have been discovered specific to older users. Inspiring examples to these are perception and definition of undesired content [17], [14] different search methods of older users [18], dealing methods and different mind mappings [4]. A recent discussion concentrates on a totally different understanding of older user's knowledge [5]. The more the scholars investigated on the issue, the more heterogenized were the results related to older users. A shift from a generalist understanding of "all the older users have similar problems" to a design for a heterogeneous aging society including diverse needs and wishes can be observed.

In accessibility field, criticisms on Web Accessibility Initiative (WAI) guidelines are emerging. As Kelly et al. stated there is an "urgent need for more investigations of evidence for the relationship between accessibility as measured by user behavior and by conformance to guidelines" [12]. A common criticism was on centralized structure, that focuses only on technology (not purpose) and on developing programmer based approaches instead of looking at social constructs [12]. Baguma and Lubega have designed a Web Design Framework for Improved Accessibility for People with Disabilities (WDFAD) [2] to overcome similar problems. They gave emphasis on issues like the "close relationship between navigation, content and user interface" for the betterment of accessibility of websites [2]. The "Web Accessibility Initiative: Ageing Education and Harmonization (WAI-AGE)" is another example who builds a solution for the issue by trying to help "developers provide Web sites that work better for people who experience changes in abilities due to ageing, as well as for people with disabilities" [1]. This initiative explores the boundaries between usability and accessibility requirements in order to gain a general understanding how accessibility for older users should be.

The term "Usable accessibility" was described to define the understanding of user centered aspects of accessibility problems. The definition of Hoel and Overby [6 on universal accessibility considers three different approaches called *syntactic accessibility*, *semantic accessibility* and *procedural accessibility* which respectively covers; first the accessibility of coding sent to the browser device, the behavior of services in the same way and third of all similar services have the same sequencing of events and the same patterns of interaction based on the information entered into a system. Testing accessibility of web services with real users are recognized to be the right way to deal with accessibility problems (e.g [19]). W3C outlined the evaluation process for this by including semi-automatic and automatic testing and usability testing. Although these intersections of two disciplines are discussed and defined long time ago, a structured methodology framework for practitioners is still missing on the area.

User centered design process on the other hand have produced numerous guidelines specific to user groups and evaluated them by using several usability evaluation techniques (summary available in [14]) The similarities of usability evaluation process and accessibility evaluation processes are also reported. (e.g.: [13]). Moreover the approach of creating a design for all users has also been discussed from many aspects, for example from *universal access* and *design for all* perspectives and also for building user interfaces for all and in the concept of unified user interfaces (e.g.: [21] [23]) Next to well known benefits of user centered research, that should apply to the future work in usability & accessibility research, problems were also reported due to lack of technical measurements and relevant methods [24]. For example, the problems due to conventional evaluation methods, like their taking too much time, can be supported by basic technical methods and these kinds of techniques can be added to programming tools [24].

As we also mentioned before [14] we believe that the knowledge and experience from user centered design can be combined with accessibility work and can be applied in a cooperative way by all stakeholders where "interface design, interaction and user experience can be designed in a universally accessible way" by testing all the steps in close cooperation of all involved stakeholders and end-users. By merging two attitudes (basic technical methods and user centered methods), we can cover all the issues that might cause a barrier for an older user, including "cognition, motivation, physical and perceptional problems" [9].The barriers and their possible solutions have been covered in many studies from usability and HCI sides (see e.g: [22] [23]).Moreover usability studies have long been concentrated on an idea of a unified solution that covers all the barrier factors (e.g: [7]). But for practitioners, it is still not clear how to deal with all reported barriers, which process to follow and how to evaluate their projects in order to see if they have reached to a real solution. Therefore, in this paper we aim to define a process framework based on ISO DIS 9241-210 norms [11] for building usable and accessible websites for all users following both user centered design principles and accessibility guidelines.

Although the ongoing research has not yet formulized a framework for practitioners on how to apply these two topics and include all stakeholders, EN ISO 9241-171(revised ISO/TS 16071:2002)[10] on "ergonomics guidance and specifications for the design of accessible software for use at work, in the home, in education and in public places" already addresses "software considerations for accessibility that complement general design for usability" For the design process ISO recommends using a user centered design norm (ISO DIS 9241-210- revised ISO 13407) [11].

3 Building a Usability Accessibility Framework for Website Engineering

In order to optimize the process of making web services accessible and usable for the widest possible majority of users, there is a need for a concrete framework of creating, developing and evaluating the products. We believe that by using a user centered framework and categorizing and applying accessibility tools and evaluation methods to the frame skeleton, we can test all the components that barriers the usage and access of these websites in one cycle. International Standard of Human-centered design processes for interactive systems ISO DIS 9241-210 [11] defines a human centered design process in four steps. These are *specification of the context of use, specification of user and organizational requirements, development of design solutions* and *evaluation vs. design goals.* Mayhew's usability engineering lifecycle [15] can be seen as an extension of the third part of ISO DIS 9241-210 to another three components. These are conceptual and structured design, evaluation and detailed design. By following ISO DIS 9241-210 and Mayhew's cycle and by iterating the phases with real users with special needs, it is possible to overcome the possible problems and barriers of a web application including accessibility aspects. By this way, accessibility evaluation methods concentrate on semi-automatic and manual evaluation techniques and user testing possibilities.

As an initial step, after finding and categorizing the problems, it is likely to share the found problems among designers, content analyzers and technical implementers to overcome them. Similarly, similar group or stakeholders are responsible for taking care of usability, technical efficiency and design problems. On our defined process, adding the components of accessibility evaluation to usability evaluation and distributing them into the relevant stakeholders decrease the amount of time and money needed for covering all aspects of accessibility assurance and increase the overall result. Additionally this framework supports the iterative and collective evaluation of design and technical solutions related to accessibility problems. Therefore this framework follows a unified problem solving approach, more than a stakeholder based approach. During the process, each stakeholder should cooperate with another one according to the constructs of the problem.

Figure 1 explains four steps of ISO DIS 9241-210. The third step of ISO DIS 9241-210 can be extended by using Mayhew's cycle. This step symbolizes the iterative development of the design solution according to the problems and recommendations found in previous steps. During this evaluation it is likely to discover new aspects while solving the other problems. In Mayhew's original lifecycle first and 2nd steps of ISO DIS 9241-210 are categorized under user requirements analysis. By collecting user requirements specific to accessibility issues next to usability issues and formulizing it in the related style guide we can integrate accessibility evaluation to this process.

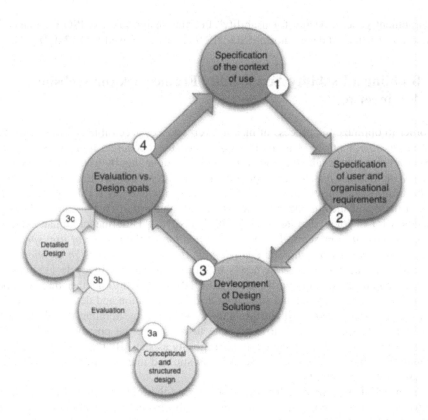

Fig. 1. ISO DIS 9241-210 (1 – 4) [10] extended by Mayhew's cycle represented by items 3a-3b[15] (re-drawn by authors of this publication)

In Figure 2 we give a close-up to the 3rd step and define relevant tools and mechanisms that might play a role in making websites accessible. By adding some components to the process, we believe that the process can include accessibility aspects.

Basically, to design technology for "usable accessibility" by following a user centered design process should be a principle, as already stated earlier in this article. The ISO DIS 9241-210 provides the basis for this framework. However, in some points a closer look needs to be taken to guarantee the "accessibility" of the resulting technology. Although the process and its steps are clear, some of these items need a closer look:

Getting to know the user and the context. A profound survey on user and context attributes need to be taken in order to find out who uses the application, where it is used and which possible factors might have an influence on usage. In these two steps of the standard ISO process designers and engineers get to know the possibilities and limitations of the users and the context, for both usability and accessibility considerations. We argue that it is important to add to this user analysis user groups that might not necessarily be in the primary focus of the application (such that need specific

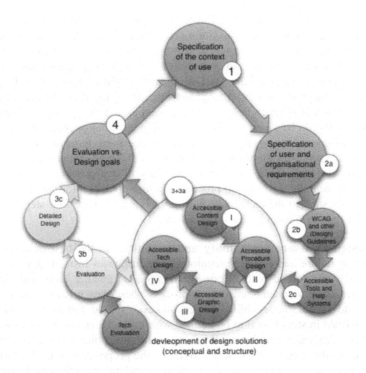

Fig. 2. Usable Accessibility Process (Based on ISO DIS 9241-210[10] and Mayhew's cycle [15])

accessible solutions). If there is no possibility to integrate these user groups directly by interviews, tests or focus groups (etc.) several guidelines published for different context and user types can be consulted. There are already guidelines published for elderly, blind, deaf or physical or cognitive impaired users [14]. Further, there are several papers on specific design solutions that deal with given accessibility problems (e.g: [1]).We believe in this (minimum) way accessibility issues might play role in finding specific design solutions from the beginning. In Figure 2 these two issues are represented by (2b) and (2c).

Finding specific design solutions. In the given ISO DIS 9241-210 the item "development of design solutions" is quite wide defined. We believe in order to guarantee a usable and accessible solution designers need to separate this design process in three different parts. Each of the following parts we believe needs to be considered at the first stage separately and then assembled into one solution:

a) Designing an Accessible Content
b) Designing an Accessible Procedure
c) Designing an Accessible Graphic Design
d) Designing an Accessible Technology Framework

This separation in subsequent steps follows the definition of Hoel and Overby [6] that define "syntactic, semantic and procedural accessibility". We argue that the development of accessible content should be the starting point. Once it is clear which information should be conveyed, it is about to put it in the right procedure and structure. For example, using click dummies and wireframes could easily do this. In general methods at this stage will not differ from any other usability methods, that are widely used in the HCI and usability field. Once the content and the procedures are drawn, graphic design should be added. At this point – as in the other ones before - guidelines could help designers finding the right solution. Once these three steps are done the last step should be the design of the technical design. Overall, the process we propose for this particular step in the "usable accessibility design process" is to start with semantics and meanings, go over to procedural and graphical information representation and finally stick to the technical solution. In Figure 2 these four steps are represented under the (3+a) point by (I), (II), (III) and (IV).

Iterate design to assure accessibility and usability. As the best design solution might contain failure and misinterpretation, iteration phases instead of waterfall design processes are needed both in prior phases among smaller tasks and later in a broader way. The "user centered design process" describes this as evaluation and iteration. And "usable accessibility design process" should follow it as well. The solutions defined in step 3 need to be iterated with users. However, to prove technical accessibility technical evaluation tools are needed to be applied. These tools provide feedback about the quality of the accessibility of the proposed technical solution. To guarantee semantic and procedural accessibility, standard (usability) evaluation tools and techniques are to be applied. In this part the proposed process differs from the standard "user centered process" as "normally" quality measurement of the code and technical solution is not a major topic for user centered design as long as the product is usable.

During this process by strengthening communication between users, different producers and especially among producers of different parts of projects & products and lastly by strictly following an iterative process including all diverse knowledge, tools and methods of included parties, a usable & accessible solution for products can easily be achieved.

4   Conclusions

In this paper we aimed to concentrate on the following points that are relevant for usable and accessible ICT services:

a.   The need of a standardized test and evaluation framework for usability and accessibility aspects of web/ICT services for practitioners
b.   The importance of balanced cooperation and more importantly optimized communication of different stakeholders in a project to ensure the best solutions for the reported problems
c.   The need to iterate all the process with real users who has diverse needs from the systems from the beginning

d. The need of a problem/barriers based definition of roadmaps, that clearly indicates the roles of different stakeholders

By following a user centered design process and extending/strengthening it with techniques from accessibility studies, we can create an efficient evaluation framework for ICT applications. Having the aging society and the increase of ICT applications in our mind, it is necessary to merge both disciplines to make technology usable and accessible at once, in a cost and time effective way.

References

1. Arch, A., Abou-Zhara, S.: How Web Accessibility Guidelines Apply to Design for the Ageing Population. In: Proceedings of Accessible Design in a Digital World Conference, York, UK (2008)
2. Baguma, R., Lubega, J.T.A.: Web design framework for improved accessibility for people with disabilities (WDFAD). In: Proceedings of ACM W4A 2008 the international cross-disciplinary conference on Web accessibility (W4A), pp. 134–140. ACM Press, New York (2008)
3. Bigham, J.P., Cavender, A.C.: Evaluating existing audio CAPTCHAs and an interface optimized for non-visual use. In: Proceedings of ACM CHI 2009 Conference on Human Factors in Computing Systems, pp. 1829–1838 (2009)
4. Fairweather, P.G.: How older and younger adults differ in their approach to problem solving on a complex website. In: Proceedings of the 10th international ACM SIGACCESS conference on Computers and accessibility, pp. 67–72. ACM, New York (2008)
5. Hanson, V.L.: Age and web access: the next generation. In: Proceedings of ACM W4A 2009 International Cross-Disciplinary Conference on Web Accessibility (W4A), pp. 7–15. ACM, New York (2009)
6. Hoel, T., Overby, E.: Access to digital information – the need for a change of paradigm, http://www.t4p.no/t4p.no/conference/programme/workshop/media/Overby-WS3-paper.pdf
7. Holzinger, A., Searle, G., Kleinberger, T., Seffah, A., Javahery, H.: Investigating Usability Metrics for the Design and Development of Applications for the Elderly. In: Miesenberger, K., Klaus, J., Zagler, W.L., Karshmer, A.I. (eds.) ICCHP 2008. LNCS, vol. 5105, pp. 98–105. Springer, Heidelberg (2008)
8. Holzinger, A.: Usability Engineering for Software Developers. Communications of the ACM 48(1), 71–74 (2005)
9. Holzinger, A., Searle, G., Nischelwitzer, A.: On some Aspects of Improving Mobile Applications for the Elderly. In: Stephanidis, C. (ed.) HCI 2007. LNCS, vol. 4554, pp. 923–932. Springer, Heidelberg (2007)
10. International Organization for Standardization. ISO DIS 9241-171:2008 Ergonomics of human-system interaction - Guidance on software accessibility. International Organization for Standardization, Geneva, Switzerland (2008)
11. International Organization for Standardization. ISO DIS 9241-210:2008. Ergonomics of human system interaction - Part 210: Human-centred design for interactive systems (formerly known as 13407:1999). International Organization for Standardization, Geneva, Switzerland (2008)
12. Kelly, B., Sloan, D., Brown, S., Seale, J., Petrie, H., Lauke, P., Ball, S.: Accessibility 2.0: people, policies and processes. In: Proceedings of ACM W4A 2007 International Cross-

Disciplinary Conference on Web Accessibility (W4A), pp. 138–147. ACM, New York (2007)

13. Lang, T.: Comparing website accessibility evaluation methods and learnings from usability evaluation methods (2003)
14. Leitner, M., Subasi, Ö., Geven, A., Höller, N., Tscheligi, M.: User requirement analysis for a railway ticketing portal with emphasis on semantic accessibility for older users. In: Proceedings of ACM W4A 2009 International Cross-Disciplinary Conference on Web Accessibility (W4A), pp. 114–122. ACM, New York (2009)
15. Mayhew, D.J.: The usability engineering lifecycle: A practitioner's handbook for user interface design. Morgan Kaufmann Publishers, San Francisco (1999)
16. Martn Garca, Y.S., Miguel González, B.S., Yelmo Garca, J.C.: Prosumers and accessibility: how to ensure a productive interaction. In: Proceedings of ACM W4A 2009 International Cross-Disciplinary Conference on Web Accessibility (W4A), pp. 50–53. ACM, New York (2009)
17. Sa-nga-ngam, P., Kurniawan, S.: A three-countries case study of older people's browsing. In: Proceedings of the 8th international ACM SIGACCESS conference on Computers and accessibility Assets 2006, pp. 223–224. ACM, New York (2006)
18. Sayago, S., Blat, J.: A preliminary usability evaluation of strategies for seeking online information with elderly people. In: Proceedings of ACM W4A 2007 International Cross-Disciplinary Conference on Web Accessibility (W4A), pp. 54–57. ACM, New York (2007)
19. Sloan, D., Gibson, L., Booth, P., Gibson, L.: Auditing accessibility of UK Higher Education web sites [Electronic version]. Interacting with Computers 14, 313–325 (2002)
20. Sloan, D., Gregor, P., Rowan, M., Booth, P.: Accessible accessibility [Electronic version]. In: Proceedings of the CUU 2000 First ACM Conference on Universal Usability. ACM, Arlington (2000)
21. Stephanidis, C.: User Interfaces for All: New perspectives into Human-Computer Interaction. In: Stephanidis, C. (ed.) User Interfaces for All - Concepts, Methods, and Tools, pp. 3–17. Lawrence Erlbaum Associates, Mahwah (2001)
22. Stephanidis, C. (ed.): HCI 2007. LNCS, vol. 4554. Springer, Heidelberg (2007)
23. Stephanidis, C. (ed.): The Universal Access Handbook. Taylor & Francis, Abington (2009)
24. Thimbleby, H.: User-Centered Methods Are Insufficient for Safety Critical Systems. In: Holzinger, A. (ed.) USAB 2007. LNCS, vol. 4799, pp. 1–20. Springer, Heidelberg (2007)
25. W3C Web Content Accessibility Guidelines 2.0, W3C Candidate Recommendation, http://www.w3.org/TR/2008/CR-WCAG20-20080430/

The Building Bridges Project: Involving Older Adults in the Design of a Communication Technology to Support Peer-to-Peer Social Engagement

Joseph Wherton[1] and David Prendergast[2]

[1] Technology Research for Independent Living (TRIL) Centre,
St James's Hospital, Dublin, Ireland
[2] Intel Digital Health Group, Leixlip, Ireland
whertonj@tcd.ie
david.k.prendergast@intel.com

Abstract. There are a variety of factors that can lead to social isolation and loneliness in old age, including decline in physical and mental health, as well as change to social environment. The Building Bridges project explores how communication technology can help older adults remain socially connected. This paper will first provide an overview of a prototype communication system designed to support peer-to-peer group interaction. A description of the user-centered design process will be provided to demonstrate the importance of involving older adults at the earliest stages. The implications for designing new technology for older adults are discussed.

Keywords: Loneliness, Social isolation, User-centered design, Voice over Internet Protocol (VoIP).

1 Introduction

Research indicates that loneliness and social isolation is closely associated with mental and physical health. Social connections might be lost due to retirement, relocation or widowhood. Engagement in social activity is also restricted by illness, depression, lack of mobility and demand to care for a significant other. The internet has the potential to enhance social connections and communication in a variety of ways, inexpensively. It also provides opportunities for meeting and interacting with new people in a flexible and autonomous way. However, there are very few social computing applications designed for inexperienced computer users, and that address specific needs and wishes of older users. This paper describes the development of a new communication system, which is designed to encourage peer-to-peer social engagement. The concept and interface was developed through a user-centered design process to ensure that the system is useful and appropriate.

1.1 The Role of Technology in Reducing Loneliness

Loneliness and social isolation are related, but distinct, concepts. Loneliness relates to a perceived lack of social contact [1,2], or the potential to socially interact with others

A. Holzinger and K. Miesenberger (Eds.): USAB 2009, LNCS 5889, pp. 111–134, 2009.

but not doing so [3]. Social isolation is a more objective term that relates to the nature of a person's social network or lack of social integration [4]. Most international research estimates that 5-16% of older adults experience frequent loneliness [5,6]. However, self-reported rates of loneliness may be an under representation of the true levels because of the stigma associated with being lonely. Loneliness and social isolation is associated with health, depression and self-efficacy [7,8]. Decline in mental and physical health is seen as a predictor as well as a consequence of loneliness. For example, restricted physical mobility can reduce engagement in social activities, which can further lead to depression or loss of appetite [9]. Drawing from these studies, Drennan et al. [10] points out that any intervention strategy needs to take into account the complexity of these factors. It should encompass the person's desire to communicate, promote good health and provide opportunities to meet people with shared interests, background or experiences.

Contact with family and friends is important for perceived social support [11,12]. However, participation in social events also plays an important role in reducing risks of depression, anxiety and cognitive impairment, as well as improving quality of life [13]. Voluntary sector befriending services have been found to be instrumental in increasing levels of happiness and reducing loneliness [14,15]. Telephone befriending services have also been found to be an effective way of connecting socially isolated older adults. For example, Monk and Reed [16] describe a befriending scheme in London that uses telephone conference calls and weekly one-to-one calls to connect older adults over the phone. They found that the users perceived an intrinsic benefit in actively engaging, or listening, to a conversation. Regular contact also provided reassurance and instrumental gains through information sharing.

A number of studies have highlighted the potential role of internet communication for reducing loneliness. White et al. [17] explored the effect of internet use in a retirement community. Fifteen older adults underwent training on a communal computer with an internet connection. Email was used primarily to communicate with family and friends. Psychosocial assessments demonstrated that reconnecting social ties decreased level of loneliness. Similarly, Groves and Slack [18] explored the impact of a computer-training program with 20 nursing home residents. Pre-post evaluations showed an increase in independence and engagement in social activities.

1.2 Involving Older Adults in Communication Technology Design

Modern technology and the internet offer new ways to help seniors remain connected with their peers and family members. However, this is often inaccessible to them due to decline in cognitive, sensory and physical abilities. Furthermore, the software is often designed for people who are familiar with using such technology. The majority of older adults are not regular computer users, and would experience problems with interface conventions (e.g. scroll bars), understanding terminology (e.g. 'File', 'Open', 'download'), and operating the system (e.g. clicking the mouse correctly) [19, 20].

Czaja, Guerrier, Nair and Landauer [21] examined the feasibility of older people using an electronic text message system to perform routine communication tasks. A 'simplified' communication system was put in the homes of 36 adults over the age of 50. The system included a text editor, basic electronic mail functions and access to information (news, weather and health information). The technology included a CRT monitor, keyboard, printer, modem and controller. The software was designed for people with little computer experience, and so operating commands were minimal. The design was specialized for message communication. It was always 'on', and there were no log-on procedures, disk operations or file access. To operate the system, the users typed the name of another participant, and the system dialed automatically. The user then pressed a boldly labeled Return key. They could then write the message. When the message was completed, the user would press a boldly labeled Send key. It was found that the participants could use the system with a minimal amount of difficulty, and all reported that they enjoyed using it and found it useful. Importantly, participants indicated that the system facilitated social interaction and a chance to meet new people. It was also noted, however, that there was a significant decline in use over time. This was due to the fact that people were busy and the system had limited functionality. This indicated that although the system was easy to use, it needed to be percieved as useful in order for it to be adopted in real contexts. The system would need to be expanded without unecessarily increasing its complexity. This would require involvment of potential users from the early stages of development.

Hawthorn [22] re-developed the Microsoft Outlook Express interface to support use by older adults. The new email system (SeniorMail) was designed through a series of focus groups, interviews and usability tests. The modifications focused on visual presentation (e.g. bigger buttons and larger font) reducing cognitive demand by simplifying navigation, and presenting a list of possible actions in a menu system.

Dickinson et al. [19] also developed an email system for seniors with no experience of internet use. Based on previous research they established guidelines for the software before development. This focused on *functionality* (e.g. each screen has a clear primary function and only a few buttons are available), *accessibility* (e.g. large clickable targets and high contrast between text and background), *user interface paradigms* (e.g. no scroll bars), *terminology*, and *personalisation* (customizable to match sensory impairment). In order to refine the design, paper prototypes of the interface were presented in a workshop with nine older people. This highlighted further requirements, such as the need to avoid formal language, and increasing the salience of icons and buttons. The final prototype was simplified by reduced functionality and minimal presentation of information on the screen. Each screen had a primary function (e.g. entering the email address of the recipient). This avoided uncertainty about moving between multiple text-entry fields and also limited mouse interactions. The 'single-purpose' page also meant that screen-specific instructions could be presented to guide users through the steps to completing the task. User testing with the final prototype demonstrated that people with no experience of the internet found it significantly easier to use than a commercially equivalent design. The positive experience of the system also led particpants to feel more confident about computer use.

These studies demonstrate how communication technology can be designed to suit the needs of older adults with little or no experience with computers. Potential users need to be involved throughout the development so that the interface is intuitive and easy to use. They also play an important role in finding a balance between increasing simplicity, without unnecessary limiting what the user can do with the system. Adoption of the technology over time will be determined by perceived usefulness and appropriatness in real contexts. The cultural gap between the researchers and older adults is particularly wide when developing social computing, as motivations and patterns in social behaviour change across the life span [23]. The concept must therefore be grounded in an understanding of what users want before the technology or interface design is considered.

This paper describes the development of a new communication system designed to support social connections among older adults and reduce risks of loneliness. Different methods were used to elicit information from potential users at each step of the design process. These methods were instrumental in developing the concept, establishing design requirements, and building the interface. This process was necessary for the development of a system that users need, want and can use.

1.3   The Building Bridges Project

The aim of the Building Bridges project is to develop communication technology that can reduce risks of loneliness and social isolation. The project is part of the Technology Research for Independent Living (TRIL) Centre, which is a collaboration between Trinity College Dublin (TCD), University College Dublin (UCD), National University of Ireland Galway, St James Hospital, Dublin, and the Intel Digital Health Group (www.trilcentre.org).

To date the Building Bridges project has developed a user friendly device for the home that provides opportunities for peer-to-peer social interaction. Older adults were involved throughout the design process, from the early stages of developing a concept to the refinement of the final prototype. The system is designed to provide opportunities to meet people and facilitate group conversations by providing a common ground through the shared experience of a broadcast (e.g. news, documentaries and stories).

This paper gives an overview of the Building Bridge system and the core design features. The design process will then be described to illustrate the importance of involving potential users in directing design efforts.

2   System Overview

The Building Bridges system is a combination of hardware and software which have been designed to work seamlessly with each other. The hardware is comprised of a 12" touch screen computer in a custom made stand, a phone handset with functioning cradle, and   speakers. The phone and speakers are used for calls and broadcasts respectively (see Figure 1).

The software uses Skype to allow communication via calls, broadcasts and messaging, but the standard Skype client is not used. Skype allows developers to create their own interface with the use of an API (Application Programming Interface). Through this a Flash based interface has been designed that allows the user to interact with the system using the touch screen.

2.1   Broadcast and Chat

During the broadcast. The user can listen to broadcasts (e.g. news, documentaries, stories and music), which are played through the speakers. The broadcasts are played daily. A guide to the broadcasts (time, day and topic) can be viewed on the left of the Main Menu screen. The broadcast schedule is updated by a main server and the

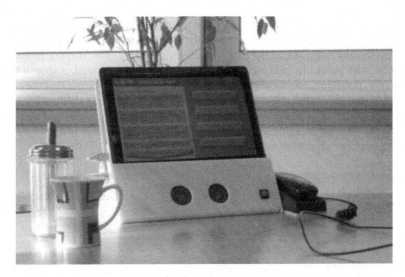

Fig. 1. The Building Bridges device showing the Main Menu Screen: On the Main Menu Screen the user can view the time, day and topic of upcoming broadcasts

broadcasts are played to each device from an admin console. At the specified time, a screen appears on the device inviting the user to listen to the broadcast. If the user wishes to listen, they press a button on the screen. Figure 2 shows the screen display during a broadcast. This provides a picture display related to the broadcast topic, which can also be used to show videos or slides. On the right of the screen, the user can see icons that represent other people who are listening. If the user wishes to leave the broadcast at anytime, they press the 'Leave Broadcast' button on the top right of the screen. At the end of the broadcast the user can join a 'group chat' with the other listeners by lifting the phone handset.

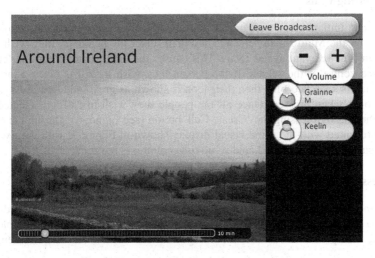

Fig. 2. The screen display during a broadcast

During the group chat. During the conference call the screen displays icons to support communication (see Figure 3). The design was based on feedback from seniors after experiencing standard conference calls with strangers. The display includes an avatar icon with names to indicate who has entered and left the call, a speech bubble to show who is talking, and a button that the user can press to indicate that they would like to interrupt the conversation. These features help overcome difficulties experienced when communicating within a group in the absence of physical and non-verbal cues. The post-broadcast chats are limited to 20 minutes. A counter is displayed at the bottom right of the screen.

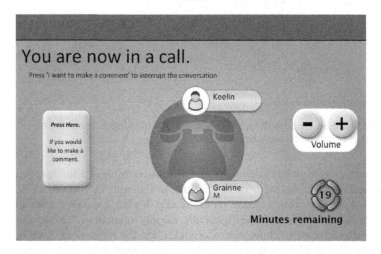

Fig. 3. Screen display during a 'group chat'. Icons are used to represent other particpants who have entered, or left, the call.

2.2 Initiating Calls

The user can initiate a call with one or more people. The user selects the button 'Create Chat' on the Main Menu screen. They then select the person(s) they wish to call by pressing the relevant avatar icons. This causes the icon to move into the 'call circle' in the centre of the screen. If the person they wish to call is not available (i.e. their device is switched off), then their icon is shown as grey and a red cross appears in front of it when pressed. Once all the people they wish to call are selected, they initiate the call by pressing the 'Create Call' button (see Figure 4). During the call the user is presented with the same visual display shown in Figure 3, with the exception that the call length is unlimted, and so no time counter is required.

2.3 Messaging

Users can write short messages (up to 160 characters). Similar to the procedure for making a call, each screen guides the user through the linear steps to complete the task. The user presses the 'Write a Message' button on the main menu screen. They

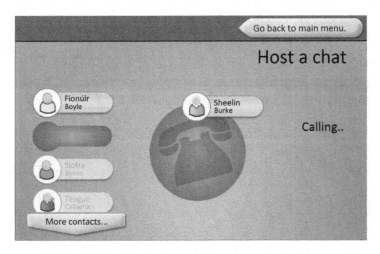

Fig. 4. The screen display when selecting people to call

then select the person(s) they wish to send the message to and press the 'Write Message' button. This leads to the next screen, which includes a touch screen keyboard (see Figure 5). The letters on the touch screen keyboard are in an alphabetical layout, so that it is easy for those unfamiliar with the standard QWERTY arrangement to use.

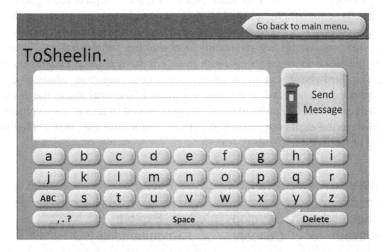

Fig. 5. The touch screen keyboard for writing messages

2.4 Tea Room

As well as talking with people after broadcasts and initiating calls, users can also enter the Tea Room for a chat, which is available any time day or night. The screen presents icons to indicate who else has entered the Tea Room. Additionally, the screen presents a 'window on the world' feature, which includes a series of images from a live webcam in various outdoor locations (see Figure 6).

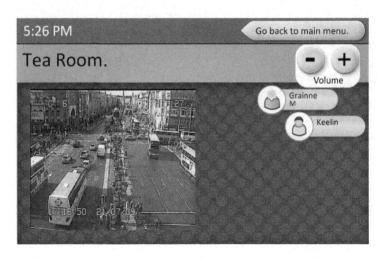

Fig. 6. The Tea Room with the 'window on the world'. On the right users can view other people who have entered the Tea Room.

3 Design Process

The design process included four main phases. Figure 7 depicts each phase in this process. Firstly, ethnography and field work was conducted to understand the problems being addressed. Second, the field notes were analysed collaboratively by the interdisciplinary research team to identify opportunities for technology. These ideas were then discussed in focus groups with older adults in order to establish a unified concept. The third phase was an iterative process involving older adults to establish design requirements and develop a usable interface. In the final phase, the device was tested in seniors' homes in order to refine the system and interface. This section of the paper will describe each phase and highlight the main outcomes that guided the development of the Building Bridges system.

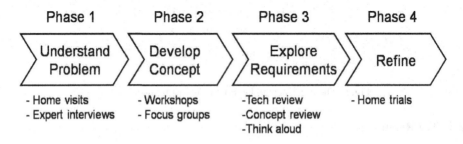

Fig. 7. A summary of the four phases in the design process and the methodology used at each step

3.1 Phase 1: Ethnography and Fieldwork

In order to develop technology that is useful and appropriate for the users, it is necessary to first define and understand the dynamics of the problems being addressed. To this end, the Building Bridges team adopted a mixed method research approach. Literature and technical reviews into loneliness and social isolation were complemented by analysis of quantitative data sets generated by the TRIL clinic cohort and large cross sectional surveys such as the Dublin Healthy Ageing Study. Qualitative insights were derived from focus groups, in home interviews with older people, and secondary analysis of databases such as Intel's Global Ageing Experience Project. This preliminary body of work clearly suggested several themes and design principles that were later taken forward within the planning and development of the Building Bridges system.

Firstly it was clear that whilst the size of social networks of older people often contract during the later phases of retirement, this is not always negative and it was important in many cases to distinguish between being alone and lonely. Subsequent research by the TRIL social connection strand developed a typology of social and emotional loneliness categories correlated to cognitive and medical biomarkers that has the potential to provide indications of risk and identify opportunities for early intervention. The original early pass at the data also suggested that whilst older people were interested in augmenting their social connections with their family, many placed greater emphasis on building relatedness with friends, neighbors and communities.

Interviews and focus groups with individuals aged between 70 and 85 years unsurprisingly revealed considerable diversity in opinions about the relevance and attractiveness of technology to the everyday lives of older people. Many participants expressed concern over the perceived complexity of modern technology and felt that whilst it might have a lot to offer them it was inaccessible "for the likes of me". As Tom, a 72 year old widower explained:

> *"...I'd love to be able to get on those sports websites. I think if they [computers] were easier looking I'd use them- they're a bit complicated looking..."*

Stories about unwanted gifts of technology from unopened DVD players to intrusive mobile phones to house alarm systems with stressful and forgettable codes frequently made an appearance during interviews. Others described suspicions about the security of online banking systems as well as worries over identity theft through public availability of personal information on websites such as Facebook, addicting games, and the ease of making foolish or expensive mistakes when shopping or booking travel online.

In contrast, awe was also often expressed at the potential of modern technologies from recognition of the utility of new telehealth offerings to opportunities to develop and showcase their own hobbies in new and interesting ways. One 80 year old male began an interview by explaining he was too old to learn how to use a computer but later grew enthusiastic as he described his cousin in England:

> *"The things she was doing with the photos on the computer! The whole picture changed. Absolutely fantastic! I would be interested in that aspect of technology in my line of work as an artist. I work from photographs you see."*

Many participants felt that advances in domestic, communication and entertainment technologies had improved their quality of life. Over 70% of the 600 older people who went through the TRIL clinic assessment owned a mobile phone, though there was considerable variation in the degree to which they were used regularly or simply kept close by in case of emergencies. As an extension of a long established technology, the leap to adoption has been facilitated by the familiarity of the concept, though several comments were made about features unused and unexplored. For instance, Mary, a 76 year old focus group participant found herself confused by her phone's complicated address book function so simply solved the problem by taping her important contact numbers on a piece of card to the back of the unit.

The importance of simplicity and familiarity became recurrent and saturated themes through our preliminary research phase with constant reference being made to the importance of the telephone, radio and television to people's daily lives and rhythms. This led the Building Bridges team to explore opportunities to adapt, expand and continue these metaphors in their work to develop an advanced communication technology designed to reduce social isolation. The design challenge of course was to do this in a manner and form factor as intuitive to this cohort as possible whilst simultaneously resisting complexity of interface and interaction.

Coincidentally in early 2008, Skype had just released one of their first stand alone VoIP phones so the building bridges team deployed several of these in the homes of four older people around Ireland for two weeks. The participants had a mean age of 73 and at the start of the pilot were unknown to each other. The purpose of the trial was to explore how and when people used the system, what technical features were useful or could be improved and how individuals found the experience of social interaction over time. To facilitate the pilot, a social anthropologist on the team arranged five conference calls on a variety of discussion topics, such as common heritage, favourite places, and personal interests, carefully moderated to draw out different modes of turn taking. This was done whilst using and comparing user experience of the Skype VoIP system vs. a conventional POTS based audio bridge.

Despite occasional technology failure and variable sound quality, all participants spoke and engaged during the five 45 minute teleconference sessions. Design insights began to emerge almost immediately. Participants found joining a group conversion on the phone highly enjoyable and novel but suggested that they were disappointed that they couldn't see who was talking. They also noted that it was frequently difficult to break into a three or more person conversation in a polite manner without access to visual cue. A means of indicating to others a desire to speak on the call was requested in order to facilitate turn taking. During exit interviews members of this early pilot described how they had looked forward to the calls and were keen to arrange a real life meeting with their co-participants in order to finally put faces to the names. Summarizing the experience of this initial exploratory deployment with off-the-shelf products, the following comments were made:

> "In principle it is great...you get to know things about people...in practice the technology is very poor..."

> "It is hard at the start...but once you learn about each other...it is like having a chat..."

> "It is a fantastic idea... it's great to chat."

"I liked it, but I think it would be better for an older person who can't get out of the house..."

On the heels of this pilot study, similar observations emerged from subsequent discussions with a range of professional and community based organizations focused on alleviating social isolation for older people. Suggestions about opportunities for developing carer networks, peer mentoring and befriending schemes as well as real time information sharing networks were forwarded as were warnings about the necessity of ensuring that such a system would be used responsibly; namely it should aim to augment and extend rather than replace social contact.

3.2   Phase 2: Developing the Concept

The second phase focused on identifying technological opportunities from the ethnographic material in order to establish the concept. This phase included three steps: Step 1 involved a collective analysis of the ethnographic material; Step 2 included focus groups with older adults to discuss technological opportunities; and Step 3 involved the development of a unified concept based on the focus group discussions. It is important to note that technical requirements and plausibility of design concepts were not considered during this phase. This was so that discussions were not limited, or biased, by knowledge of existing technologies.

Step 1: Identifying opportunities for technology. The first step was to establish themes from the ethnographic material. This was a collaborative process involving a multidisciplinary research team (social scientists, engineers, computers scientists, designers and clinicians).

The ethnographers presented the material to the team. During these presentations all members wrote down key points (e.g. quotes, ideas and questions), that they considered important, onto post-it notes.

Once all the ethnographic material was presented, the post-it notes were collated and stuck onto a large whiteboard. The researchers collectively grouped related post-it notes together to form categories. Once categories had been identified, these were further grouped to form broader themes. Six themes emerged:

(i) *Learning curve* (e.g. training support, avoid dependency)
(ii) *Privacy and intrusion* (e.g. security, speaking with strangers)
(iii) *Joining conference calls* (e.g. timing/scheduling, reluctance to connect)
(iv) *Making it interesting* (e.g. gaming, competition, sharing)
(v) *Visualisation of others* (e.g. simulate physical presence, who is talking)
(vi) Group generation (e.g. common factor, snowballing contacts)

The team was then divided into three groups. Each group was given two of the themes, and they were required to build an idea or concept related to each category. In order to stimulate discussion, the groups were required to state: a) the problem being addressed; b) the solution to the problem; and c) a metaphor for the solution. Each of these three points were written on a post-it note and attached to the corners of a triangular sheet of paper. In the centre of the triangle, the group had to draw a picture to describe the idea or concept. These were used to present ideas to the other groups in the research team. See Figure 8 for example photos during the formation of categories and concepts during these workshops.

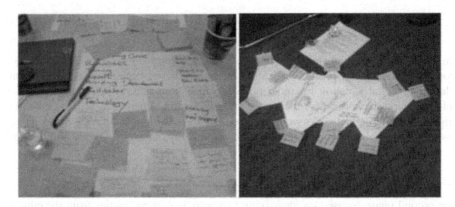

Fig. 8. Example photos taken during formation of categories through the grouping of post-it notes (left) and concepts developed around these categories (right)

Step 2: Reviewing concept ideas. The opportunities for technology were reviewed in focus groups with older adults. There were six focus groups in total. Four took place at Active Retirement Groups in Dublin (each including 10-20 participants). Two focus groups took place at St James's Hospital, Dublin (each including 5 participants), in which participants were recruited through the TRIL clinic.

At the start of the focus group, the researchers introduced themselves and explained the aim of the project. Each idea was presented to the participants using a 'storyboard', which included 4 to 6 frames on a piece of board (42x32cm). The scenario for each storyboard was structured so that the first frame described the user and the last frame highlighted how the technology benefited the user. The middle frames described the concept. Figure 9 shows an example storyboard.

After each storyboard was presented, the researcher asked participants what they thought about the idea, how they would use it, what they liked or disliked about it and how it might be improved. There were 10 storyboards in total. The focus groups were audio recorded and lasted approximately one hour.

The storboards were used as probes for stimulating discussion. It focused on the concept and how it would be used, as opposed to the technology involved. In this way the discussions were open-ended in order to reveal requirements for social computing and design issues that were not previously considered. For example, the main theme captured in the scenario presented in Figure 9 includes the linking of strangers through shared interests. In the subsequent discussion, particpants commented that linking people in this way was limited. Many also found it difficult to think of a hobby or personal interest that they would want to discuss with a stranger. It was however, highlighted that a common ground is needed in order to interact with strangers in a meaningful way. Conversations based around shared experiences, circumstances and events were considered to be more natural, informal and less limited:

> *"I don't have any interests."*

> *"That's one thing older people are good at, talking about old*
>
> *memories."*

Phone-Pal

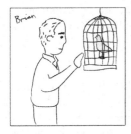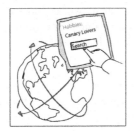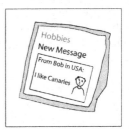

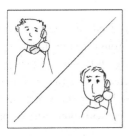

Fig. 9. Example storyboard, 'Phone Pal': This scenario focused on connecting people with shared interests. Frame 1 introduces the character, who has an interest in canaries. In Frame 2 he registers his profile on system, including his personal interests. In Frame 3 he gets a response from someone in America who is also interested in canaries and would like to have a chat. Frame 4 describes them having a chat and sharing tips on looking after canaries.

The example storyboard in Figure 9 also cued discussion around keeping the system 'community contained'. There was a preference to limit the system to people in the same community, rather than linking people from around the world. They felt that this would provide opportunities for face-to-face contact once a friendship has been developed.

> *"I would prefer community contained, more local."*

> *"The option to meet people face to face would be good."*

Furthermore, it triggered discussions regarding security. One aspect of the storyboard they did not like was the openness to the public. There was a clear preference for a 'closed system', controlled by an organization (e.g. local club or active retirement group).

> *"The internet and chat rooms are very open to abuse."*

> *"There should be a centre, someone in charge."*

> *"You have to be careful who you are talking to, giving address."*

The storyboards were designed to stimulate discussion and so were structured to be short, simple and ambiguous with regard to technology. This was to ensure that contributions made in the focus groups were not limited or biased by perceived knowledge or anxieties about computers. The ten storyboards used were broad and ranged from recreational interaction (e.g. games) to more instrumental interaction, such as peer-support (e.g. caregiver network) and formal health consultations (e.g. collaborative health check with consultants and family members). Key points raised during the focus groups were recorded in order to guide the design towards a unified concept.

Step 3: Establishing a unified concept. The third step in this phase was to establish a technological concept based on the focus group discussions. The researchers documented the positive and negative comments associated with each storyboard. This provided a summary of the participants' perspectives about important design issues. Listed below are some of the key points that emerged:

i) *The need for common ground*: Particpants emphasized the need to have something to talk about. Connecting people through shared hobbies or interests was too limited, and some found it difficult to think of personal interests that they would be motivated to discuss with strangers. They felt that many social interactions centre on shared experiences (e.g. visiting same place), common ground (e.g. speaking with other stroke patients), or reminiscence.

ii) *Concerns about social obligation:* Participants expressed concerns about being 'trapped' in a conversation with someone. They believed that different people require different degrees of social contact. The system should provide opportunities for meeting, but avoid feelings of social obligation or fear of intruding others.

> *"I have one person who calls me every morning you can't get away."*

> *"You could get someone who is not getting off the line, and the other person doesn't know what to do."*

> *"There should be a time limit on the calls."*

iii) *Security:* They raised the need for a 'closed system' that is controlled by an organization (e.g. local club or active retirement group). This approach would be in contrast to most social computing and networking systems, whch are open to the public:

> *"There should be a centre, someone in charge."*

> *"It must not go out to all in sundry, but to a limited circle."*

iv) *Bringing outdoor events into the home:* There was a positive response to concepts that provided something educational (e.g.' health lectures'), as they felt this was an added benefit to meeting people. It was pointed out that they should not be too formal and there should still be a social element to these events:

"Helpful as a lot of elderly people wouldn't be able to dream of going to them."

"You do pick up a lot of information from other people."

Main outcomes. Feedback from older adults during the focus groups was instrumental in directing design efforts. It was evident that social interaction with strangers should be supported by providing a common ground. The social encounters would need to be flexible and unobtrusive.

As participants felt that educational and informative broadcasts would be beneficial to them, it was decided that this would be a useful channel for people to meet and have something to talk about. Hence, it was decided that a core feature in the design would be to provide broadcasts, which would be followed by a group chat. This would allow opportunistic social interaction, as well as provide common ground through the shared experience of the broadcast.

3.3   Phase 3: Developing the System and User Interface

After establishing the core features, the technical requirements for hardware and software were established in order to begin devloping the prototype. It was decided that the main features (broadcasts, group calls and messaging) could be achieved through Skype, which allows developers to create interfaces with an API   (Application Programming Interface). It was also decided that the user would interact with a Flash based interface though a touch screen. As the touch screen input device is also the output device, it is easy to learn and more suited for older adults with little experience with using a mouse or keyboard [24].

Existing design guidelines for accessible systems for the older people provided a useful starting point [19,20,25,26]. These related to *vision* (e.g. text should be in sentence case, Arial font greater than 14-point, and high colour contrast to the background), *dexterity* (e.g. no double clicks and large buttons), *attention* (e.g. no moving text or animations, provide ample time to read text and do not use pop-up widows), *cognition* (e.g. use bold navigation tools, limit functionality and number of buttons per screen, avoid hierarchical structure and drop-down menus), and *computer knowledge* (e.g. avoid technical terminology). As many of these recommendations relate to existing applications (e.g. email) with standard keyboard and mouse, it was necessary to explore requirements specific to our touchscreen interface.

Six of the participants who took part in the focus groups were visited in their own homes. During the visit the researcher described the final concept, which was presented in the same 'storyboard' format described in Section 3.2. The concept was then discussed to understand how the participants would use it and what difficulties or concerns they would have.

They were then shown different interface designs on a touchscreen. The researcher conducted a 'think aloud' interview. This involved giving participants specific goals (e.g. send a message) without providing instructuctions on how to perform the task. At points where they appeared to struggle, or made a mistake, the researcher would encourage them to say what they were trying to do This observation technique helps reveal aspects of the interface that are not intuitive to novel users.

Main outcomes. The 'think-aloud' interviews provided insight into how the interface needed to be structured so that it was easy to use. Key design decisions are discussed in Section 4.3. In addition to the interface design, the semi-structured interviews also highlighted requirements regarding system use. In an earlydesign users would be required to specify broadcasts they wanted to listen to in advance, and choose a time and day for it to be played. However, this approach raised concerns about feeling committed to meet the scheduled time:

> *"Suppose you say you're listening into it and then something happens.*
>
> *...If you make a commitment, you should at least attend."*

Consequently it was decided to take a top-down approach for scheduling broadcasts. Similar to that of a radio, the broadcast schedule was pre-set. If the user wishes to listen to a specific broadcast they would need to make the scheduled time. Although this reduced their control over broadcast shedule, it did provide a greater sence of flexibility in that they did not feel committed to listening.

The interviews also highlighted requirements for the messaging feature. In the initial design users wrote messages directly onto the screen using a stylus. Although this was popular with many, some raised concerns about how their handwriting appeared to other people.

> *"My writing is a lot better than that on paper...that looks*
> *like it's been written by a four-year old."*

As a result it was decided that a touch screen keyboard was more inclusive. Additionally, the alphabetical layout of keys was included in the design as some particpants who were unfamiliar with the standard QWERTY arrangements found it difficult to find the correct keys.

Involving older adults during this phase of the design helped develop a prototype that was intuitive and matched their preferences and expectations about how it should be used. However, conducting one-off interviews in the home presents limitations. Firstly, interactions with the interface during the 'think aloud' interview were at the request of the researcher, and so the task being performed had little meaning to the participant. Second, the participants were not very familiar with the system, and so their contributions were limited, and they would feel less confident in criticising the design. Third, more subtle problems would only emerge from use over time and in real situations. Therefore, in the final phase of the design process, older adults used the system over a number of weeks to understand how the prototype could be refined to suit real cotexts.

3.4 Phase 4: Refining the Design through Home Trials

In the final phase the prototype devices were deployed in 15 homes in two separate home trials. *Home trial 1* focused on usability and dependability, and *home trial 2* focused on the experience and use of the system. After home trial 1, modifications were made to the device, based on outcomes from the trial, before running home trial 2.

All participants were over 60 and lived in the Dublin area. Four of the participants used a computer and the internet, and 11 did not use a computer. The prototype used for the trial included the broadcast, group calls and messaging features described in Section 2.

Home Trial 1. Five participants were given the device for 4 weeks. The trial involved two home visits, both lasting approximately one hour. During home visit 1 the device was installed in the house. It was located in a room of the participant's choosing (e.g. lounge, bedroom or kitchen). The researcher first explained the main features (broadcasts, calls and messaging). A 'think-aloud' interview was then conducted, followed by a semi-structured interview, focusing on their initial thoughts, concerns and expectations about the device.

At the end of the 4-weeks, the researcher re-visited the participants. A second 'think-aloud' and semi-structured interview was conducted, focusing on problems experienced and their perspective on how the device could be improved.

A video camera was used to record their interactions with the screen during the 'think aloud' interview. The semi-structure interviews were audio recorded.

Home Trial 2. The second home trial lasted for 6 weeks and focused on users' experience and usage. The trial included two separate groups of five people. Group 1 consisted of five strangers and Group 2 consisted of five members of an Active Retirement Groups (ARG). This allowed system use to be explored under two different social contexts.

The home visit procedure was the same as that used in home trial 1. Additionally the semi-structured interview included issues around communication with other users (e.g. reasons for calling other people and what they talked about), usage (e.g. when they use it), and how it fitted into daily routines (e.g. reasons for switching it off).

The 'think aloud' interviews were recorded using a video camera, and the semi-structure interviews were audio recorded. Participants' usage (time, frequency and duration) of each feature and screen presses were logged remotely on a server.

Main outcomes. The analysis provided insight into how the device was used in real contexts and revealed additional design issues that did not emerge through one-off home visit interviews.

Use of the system: The remote log data collected in trial 2 provided insight into how the system was used and incorporated into daily routines. Across the two groups, 156 calls were initiated. However, only 53 (34%) of these were answered by the recipient, and so nearly two thirds of calls made were unanswered. This problem was also reported in the exit interviews:

> "When I did ring both of them, it seemed to ring out or I
> was wondering if they were out a lot and I sent them mes-
> sages instead."

The exit interviews revealed that this was due to the fact that many participants kept the device 'on' when they left the house. A related problem was that participants turned the device 'off' when they were in the house. One particpant turned her device 'off' when she saw that people in her address book were not available:

> *"Everyone was [not available], so they were obviously off so
> I switched mine off too."*

Encouraging users to switch the device 'off' when they leave the house, and 'on' when they get back in is an important design issue. Subsequent to this it was decided to locate the device in a prominent location of the house, and use it as a digital photo frame when not in use. Subsequent home trials will explore wether this encourages the routine of turning the device 'on' and 'off' at the appropriate times.

As participants became familiar with the system over time, they became more confident in suggesting how it should be improved to suit real situations. They requested a loud audio cue when a message was received, or when a broadcast was about to start, so that they could be alerted when away from the device. They also requested added functionality in the messaging. For simplicity the messaging feature only allowed for one-to-one messages. During trial 1 participants suggested that group messages should also be allowed, mainly because they often used it to inform others of their availability to chat. The option to send group messages was included in the prototype used for trial 2. Remote logs confirmed the instrumental value of using group messages for scheduling chats. In total, eighty-five messages were sent during trial 2. The majority of these messages were *greetings* (e.g. "Hi are you home? if so how are you?"), which constituted 35% of the all messages. The second most common centered on *scheduling* (e.g. "Hi. How are you today, would you like to come to bowls tonight?), and *availability* (e.g. "I will not be around this afternoon"), which constituted 29% of all messages. Other messages included *device problems* (16%), *broadcasts* (12%), and discussing *daily activities* (7%). Within Group 1, ten multi-person messages were sent. Within Group 2, only one multi-person message was sent. All multi-person messages were used to send out greetings (55%), and scheduling or informing other about availability (45%). These logs confirm the need to include both one-to-one and multi-person messaging, as it provided a channel for lightweight group interaction among the strangers and was instrumental in arranging times to talk.

Usability. The exit interviews highlighted a number of subtle usability problems. At the end of the trials most participants adopted the use of a stylus (e.g. using a pencil or chopstick) to interact with the screen as they found this easier than using their finger:

> *"I use this chopstick to type messages, it makes it much easier.
> You can also see what letters are being pressed because your
> finger isn't covering the button."*

Problems with the location of buttons were also revealed. When using one of the features (e.g. writing a message) the 'Go Back to Main Menu' button was located at the bottom of the screen. When interacting with the screen (e.g. writing a message) participants would inadvertently press this button with their knuckle of wrist.

> *"I would occasional hit the 'Go Back to Main Menu' button,
> so that would be better positioned somewhere else, maybe
> the top-right corner."*

To overcome this all navigation buttons were placed at the top of the screen so that they would not be pressed by mistake.

It was also observed that particpants attempted to call contacts that were offline. In the contact list off-line contacts were greyed out. However, during exit interviews, some particpants still attempted to select an offline contact when making a call, and were confused as to why the system did not respond. This indicated that they did not know that the grey meant that the person was offline. This was rectified so that if the user presses an offline contact the words 'offline' appear infront of the contact avatar.

Usability issues were also identified through remote logging of screen presses. It emerged that icons and arrows located on buttons were distracting the users. For example, in the original design the 'Back to Main Menu' button had an arrow on the left edge. However, the arrow often became the hit target, which frequently led to a lack of response from the system when particpants pressed the edge of the button. This is illustrated in Figure 10 which shows the different clusters of screen presses on the touch screen keyboard. As a result icons were removed from all buttons.

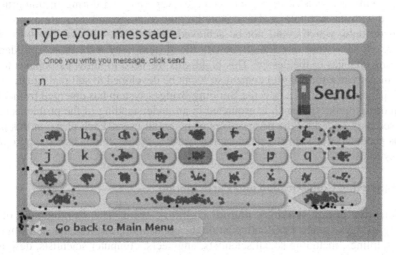

Fig. 10. Screen presses on the touch screen keyboard during trial 2: Each dot indicates the participant's screen press. Presses on the 'Go Back to Main Menu' button (bottom left) cluster around the arrow icon on the left side of the button.

4 Discussion

4.1 A Bottom-Up Approach

In order to design technology that is useful and appropriate for the users it is necessary to involve them throughout the design process. This not only means involving them in the evaluation of new technologies, but to include them at the earliest stages in order to direct design efforts. Each phase in the development of the Building Bridges technology has been necessary to ensure that the system matches what users need and want.

The first phase helped understand the problems being addressed. Home visits and expert interviews revealed the benefits of peer-to-peer social engagement and the role of the telephone in reducing feelings of loneliness.

The second phase involved the identification of technological opportunities based on the ethnographic data. The multidisciplinary research team collectively analysed the material to generate a large quantity of ideas that would stimulate discussions with older adults during focus groups. The storyboards used during the focus groups allowed these ideas to be communicated to seniors with different levels of experience with technology in order to establish unified concept.

The third phase involved home visits to identify design requirements. The 'think aloud' interviews guided the design towards an intuitive interface that could be easily used by older adults with little or no computer experience. The semi-structured interviews also ensured that the design was sensitive to how potential users would want to use the system in the home setting.

The final phase allowed users to contribute to the design after using the device for a number of weeks. This was important for refining the protype and revealing subtle but important design issues that only emerge over time and during meaningful engagement with the technology. The remote logging of usage and interactions provided naturalistic data, which could not be achieved through one-off usability tests. Furthermore, as they were more familiar with the system, they were more confident in suggesting changes to the design. This highlights the need to allow particpants to use the technology in a meaningful context so it can be developed to suit real situations. .

This paper demonstrates how the Building Bridges system has emerged from a bottom-up design process, which is grounded in an understanding of the problems being addressed and guided by the perspectives of potential users. Each phase in this process was necessary for focusing the design towards a system that is useful, appropriate and easy to use.

4.2 Supporting Collaboration and Participation

Collaborative design within a multidisciplinary team. This development of the Building Bridges system was contingent on the contributions of researchers from multiple disciplines, including social scientists, engineers, computer scientists, designers, and clinicians. The project relied on effective communication across these disciplines. In phase 2 a collective analysis of ethnographic data was achieved. The collaborative approach of grouping post-it notes, which individuals had recorded key points onto, to form categories and themes was an effective way of drawing from different perspectives. The method reflects a collective approach to Grounded Theory Analysis (GTA) [27], which involves the steps of identifying key points ('open coding'), grouping these together to form categories ('axial coding'). Categories are then linked together to form broader themes ('selected coding'). The design workshops took a collaborative approach to this method in which individual members of the team recorded key points on post it notes, collated them, and collectively grouped them to form meaningful categories and themes. Establishing the themes provided direction for discussing specific problems to be addressed and possible solutions for each problem.

Participatory design with older users. Others have highlighted the difficulties in involving older adults in design. The majority of older adults have little knowledge of computers and so communication with the researcher and other members of the focus group can be difficult Anxiety around technology and reluctance to learn also increases assumptions that the technology is no use to them [28, 29].

Each phase in the design process involved different methods for eliciting information from potential users. The storyboards used during focus groups in phase 2 were effective in stimulating discussion about the concepts and revealing design issues that were not initally considered. The frames were structured to focus on the use of the system as opposed to the technology involved. This helped centre the discussion on issues related to the concept (e.g. security, concerns around social obligation and need for common ground).

Phase 3 focused more on system use and design requirements. Conducting one-to-one interviews in participants' homes allowed them to relate the proposed technology to their daily lives. The 'think aloud' interviews included numerous interface designs to encourage broad discussion. This also reinforced the message that development was at the early stages, so that they would feel comfortable stating what they disliked.

In the final phase, a prototype was left in particpants' own homes. This revealed more subtle design issues that did not emerge through one-off interviews and evaluation sessions. After using the system over a period of weeks, participants felt more confident in highlighting problems and recommending how it should be improved. This phase was therefore important for establishing the balance between simplicity and functionality. Naturalistic data through remote logging also provided insigh to into interaction errors after prolonged use and difficulties that arise during meaningful engagement in real settings.

The outcomes from each phase highlights the importance of using different elicitation methods to guide the research towards development of a system that is perceived as useful, easy to use, and has sufficient functionality.

4.3 Implications for Interface Design

Design phases 3 and 4 focused on developing a usable touch screen interface for older adults with little or no computer experience. Listed below are some of the key design decisions, which also have implications for other touch screen designs for older users.

-   *Press, not drag:* In an initial design the user was required to drag and drop avatar icons into the 'call circle. They found this difficult as it required them to maintain pressure to the screen as they dragged the icon. The design was changed so that they only had to press the icon, which would then automatically move into the 'call circle.'
-   *Position buttons at top of the screen:* Having larger buttons makes it easier to press them. However, this also increases the chances of inadvertently pressing them. When navigation buttons were positioned at the bottom of the screen (e.g. 'Go Back to Main Menu' button), particpants would hit it with their knuckle or wrist. Moving the button to the top of the screen reduced this problem.
-   *Button affordance:* As all interactions are directly the screen, effort should be made to ensure that the user can easily recognize buttons. This is achieved by giving them a three-dimensional appearance and representing them consistently (shape and colour). In addition, boxed text should be avoided (e.g. screen titles) so that they do not resemble buttons.

- *Button feedback:* In the absence of using a keyboard or a mouse, the need for salient visual and audio cues are even greater to provide confirmation that the button has been pressed.
- *Avoid redundancies:* When presented with a new interface, participants attended to all of the information on the screen. Information that does not support interaction should be removed.
- *Avoid symbols/icons on buttons:* Icons should not be used on buttons as these become hit targets reducing the target size. Button functionality should be represented using text.

4.4 Future Work

The next step in the Building Bridges project is to conduct an intergenerational study that supports connections with family and friends, in addition to peer-to-peer social engagement. The prototype will include the four features described in Section 2 (broadcasts, calls, messaging and Tea Room). Twenty seniors will use the device. In addition, each senior can nominate friends and family members to have a PC client version of the software that can be installed on their own computer. This will allow the older adults to engage in peer-to-peer social engagement, but also sustain their existing social network. This requirement emerged from the previous trials in which participants expressed a desire to include existing contacts and distant relatives in their contact list. During this trial the nominees can also send digital photos to the older participants own device, which are then incorporated into the digital photo frame feature described in Section 4. The project will measure impact on loneliness, perceived social connectedness, as well as patterns of usage over time.

5 Conclusion

This paper provides an overview of the Building Bridges project, which explores how communication technology can be developed to help seniors remain socially connected and reduce risks of loneliness. The paper illustrates the need to involve older adults at every step in the design process so that the technology is grounded in an understanding of what people need and want.

The broadcast feature is a key component in the design as this provides a context for meeting people and common-ground through a shared experience. This was based on the perspectives of potential users, who highlighted the importance of engaging in a flexible and non-obtrusive way, and the need to have something to talk about when meeting new people.

The iterative design process highlighted key design requirements for touch screen interfaces for older adults with little or no computer experience. One-off interviews and observations guided the design towards an intuitive design. However, collecting naturalistic data during home trials was also necessary for identifying more sublte requirements.

This paper illustrates the need to include potential users at different stages of the design process. It also demonstrates the benefits of using different methods for eliciting information. A similar approach should be taken for developing ICT for other user groups at risk of loneliness and social isolation.

Acknowledgements. Thanks are due to our colleagues, especially Brian Lawlor, Ben Arent, James Brennan, Vanessa Buckley, Julie Doyle, Ronan McDonnell, Blaithin O'Dea, Simon Roberts, Cormac Sheehan, David Singleton, Claire Somerville, Zoran Skrba, Susan Squires, Maurice ten Koppel, Flip van den Berg and Ciaran Wynne.

References

1. Weiss, R.: Loneliness: The Experience of Social and Emotional Loneliness. MIT Press, Cambridge (1973)
2. Rook, K.S.: Research on social support, loneliness and social isolation, towards an integration. In: Shaver, P. (ed.) Review of Personality and Social Psychology, vol. 5, pp. 239–264. Sage, Beverley Hills (1994)
3. Shalev, S.: On loneliness and alienation. The Israel Journal of Psychiatry and Related Studies 25(3-4), 236–245 (1988)
4. Wenger, G.C., Davies, R., Shahtahmasebi, S., Scott, A.: Social isolation and loneliness in old age: Review and model refinement. Ageing Society 16(3), 333–358 (1995)
5. Pinquart, M., Sorensen, S.: Influences on loneliness in older adults: A metaanalysis. Basic and Applied Social Psychology 23(4), 245–266 (2001)
6. Victor, C., Scambler, S., Bond, J., Bowling, A.: Being alone in later life: Loneliness, social isolation and living alone. Reviews in Clinical Gerontology 10, 407–417 (2000)
7. Luanaigh, C.O., Lawlor, B.A.: Loneliness and the health of older people. International Journal of Geriatric Psychiatry 23(12), 1213–1221 (2008)
8. Holmen, K., Furukawa, H.: Loneliness, health and social network among eldery people: A follow-up study. Archives of Gerontology and Geriatrics 35(3), 261–274 (2002)
9. Tijhuis, M.A.R., de Jong-Gierveld, J., Feskens, E.J.M., Kromhout, D.: Changes in and factors related to loneliness in older men: The Zutphen Elderly Study. Age and Ageing 28(5), 491–495 (1999)
10. Drennan, J., Treacy, M., Butler, M., Byrne, A., Fealy, G., Frazer, K., Irving, K.: The experience of social and emotional loneliness among older people in Ireland. Ageing and Society 28(8), 1113–1132 (2008)
11. Bowling, A.: The most important thing in life: Comparisons between older and younger population age groups by gender. International Journal in Health Sciences 6(4), 169–175 (1995)
12. Sidell, M.: Death, dying and bereavement. In: Bond, J., Coleman, P., Peace, S. (eds.) Ageing in Society: An Introduction to Social Gerontology. Sage Publications, London (1993)
13. Golden, J., Conroy, R.M., Lawlor, B.: Social support network structure in older people: Underlying dimensions and association with psychological and physical health. Psychology, Health and Medicine 14(3), 280–290 (2009)
14. Andrews, G.J., Gavin, N., Begley, S., Brodie, D.: Assisting friendships, combating loneliness: Users' views on a 'befriending' scheme. Ageing and Society 23(3), 349–362 (2003)
15. McNeil, J.K.: Effects of non-professional home visit programmes for subclinically unhappy and unhealthy older adults. Journal of Applied Gerontology 14(3), 333–342 (1995)
16. Monk, A.F., Reed, D.J.: Telephone conferences for fun: Experimentation in people's homes. In: HOIT, Chennai, India, pp. 201–214. Springer, Heidelberg (2007)

17. White, H., McConnell, E., Clipp, E., Bynum, L., Teage, C., Navas, L., Craven, S., Halbrecht, H.: Surfing the net in later life: A review of the literature and pilot study of computer use and quality of life. Journal of Applied Gerontology 18(3), 358–378 (1999)
18. Groves, D.L., Slack, T.: Computers and their application to senior citizens therapy within a nursing home. Journal of Instructional Psychology 21(3), 221–227 (1994)
19. Dickinson, A., Newell, A.F., Smith, M.J., Hill, R.L.: Introducing the Internet to the over-60s: Developing an email system for older novice computer users. Interacting with Computers 17(6), 621–642 (2005)
20. Inoue, M., Suyama, A., Takeuchi, Y., Meshitsuka, S.: Application of a computer based education system for aged persons and issues arising during the field test. Computer Methods and Progress in Biomedicine 59(1), 55–60 (1999)
21. Czaja, S.J., Guerrier, J.H., Nair, S.N., Landauer, T.K.: Computer communication as an aid to independence for older adults. Behaviour and Information Technology 12(4), 197–207 (1993)
22. Hawthorn, D.: How universal is good design for older people? In: Proceedings of the ACM Conference on Universal Usability, Vancouver, Canada, pp. 38–45 (2003)
23. Carstensen, L.L.: Motivation for social contact and life span: A theory of socioemotional selectivity. In: Jacobs, J.E. (ed.) Nebraska symposium on motivation: Developmental Perspectives on Motivation, vol. 40, pp. 209–254. University of Nebraska Press, Lincoln (1992)
24. Holzinger, A.: Finger instead of Mouse: Touch screens as a means of enhancing universal access. In: Carbonell, N., Stephanidis, C. (eds.) UI4ALL 2002. LNCS, vol. 2615, pp. 387–397. Springer, Heidelberg (2003)
25. Holt, B.J., Morrell, R.W.: Guidelines for web site design for older adults: The ultimate influence of cognitive factors. In: Morrell, R.W. (ed.) Older Adults, Health Information and the World Wide Web, pp. 109–132. Lawrence Erlbaum Associates, Mahwah (2002)
26. Westerman, S.J., Davies, D.R., Glendon, A.I., Stammers, R.B., Matthews, G.: Age and cognitive ability as predictors of computerised information retrieval. Behaviour and Information Technology 14(5), 313–326 (1995)
27. Strauss, A.L., Corbin, J.: Basics in qualitative research. Sage, London (1990)
28. Newell, A.F., Carmichael, A., Morgan, M., Dickinson, A.: The use of theatre in requirements gathering and usability studies. Interacting with Computers 18(5), 996–1011 (2006)
29. Rice, M., Newell, A.F., Morgan, M.: Forum theatre as a requirements gathering methodology in design of home telecommunication systems for older adults. Behaviour and Information Technology 26(4), 323–331 (2007)

Cultural Specific Effects on the Recognition of Basic Emotions: A Study on Italian Subjects

Anna Esposito[1,3], Maria Teresa Riviello[3], and Nikolaos Bourbakis[2]

[1] Second University of Naples, Department of Psychology, Italy
[2] Wright State University, Dayton, OHIO, USA
[3] International Institute for Advanced Scientific Studies (IIASS), Vietri sul Mare, Italy
iiass.annaesp@tin.it, nikolaos.bourbakis@wright.edu

Abstract. The present work reports the results of perceptual experiments aimed to investigate if some of the basic emotions are perceptually privileged and if the cultural environment and the perceptual mode play a role in this preference. To this aim, Italian subjects were requested to assess emotional stimuli extracted from Italian and American English movies in the single (either video or audio alone) and the combined audio/video mode. Results showed that anger, fear, and sadness are better perceived than surprise, happiness in both the cultural environments (irony instead strongly depend on the language), that emotional information is affected by the communication mode and that language plays a role in assessing emotional information. Implications for the implementation of emotionally colored interactive systems are discussed.

Keywords: Perceptually privileged emotions, cultural specificity, effect of communication modes.

1 Introduction

Emotion is a topic that has received much attention during the last few years, in the context of Human Computer Interaction (HCI) field that involves research themes related to speech synthesis, as well as automatic speech recognition, interactive dialogues systems, wearable computing, embodied conversational agent systems, and intelligent avatars that are capable of performing believable actions and naturally reacting to human users [5, 11, 48]. Along these application requirements, research on emotions plays a fundamental role.

It is evident that the same words, the same facial expression, and/or the same gestures may be used as a joke, or as a genuine question seeking an answer, or as an aggressive challenge. Knowing what is an appropriate continuation of the interaction depends on detecting the register that the addresser is using, and a machine communicator that is unable to acknowledge the difference will have difficulty managing a natural-like interaction.

In the HCI field, therefore, the research objectives are to identify methods and procedures capable of automatically identifying human emotional states exploiting the multimodal nature of emotions. This requires the consideration of several key aspects, such as the development and the integration of algorithms and procedures for applications in

A. Holzinger and K. Miesenberger (Eds.): USAB 2009, LNCS 5889, pp. 135–148, 2009.

communication, and for the recognition of emotional states, from gestures, speech, gaze and facial expressions, in anticipation of the implementation of intelligent avatars and interactive dialog systems that could be exploited to improve the learning and understanding of emotional behavior and facilitate the user's access to future communication services.

Given the complexity of the problem, there has been a branching of the engineering approach toward the improvement and the development of video-audio techniques, such as video and image processing [24, 36, 41], video and image recognition [28-29], synthesis [23, 37-38] and speech recognition [1-2, 25], object and features extraction from audio and video [3-4, 13], with the goal to develop new cutting age methodologies for synthesizing [12, 14, 18, 40-41] analyzing [26, 30] and recognizing emotional states from faces [32, 39, 43-44], speech [1-2, 27, 31] and/or body movements [6, 48].

Yet, so far, there is little systematic knowledge about the details of the decoding process, i.e. the precise cues the addressees use in inferring addressers emotional state. Among the facets of the decoding process that call for stricter investigations are questions on whether some of the basic emotions are perceptually privileged and whether the cultural environment and the perceptual mode play a role in this preference. To this aim, current research on emotions is addressing studies on the cross modal analysis of multimodal signals through the development of a digital video-audio database of spontaneous, cross-cultural emotional transactions attempting to clarify the basic mechanisms of emotional processes both in typical and impaired conditions [7-8, 12, 19, 21-22]. Such a database would be of great interest both for the identification of the relationships and the shared information conveyed by the audio and visual communication channels, and as a benchmark, for comparing and evaluating the several research approaches, as well as for identifying cross-cultural differences among emotional expressions. Moreover, the database should allow the cross-modal analysis of audio and video recordings for defining distinctive, multi-modal, and cultural specific (loudness, pitch, and timing)[1] emotional features, and identifying emotional states from multimodal signals as well as for the definition of new methodologies and mathematical models for the automatic modeling and implementation of naturally human-like communication interfaces.

In specifying the experimental set-up for facing the above theoretical issues, the authors ended up with a collection of audio and video stimuli extracted from Italian and American English movies. The stimuli may result useful for any practical application related to the implementation of automatic emotional colored systems that exploit vocal and facial expression of emotion. The general specification and the characteristic of the collected set of stimuli are reported below.

2 Materials

The collected data are based on extracts from Italian and American English movies whose protagonists were carefully chosen among actors and actresses that are largely

---

[1] Natives rely on paralinguistic and suprasemental information that is strictly related and unique to their own language. In the case of Italian, it should be emphasized that cultural specificity is also carried in the language due to the strong dialectal influence that affects Italian speakers (the actors/actresses protagonist of the video clips) speaking standard Italian.

acknowledged by the critique and considered capable of giving some very real and careful interpretations. The final database consists of audio and video stimuli representing 6 basic emotional states: *happiness, sarcasm/irony, fear, anger, surprise,* and *sadness*. For each of the above languages and listed emotional states, 10 stimuli were identified, 5 expressed by an actor and 5 expressed by an actress, for a total of 120 video-clips (60 for Italian and 60 for American English) each acted by a different actor and actress to avoid bias in their ability to portray emotional states. The stimuli were selected short in duration (the average stimulus' length was 3.5s, SD = ± 1s). This was due to two reasons: 1) emotion cannot last more than a few seconds [42]; 2) longer stimuli may produce overlapping of emotional states and moods, and confuse the subject's perception. Consequently, longer stimuli do not increase the recognition reliability.

The use of video-clips extracted from movies allowed to overcome two critiques generally moved to perceptual studies of the kind proposed: 1) the stillness of the pictures in the evaluation of the emotional visual information. The still image usually captures the apex of the expression, i.e. the instant at which the indicators of emotion are most marked. However, in daily experience, emotional states are intrinsically dynamic processes and associated facial expressions also vary along time. 2) even though, the emotions expressed in the video-clips were simulations under studio conditions (and may not have reproduced a genuine emotion but an idealization of it), they were able to catch up and engage the emotional feeling of the spectators and therefore we were quite confident of their perceptual emotional contents.

Moreover, the video-clip's protagonist is acting according to the movie script and the movie director (supposed to be an expert) has assessed his/her performance as appropriate to the required emotional context.

Care was taken in choosing video clips where the protagonist's face and the upper part of the body were clearly visible. Care was also taken in choosing the stimuli such that the semantic meaning of the sentences expressed by the protagonists was not clearly expressing the portrayed emotional state and its intensity level was moderate. For example, stimuli of sadness where the actress/actor were clearly crying or stimuli of happiness where the protagonist was strongly laughing were not included in the data. This was because we wanted the subjects to exploit emotional cues that could be less obvious but that were generally employed in every natural and not extreme emotional interaction.

From each complete video-clip, the audio and the video alone were extracted summing up with a total of 180 Italian (60 stimuli only audio, 60 only video, and 60 audio and video) and 180 American English (60 stimuli only audio, 60 only video, and 60 audio and video) emotional stimuli.

The emotional labels assigned to the stimuli were given first by two expert judges and then by three naïve judges independently. The expert judges made a decision on the stimuli carefully exploiting emotional information on facial and vocal expressions such as frame by frame analysis of changes in facial muscles, and F0 contour, rising and falling of intonation contour, etc, as reported by several authors in literature [4, 9, 15, 16-17, 33-34, 45, 47] and also exploiting the contextual situation the protagonist is interpreting. The naïve judges made their decision after watching the stimuli several times. There were no opinion exchanges between the experts and naïve judges and the final agreement on the labeling between the two groups was 100%. The stimuli in each set were then randomized and proposed to the subjects participating at the experiments. The collected stimuli, being extracted from movie scenes containing environmental noise are also useful for testing realistic computer applications.

2.1 Participants

A total of 180 subjects (90 for the Italian and 90 for the American English) participated at the perceptual experiments. For each language, 30 were involved in the evaluation of the audio stimuli, 30 in the evaluation of the video stimuli, and 30 in the evaluation of the video and audio stimuli. The assignment of the subjects to the task was random. Subjects were required to carefully listen and/or watch the experimental stimuli via headphones in a quite room. They were instructed to pay attention to each presentation and decide as quickly as possible at the end of the presentation, which emotional state was expressed in it. Responses were recorded on a matrix paper form 60x8 where the rows listed the stimuli's numbers and the columns the emotional states of *happiness, sarcasm/irony, fear, anger, surprise,* and *sadness,* plus an option for *any other emotion* (where subjects were free to report a different emotional label than the six listed), and an option of *no emotion* that was suggested when according to the subject's feeling the protagonist did not show emotions. Each emotional label given by the participants as an alternative to one of the six listed was included in one of the listed emotional classes only if criteria of synonymity and/or analogy were satisfied. The extra requirement for the subjects involved in the assessment of the American English stimuli was the lack of familiarity with American English language. The participants in each group were equally distributed between females and males.

3 Stimuli Assessment

Tables 1 and 2 report for each emotion the percentage of agreement expressed by the Italian subjects participating to the experiments for the Italian and American English stimuli respectively. Figures 1a, and 1b provide histograms of the same data for a better visualization. On the x-axis of the figures are the basic emotions under consideration and on the y-axis is reported (for each emotion) the percentage of correct agreement under the three experimental conditions.

An ANOVA analysis was performed for Italian stimuli, considering *condition* as a between subject variable and *emotions and gender* as within subject variable. *Condition* plays a significant role for the perception of emotional states [(F(2, 12) = 7.701, ρ=.007) and does not depend on the emotion (F(5, 60) = .938, ρ=.46).

In the case of Italian, significant differences were found between the video and the combined audio-video condition (F(1, 8) = 10.414, ρ=.01) in particular for **sadness** (F(1, 8) = 5.548, ρ=.04), and between the video and audio condition (F(1, 8) = 13.858, ρ=.005), in particular for **sadness** (F(1,8) = 8.941, ρ=.01), **fear** (F(1,8) = 7.342, ρ=.02), and **anger** (F(1,8) = 9.737, ρ=.01). No differences were found between the audio and the combined audio and video (F(1, 8) = .004, ρ=.95).

The ANOVA analysis for American stimuli is in progress.

Table 1. Percentages of accuracy in the emotion recognition obtained by three groups each of 30 Italian subjects, tested separately in recognizing emotions through the audio, the video, and the audio and video combined in an Italian cultural context

EMOTIONS	Italian Stimuli		
	AUDIO	VIDEO	AUDIO/VIDEO
Happiness	48,4	60,7	56,4
Fear	60,3	58,7	47,7
Anger	77	67,9	60,1
Irony	75,4	48,6	64,3
Surprise	37	37,2	54
Sadness	66,9	47,9	75,4

Table 2. Percentages of accuracy in the emotion recognition obtained by three groups each of 30 Italian subjects, tested separately in recognizing emotions through the audio, the video, and the audio and video combined in an American English cultural context

EMOTIONS	American English Stimuli		
	AUDIO	VIDEO	AUDIO/VIDEO
Happiness	40	63,35	61
Fear	49	68,7	74,7
Anger	76,3	92	89,7
Irony	27,3	56	47,3
Surprise	32,3	53,3	58
Sadness	44,7	71	70

The data in the tables and figures show that, independently form the language and the communication mode, anger is the emotion better recognized among the six proposed. Scherer et al. [46]and van Bezooijen [49] reported a similar result on subjects tested on the vocal expressions of emotions, supporting our study that is displaying something more, i.e. that anger recognition does not depend on the communication mode, and on the cultural environment. Italian subjects are able to recognize with high accuracy anger both when it is expressed in native and in a foreign context. As it is expected, Italian subjects are able to perceive irony very well in their own language exploiting through the audio any subtle change in the prosodic and paralinguistic features transmitted in the speech, but are less good in doing so using only visual information. Moreover, they hardly recognize irony in a foreign language or in foreign facial expressions. Italian recognize fear very well in the audio when their native language is used and are less capable of doing that when fear is expressed by video or by audio and video combined. On the contrary they recognize fear very well in foreign video-clips (either mute or with audio). Surprise is not very well recognized both in the native and nonnative cultural context (no matter which communication mode is

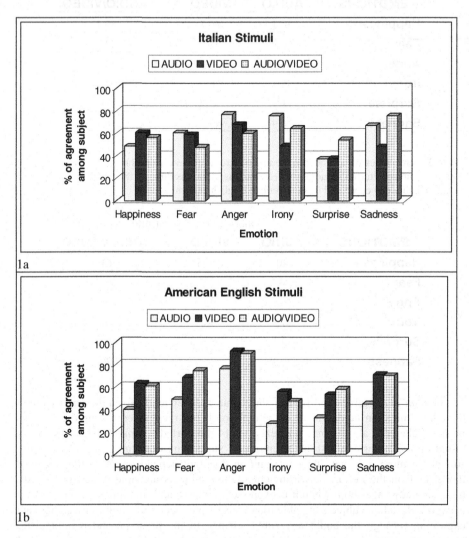

exploited). Happiness is better identified in the video alone than in the audio and in the audio and video combined in both the sets of stimuli (Italian and American English). Sadness is very well identified in the audio and audio and video for the Italian stimuli, whereas for the American English, the preferred communication modes are the video alone and the audio and video combined.

Fig. 1. Overall results in emotion recognition on the Italian (1a) and American English (1b) stimuli. In each figure (1a, 1b) the histograms refer to the percentage of correct recognition obtained by three groups, each of 30 Italian subjects, tested separately on the audio, the video, and the audio and video combined.

Figures 2 and 3 show, for the two different cultural contexts (Italian and American English), the percentages of emotion recognition accuracy according to the gender. White bars refers to emotional stimuli portrayed by actresses and black bars to stimuli portrayed by actors.

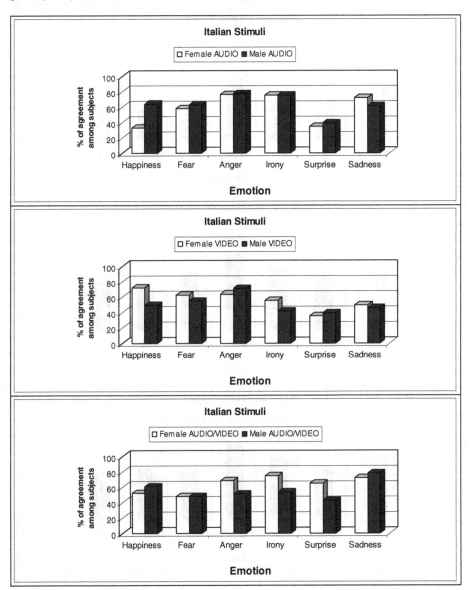

Fig. 2. Percentages of emotion recognition accuracy according to the gender in the Italian cultural context. White bars refers to emotional stimuli portrayed by actresses and black bars to stimuli portrayed by actors.

It appears that there are no significant differences, both in the audio and video alone, between emotional stimuli portrayed by males and by females except for happiness.

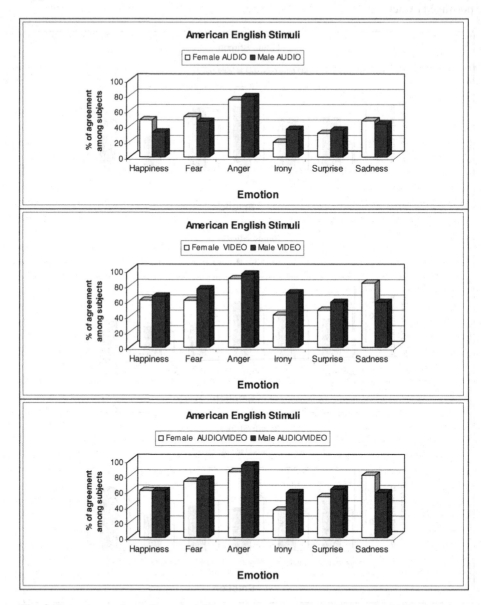

Fig. 3. Percentages of emotion recognition accuracy according to the gender in the American English cultural context. White bars refers to emotional stimuli portrayed by actresses and black bars to stimuli portrayed by actors.

Interestingly, happiness is better identified in females when the communicative mode is the audio and in males when it is the video alone. In the audio and video combined, these discrepancies disappear. However, in the combined communication modes, irony, anger, and surprise are better identified for female emotional stimuli. This is the case for Italian cultural context.

In the American English cultural context, female stimuli of irony are better identified than male stimuli in all the three communication modes, whereas gender made a difference for sadness in the video and the audio and video combined, since stimuli portrayed by females are better perceived than those portrayed by males.

4 Discussion and Conclusions

The data discussed above, show that, among the primary human emotions that have been evolved to enhance the adaptation and the survival of the species (see [10, 35]) anger plays a special role, since no matter the cultural context and the communication modes, its recognition is always very high.

Why is that? We can speculate that the experimental set up proposed is testing the capability of the subjects to infer emotional cues from the others. Identifying anger in the interlocutor may trigger cognitive self-defense mechanisms that are critical for the perceiver's survival, and therefore humans may have a high sensitivity to recognize it independently from the cultural environment.

The data also show that audio is favoured in the native cultural context, whereas video and audio and video combined are favoured in the non native cultural context.

In general, Italian subjects are good in recognizing the proposed emotions both in the Italian and the American English cultural context, even though they rely on audio information when they are native speakers of the languages and on visual information when a non native language is used being able to obtain the same performance even through different communication modes. The results reveal that the audio and visual components of emotional messages convey much the same amount of information either separately or in combination, hence suggesting that each channel performs a robust encoding of the emotional features. Redundancy probably facilitates the recovery of emotional information in case one of the channels is impaired. This conclusion is challenged by language cultural specificity, since when tested on a foreign language the addressers rely more on visual information (see [19-21]).

The biggest difference in the recognition accuracy is for irony that is very well identified in the native cultural context (mostly in the audio) probably because the expressions of this emotion are strictly linked to the cultural context.

As for gender differences in the ability to portray emotional states, in the American English cultural context, females appear to better encode visual emotional cues of sadness, and both audio and visual emotional cues of irony, whereas, in the Italian cultural context, females better encode emotional cues of irony, anger, and surprise in the combined audio and video communication mode.

The data presented can be of great utility in helping researchers both to develop new algorithms for vocal and facial expression recognition and for cross cultural comparison of emotional decoding procedures.

Why is that? The data show that subjects' perception of emotional states involves embodiment, intended here as the mutual influence of the physical environment and the human activities that unfold within it. The underlying idea is that embodiment emerges from the interaction between our sensory-motor systems and the inhabited environment (that includes people as well as objects) and dynamically affects /enhances our reactions/actions, or our social perception. Several experimental data seem to support this idea [50-53]. Context interaction, therefore – the organizational, cultural, and physical context – plays a critical role in shaping social conduct providing a means to interpret and understand individuals' choices, perception, and actions. These effects must be taken into account in "*every interaction a user perform with an interface*" as reported in Stickel et al. [54].

In addition, these results will lead to new mathematical models describing human interaction, thus permitting new approaches to the psychology of the communication itself, as well as to the content of any interaction, independently from its overt semantic meaning.

In fact, in an attempt to quantify how well signals encode meaningful information and how well systems process the received information, it clearly appears, that the mathematical models proposed in the literatures, such as *entropy, joint entropy,* and *mutual information* [55], do not take into account concurrently, the informative value of the source (i.e. the meaning the signal can convey) and what the receiver assumes to be informative about the received signal. These models do not consider cases where the source can be only noise, and/or cases where extraneous information can be exploited by the receiver (as in our case).

In seeking for the mathematical modeling of the above experimental data, therefore, these models must be disregarded because cannot explain why by combining the audio and video channels, the information about the emotional states does not increases and cannot explain the performance of Italian subjects with respect to close (Italian video clips) and distant (American English videoclips) cultural backgrounds in the perception of emotional states.

The *information transfer ratio* proposed by Sinanović and Johnson [56] seems to be a more appropriate and adequate model since it quantifies how the receiver affects the received information by measuring the distance between the actions performed by the receiver for given received inputs and the received inputs. Assuming that the emotional information encoded through the audio and the video represents the input to a processing system, the information transfer ratio value is the ratio of the distances between the information transmitted by the sources and the distances between the outputs (for those sources) of the processing system. The information transfer ratio is described by the following equation:

$$\gamma_{XY,Z}(\alpha_0, \alpha_1) \equiv \frac{d_Z(\alpha_0, \alpha_1)}{d_X(\alpha_0, \alpha_1)} + \frac{d_Z(\alpha_0, \alpha_1)}{d_Y(\alpha_0, \alpha_1)} \tag{1}$$

Where $\alpha 1$ indicates the changes in the emotional contents of the sources with respect to a reference point α_0, which depends not on the signals themselves but on their probability functions $p_X(x; \alpha_0)$, $p_X(x; \alpha_1)$, $p_Y(y; \alpha_0)$, $p_Y(y; \alpha_1)$, and $p_Z(z; \alpha_0)$, $p_Z(z; \alpha_1)$. X and Y are the sources (audio and video), Z the processing systems, and $d(...)$ indicates is the Kullback-Leibler distance [58] or any information theoretic distance.

However, any information theoretic distance generally obeys to the Data Processing Theorem [55], which roughly states that the output of any processing system cannot contain more information than the processed signal. This may not be true if the receiver is a human being since the filtering actions of humans is generally arbitrary and the corresponding transfer function is unknown. Due to these difficulties, a more appropriate distance measure is suggested here based on fuzzy membership functions [57]. Fuzzy membership functions are more appropriate to model human categorization processes and allow inferring the emotional information exploiting the number of the subject's correct answers.

Acknowledgments. The paper has been partially supported by COST Action 2102: "Cross Modal Analysis of Verbal and Nonverbal Communication" (http:// cost2102.cs.stir.ac.uk/) and by Regione Campania, L.R. N.5 del 28.03.2002, Project ID N. BRC1293, Feb. 2006. Acknowledgment goes to Tina Marcella Nappi for her editorial help.

References

1. Apolloni, B., Aversano, G., Esposito, A.: Preprocessing and classification of emotional features in speech sentences. In: Kosarev, Y. (ed.) Proceedings, IEEE Workshop on Speech and Computer, pp. 49–52 (2000)
2. Apolloni, B., Esposito, A., Malchiodi, D., Orovas, C., Palmas, G., Taylor, J.G.: A general framework for learning rules from data. IEEE Transactions on Neural Networks 15(6), 1333–1350 (2004)
3. Apple, W., Hecht, K.: Speaking emotionally: The relation between verbal and vocal communication of affect. Journal of Personality and Social Psychology 42, 864–875 (1982)
4. Banse, R., Scherer, K.: Acoustic profiles in vocal emotion expression. Journal of Personality & Social Psychology 70(3), 614–636 (1996)
5. Bartneck, C.: Affective expressions of machines. StanAckerman Institute, Eindhoven (2000)
6. Bryll, R., Quek, F., Esposito, A.: Automatic hand hold detection in natural conversation. In: Proceedings of IEEE Workshop on Cues in Communication, Hawai, December 9 (2001)
7. Bourbakis, N.G., Esposito, A., Kavraki, D.: Multi-modal interfaces for interaction-communication between hearing and visually impaired individuals: Problems & issues. In: Proceedings of the International Conference on Tool for Artificial Intelligence, Patras, Greece, October 29-31, pp. 1–10 (2007)
8. Bourbakis, N.G., Esposito, A., Kavraki, D.: Analysis of invariant meta-features for learning and understanding disable people's emotional behavior related to their health conditions: A case study. In: Proceedings of 6th International IEEE Symposium BioInformatics and BioEngineering, pp. 357–369. IEEE Computer Society, Los Alamitos (2006)
9. Cacioppo, J.T., Berntson, G.G., Larsen, J.T., Poehlmann, K.M., Ito, T.A.: The Psychophysiology of emotion. In: Lewis, J.M., Haviland-Jones, M. (eds.) Handbook of Emotions, 2nd edn., pp. 173–191. Guilford Press, New York (2000)
10. Campos, J.J., Barrett, K., Lamb, M.E., Goldsmith, H.H., Stenberg, C.: Socioemotional development. In: Haith, M.M., Campos, J.J. (eds.) Handbook of Child Psychology, 4th edn., vol. 2, pp. 783–915. Wiley, New York (1983)

11. Cassell, J., Vilhjalmsson, H., Bickmore, T.: BEAT: the Behavior Expression Animation Toolkit. In: Proceedings of SIGGRAPH (2001)
12. Chollet, G., Esposito, A., Gentes, A., Horain, P., Karam, W., Li, Z., Pelachaud, C., Perrot, P., Petrovska-Delacrétaz, D., Zhou, D., Zouari, L.: Multimodal Human Machine Interactions in Virtual and Augmented Reality. In: Esposito, A., et al. (eds.) Multimodal Signals: Cognitive and Algorithmic Issues. LNCS, vol. 5398, pp. 1–23. Springer, Heidelberg (2009)
13. Cosmides, L.: Invariances in the acoustic expressions of emotions during speech. Journal of Experimental Psychology, Human Perception Performance 9, 864–881 (1983)
14. Doyle, P.: When is a communicative agent a good idea? In: Proceedings of Inter. Workshop on Communicative and Autonomous Agents, Seattle (1999)
15. Ekman, P.: Facial expression of emotion: New findings, new questions. Psychological Science 3, 34–38 (1992)
16. Ekman, P., Friesen, W.V.: Facial action coding system: A technique for the measurement of facial movement. Consulting Psychologists Press, Palo Alto (1978)
17. Ekman, P., Friesen, W.V.: Manual for the Facial Action Coding System. Consulting Psychologists Press, Palo Alto (1977)
18. Elliott, C.D.: The affective reasoner: A process model of emotions in a multi-agent system. Ph.D. Thesis, Institute for the Learning Sciences, Northwestern University, Evanston, Illinois (1992)
19. Esposito, A.: The Perceptual and Cognitive Role of Visual and Auditory Channels in Conveying Emotional Information. Cognitive Computation Journal 2, 1–11 (2009)
20. Esposito, A.: Affect in Multimodal Information. In: Tao, J., Tan, T. (eds.) Affective Information Processing, pp. 211–234. Springer, Heidelberg (2008)
21. Esposito, A.: The amount of information on emotional states conveyed by the verbal and nonverbal channels: some perceptual data. In: Stylianou, Y., Faundez-Zanuy, M., Esposito, A. (eds.) COST 277. LNCS, vol. 4391, pp. 249–268. Springer, Heidelberg (2007)
22. Esposito, A.: COST 2102: Cross-modal analysis of verbal and nonverbal Communication (CAVeNC). In: Esposito, A., Faundez-Zanuy, M., Keller, E., Marinaro, M. (eds.) COST Action 2102. LNCS (LNAI), vol. 4775, pp. 1–10. Springer, Heidelberg (2007)
23. Ezzat, T., Geiger, G., Poggio, T.: Trainable videorealistic speech animation. In: Proceedings of SIGGRAPH, San Antonio, Texas, July 2002, pp. 388–397 (2002)
24. Fasel, B., Luettin, J.: Automatic facial expression analysis: A survey. Pattern Recognition 36, 259–275 (2002)
25. Friend, M.: Developmental changes in sensitivity to vocal paralanguage. Developmental Science 3, 148–162 (2000)
26. Frick, R.: Communicating emotions: the role of prosodic features. Psychological Bulletin 93, 412–429 (1985)
27. Fulcher, J.A.: Vocal affect expression as an indicator of affective response. Behavior Research Methods, Instruments, & Computers 23, 306–313 (1991)
28. Fu, S., Gutierrez-Osuna, R., Esposito, A., Kakumanu, P., Garcia, O.N.: Audio/visual mapping with cross-modal Hidden Markov Models. IEEE Transactions on Multimedia 7(2), 243–252 (2005)
29. Gutierrez-Osuna, R., Kakumanu, P., Esposito, A., Garcia, O.N., Bojorquez, A., Castello, J., Rudomin, I.: Speech-driven facial animation with realistic dynamic. IEEE Transactions on Multimedia 7(1), 33–42 (2005)
30. Hozjan, V., Kacic, Z.: A rule-based emotion-dependent feature extraction method for emotion analysis from speech. Journal of the Acoustical Society of America 119(5), 3109–3120 (2006)

31. Hozjan, V., Kacic, Z.: Context-independent multilingual emotion recognition from speech signals. International Journal of Speech Technology 6, 311–320 (2003)
32. Huang, C.L., Huang, Y.M.: Facial expression recognition using model-based feature extraction and action parameters Classification. Journal of Visual Commumication and Image Representation 8(3), 278–290 (1997)
33. Izard, C.E., Ackerman, B.P.: Motivational, organizational, and regulatory functions of discrete emotions. In: Lewis, J.M., Haviland-Jones, M. (eds.) Handbook of Emotions, 2nd edn., pp. 253–264. Guilford Press, New York (2000)
34. Izard, C.E.: The maximally discriminative facial movement coding system (MAX). Unpublished manuscript. Available from Instructional Resource Center, University of Delaware (1979)
35. Izard, C.E.: Human Emotions. Plenum Press, New York (1977)
36. Kähler, K., Haber, J., Seidel, H.: Geometry-based muscle modeling for facial animation. In: Proceedings of the International Conference on Graphics Interface, pp. 27–36 (2001)
37. Kakumanu, P., Esposito, A., Garcia, O.N., Gutierrez-Osuna, R.: A comparison of acoustic coding models for speech-driven facial animation. Speech Commumication 48, 598–615 (2006)
38. Kakumanu, P., Gutierrez-Osuna, R., Esposito, A., Bryll, R., Goshtasby, A., Garcia, O.N.: Speech Dirven Facial Animation. In: Proceedings of ACM Workshop on Perceptive User Interfaces, Orlando, November 15-16 (2001)
39. Kanade, T., Cohn, J., Tian, Y.: Comprehensive database for facial expression analysis. In: Proceedings of the 4th IEEE International Conference on Automatic Face and Gesture Recognition, pp. 46–53 (2000)
40. Koda, T.: Agents with faces: A study on the effect of personification of software agents. Master Thesis, MIT Media Lab, Cambridge (1996)
41. Morishima, S.: Face analysis and synthesis. IEEE Signal Processing Magazine 18(3), 26–34 (2001)
42. Oatley, K., Jenkins, J.M.: Understanding emotions. Blackwell, Oxford (1996)
43. Pantic, M., Patras, I., Rothkrantz, J.M.: Facial action recognition in face profile image sequences. In: Proceedings IEEE International Conference Multimedia and Expo., pp. 37–40 (2002)
44. Pantic, M., Rothkrantz, J.M.: Expert system for automatic analysis of facial expression. Image and Vision Computing Journal 18(11), 881–905 (2000)
45. Scherer, K.R.: Vocal communication of emotion: A review of research paradigms. Speech Communication 40, 227–256 (2003)
46. Scherer, K.R., Banse, R., Wallbott, H.G., Goldbeck, T.: Vocal cues in emotion encoding and decoding. Motiation and Emotion 15, 123–148 (1991)
47. Scherer, K.R.: Vocal correlates of emotional arousal and affective disturbance. In: Wagner, H., Manstead, A. (eds.) Handbook of social Psychophysiology, pp. 165–197. Wiley, New York (1989)
48. Stocky, T., Cassell, J.: Shared reality: Spatial intelligence in intuitive user interfaces. In: Proceedings of Intelligent User Interfaces, San Francisco, CA, pp. 224–225 (2002)
49. Van Bezooijen, R.: The Characteristics and Recognizability of Vocal Expression of Emotions. Foris, Drodrecht, The Netherlands (1984)
50. Schubert, T.W.: The Power in Your Hand: Gender Differences in Bodily Feedback from Making a Fist. Personality and Social Psychology Bulletin 30, 757–769 (2004)
51. Bargh, J.A., Chen, M., Burrows, L.: Automaticity of Social Behavior: Direct Effects of Trait Construct and Stereotype Activation on Action. Journal of Personality and Social Psychology 71, 230–244 (1996)

52. Stepper, S., Strack, F.: Proprioceptive Determinants of Emotional and Nonnemotional Feelings. Journal of Personality and Social Psychology 64, 211–220 (1993)
53. Esposito, A., Carbone, D., Riviello, M.T.: Visual Context Effects on the Perception of Musical Emotional Expressions. In: Fierrez, J., et al. (eds.) Biometric ID Management and Multimodal Communication. LNCS, vol. 5707, pp. 81–88. Springer, Heidelberg (2009)
54. Stickel, C., Ebner, M., Steinbach-Nordmann, S., Searle, G., Holzinger, A.: Emotion Detection: Application of the Valence Arousal Space for Rapid Biological Usability Testing to Enhance Universal Access. In: Stephanidis, C. (ed.) Universal Access in HCI, Part I, HCII 2009. LNCS, vol. 5614, pp. 615–624. Springer, Heidelberg (2009)
55. Gallager, R.G.: Information theory and reliable communication. John Wiley & Son, Chichester (1968)
56. Sinanović, S., Johnson, D.H.: Toward a theory of information processing. Signal Processing 87, 1326–1344 (2007)
57. Massaro, D.W.: Perceiving talking faces. MIT Press, Cambridge (1998)
58. Ali, S.M., Silvey, S.D.: A general class of coefficients of divergence of one distribution from another. Journal of Royal Statistic Society 28, 131–142 (1996)

Digital Literacy – Is It Necessary for eInclusion?

Denise Leahy and Dudley Dolan

School of Computer Science and Statistics,
Trinity College,
Dublin 2, Ireland
denise.leahy@cs.tcd.ie, dudley.dolan@cs.tcd.ie

Abstract. In order to live and work in today's technological world, it is important to be able to use information and communications technology. More and more of us are communicating with family and friends using technology; business is carried out using technology; in the work environment companies use intranets to communicate with staff; governments are moving towards interacting with citizens online. While accessibility and usability in technology are absolutely necessary, is digital literacy a pre-requisite to benefit from what the Information Society can offer? The EU has recognised the need for digital literacy and has included this in the definition of eInclusion [1]. This paper examines definitions of digital literacy and suggests that digital literacy is necessary for a person to take a full part in today's Information Society.

Keywords: Digital literacy, accessibility.

1 Introduction

Developments in Information and Communications Technology (ICT) have changed how people work and live today. We use technology daily – mobile phones, iPods, PDAs, etc and we are now living in an Information Society. This could lead to a "digital divide", where people who cannot access or use technology are at a disadvantage. ICT is creating new opportunities, connecting people to each other in new and immediate ways, providing information at the touch of a button, allowing us to compare our lives and communicate with people we may never meet. It may give access to better paid jobs, to government services, and may increase consumer power and access to political debate and decision making. "We are finding ourselves at the new frontier of civil rights" according to Wilhelm [2]. We use ICT increasingly in our day to day lives – to communicate, to carry out business, to acquire information and to socialize. Today's Information Society is becoming more dependent on technology and sometimes we are not even aware of this.

ICT is affecting all of our lives and this is encouraged by many Governments worldwide [3]. How do we ensure that ICT is not a barrier to gaining the benefits from the Information Society? The technology has to be usable and the technology has to be accessible – but we also need to know how to use the technology. There can be risks if the technology becomes so usable that we do not understand what we are doing. What do we need to know in order to be part of this society – is digital literacy the answer? If so, what do we mean by this - how do we define Digital Literacy?

A. Holzinger and K. Miesenberger (Eds.): USAB 2009, LNCS 5889, pp. 149–158, 2009.

This paper examines the definition of digital literacy by academic writers over the past 20 years, the present need for digital literacy and looks at particular accessibility and usability issues which can cause a barrier to full participation and could exclude some groups in the Information Society.

2   eInclusion and Digital Literacy

2.1   Today's Society

Being able to use technology is necessary for employment and is becoming more important in all aspects of daily living. The European Union recognises this in many initiatives including i2010 – "A European Information Society for growth and employment". [4] This initiative promotes a European Information Society for all citizens. Actions have been defined in this initiative to ensure that the benefits of technology can be enjoyed by everyone. "Inclusion, better public services and quality of life" is one of the main areas of this initiative. The eInclusion policy covers ageing, eAccessibility, broadband gap (digital divide), inclusive eGovernment, digital literacy and culture [5].

Governmental Policy in many countries of the world is to increase its communications with its citizens and increase the services available via the Internet. This "eGovernment" means that, increasingly, government information and services will be available online. This is a move to Rheingold's "Citizen based democracy" [6] and people who do not have access to the Internet will be at serious disadvantage.

Businesses are using Web 2 functionality, for example using social networking sites for sales promotions and opportunities and for communicating with staff and business partners [7]. Job opportunities are offered on line and electronic social networking is becoming an everyday part of people lives.

Why is eInclusion so vital? "As our society is evolving to an Information Society, we are becoming intrinsically more dependent on technology-based products and services in our daily lives. Yet poor accessibility means many Europeans with a disability are still unable to access the benefits of the information society." [8] According to the EU "more than one in three Europeans do not fully benefit from these opportunities." [9]

The European Union member States have committed to targets in the area of eInclusion in the Riga Ministerial Declaration [10]. This declaration states that "ICT contributes to improving the quality of everyday life and social participation of Europeans, facilitating access to information, media, content and services, to enhanced and more flexible job opportunities, and to fight against discrimination. Improving ICT access for people with disabilities and elderly is particularly important."

Castells [11] speaks of the Network Society in which we now live and defines a Network Society as one where a "social structure is made up of networks powered by micro-electronics –based information and communication technologies". In order to be included in this society we need to know how to use the technology. What does this mean and how can a person be helped? According to the Danish Technological Institute [12] "Digital literacy is needed by all citizens, for example in order to:

- ensure better service access and use
- ease citizens' daily life burdens (such as engaging with public administrations)
- obtain better access to education, training, work, and jobs
- improve each citizen's personal capacity (quality of life and life chances)
- enhance citizens' social networks and participation. "

It is vital to ensure that technology is not part of the barrier to inclusion. Therefore, in order to be included, the following must be in place:

1. The person must know how to use the technology
2. The technology must be accessible
3. The technology must be usable

2.2 Why Do We Need Digital Literacy?

Why do we need to be digitally literate? It is important to understand what we are doing with technology. If we do not, we can believe information we do not understand and which may be incorrect; we can expose our information to others, we can reveal information by accident, we can expose our systems to malicious attacks. Can you be too usable?   Caldwell [13] puts the argument "if users are led to believe that they do not need to spend time learning or developing expertise with the ICT systems that they buy, these users are in fact becoming more detached from the ICT and its influences on the Information Society."

If we believe that just pushing a button can deliver what we need, what happens if it goes wrong? What happens if we do not know it is going wrong and continue using it, for example, not noticing that there is a virus running, using data which is incorrect, but believing it. We need to understand and be able to interpret what we find when using technology - as Holmes says "information is not knowledge" [14]. If we do not understand where data is coming from it could lead to believing bad, incorrect or incomplete information. We might act on incorrect data in our personal lives (friends, purchasing, etc) and business lives (in scientific investigation, business analytics, etc). Therefore it is important to be able to assess the validity of the information we find. Security can be a major issue in using technology; we need to understand about computer virus programs and other forms of malicious software; we need to understand when our systems can be exposed to hacking or interception.

We must learn how to interpret the information retrieved and how to use technology efficiently. According to research by Smith-Gratto [15], we tend believe what we read if it is written in a scientific manner. We often do not use our intelligence – it is "Easier to Google a 2nd or 3rd time than to remember" [16].

What would we miss if we are not digitally literate? We might not take full advantage of or understand the benefits of technology. We might not see opportunities in our personal and business lives. We would lose out on all that can be offered by Web 2 and social networking, including job opportunities and keeping in touch with friends and business partners. In order to be included in the Information Society we need digital literacy.

2.3   eInclusion and Digital Literacy

The term "digital literacy" is used by the European Union in "Digital Literacy: Skills for the Information Society", where it is stated that "Information and communications technologies (ICTs) affect our lives every day - from interacting with our governments to working from home, from keeping in touch with our friends to accessing healthcare and education" [1]. According to the EU *"Digital literacy involves the confident and critical use of Information Society Technology (IST) for work, leisure and communication. It is underpinned by basic skills in ICT: the use of computers to retrieve, assess, store, produce, present and exchange information, and to communicate and participate in collaborative networks via the Internet."*

There have been many definitions of digital literacy since the early days of computing; these identified skills ranging from those needed by IT professionals to those required by the average citizen in the Information Society. Historically these terms have been used:

- Computer literacy – initially used for IT/computer professionals who were technical people
- Digital literacy – used today, but with different and evolving meanings
- Information literacy – often used to include the ability to verify, interpret and validate the information
- Cyber literacy – was used when the use of the Internet became prevalent

In the 60s and 70s a person was computer literate if he or she knew how to program a computer; this person was usually a computer professional. As computers began to be used widely in business, there was a requirement for the business user to become competent in using systems – usually related to the specific task or job. The term "computer literacy" appeared in writings in the 70s [17]. At this time, there was a clear separation of the role of the technical person and the computer user. In the 80s, with the arrival of the PC, people could use tools to develop small systems – word processing, spreadsheets and small databases were available to all. This was the start of what was called "end user computing ". The term computer literacy, evolved during the 1980s, as end users began to use computing, to include the use of personal computers by the non technical person. In 1983, Van Dyke [18] stated "if the vernacular of the term computer literacy is assured, its meaning is not". During the 90s, the term "digital literacy" began to appear.

Paul Gilster, in 1997, suggests that to be digitally literate a person should be able to find information on line and evaluate it and suggests that the skills of such a person would include use of email and search engines and the ability to evaluate a Web Site, other on line resources and other information resources. [19]

Digital literacy is often used to include the ability to interpret information. According to Wilhelm in Digital Nation [2], to be digitally literate you should be able to "Access, manage, integrate, evaluate and create information". The work of Eshet-Alakali et al finds that "Having digital literacy requires more than just the ability to use software or to operate a digital device; it includes a large variety of complex skills such as cognitive, motoric, sociological, and emotional that users need to have in order to use digital environments effectively." [20]

In this paper, digital literacy is used to refer to the use of information technology by non IT professionals; that is, by all members of society, for personal, social, educational and business use. This includes the use of pervasive and ubiquitous technology for daily life by all citizens and includes school leavers, students, researchers, older people and people with disabilities.

2.4 A Definition of Digital Literacy for Today

Today, digital literacy includes the ability to use a computer, send e-mail, prepare material using the computer, search for information on the web and use other personal computer based tools. Other technologies include use of mobile devices and electronic equipment in the home. The use of technologies, especially mobile technologies, is likely to grow – it is important that the digitally literate person understands the changing world. According to Microsoft's Digital Literacy curriculum (http://www. microsoft.com) "The goal of Digital Literacy is to teach and assess basic computer concepts and skills so that people can use computer technology in everyday life to develop new social and economic opportunities for themselves, their families, and their communities."

A definition of digital literacy today would include the awareness of what information technology can do, coupled with the skills to perform tasks and the competence to work alone and to know when help is needed. In summary, it is important to be comfortable with using technology, to be able to use a computer or mobile device to communicate with friends, both in the home and in work environments, and be aware that technology is changing and need not be feared.

2.5 Standards for Digital Literacy

If digital literacy is necessary, how can a person become digitally literate if the means to become so are inaccessible or unusable? The European Computer Driving License (ECDL) is one standard of digitally literacy. There are other standards, including Microsoft, Certiport Internet and Computing Core Certification (IC³).

ECDL had as its major objective in 1995 "to raise the level of IT competence.....within the European population" [21]. The other objectives included to help in re-skilling the unemployed and to provide a means to reduce the gap between the "haves" and "have-nots" in the Information Society.

ECDL was an EU project which started in 1995 with the objectives stated above. [22] The project was an initiative of the Council of European Professional Informatics Societies (CEPIS) and was based on a model which was already successful in Finland [23]. A target of reaching10 million people was declared in 1997. In 2008, José Manuel Barroso, President of the European Commission, accepted the 9th millionth ECDL Skills card.

Initially, accessibility was not built into ECDL, causing problems for many in the population. In 2001, a project was set up to investigate the accessibility issues in ECDL. The outcome of this project was the definition of "reasonable adjustments" in testing and slight procedural changes with regard to how the tests were defined and administered. It was not necessary to change the syllabus, but it was necessary to take into account how people use computing in very different ways [24].

This confirms Shawn Henry's observation "Designing for accessibility doesn't require a whole new design process; it generally involves only minor adjustments to your existing design process" [25].

3   The Need for Accessibility and Usability

Technology should help people rather than pose a further barrier. However, even those who are digitally literate can face problems in trying to work with technology. Initially attempting to access some web sites can be a problem and then navigating within a site can cause further problems. If Information Technology is not accessible who is being excluded and what are the implications?

It is vital that Web sites are accessible in order to provide equal access and equal opportunity to all. According to Raman "an increasing part of our social interaction happens via the Web" [26]. However the web is not always accessible. AbilityNet [27] carried out a survey in 2008 and found that most social networking websites on the Internet were "either difficult or impossible for disabled people to use – in many cases a user is not even able to register with the website." A serious problem with trying to access a website is the use of the CAPTCHA when trying to log in (CAPTCHA – Completely Automated Public Turing test to tell Computers and Humans Apart). Screen readers cannot read this and a screen reader user can be locked out at this stage.

Technology can change the lives of people with disabilities. Assistive technologies such as screen readers, magnifiers, alternate input devices and many other items of hardware and software are now in common use. However, the systems or web site to be accessed by these assistive technologies must be written to interface with them.

Older people have particular needs with regard to the accessibility and usability of technology. They have grown up in an era without technology and often cannot see the benefits of using technology. Social networking sites may be alien to them. However, the ageing population could benefit from better communication with distant family and friends, access to more information and even in healthcare. This group of the population are major users of healthcare services and in the future there may be difficulties providing the level of care required to ensure a reasonable quality of life for this growing population. It is possible that technology could provide information and, perhaps, some services [28]. "In order to prepare the elderly population to live longer and more independent lives with the help of information technology, we must first introduce them not to any particular device but to the concept of modern engineering." [37]

Zajicek [29] identifies the importance of accessibility on the web - "Those for whom the Web is inaccessible for whatever reason will become increasingly excluded from mainstream life if it is not made accessible to them." Technology must be accessible and it must also be usable and "fit for purpose". Zajicek [29] continues the definition of accessibility to include usability "An accessible Web means that the Web can be used by all, but it must also mean that it is easy to use by all and should not be labor intensive or arduous." To develop usability into web sites, the designer must understand how a person will use the site. This is important for everyone, but especially for a person with any disability; a person using a screen reader will need the web site to be readable with graphics identified, a person with a hearing impairment will find a site with less text and clear graphics to be more usable, etc.

"Usability measures the quality of a user's experience when interacting with a product or system - whether a Web site, a software application, mobile technology, or any user-operated device" [30]. Nielsen defines usability as a "quality attribute" which can assess how easy a site or product is to use and he states that once in a site or product it must behave as expected and should be able to achieve what is intended [31]. All people have a requirement for usability. If the web site or system is not easy to use, it will not be used; there are implications for business in this regard.

4   Issues to Be Considered

Technology is evolving: A problem with the continual development and innovation in technology is that the functionality and interfaces are changing all the time. The number of features in new technology is growing; some of these features are irrelevant or unnecessary – users should understand this and be able to select what is appropriate to their needs.

Voluntary codes: Standards for accessibility have been published (e.g. WAI WCAG). These are generally voluntary codes and are often not followed. While there are many laws recognising accessibility issues, there are often exemptions to these. It will probably take test cases to enforce the laws.

Different needs: People access and use technology in different ways. A screen reader user does not require graphics and any graphics used should have descriptions attached. A person with a hearing impairment will prefer less text and more graphics. For people whose first language is not the local one, the use of plain language is necessary. There are other requirements which can be implemented by technology, but are often ignored due to cost or sometimes simply lack of awareness

User Generated Content (user created content): Web 2.0 as a social networking system consists of much content created by its users. Web 2.0 tools are usable once you can get in, they are not intuitive for older people and generally do not work with assistive technologies for people with disabilities.The use of social networking sites is growing worldwide. Facebook had 223 million unique visitors by early 2009, MySpace had 125 million [32]; the use of other sites such as MySpace, Bebo and Twitter is growing and the world-wide use of all of these sites is increasing. Users are becoming more involved in created content for the web - about 150 million pieces of content have been created under Creative Commons licences by December 2008 [33].

Ageing: The number of people over 80 years of age in Europe is expected to double by 2050 [34]. By 2020 it is expected that 25% of the population will be over 60 years of age. It is estimated that 21% of the population of Europe have a disability and with the increasing age profile of the population this figure is likely to increase [35]. The European Commission believes that older people should be getting more benefits from the digital age. According to Frans de Bruïne, (Director, European Commission), "By 2013, the Commission plans to invest one billion Euros in researching and piloting digital technologies that make the lives of older citizens easier" [36] and that these initiatives could "turn the silver challenge into a golden opportunity".

Privacy and Security: People can be concerned about privacy when using technology and may be afraid to discuss personal matters or to put personal details online. Digital literacy could help to educate about security, to make people aware of where they could be exposed and to help to ensure that proper procedures are followed.

5 Conclusions

It is necessary to have a level of digital literacy to benefit from all that technology can offer in today's Information Society. There are many benefits in using technology. The Information Society can help people to keep in touch with friends with social networking sites, can provide information for those seeking employment, can give people access to information, can be used for learning and can allow a person to be part of digital living.

Technology should be accessible and usable. This has benefits for all and will increase inclusion and equality in business, eGovernment and everyday life. Awareness of usability and accessibility issues is important for designers and developers of systems and web sites, and should be part of all development practices. There are problems when sites and systems are not accessible and this greatly affects people with disabilities or people who are older and have not grown up with technology. There are problems when sites and systems are not usable and this affects all potential users. Usability is an issue for all computer system and web site designers and owners. If a system or site is not usable, it has little purpose or value.

It is important that a person does not fear technology and can understand how it can be used. "Digital literacy is about mastering ideas, not keystrokes." [19] To be digitally literate a person should be able to use the technology with confidence, know what a system should look like when it is working properly, know what to do when things go wrong and when to ask for help, and understand possible risks in using technology.

There are dangers for those who are not digitally literate. While it is vital that technology is accessible to all, usable and fit for its purpose, there is a risk in making systems appear so simple that there is no need for thought and responsibility - digital literacy is needed to ensure the safe use of technology.

References

1. Digital Literacy: Skills for the Information Society,
   http://ec.europa.eu/information_society/tl/edutra/skills/
   index_en.htm (accessed July 20, 2009)
2. Wilhelm, A.G.: Digital nation: toward an inclusive information society. MIT Press, Cambridge (2004)
3. Europe's Information Society: E-Inclusion,
   http://ec.europa.eu/information_society/policy/
   accessibility/index_en.htm (accessed July 2, 2009)
4. i2010 - A European Information Society for growth and employment,
   http://ec.europa.eu/information_society/eeurope/i2010/
   index_en.htm (accessed July 2, 2009)

5. Social inclusion, better public services and quality of life, http://ec.europa.eu/information_society/eeurope/i2010/inclusion/index_en.htm (accessed July 3, 2009)

6. Rheingold: In: Hand, M. (ed.) Making digital cultures: access, interactivity, and authenticity, Aldershot, Ashgate (2008)

7. McKinsey Quarterly: How Businesses are using Web 2.0: A McKinsey Global Survey (March 2007), http://www.mckinseyquarterly.com/information_technology/management/how_businesses_are_using_web_20_a_mckinsey_global_survey_1913 (accessed July 19, 2009)

8. Communication from the Commission to the European Parliament, The Council, The European Economic and Social Committee and the Committee of the Regions: Towards an accessible information society, Brussels (2008)

9. e-Inclusion: Be Part of It!, http://ec.europa.eu/information_society/activities/einclusion/bepartofit/index_en.htm (accessed July 20, 2009)

10. Ministerial Declaration approved on 11th June 2006, Riga, Latvia, http://ec.europa.eu/information_society/events/ict_riga_2006/doc/declaration_riga.pdf (accessed July 2, 2009)

11. Castells, M.: The network society: a cross-cultural perspective. Edward Elgar, Cheltenham (2005)

12. Supporting Digital Literacy, http://www.digital-literacy.eu/ (accessed July 19, 2009)

13. Caldwell, B.S.: Towards improved concepts of appropriate usability. In: Proceedings of IADIS International Conference ICT, Society and Human, Portugal (2009)

14. Holmes, W.N.: Computers and people. Wiley-IEEE Computer Society, Chichester (2006)

15. Smith-Gratto: In: Huerta, E., Sandoval-Almazan, R. (eds.) Digital Literacy: Problems Faced by Telecenter users in Mexico, Information technology for development (2007)

16. Carr, N.G.: The big switch: rewiring the world, from Edison to Google. W. W. Norton, New York (2008)

17. Gupta, G.K.: Computer literacy: essential in today's computer-centric world. SIGCSE Bull. 38, 115–119 (2006)

18. Van dyke, C.: Taking "computer literacy" literally. Communications of the ACM 30, 366–374 (1987)

19. Gilster, P.: Digital literacy. John Wiley, Chichester (1997)

20. Eshet-Alakali, Y., Amichai-Hamburger, Y.: Experiments in Digital Literacy. Cyber Psychology and Behavior 7, 421–429 (2004)

21. Dolan, D.: The European computer driving licence. In: Marshall, G., Ruohonen, M. (eds.) Capacity Building for IT in Education in Developing Countries. Chapman & Hall, Harare (1997)

22. Carpenter, D., Dolan, D., Leahy, D., Sherwood-Smith, M.: ECDL/ICDL: a global computer literacy initiative. In: 16th IFIP Congress ICEUT 200, educational uses of information and communication technologies, Beijing, China (2000)

23. The Finnish Information Processing Society, http://www.ttlry.fi/yhdistykset/tietotekniikan_liitto/in_english/ (accessed July 18, 2009)

24. Petz, A., Miesenberger, K.: ECDL- PD — Using a Well Known Standard to Lift Barriers on the Labour Market. Springer, Heidelberg (2002)

25. Henry, L.S.: Just Ask: Integrating Accessibility Throughout Design. Madison, W. (2007) ISBN 978-1430319528, http://www.uiAccess.com/JustAsk/ (accessed July 19, 2009)
26. Raman, T.V.: Toward 2w, Beyond Web 2.0. Communications of the ACM 52(2) (2009)
27. AbilityNet: State of the eNation Reports: Social networking sites lock out disabled users (2008), http://www.abilitynet.org.uk/enation85 (accessed July 2, 2009)
28. EU Brussels, 14.6.2007 COM (2007) 332 final "Ageing well in the Information Society", An i2010 Initiative, Action Plan on Information and Communication Technologies and Ageing, {SEC (2007)811},
    http://eur-lex.europa.eu/LexUriServ/
    LexUriServ.do?uri=COM:2007:0332:FIN:EN:PDF (accessed July 19, 2009)
29. Zajicek, M.: Web 2.0 Hype or Happiness. In: Proceedings of the 2007 international cross-disciplinary conference on Web accessibility, W4A (2007), http://portal.acm.org/citation.cfm?id=1243441.1243453 (accessed July 19, 2009)
30. Your guide to developing usable and useful web sites, http://www.usability.gov/basics/whatusa.html (accessed July 19, 2009)
31. Nielsen: Introduction to Usability,
    http://www.useit.com/alertbox/20030825.html (accessed July 19, 2009)
32. Facebook Now Nearly Twice The Size Of MySpace Worldwide,
    http://www.techcrunch.com/2009/01/22/
    facebook-now-nearly- twice-the-size-of-myspace-worldwide/
    (accessed July 20, 2009)
33. Creative Commons: Metrics, http://wiki.creativecommons.org/Metrics (accessed July 2, 2009)
34. EU Brussels, 14.6.2007 COM (2007) 332 final "Ageing well in the Information Society", An i2010 Initiative, Action Plan on Information and Communication Technologies and Ageing, {SEC (2007)811},
    http://eur-lex.europa.eu/LexUriServ/
    LexUriServ.do?uri=COM:2007:0332:FIN:EN:PDF (accessed July 20, 2009)
35. Wintlev-Jensen, P.: EU IST Event (2006),
    http://ec.europa.eu/information_society/istevent/2006/cf/
    people-detail.cfm?id=1758 (accessed July 19, 2009)
36. Turning the silver challenge into a golden opportunity,
    http://sap.info/archive/interviews/
    int_Interviews_Turning_the_Silver_Challenge_into_a_Golden_
    Opportunity_01.08.2007.html (accessed July 20)
37. Holzinger, A., Searle, G., Kleinberger, T., Seffah, A., Javahery, H.: Investigating Usability Metrics for the Design and Development of Applications for the Elderly. In: Miesenberger, K., Klaus, J., Zagler, W.L., Karshmer, A.I. (eds.) ICCHP 2008. LNCS, vol. 5105, pp. 98–105. Springer, Heidelberg (2008)

Enhancing Wikipedia Editing with WAI-ARIA

Caterina Senette[1], Maria Claudia Buzzi[1], Marina Buzzi[1], and Barbara Leporini[2]

[1] IIT – CNR, v. Moruzzi, 1, 56124 Pisa, Italy
[2] ISTI – CNR, v. Moruzzi, 1, 56124 Pisa, Italy
{Caterina.Senette,Claudia.Buzzi,Marina.Buzzi}@iit.cnr.it
Barbara.Leporini@isti.cnr.it

Abstract. Nowadays Web 2.0 applications allow anyone to create, share and edit on-line content, but accessibility and usability issues still exist. For instance, Wikipedia presents many difficulties for blind users, especially when they want to write or edit articles. In a previous stage of our study we proposed and discussed how to apply the W3C ARIA suite to simplify the Wikipedia editing page when interacting via screen reader. In this paper we present the results of a user test involving totally blind end-users as they interacted with both the original and the modified Wikipedia editing pages. Specifically, the purpose of the test was to compare the editing and formatting process for original and ARIA-implemented Wikipedia user interfaces, and to evaluate the improvements.

Keywords: WAI-ARIA, Wikipedia, user testing, accessibility, usability, blind users.

1 Introduction

In recent years wikis have enjoyed increasing popularity as collaboration tools in many areas. The most famous one is Wikipedia, the on-line Encyclopedia, which contains articles written collaboratively by volunteers from all around the world [22]. Building a single product in this way leads to a result with more integrated content [3]. In environments that allow many users to contribute to the creation of content, accessibility and usability are essential for universal participation. Wikis are a great opportunity for blind users, but the interactive environment and contents must be properly designed and delivered. Interacting with a wiki system can be difficult for a blind user since interaction requires the aid of assistive technology, adding a considerable degree of complexity.

We believe that an ARIA (Accessible Rich Internet Applications)-based editing interface would overcome many of the accessibility and usability problems that prevent blind users from actively contributing to Wikipedia.

In previous phases of this study we discussed difficulties experienced by blind users when interacting with Wikipedia [5] and proposed applying the ARIA suite to enhance the usability of the editing page [4]. In this paper we compare the original Wikipedia Editing Page (WEP) and the proposed ARIA-based WEP in order to evaluate whether the latter simplifies editing and formatting. This comparison was

A. Holzinger and K. Miesenberger (Eds.): USAB 2009, LNCS 5889, pp. 159–177, 2009.
© Springer-Verlag Berlin Heidelberg 2009

carried out by means of a user test on both the editing pages involving totally blind end-users.

The paper is structured as follows: in Section 2 we present related works, in Section 3 we briefly summarize the problems of interacting via screen reader with the original WEP and describe changes to the HTML source file to improve accessibility/usability; Section 4 describes the user test environment and results. Lastly, conclusions and future work are presented.

2   Related Works

In recent years Wiki systems have become very popular as collaboration tools in several areas including eLearning, where Wikis are increasingly used as educational tools and/or integrated in Learning Management Systems (LMSs). However the effectiveness of Wiki-based systems as learning tools is still controversial: various studies have confirmed the effectiveness of Wikis in education [2], [3], [18] while others have revealed important limits [7], [8].

Soo-Hwan et al. [18] found that learning programming is more effective in the community setting than in a content-centered setting, and collaborative learning via Wikis is more valuable when learning requires problem-solving skills or the process of elaborating knowledge.

By analyzing the use of two wikis in two Masters in IT, Bower et al. [3] verified that these collaborative tools can facilitate multi-user asynchronous creation, editing and restructuring of information.

To remedy the lack of interaction noted in online discussion groups, and to stimulate the collaborative environment, Augar et al. [2] adapted a traditional icebreaker exercise used in classrooms for use on a wiki, with good results: in the two-week exercise, the number of pages of the wiki increased steadily each day.

In contrast, other studies pointed out that wiki ideas and principles did not work in some learning environments, due to students' lack of motivation, no "community feeling", and poor usability [7], [8]. Specifically Ebner et al. [8] carried out two studies in higher education to investigate Wiki usage (student participation was voluntary, that is, users were not forced to utilize the system), highlighting "difficult to use" as one of the main causes of low active use of Wikis (inserting new content).

However, it is important to note that results of user tests directly depend on accessibility and usability of the UIs of the selected Wiki.

The design and implementation of wiki-based learning tasks can greatly affect their success. Bower et al. [3] recommend a set of 12 principles for improving their effectiveness. For instance, these authors observed that tasks requiring a single product produce a wiki containing more integrated content. This is the case of Wikipedia, where each encyclopedia entry requires contributions by multiple authors, which are then integrated into a single description.

Usability is essential for the collaborative Web. Wikis' usability can be studied both by analyzing user navigation throughout pages (looking for the desired information) and by evaluating user interaction with the editing page (inserting/updating new content). In the latter case it was observed that in the initial life of wiki systems, an exponential growth of content starts only after an initial (and sometimes long) linear trend [7].

Wikis and e-Learning systems are a great opportunity for blind persons with mobility problems. However, electronic barriers can impede access to on-line resources. Accessibility guarantees that anybody can access Web content, regardless of any disability. This implies that different channels (visual, auditory, tactile) should be used to present the same content to the differently-abled.

The World Wide Web Consortium promotes accessibility on the Web through its Web Accessibility Initiative (WAI). Recently (Dec 2008) the WAI group produced a new version of the Web Content Accessibility Guidelines - WCAG 2.0 [23], which greatly improves the 1.0 version, and includes usability as a key factor, to be closely coupled with accessibility.

In order to verify Web page accessibility Takagi et al. suggest spending more time on the practical aspects of usability rather than focusing on the syntactic checking of Web pages. Indeed, some aspects are difficult to evaluate automatically, such as ease of understanding page structure and interface navigability [19].

To fill this gap, the WAI group is working on the Accessible Rich Internet Applications specification (WAI-ARIA) to make dynamic web content and applications (developed with Ajax, (X)HTML, JavaScript) more accessible to people with disabilities [24]. Using WAI-ARIA web designers can define roles to add semantic information to interface objects, mark regions of the page so users can move rapidly around the page via keyboard, etc. [24]. Useful examples of ARIA code are available on-line [25].

As previously mentioned, the design of any User Interface (UI) should include usability; a clear definition of usability is provided by the ISO 9241 standard [11]: "The effectiveness, efficiency and satisfaction with which specified users achieve specified goals in particular environments". There are many methods for evaluating usability, including heuristics, cognitive walkthroughs, guidelines, and usability testing.

In the study reported in this paper we describe a remote user testing conducted with a group of blind individuals in order to evaluate a modified Wikipedia editing page implemented with ARIA. Remote evaluation greatly reduces the cost of usability testing: in this type of usability evaluation, the evaluator performs all observation and analysis from a distance [10].

Different technologies for monitoring user behavior and capturing data can be applied, as shown in [17], [9] and [10], including videoconferencing, automatic logging of user paths and tasks, or others specific tools.

Recent studies performing a comparative analysis have shown that during remote testing, users take a bit longer to complete tasks due to the communication overhead, but the results are as effective as, if not better than, traditional testing performed in the laboratory [21].

In contrast, Petrie et al. [16] conducted two case studies with disabled users (including totally blind and visually-impaired persons) to explore asynchronous remote evaluation techniques, and showed that while quantitative data were comparable, local evaluations collected richer qualitative data. However, these authors also argued that experienced specialists often lack a thorough understanding of how people with disabilities use their assistive technologies; thus perhaps the proposed questionnaire did not sufficiently reflect their needs and problems.

3 Modifing the Wikipedia Editing Page (WEP)

3.1 Interaction via Screen Reader with the WEP

Blind users usually interact with computers (or other electronic devices) using assistive technology in the form of a screen reader. A screen reader is software that identifies and interprets the content being displayed on the screen, reproducing it through vocal synthesis (or rarely, by a Braille display). The screen reader reads a web page sequentially, one line at a time. When it works in "virtual mode" it is able to perceive that a browser is working, then tries to interpret the original Web page structure and give the user the navigation keyboard control. In this way blind users can halt the screen reading to scan a page with keyboard commands such as Tab key, from link to link, or via arrow keys to explore content line by line.

In the following we refer to the JAWS screen reader with vocal synthesis since it is the most frequently used by the blind users in Italy [1].

The editing page of Wikipedia presents three main usability issues for totally blind users:

1. The formatting toolbar is difficult to perceive, access and use.
   The widgets of the Wikipedia toolbar are graphic icons, generated by JavaScript. The browser is unable to recognize these widgets as active elements (such as links, buttons, boxes, etc.) so they are skipped (never receive the focus) when the user explores the page via Tab key. Consequently, in this type of navigation the user never perceives the presence of a toolbar on the page. Instead, if the user explores the page sequentially (via arrow keys), the screen reader announces these widgets with the alternative description associated with the icons (for instance "graphic bold clickable"). However the user must be aware that each description/icon is associated with a formatting function and know how to activate it. This may be difficult for unskilled users. Another complex way to find a specific widget is to use the "find" command on the page. It is also possible to use other advanced screen reader commands but most users only utilize basic commands and are not even aware of this possibility [20].

2. It is difficult to select special characters and symbols.
   To insert a special character or symbol, Wikipedia offers a combo-box for selecting an alphabet. After the selection, a list of links of the corresponding alphabet characters is shown. Visually, this list is rapidly scanned, but since some alphabets contain more than one hundred links, it is not suitable for navigation via Tab key. Having many links makes the navigation long and users become disoriented. Furthermore, JAWS does not recognize uncommon symbols or characters, so it produces ambiguous text. For instance JAWS announces "link e" for each character in the group e, é, è, È and É. To distinguish each character, a more descriptive text should be associated (e.g. "e with acute accent") for enhancing usability.

3. Focus issue.
   In the WEP the focus is managed via JavaScript: when one or more words in the text area are selected, all related parameters (including the focus) are stored by the script in order to apply the formatting correctly. However, when interacting via screen reader a blind user may not correctly understand how the focus is

processed since the screen reader provides a "virtual focus", and this may not coincide with the system focus. This problem could be quite important since to format a portion of text in the original WEP, the user must switch between editing and navigation modalities several times (see [4] for further details).

The screen reader is only one of the elements involved in the process of interaction between a blind user and a web page. In this process, blind people must understand the browser, the screen reader and finally the web page [20]. Visually-impaired people must make a great effort to obtain a good mental model of each of these three elements, especially if one of them is relatively unknown to the user. This problem is probably less relevant when they have to interact with desktop applications, but it becomes enormous when they navigate through the Web.

3.2 New Wikipedia Editing Page

To improve interface usability and solve the three issues described above, we introduced ARIA in the WEP UI source code. ARIA adds semantic information that communicates the object role (for instance role = "button") to the screen reader and so to the user. In this way a graphic icon can be recognized as a control element.

In this context the use of ARIA greatly enhances interface usability compared to using only standard (X)HTML elements (i.e. input element), making interaction via keyboard easier and more comfortable, as discussed in the following:

1. Formatting toolbar
   The Wikipedia formatting toolbar, originally created with JavaScript, may be replaced with standard XHTML input elements with associated images (i.e. buttons), maintaining the graphical appearance of the original but providing accessible widgets. Access keys may be associated with each toolbar element to make it faster to apply formatting functions. However, memorizing 22 shortcuts (corresponding to the toolbar elements) costs the user significant cognitive effort, also because browsers and screen readers provide numerous shortcuts as well. Alternatively, several Tab key pressures are necessary in order to navigate the entire toolbar, so the UI is accessible, but navigation is still quite long and tedious. In order to simplify interaction, we have defined the formatting toolbar using the ARIA "toolbar" and "button" roles. The *activedescendant* attribute makes the toolbar navigable via arrow keys. Once the toolbar receives the focus via Tab key, the child elements -- i.e. each widget -- can be accessed by up and down arrows, and can be activated by pressing the ENTER key, which applies the associated formatting function (e.g. Bold, Italics, etc.).
2. Special characters and symbols
   In the new UI we aggregate all characters of each alphabet in a second combobox located close to the alphabet combobox, as shown in Fig. 2 (right). Users first choose a 'language' and then select the desired character of that language.
   This compact solution is faster for blind users since when navigating the combobox with arrow keys, the screen reader announces the character name directly while in the original WEP every character read is preceded by the word 'link'. In addition when a user is in exploration modality, (s)he can skip/exit the combobox pressing a Tab key once, while in the original WEP it is necessary to cross/visit all

the links. Lastly, the many links on a page make it difficult to use the special JAWS command Insert + F7 that gives the list of all the links in the page.

To simplify selection of a special character, we also specified a clear label attribute for each <option> item of the second combo-box, so the screen reader can announce a clear description of the selected character.

3. Focus

The focus problem is partially resolved by our new WEP. With the JAWS English version 9, the new interface allows users to insert and edit text without having to switch to navigation modality in order to find the active elements (widgets and comboboxes). The user activates the editing modality and it remains for the entire editing/formatting process, reducing the number of steps needed to complete the whole task. Instead with the JAWS Italian version 9 the focus is in the correct position but JAWS loses the editing modality. Indeed Jaws 10 automatically enables the editing mode when the virtual focus is in a text box (Auto Forms Mode) and a vocal tone is provided to the user to indicate the editing modality (Forms Mode on). Exiting the control element, the user automatically returns to the navigation modality. This makes interaction with form fields simpler and faster.

The ARIA *activedescendant* attribute (associated with the toolbar) allowed us to exploit the Wikipedia Javascript, which in the original UI was activated by the mouse click. Once the keypress event of a formatting button is captured, this Javascript applies the related function and moves the focus back to the text box.

4   User Test

In order to evaluate the new Wikipedia Editing interface developed by applying our proposed solution, we conducted a user test with a group of blind people. Specifically, our evaluation aims to answer the following questions:

- Is the editing/formatting effectively simplified?
- Does the user perceive the editing/formatting task more quickly?
- Is the presentation of interface elements (combobox, labels) clearer?
- Which UI changes (i.e., ARIA toolbar or comboboxes) are more valuable for users?

Nielsen suggests that the following criteria are the most significant measures for evaluating a usability test [14]:

- performance (that is, the time required to perform a task)
- success rate (which measures whether users can perform the task at all)
- error rate
- users' subjective satisfaction.

In this study usability was analyzed based on the user's effectiveness and efficiency in carrying out a given task by blind users. Regarding performance, we only measured the total time required by the user to complete each of two tasks on one of the WEPs (by using time-stamps server-side).

4.1 Design of the Test

4.1.1 Method

To carry out the test we developed an environment that reproduced prototypes of both the original and the modified Wikipedia user interfaces. The environment also includes SW for recording and collecting useful information for the analysis of the user test results. The pages were developed in XHTML, PHP and Javascript. The system is mainly composed of the following components:

- A login page where the user can enter her/his name or nickname.

  This (nick)name allowed all participants to be as anonymous as possible, which was greatly appreciated by the test subjects, who preferred not to be identified, and it allowed us to match together the test results with two questionnaires filled in by the users (described in the following).

  The combination of recorded data with the users' subjective information (extracted by questionnaires) allowed us to better analyze the collected data.

  The login page contained two buttons, one for the original and one for the modified UI, so the user could easily reach the two UIs (Fig. 1).

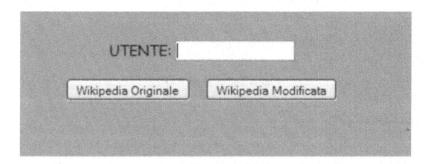

Fig. 1. Login Test Page

- Two Web pages reproducing the two WEPs – the original (Fig. 2) and the modified one (Fig. 3) – to be used for carrying out the tasks.

  Since the main aim of our test was to compare user interaction with the editing field, the toolbar and the combobox, we had decided to remove additional text and links from the page, in order to focus users' attention on the features being evaluated. In this way we probably underestimate the advantage of ARIA that is particularly useful in complex UI.

  For testing with Italian blind users, we used the Italian version of Wikipedia, downloaded on 2009 January (http://it.wikipedia.org/w/index.php? title= Wikipedia:Pagina_delle_prove&action=edit).

- A logging module to capture and record information on the test when the user navigated through the two WEPs.

  The test produces two files for each participant: one concerning the interaction with the original WEP and one related to the modified one.

Figure 4 shows a snippet of the log file. Each time the user clicks on the "Save page", "Show Preview" or "End" buttons, the content of the text areas and a timestamp are memorized.

We added the "End" button to both the WEPs to force the user to register the server-side time before leaving the pages. This data is used to analyze how much time the user spent performing a task on a WEP.

Fig. 2. The original WEP

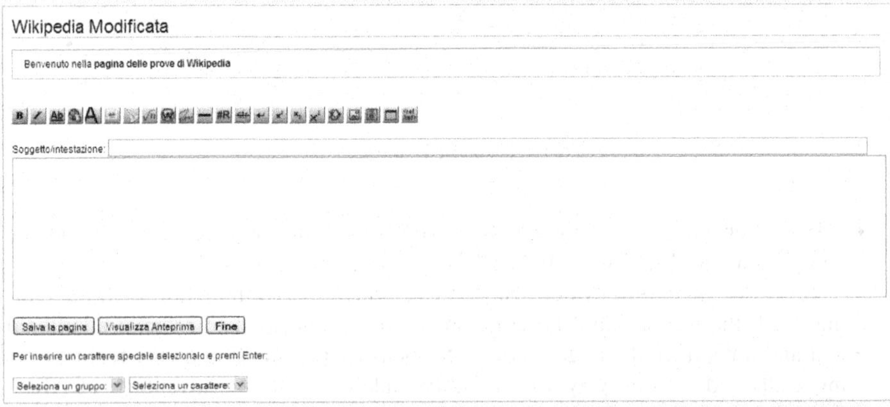

Fig. 3. The modified WEP

The test given to the blind users consisted of three parts, available in electronic format. The details about the test were sent to participants by email while tasks were executed via web, i.e. each user loaded from our server the original and modified UIs on their client via browser. In detail, the tests comprised three phases.

1. The first step of the test was sending the users a preliminary questionnaire. This questionnaire aimed to collect information about participants, investigating their technical expertise, age, gender, computer environment (OS and screen reader), and use of Wikipedia.

   Each participant had to choose a nickname for the identification.

   Contextually we also sent user a URL for downloading and installing the Firefox 3.0.5 browser (being ready for the test).

2. The second step of the test was sending the users a document (Test Description Document) containing the test URL and directives for executing the test.

   The test, executed by the user on his/her home computer (remote test), included two tasks to be performed on each WEP.

   A task was considered finished when the user pressed the "save page" or "end" buttons. Data was appended in the file and elaborated after the test.

3. Last, user feedback was collected with a post-test questionnaire, consisting of 16 questions about:

   (1) difficulties in editing and formatting text
   (2) information about the subject's experience performing the assigned tasks
   (3) the users' subjective satisfaction

The post-test questionnaire was sent to the users together with the document describing the remote test.

```
...
    User name
...
    Text area content
...
    Text area end
Subject
...
    IP address
    82.57.143.XXX
    Request time
    25-01-2009 23:47:12
    Browser
    Mozilla/5.0 (...rv:1.9.0.5)...
    Firefox/3.0.5
...
```

Fig. 4. Snippet of the log file

Users were free to interact with the environment developed for the test (original and modified WEP) as they liked before the test, but we required them to perform each of the two parts of the test in one sitting (each part consisted of two tasks that were performed twice, on different WEPs). They could relax after completing each part in one of the WEPs and before starting the second part.

Users were divided into two groups (A and B) and each group began the test with a different WEP, in order to balance the average time spent on each WEP, because it is possible to assume that interaction with the second WEP assigned might be faster than the first. So we created two versions of the Test Description Document, and two of the post-test questionnaire, inverting the order of the WEP interaction. Since we did not know the number of the users participating in the test phase, we did the group assignment in progress, deciding on which group to assign a user only after (s)he sent back the preliminary questionnaire, and taking care to balance the groups.

4.1.2 Remote Testing

We decided to set up a test where the tester and users were not co-located, i.e., remote testing as defined in [12]. According to Petrie et al. [16] classification, the remote testing was carried out asynchronously (i.e., the participant and the evaluator do not participate at the same time) guaranteeing participant independence (i.e., users undertake the evaluation independently).

The validity of remote testing, in comparison to classic laboratory usability testing, is a topic that frequently comes up in the literature. Both techniques have advantages and disadvantages, as discussed in [15] where the authors also suggest a "mixed" solution. We were forced to do remote testing since even a small change in the blind users' hardware/software can dramatically impact on performance and thus on test results. In addition, with remote user testing we could easily recruit people from several Italian cities.

Furthermore, most of the subjects participating in the remote test reported that they did not feel comfortable and free to work if observed or monitored in any way during execution of the task. For this reason we choose a middle way, only recording times per task on each WEP. Data was created with server timestamps. It should be noted that performance measures require the homogeneity of the user hardware/software configuration and full control over user actions for test feasibility and validity of results, while qualitative testing is conceived for understanding user satisfaction and highlighting any problems. However, the test was based on the repetition by each user of the same task in both the UIs (the original and the modified) and on its evaluation.

This means that although executed in different environments (O.S. and screen reader version), the result is significant since the subjective improvement/worsening of any users in her/his interaction environment (user performance and satisfaction for the same task in the original and new UI) is evaluated.

4.2 The Test

To complete the test, each participant needed to connect to a URL (http://test-utenti.iit.cnr.it/) where they found a simple page with a login text box (password is not required) and the two buttons to the original and the modified WEPs (Fig. 1). The test consisted of two tasks to perform on both the UIs: (I) editing process using a special character; and (II) the use of a formatting function. Each task was split into a few steps to encourage the user to press a push button in order to allow us to register server-side a time-stamp in the logging file associated to each participant.

Tasks were balanced between users: half the people were asked to utilize first the original WEP and then the modified interface, and vice-versa for the other group. Table 1 contains the steps assigned to the users for the two tasks to perform in both the interfaces.

The right sequence of steps for each group was specified in the test instructions (Test Description Document). Without any temporal constraint, users were able to perform the test comfortably and without stress. Freedom to write any comment or observation, in addition to the multiple-choice answers of our questionnaire, added very useful information to the analysis.

After preparing a preliminary version of the documents (Test Description Document and questionnaires) a pilot test set up by one of the authors of this paper, who has been totally blind since childhood, was performed. Other sighted authors also performed the test independently (with PC screen turned off), and afterwards outcomes were compared and discussed.

Thus, issues that might occur while performing the test (due to confusing descriptions/directives) were identified and fixed. The pilot test was an iterative process leading to the appropriate modifications to create an easier version of the test in relation to comprehension, set up and on-line access.

Table 1 shows test steps. Blind users had to write a simple article, the title was: "L'Italia" and the text was: "É una Repubblica" inserting the special character "É" from the combobox (task 1), and applying the formatting function Bold to the word: "Repubblica" (task 2).

We tested the interfaces with MS IE and Mozilla Firefox. We would favor the use of IE since test participants are familiar with this browser. Unfortunately, at the time of our test (January 2009) the new ARIA-based WEP was not correctly interpreted by IE v. 8 Beta while Mozilla Firefox v. 3.0.5 fully supports ARIA, so we required the use of the latter (Firefox). We tested the WEP with the Jaws screen reader v. 9.0. and v.10.

Table 1. Test description: steps of the tasks

T1 Editing task	
Step 1	Insert the word "L'Italia" in the Editing summary
Step 2	Select and insert in the Editing field the special character (È) using the combobox
Step 3	Continue to write the phrase: " una Repubblica"
Step 4	Press the "Save page" button
T2 Formatting task	
Step 5	Apply bold formatting at the word Repubblica
Step 6	Press the "End" button

4.3 Participants

The user test was directly carried out with blind people, although it has been observed that working with sighted persons who have a certain expertise in computing and in using a screen reader could be a very effective method for testing accessibility problems [13]. In fact, anyone who regularly uses an assistive technology and perceives the content in a specific way can easily appreciate certain differences and features. However, we believe that a user interface developed for improving interaction by screen reader requires feedback from users who really interact with that assistive technology. In addition, the interface evaluation by usability experts may not be adequate, since blind users use the interface by responding to a different set of stimuli and criteria. For example, aural perception by a blind person is probably better than that of a sighted user, since evaluation of sounds and tones may be more accurate. Therefore, in our opinion it is necessary to perform the evaluation with a group of blind users who actually interact with assistive technologies.

The participants were contacted through the Italian Association for the Blind, to which one of the authors also belongs. She initially contacted potential users via phone and email to describe the project and the aim of testing the new interface. In this way, 30 persons, completely blind since birth, took part in the first phase by filling out the preliminary questionnaire while 15 persons went on to participate in the entire test. In the following we will only refer to the 15 users who took the test.

4.4 Results

4.4.1 The Preliminary Questionnaire

Evaluating user feedback on a preliminary questionnaire is a basic procedure that can help to better understand the test results.

Data from the preliminary questionnaire provided a characterization of the sample. The 15 blind subjects comprised 5 women and 10 men, with age ranging from 18-24 years to more than 75 years (only 1 person) as shown in Figure 5.

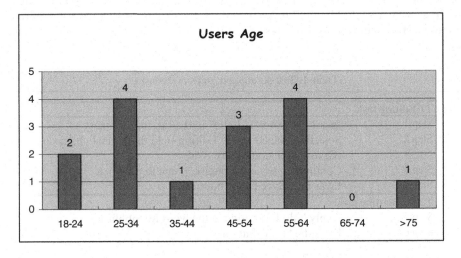

Fig. 5. Users' Age

Concerning the use of the Internet, 20% are beginners, 47% intermediate, and 33% had considerable experience. All the sample was using JAWS (from v. 6 to v. 9) on Windows (all use Windows XP; 3 of them also use Windows Vista).

In the test instructions we pointed out the need to use JAWS version 9.0 in order to benefit of the ARIA suite, but some people used a different version. For blind people in fact, it difficult to use a new version of assistive technology (different from their usual one), since most of them usually customize (with great difficulty) the screen reader according their specific needs or preferences.

It is obvious that different screen readers, as well as different versions of the same screen reader, may have different features, but their basic behaviors are similar. Furthermore, since evaluation of both the original and modified UIs was performed by each user in the same environment, the results are comparable and the subjective evaluation has significance.

Regarding the use of JAWS advanced commands (for example: advanced command 'INSERT+F7' to have the link list, 'INSERT+F6' to have the heading list; 'N' to skip links), 40% of subjects use them always or frequently, 47% never or nearly never, 13% know only a few advanced commands.

Another of the questions included in the preliminary questionnaire was about the subjects' degree of knowledge of Wikipedia interfaces; answers highlighted that 20% of the sample don't know Wikipedia or know it only superficially, 40% are somewhat familiar with Wikipedia and 40% know it well. It is important to note that only four users (27% of the sample) have occasionally tried to use the Wikipedia editing page, which is the object of the test.

4.4.2 User Performance

We consider a test concluded if the user executed both the tasks regardless of correctness (e.g. applied the bold but inserted è instead of È). A total of 47% of the sample completed the test in the original WEP compared to 80% on the modified UI (Fig. 6).

A test was successful if the user concluded both tasks correctly in a WEP. The main observation is that 13% executed the test successfully in the original WEP compared to 33% on the modified UI (Fig. 6).

Figure 7 and Figure 8 show completeness and success of the two tasks.

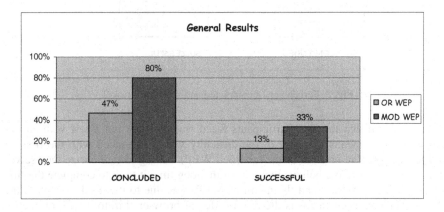

Fig. 6. Percentage of completed and successful tests

These data indicate that the proposed UI appears to simplify interaction.

Regarding the execution times expressed in minutes, Figure 9 shows the average execution time for the entire test. Participants who completed the test reduced their execution time by 10% in the modified UIs.

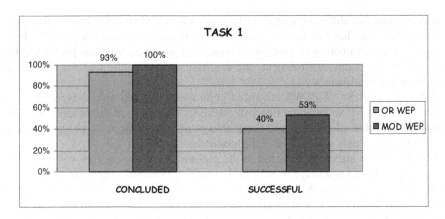

Fig. 7. Percentage of completed and successful task 1

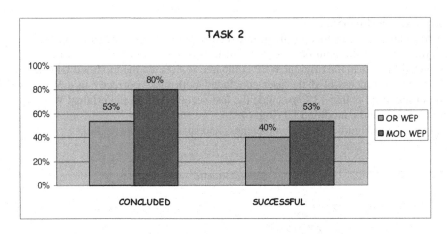

Fig. 8. Percentage of completed and successful task 2

One problem that most of participants faced was carrying out a test with an unknown UI. This means that part of the difficulty was experienced with the first UI used for the test (the original or the modified WEP), having to familiarize themselves with form elements. We believe that part of the long time it took to complete the first task (in both the original and the modified WEP) was due to the need to explore the UI. Another important factor is the use a different browser (Firefox) with respect to the usual navigation environment (IE).

It should be observed that in our test environment we only reported a small number (20) of all characters of the Latin alphabet actually present in Wikipedia (more than 150). For coherence of the test we restricted this number of characters to 20, and in the original WEP as well. This facilitates interaction of the original WEP compared to the editing page of en.wikipedia.org. The latter presents more difficulties, thus the real advantage of the proposed combobox should be even greater.

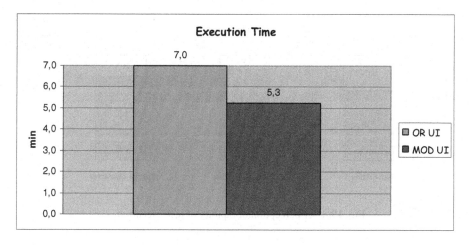

Fig. 9. Test execution time

Results in terms of user performance must be evaluated by looking at the data test and at the feedback that users gave us. To interpret results correctly it is necessary to understand when and how the participants performed the test, and also to consider all the factors involved, objective and psychological, when a person performs a test:

- 50% of the participants did the test at night; this may indicate that users needed a quieter environment but also implies that they may be tired or in a hurry;
- 80% of the sample did not experiment with the WEP before the test, possibly due to fear of interacting with the WEP, or to lack of time or interest.

Regarding the psychological aspect, which of course had great impact on perform-ance, we can hypothesize following elements:

1. the user believes him/herself (and not the interface) to be the object of the ex-amination. This explains why some users praise the modified interface although they have performed the tasks badly;
2. lack of self-confidence, probably due to inadequate feedback given to the user from the three software elements involved in the interaction: browser, screen reader and UIs (WEPs);
3. lack of naturalness while performing the tasks, since the user probably knows that someone is monitoring his/her behavior.

4.4.3 The Post-Test Questionnaire
The post-test questionnaire was formulated in a neutral way in order to avoid influ-encing the users, with the same question presented in two versions: one referred to the original and one to the modified WEP.

The post-test questionnaire reveals the user perception of the interaction with the WEPs and the user subject satisfaction. Of the sample, 60% found some differences while 40% found many differences between the original and modified WEPs.

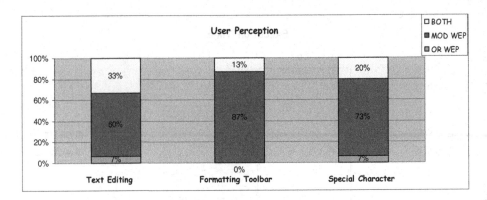

Fig. 10. User perception of rapidity of task execution

Concerning difficulties with the test execution 73% found some difficulties, 20% many difficulties and only 7% no difficulties.

Some questions regard the user perception of rapidity of task execution: 1) editing text, 2) applying a formatting function 3) selecting a special character, as shown in Figure 10.

Those results revealed that most users appreciated the interaction with the modified UIs. Specifically, 60% of subjects declared that text entry was faster in the modified WEP, 33% in the original, and 7% found both interfaces equivalent.

A total of 87% of the participants declared that using the toolbar was faster in the modified WEP while 13% believed they were equivalent.

A total of 73% of subjects perceived the selection of a special character via combobox (instead of links) to be more efficient, 7% perceived the selection via links in the original WEP to be more efficient and 20% declared they were equivalent.

5 Discussion

In this paper we presented and discussed a usability test involving totally blind end-users regarding a proposed new Wikipedia editing page aimed at simplifying interaction via screen reader. The main purpose of our testing was comparing interaction via the screen reader JAWS with the original and new UIs developed using ARIA.

In this test we only evaluated two proposed changes in the original UI: an ARIA-based formatting toolbar and an additional combobox for selecting special characters.

Results of the test showed that interaction was simplified, since the number of completed tests is higher for the modified Wikipedia editing page. In the original editing page 47% of users concluded the test while the percentage increased to 80% in the modified one. Regarding correctness, 13% of the users concluded the test successfully in the original Wikipedia editing page while 33% of the sample did so in the modified interface. The interaction seems to be faster in the modified UIs, with a decrease in test execution time of 10%. Specifically, ARIA allowed more users to successfully complete the test and improved user performance.

However, the new UI would be expected to work much better than the original one, but results do not show great differences between the two WEPs. One problem is that we are unable to verify whether some users did not follow our instructions closely, because we only measured users' final actions. In fact, we need to monitor all the events performed by the user (i.e. keyboard key or key combination press), in order to have real and total control of the experiment. Furthermore we forced many users to use an unknown browser (Mozilla Firefox) on a unknown UI (only 27% of users had previously used the Wikipedia editing page), with undoubted consequences for the results of the usability test.

User perception revealed that most users appreciated interacting with the modified WEP. Specifically 87% of the participants declared that using the toolbar is faster in the modified WEP while 13% declared they were equivalent. A total of 73% of the sample also perceived the selection of a special character via combobox to be more efficient than links.

6 Conclusions and Future Work

ARIA is an emerging technology that simplifies interaction for the differently-abled. Especially blind persons who interact via screen reader and voice synthesizer and the cognitively impaired may benefit to manage small portions of content anytime.

In the design of UIs all physical and cognitive resources required for the user interaction with all HW/SW components would be carefully analyzed. We believe it is crucial for designers to incorporate WAI-ARIA when developing user interfaces, to enhance usability via assistive technologies.

In this initial user test, we only worked on the main part of the Wikipedia Editing Page, removing additional text and links in order to focus users' attention on the features being evaluated. We have also used a restricted set of alphabets and characters, greatly simplifying the UI.

As a further step of this research we have completed the WEP with text, links, and special/alphabets characters, and we have added ARIA regions. In this new configuration, we anticipate considerable improvement in simplifying interaction with the Wikipedia editing page for the blind, since the current page layout is complex and crowded with active elements, making very useful for the blind users have a page overview (the list of the page regions) and be able to jump directly to the desired part of the UI (main contents), skipping navigation bar and menu (see [6] for a scenario of use)

However, at the moment we are unable to carry out a new test to evaluate our hypothesis, since JAWS v. 10, which supports ARIA regions, is not widespread among our test participants.

In the future, we intend to further utilize WAI-ARIA specification in other collaborative software as well, such as blogs and social networking sites.

References

1. Andronico, P., Buzzi, M., Castillo, C., Leporini, B.: Improving Search Engine Interfaces for Blind Users: a case study. Universal Access in the Information Society (UAIS) 5(1), 23–41 (2006)
2. Augar, N., Raitman, R., Zhou, W.: Teaching and learning online with wikis. In: 21st ASCILITE Conference, pp. 95–104 (2004),
   `http://ascilite.org.au/conferences/perth04/procs/pdf/augar.pdf`
3. Bower, M., Woo, K., Roberts, M., Watters, P.: Wiki Pedagogy - A Tale of Two Wikis. In: Information Technology Based Higher Education and Training Conference (ITHET 2006), pp. 191–202 (2006), doi:10.1109/ITHET.2006.339764
4. Buzzi, M.C., Buzzi, M., Leporini, B., Senette, C.: Making Wikipedia Editing Easier for the Blind. In: ACM NordiCHI 2008, pp. 423–426. ACM, New York (2008)
5. Buzzi, M., Leporini, B.: Is Wikipedia usable for the blind? In: ACM W4A Workshop, pp. 15–22. ACM, New York (2008)
6. Buzzi, M., Leporini, B.: Editing Wikipedia content by screen reader: Easier interaction with the Accessible Rich Internet Applications suite. Informa healthcare. Disability and Rehabilitation: Assistive Technology 4(4), 264–275 (2009)
7. Ebner, M., Zechner, J., Holzinger, A.: Why is Wikipedia so successful? Experiences in establishing the principles in Higher Education. In: International Conference on Knowledge Management (iKNOW), Knowledge Sharing in Research and Higher Education (KSR 2006), pp. 527–535 (2006)
8. Ebner, M., Kickmeier-Rust, M.D., Holzinger, A.: Utilizing Wiki-Systems in higher education classes: a chance for universal access? Universal Access in the Information Society 7(4), 199–207 (2008)
9. Hartson, H.R., Castillo, J.C., Kelso, J., Neale, W.C.: Remote evaluation: the network as an extension of the usability laboratory. In: ACM CHI 1996, pp. 228–235. ACM, New York (1996)
10. Hartson, H.R., Castillo, J.C.: Remote evaluation for post-deployment usability improvement. In: Working conference on Advanced visual interfaces, pp. 22–29 (1998), doi:10.1145/948496.948499
11. International Organization for Standardization, Geneva: ISO 9241-11: Ergonomic Requirements for Office Work with Visual Display Terminals (VDTs), Part 11: Guidance on Usability, 1st edn., 1998-03-15 (1998)
12. Ivory, M.Y., Hearst, M.A.: The state of the art in automating usability evaluation of user interfaces. Computing Surveys 2001(4), 470–516 (2004)
13. Mankoff, J., Fait, H., Tran, T.: Is your Web page accessible? A comparative study of methods for assessing Web page accessibility for the blind. In: SIGCHI conference on Human factors in computing systems (2005), doi:10.1145/1054972.1054979
14. Nielsen, J.: Alertbox. Usability Metrics (January 21, 2001),
    `http://www.useit.com/alertbox/20010121.html`
15. Norman, K.L., Panizzi, E.: Levels of automation and user participation in usability testing. Interacting with Computers 18(2), 246–264 (2006)
16. Petrie, H., Hamilton, F., King, N., Pavan, P.: Remote Usability Evaluations with Disabled People. In: SIGCHI conference on Human Factors in computing systems, pp. 1133–1141 (2006), doi:10.1145/1124772.1124942
17. Scholtz, J.: Adaptation of traditional usability testing methods for remote testing. In: HICSS 2001, pp. 1–9. IEEE, Los Alamitos (2001)

18. Kim, S.-H., Han, H.-S., Han, S.-G.: The Study on Effective Programming Learning Using Wiki Community Systems. In: Nejdl, W., Tochtermann, K. (eds.) EC-TEL 2006. LNCS, vol. 4227, pp. 646–651. Springer, Heidelberg (2006)
19. Takagi, H., Asakawa, C., Fukuda, K., Maeda, J.: Accessibility designer: visualizing usability for the blind. In: 6th international ACM SIGACCESS conference on Computers and accessibility, pp. 177–184 (2004)
20. Theofanos, M.F., Redish, G.: Bridging the gap: between accessibility and usability. Interaction 10(6), 36–51 (2003)
21. Thompson, K.E., Rozanski, E.P., Haake, A.R.: Here, there, anywhere: remote usability testing that works. In: 5th conference on Information technology education table of contents, pp. 132–137. ACM Press, New York (2004)
22. Wikipedia. Wiki, http://en.Wikipedia.org/wiki/Wiki
23. W3C. Web Content Accessibility Guidelines 2.0 (December 5, 2008), http://www.w3.org/TR/WCAG20/
24. W3C. WAI-ARIA Overview, http://www.w3.org/WAI/intro/aria.php
25. W3C. WAI-ARIA Best practices, http://www.w3.org/TR/wai-aria-practices/

Seeing the System through the End Users' Eyes: Shadow Expert Technique for Evaluating the Consistency of a Learning Management System

Andreas Holzinger[1], Christian Stickel[2], Markus Fassold[2], and Martin Ebner[2]

[1] Medical University Graz, A-8036 Graz, Austria
Institute for Medical Informatics (IMI), Research Unit HCI4MED &
Graz University of Technology, A-8010 Graz, Austria
Institute for Information Systems and Computer Media (IICM)
a.holzinger@tugraz.at
[2] Graz University of Technology, A-8010 Graz, CIS/Department of Social Media
{stickel,martin.ebner}@tugraz.at

Abstract. Interface consistency is an important basic concept in web design and has an effect on performance and satisfaction of end users. Consistency also has significant effects on the learning performance of both expert and novice end users. Consequently, the evaluation of consistency within a e-learning system and the ensuing eradication of irritating discrepancies in the user interface redesign is a big issue. In this paper, we report of our experiences with the Shadow Expert Technique (SET) during the evaluation of the consistency of the user interface of a large university learning management system. The main objective of this new usability evaluation method is to understand the interaction processes of end users with a specific system interface. Two teams of usability experts worked independently from each other in order to maximize the objectivity of the results. The outcome of this SET method is a list of recommended changes to improve the user interaction processes, hence to facilitate high consistency.

Keywords: Consistency, Shadow Expert Technique, Usability Test, Methods, Performance, Measurement.

1 Introduction and Motivation for Research

It is generally known that the acceptance and usability of software is significantly related to its user interface quality [1] and the first of Ben Shneidermans' Golden Rule of Interface Design is "Strive for Consistency" [2]. Consistent sequences of actions are required in similar situations; identical terminology should be used; consistent color, layout, fonts, etc. should be used throughout the complete system. This not only enhances accessibility, but it is of benefit to every user.

Consequently, for a long time the most important design guideline has been: Build consistent human interfaces [3], yet often this guideline is ignored by designers [4]. Moreover, previous studies on Learning Management Systems (LMS, e-Learning systems) show that the user interface consistency has significant effects on the learning

A. Holzinger and K. Miesenberger (Eds.): USAB 2009, LNCS 5889, pp. 178–192, 2009.

performance. Experienced end users make more errors than novices and their satisfaction level is lower when using a physically inconsistent user interface, whereas conceptually consistent user interfaces facilitate performance and satisfaction [5].

These facts have been the motivation for the work described here: At Graz University of Technology approximately 10,000 students and teachers work daily with the TeachCenter software, which is a large LMS, consisting of a number of applications, i.e. Classroom Pages, Chat rooms, Forums, Blogs, Polls, FAQ's, Plagiarism Tests etc. All these functions facilitate the daily teaching and learning of the students and teachers. However, the efficient use of those functions depends highly on the acceptability of the system and in previous usability studies it was found that the design of the system is lacking consistency. In order to carefully identify these inconsistencies, we decided to apply a new usability testing method called the Shadow Expert Technique (SET), which is basically a mixture of existing usability test methods.

2 Theoretical Background and Related Work

This section provides a short overview about the basic concept of consistency and describes two usability testing methods: Focused Heuristic Evaluation and the NPL Performance Measurement, which have been in use individually prior to their inclusion in the Shadow Expert Technique.

2.1 The Three-Dimensional Model of User Interface Consistency

Interface consistency has been studied for quite a long time, actually since Graphical User Interfaces (GUIs) began to be used widely, under the premise that a worker who is able to predict what the system will do in any given situation and can rely on the rules will be more efficient [6]. Consequently, the focus of research was on worker's productivity in order to achieve higher throughput and fewer errors. As a result of this goal, most early studies were on job performance of office workers, i.e. error rate and time to perform a task. The latter is the typical Human–Computer Interaction (HCI) approach and is usually considered in a transfer paradigm in which: *the higher the similarity between two tasks, the higher the transfer, hence the consistency* [7].

However, a strict establishment of the primary places of where consistency is most necessary, is difficult. Grudin (1989) [4] separated consistency into *internal* interface consistency and *external* interface consistency, wherein internal refers to consistency within a task and external means consistency among various tasks. Ozok & Salvendy (2000) [8] classified it into three sub types, establishing the *three-dimensional model of interface consistency:*

1) conceptual consistency (language, stereotypes, task concept, skill transfer, output consistency, hierarchical order of concept, etc.);
2) communicational consistency (moving between screens, menus, user conventions, between-task consistency, distinction of tasks and objects, etc.); and
3) physical consistency (color, size, shape, location, spacing, symbols, etc.).

Ad 1) *Conceptual consistency* can be defined as the consistency of metaphor applied to an interface feature or an action that is embodied within a feature. Frequent and inconsistent use of synonyms, instead of using the same words for the same items, is unhelpful. Leaving something to students' conception and interpretation due to lack of explicitness is also regarded as conceptual inconsistency [4], [8].

Ad 2) *Communicational consistency* can be defined as the consistency of both input and output of the interface. It deals with how the user interacts with the computer interface and whether the means of interaction are consistent for fulfilling the same or similar tasks.

Ad 3) *Physical consistency* can be defined as the consistency of the visual appearance of an interface feature and indicates that the features are supposed to be consistent with the users mental models [9].

Although this has been known for quite a long time, research on the relationship between *consistency and human learning processes* has only recently been documented, and Satzinger & Olfman (1998) [10] pointed out that very few studies have investigated the effects of interface consistency on learning performance. Many questions still remain as to the effectiveness of interface design in enhancing learning and since designers are currently able to include a wide range of various visual elements, the complexity of design decisions is steadily increasing and most design decisions are not made on a scientific basis. To design an appropriate user interface demands insight into the *behaviour of the end users* and the application of user centered development [11], [12], [13], in order to achieve a true interaction. This is definitely important, since learning with interactive media is generally highly demanding from the perspective of the limited cognitive processing capabilities of the end users [14], [15]. Daily practice shows that many end users have difficulty learning with electronic systems, since they are often unable to form a mental model of the system and their current position within its complexity. However, when striving for a design following the "principle of the least surprise", we are faced with the problem that designers and developers rarely are able to predict exactly what the end users really expect (remember Steve Krug [16]: "Don't make me think!").

2.2 Focused Heuristic Evaluation

A Heuristic evaluation (HE) is an *inspection* method (for a overview on methods see [17]) to improve the usability of an interface by checking it against established standards [18], [19] [20]. The basic idea is to have usability experts examine the interface of a system according to a list of pre-determined heuristics. Each usability expert has to perform the evaluation with complete independence from each other.

They do not share their results or findings until they are all finished with their respective evaluations. The purpose of this independence is to assure an objective and unbiased evaluation. During an evaluation process each evaluator goes through the entire interface and checks if the interface complies with the pre-determined list of heuristics. The number of necessary evaluations is still debated, however, Nielsen (1992) [21] recommends to use from three to five evaluators. So far the outcome depends on the used list of heuristics. Usually these heuristics cover diverse or general design issues and system behavior. In the case of a **Focused** Heuristic Evaluation, one single issue (here consistency) is chosen and a list of appropriate heuristics is generated and used for evaluation [22].

2.3 NPL Performance Measurement Method

A performance test is a rigorous usability evaluation of a working system [5], [23]. In order for the performance test to gather realistic and precise information of the working system, the performance test must take place under realistic conditions (ideally in the real context, see figure 1) with real end users. Usually 12 to 20 test persons are sufficient to get reliable data [24]. Each trial of the test is video recorded and screen captures in order to provide a good documentation for the gathered data. A Performance Test identifies issues that influence the performance of an end user, including time, effectiveness and user efficiency [25]. This enables the comparison of different designs or design steps in an iterative development circle. Usually the Performance Test also addresses user satisfaction with the current system.

The NPL (National Physical Laboratory) Performance Measurement Method focuses on the quality and degree of work goal achievement in terms of task performance achievement of frequent and critical task goals by end users in a context simulating the work environment [26], [27], [28], [29], [30]. User performance is specified and assessed by measures including task effectiveness (the quantity and quality of task performance) and User efficiency (effectiveness divided by task time). Measures are obtained with users performing tasks in a context of evaluation which matches the intended context of use (figure 1) [29], [31]. Casually speaking, the test person

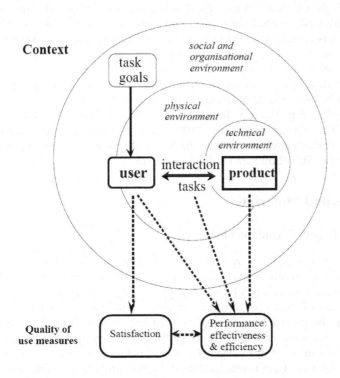

Fig. 1. According to Nigel Bevan (1995) [35] Performance consists of Effectiveness and Efficiency and is directly related with satisfaction

performs tasks, whereby the time is measured and a video is taken. Test persons are not allowed to talk with the facilitator, instead they are instructed to accomplish the tasks as fast as possible. Measures of core indicators of usability can be obtained, as defined in ISO 9241-11 [26], [32], [33], [34] e.g. user effectiveness, efficiency and satisfaction. It is possible to compare these measures with the requirements. These measures are directly related to productivity and business goals. In this study the metrics Task Effectiveness, User Efficiency, Relative User Efficiency and User Satisfaction were derived. Task Effectiveness (TES) determines how correctly and completely the goals have been achieved in the context of the task. In most cases there's more than one way to accomplish a task and every task has several steps, as it's not meaningful to test single click actions - instead the use of the systems main functions is compiled in a task. TES is a function of quantity and quality of the task.

Quantity is measured objectively as the percentage of the control parameters, which have been altered from their default values by the end of the task. Quality consists of the definition of an optimal path, with weighted alternatives and penalty actions (e.g. help or explorative search). Quantity and Quality are measured as percentage values, so the resulting TES is also a percentage value. The value of TES is obtained by measuring quantity and quality and application of the formula TES = 1/100 (Quantity x Quality). User Efficiency (UE) relates effectiveness to costs in terms of time, e.g. if a task can be completed in a high quality AND fast, then the efficiency is high. UE provides here the absolute measure for the comparison of the five tasks of this study, carried out by the same users, on the same product in the same environment. It is calculated as the ratio between the effectiveness in carrying out the task and the time it takes to complete the task using UE = Task Effectiveness / Task Time. The Relative User Efficiency (RUE) is a metric that can be employed by the relation of a particular group of users compared to fully trained and experienced user of the product being tested. It is defined as the ratio of the efficiency of any user and the efficiency of an expert user in the same context RUE = (User TES / Expert TES) * (Expert Task Time / User Task Time) *100. The User satisfaction is derived with a standardized questionnaire, for example the SUMI (Software Usability Measurement Inventory) [36] or SUS (Software Usability Scale) [37].

3   Methods and Materials

3.1   Shadow Expert Technique Flow

The first step (see flowchart figure 2) was to analyze the interface of the system in the role as consistency experts in order to find as much inconsistencies as possible. The Focused Heuristic Evaluation (FHE) was applied - the focus being on consistency. The result of the FHE was a list of general inconsistency issues, ordered by severity.

Considering the most severe inconsistency issues, as well as the LMS main features, tasks for the performance test were gathered. Two independent teams derived these tasks. The reason for this independency is to obtain more objective results from the evaluators later on. Both teams conducted the performance test with seven different subjects each. Subsequently, they analyzed the tests to determine a subject with average results. For the SET an end user with average results is needed in order to

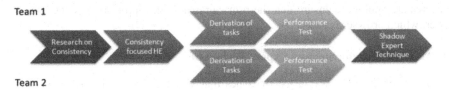

Fig. 2. The way from the research to the Shadow Expert Technique

provide a representative end user behavior. Once this was achieved the two teams exchanged the video and screen records of this subject and carried out the SET.

3.2 Focus on Consistency

Five evaluators examined the interface of the LMS based on a defined heuristic list. The output of this process was a list of issues that violated the consistency heuristics. The following section will outline the different relevant viewpoints on consistency, which lead to a set of applicable heuristics. A short table form of the heuristics can be found at the end of this section (see figure 3).

3.2.1 Principle of Least Surprise (POLS)

A golden rule in interface design is the Principle of Least Surprise (POLS). According to Geoffrey James "A user interface should be arranged in a way that the user experiences as few surprises as possible". It is a psychological fact, that humans can pay considerable attention only to one thing at one time (locus of attention) [38]. In many cases this is difficult for the software engineers, since they usually think in functional terms of the system and have difficulty putting himself in the end user's position (often the end users are not known). Moreover, different users have varying expectations.

3.2.2 Expectation Conformity (Playful Consistency)

This means that already learned techniques can likewise be applied anywhere in an application. One could also say that 'everything' must be conclusive (see DIN ISO 9241-10 Ergonomic demands for office activities with screen devices – part 10: principles of dialogue formation, expectation conformity) [39]. Accordingly a dialogue is conform to expectations if it is consistent and matches the characteristics of the user (user mental models, previous knowledge, expertise, education, literacy, experience etc.) as well as common acknowledged conventions. Operation cycles, symbols and the arrangement of information should be consistent within the application, match the gained knowledge of the user and should thus be conform to expectations. For example status declarations of the dialogue system are emitted at the same place or pressing the same button ends a dialogue. So, the dialogue behavior and information display are uniform within the dialogue system and thus consistent.

3.2.3 Browser Consistency

Concerning the UI design of websites and web applications, it is particularly the varied display in the different browsers, which plays an important role. The continuous uniform appearance as well as the same reaction to a given action (in all different kinds of browsers) could be subsumed under the term browser consistency. These measures are applied to ensure that the user can handle the application or the site, no matter, which browser is used.

3.3 Materials for the Shadow Expert Technique

The output of the FHE was a list of issues that violated the consistency heuristics. From the list of issues we selected the most severe ones and used them to derive tasks for a performance test. This approach enables insight into the influence of these issues in a realistic context and get as much relevant results as possible. The subjects had to be also as realistic as possible, which is why we defined a test subject profile. As the learning platform is targeted at the use at university level, we set the profile for our test subjects according, to be students with some basic IT knowledge.

Consistency	Description	Evaluation
Expectation conformity (playful consistency)	I expect to be logged out if I click on "logout" – in the entire application, no matter in which context.	1 – 5 (fully met - not met)
Visual consistency	The design (typeface, colors, styles etc.) should be consistent within the application.	1 – 5 (fully met - not met)
Hyperlink consistency	Hyperlinks should not be a dead-end-street ("death links"). Furthermore, links should always behave the same way: this means, for example, that external links should always be opened in a new window, while internal links should always be opened in the same window.	1 – 5 (fully met - not met)
Linguistic consistency	If the application is available in several languages, there should be no mixture of languages.	1 – 5 (fully met - not met)
Browser consistency	The used browser should not limit the application. Furthermore, the browser should not significantly alter the appearance of the application (typefaces, colors, positioning of the different elements).	1 – 5 (fully met - not met)

Fig. 3. List of Consistency Heuristics

It is important, that the test users corresponded to the target group to avoid rough outliers in the analysis phase. Before deriving the tasks we divided our team into two groups in order to work completely independent from each other. This also meant that the two groups had a different set of tasks that were to be used on the performance test, and that both groups had absolutely no knowledge of each others tasks. Each group tested the system on seven subjects. The tasks were chosen so that the complete set of tasks would take the user no longer than 15 minutes. At the beginning of the test each subject was briefed on the process. They had a limited amount of time for each task, and did not receive any assistance whatsoever from our part. If a subject would exceed the time limit, they were told to move to the next task.

The user test environment was a Laptop with Windows XP, standard mouse and keyboard. As the learning management system is of course an online product, we used Internet Explorer 6 as browser.

All 14 trials of the performance test were recorded with webcam and screen recorder software. Techsmith Camtasia Studio [40] (http://ww.techsmith.com) was used. This tool synchronically recorded the computer screen during the test, as well as the test subjects upper body and face. Later on this allowed screening the subjects expressions with a Picture-in-Picture (PnP) view as can be seen in Fig. 2.

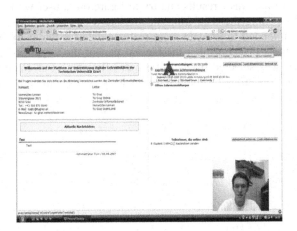

Fig. 4. Example screen recording with picture-in-picture

3.4 Methodology

The SET method has three phases: 1) preparation, 2) discussion and 3) analysis. SET is a multilevel-method in which two teams of experts try to understand the interaction processes of an end user, in order to derive suggestions for improvement. The primary goal of SET is to explore the users behavior by observation and discussion. Therefore synchronized screen recordings and video material of the user were used, without sound in order to recognize the end users inner state (e.g. frustration) from mimic, gestures and interactions with the systems. This enables the evaluator to see the system through the end users eyes and provides an in-depth understanding of occurring problems. Through iterative stop&go video review and discussion, this understanding grows to a point where simple and efficient solutions were gained during the discussion. The videos from the average users had a length of approximately 15 minutes. During the SET discussion session we produced four videos of the expert reviews and discussions (two reviews per group) that were transcribed in a final step. The length of the session videos varies, depending on the actual pass: The first round takes app. as long as the video from the average user (15 minutes), while the second round took in our case about 30 minutes. The entire SET discussion session lasted 4 hours including preparation time and debriefing.

3.4.1 SET Preparation Phase

In the preparation phase each expert-team must run a performance test as described in the section before. Both teams define the tasks for the performance test separately on base of a heuristic evaluation. The subjects should meet the requirements of the target user profile. Important is that screen records and videos of the subjects face are done during the performance test. We recommend using synchronized picture-in-picture screen recording.

These recordings will be exchanged between the groups later. After conducting the test both teams evaluate their results and try to figure out a user with average overall efficiency results. Using the data from an average user rather from a very good or very bad user is intended to provide more realistic data for the analysis than outliers and thus covers most problems that the biggest part of the target group would have. The average user was selected by the total user efficiency. For calculating the total user efficiency and selecting the data for the analysis we used the following formulas:

$$user\ efficiency\ task_x = \frac{effectivness}{t_{task}/t_{max}}$$

$$total\ user\ efficiency_x = \sum_{i=1}^{\sum tasks} user\ efficiency\ task_{x_i}$$

$$user\ efficiency\ intersection = \frac{\sum_{i=1}^{\sum user} efficiency_i}{number\ of\ users}$$

The *effectiveness* describes the success per task in % (e.g. Log in 30%, Find the chat and send a message via it 60%, Go back to the start screen 10% != 100%). If a user failed a partial task like "Go back to the start screen", he got a point deduction - in that case 10%.

The value t_{task} corresponds to the time the user needed for the task, and the value t_{max} corresponds to the maximum time for the task. The intersection task efficiencies results in the *total user efficiency* for every user. The *user efficiency intersection* calculates the average efficiency over all users. The subject with *total user efficiency* nearest to the *user efficiency intersection* was selected for SET screening. After these initiatory steps the discussion phase of the Shadow Expert Technique can be executed. For this purpose, both teams need to take a session together.

3.4.2 SET Discussion Phase

The technical requirements for the discussion phase are a laptop for replaying the recordings, a beamer for better review of the expert team and a video camera for recording the SET discussion session, thus collecting all discussed problems and solutions. Additional, we recommend a screen recording of the session on the laptop, in order to be able to understand what was spoken about, when the SET session is transcribed and analyzed later on. The roles of the discussion team are moderator, 2-4 experts and a scribe. These roles and tasks of the participants change during the discussion session.

In the first step, the teams exchange the videos of their average user. Now the first team starts with the review of the video from the other team. The review team must consist of 2-4 persons. During the whole session every reviewer first guesses the task, then commentates problems and anticipates following actions in the interaction process.

One external person must take over the role of the moderator in order to lead the discussion to a productive point. While the review team analyzes the video, at least one of the other team must log the main predicates of the session. The discussion is recorded on video for later transcription. As mentioned before, no one of the review team knows the tasks from the other team, and so in the first round the SET discussion is focused on the task detection. The PnP screen record of the average user is thereby viewed one time and without sound. If the review team can't identify a task in the first round, the other team explains the task in the next pass. It also must be said, that the number of the session passes is not limited, but at least two are required. The more passes are recorded, the more insights may be won. In our case, we recorded two passes per team. An important role during the sessions takes the moderator. In the first round, he has to guide the discussion towards the task detection, and to summarize the possible task.

In the second round the SET discussion should specifically pay attention to the behavior and expressions of the user, to get more information about his expectations, intentions and thoughts during the task completion - especially when he has a problem. Another question that arises at this point is: Has the user completed the task or not? If the second round doesn't generate satisfactory results, this process can be repeated as often as necessary. In this round(s), the moderator has to lead up the discussion towards some problem solving approaches. So the moderator has a continually steering function, and he is also responsible for ensuring that the team will not waste too much time on one problem.

A help for the reviewers to comment and anticipate the interactions may be first problem oriented statements like *The user does ... because he thinks / perceives / feels ...* These statements may then be reversed in order to generate solutions, e.g. *In order to prevent that the user ... thinks / perceives / feels etc. ...* Another solution oriented statement could be *In order to support the user ... thinking / perceiving / feeling etc. a possible solution would be...* and so on.

The result of this iterative review process is a list of improvements for single steps in an interaction process. From the detailed review of single steps may also general improvements derived. However the generated solutions still need to be refined from the scribe's notes and the video recordings of the discussion session. The teams change their actions after team 1 finishes step 2 of the discussion, thus team 2 analyzing the data of team 1 now, while team 1 takes notes. Figure 5 summarizes the actions to be taken in the different steps.

3.4.3 SET Analysis Phase

The last step in the SET method is the analysis phase. Here the video recordings of the discussion phase are transcribed in order to refine and consolidate the findings from the discussion. Significant statements are investigated further. Each group transcribes the video of the other group, thereby analyzing their own data. The outcome is a list of problems and recommendations. This list should give the developers an insight into the thoughts of the user, to improve the system in a further consequence. In the most optimal case, developers are part of the evaluation teams.

Team	Roles	Discussion Step 1	Discussion Step 2	Analyse
Team 1	Expert 1 Expert 2 Expert 3	First review of video from team 2, find out unknown tasks	second review of video, comment behavior, anticipate interactions	
Team 2	Expert 1 Expert 2 Expert 3	scribe, take notes of guesses for tasks, no help for guesses at this point	scribe, help with task definitions, take notes of main discussion points	Transcribe session from video of discussion, refine results
	Moderator	focus discussion on task identification, summarize, conclude	focus discussion on problems and solutions, observable behavior, summarize, conclude	

Fig. 5. Summary of actions in the SET discussion and analysis phase

4   Results and Discussion

According to a predefined user profile it was limited to the areas and tasks, which are accessible by students. FHE revealed a comprehensive list of issues according to the predefined heuristics (see an sample extract in figure 6). Naturally these issues are based on assumptions and thus provide only hypothetical and limited insight into the underlying problems.

However, they provided a starting point for further investigation, as we used them for defining tasks for the following performance test. The performance test provided us with screen recordings and video records of the subjects during the trials. Selected records of average users were then reviewed, commented and analyzed.

While the Focused Heuristic Evaluation anticipates and explains general possible issues, the Performance Test shows real issues, however without explanation. The Shadow Expert Technique reveals the reason for real issues and provides solutions. Problems and flaws in the interaction design become visible. The art of discussing the users inner states while observing his behavior, combined with the possibility to review the actions again and in detail may prove valuable for user experience design. The outcome of the SET was a comprehensive discussion of problems and a list of tiny but effective improvements that should satisfy the needs and expectations of the biggest part of the users. We expected to discuss in the SET at least some of the issues detected in the Focused Heuristic Evaluation, however we found that the SET reveals problems and solutions on a deeper and more detailed level than the generalized assumptions of the FHE. Compared to the Thinking Aloud Method the SET reveals

Nr.	Title	Description	Image	Severity
1	Logout	The way to logout is always different.	1,2,3,4,5,6	3
2	RSS	The RSS button is in a different place in every room.	1,2,3,4,5,6	2
3	Position Sidebar	The Sidebar is not in a constant place.	1,2,3,4,5,6	3
4	Right Sidebar	The right sidebar is only available in the course main page.	1,3,4,5,6	1
5	SMS	The SMS button is only available in the course main page.	1,3,4,5,6	2
6	Mobiler Zugang	The Mobiler Zugang button is only available in the course main page.	1,3,4,5,6	1
7	Back Course Page	This link disappears on the FAQ room and on the chat room.	5,6	3
8	Hauptmenü Button	The button does the same, but is described differently.	5,6	2

Fig. 6. A sample extraction of the list of problems found

more objective data as tiny parts of an interaction process are reviewed in depth. While Thinking Aloud provides information on subjective experiences and recommendations from users, the SET method is based on objective observation of behavior and subjective simulation of the users inner states, in order to anticipate emotions and further courses of interaction.

5 Conclusion and Future Research

In this paper, we have presented a new usability test method called Shadow Expert Technique (SET). We described the path from our research on consistency to the results for the developers. One of the biggest advantages is the more natural and less intrusive interaction of the user with the system in comparison to more conventional methods, such as the thinking aloud test. Advantages include: its timesaving properties, the performance test only lasts 15 minutes per person, subjective properties, it enables you to see the system through the users eyes and to get a feeling for their expectations. Consequently, developers can gain helpful insight on user issues by stepping through single interaction processes of the system. Optimizing these interactions result in a significantly improved usability and acceptability.

Future research on the SET may include the data resulting from a Thinking Aloud Method as well as a Performance Test. Thereby enabling the comparison of comments by the experts calmly reviewing the video in retrospect, and the comments of the user thus revealing the degree of discrepancy between the users' perception and the expert reviewing the users' actions.

This combination of the users' and the experts' comments, issues and solutions, provides the foundation of improvement, leading to successful interaction, increased accessibility and an eventual increase in learners acceptance.

Acknowledgements

We cordially thank the following students of the lecture 706.046 "AK Human-Computer Interaction: Applying User Centered Design" for their enthusiasm in carrying out the evaluations: Claus Bürbaumer, Marco Garcia, Daniela Mellacher and Thomas Gebhard.

References

1. Chu, L.F., Chan, B.K.: Evolution of web site design: implications for medical education on the Internet. Computers in Biology and Medicine 28(5), 459–472 (1998)
2. Shneiderman, B.: Designing the User Interface. Strategies for effective Human-Computer Interaction, 3rd edn. Addison-Wesley, Reading (1997)
3. Rubinstein, R., Hersh, H.: The human factor. Digital Press, Bedford (1984)
4. Grudin, J.: The Case against User Interface Consistency. Communications of the ACM 32(10), 1164–1173 (1989)
5. Rhee, C., Moon, J., Choe, Y.: Web interface consistency in e-learning. Online Information Review 30(1), 53–69 (2006)
6. Nielsen, J.: Coordinating User Interfaces for Consistency. The Morgan Kaufmann Series in Interactive Technologies. Morgan Kaufmann, San Francisco (2001)
7. Tanaka, T., Eberts, R.E., Salvendy, G.: Consistency of Human-Computer Interface Design - Quantification and Validation. Human Factors 33(6), 653–676 (1991)
8. Ozok, A.A., Salvendy, G.: Measuring consistency of web page design and its effects on performance and satisfaction. Ergonomics 43(4), 443–460 (2000)
9. Satzinger, J.W.: The effects of conceptual consistency on the end user's mental models of multiple applications. Journal of End User Computing 10(3), 3–14 (1998)
10. Satzinger, J.W., Olfman, L.: User interface consistency across end-user applications: the effects on mental models. Journal of Management Information Systems 14(4), 167–193 (1998)
11. Norman, D.A., Draper, S.: User Centered System Design. Erlbaum, Hillsdale (1986)
12. Holzinger, A.: User-Centered Interface Design for disabled and elderly people: First experiences with designing a patient communication system (PACOSY). In: Miesenberger, K., Klaus, J., Zagler, W.L. (eds.) ICCHP 2002. LNCS, vol. 2398, pp. 33–41. Springer, Heidelberg (2002)
13. Norman, D.A.: Cognitive engineering. In: Norman, D., Draper, S. (eds.) User Centered System Design: New Perspectives on Human-Computer interaction. Erlbaum, Mahwah (1986)
14. Holzinger, A., Kickmeier-Rust, M., Albert, D.: Dynamic Media in Computer Science Education; Content Complexity and Learning Performance: Is Less More? Educational Technology & Society 11(1), 279–290 (2008)
15. Holzinger, A., Kickmeier-Rust, M.D., Wassertheurer, S., Hessinger, M.: Learning performance with interactive simulations in medical education: Lessons learned from results of learning complex physiological models with the HAEMOdynamics SIMulator. Computers & Education 52(2), 292–301 (2009)

16. Krug, S.: Don't Make Me Think: A Common Sense Approach to Web Usability. New Riders, Indianapolis (2000)
17. Holzinger, A.: Usability Engineering for Software Developers. Communications of the ACM 48(1), 71–74 (2005)
18. Nielsen, J., Molich, R.: Heuristic evaluation of user interfaces. In: CHI 1990, pp. 249–256. ACM, New York (1990)
19. Kamper, R.J.: Extending the usability of heuristics for design and evaluation: Lead, follow get out of the way. International Journal of Human-Computer Interaction 14(3-4), 447–462 (2002)
20. Hvannberg, E.T., Law, E.L.C., Larusdottir, M.K.: Heuristic evaluation: Comparing ways of finding and reporting usability problems. Interacting with Computers 19(2), 225–240 (2007)
21. Nielsen, J.: Finding usability problems through heuristic evaluation. In: CHI 1992, pp. 373–380 (1992)
22. Javahery, H., Seffah, A.: Refining the usability engineering toolbox: lessons learned from a user study on a visualization tool. In: Holzinger, A. (ed.) USAB 2007. LNCS, vol. 4799, pp. 185–198. Springer, Heidelberg (2007)
23. Bailey, R.W., Wolfson, C.A., Nall, J., Koyani, S.: Performance-Based Usability Testing: Metrics That Have the Greatest Impact for Improving a System's Usability. In: Kurosu, M. (ed.) Human Centered Design HCII 2009. LNCS, vol. 5619, pp. 3–12. Springer, Heidelberg (2009)
24. Virzi, R.A.: Refining the test phase of usability evaluation: how many subjects is enough? Human Factors 34(4), 457–468 (1992)
25. Nielsen, J.: Usability Metrics: Tracking Interface Improvements. IEEE Software 13(6), 12–13 (1996)
26. Bevan, N.: Measuring Usability as Quality of Use. Software Quality Journal 4(2), 115–130 (1995)
27. Thomas, C., Bevan, N.: Usability Context Analysis: A Practical Guide. National Physical Laboratory, Teddington (1996)
28. Bevan, N.: Quality in Use: Incorporating Human Factors into the Software Engineering Lifecycle. In: 3rd International Software Engineering Standards Symposium (ISESS 1997), pp. 169–179 (1997)
29. Macleod, M., Bowden, R., Bevan, N., Curson, I.: The MUSiC performance measurement method. Behaviour & Information Technology 16(4-5), 279–293 (1997)
30. Bevan, N.: Extending Quality in Use to Provide a Framework for Usability Measurement. In: Kurosu, M. (ed.) Human Centered Design HCII 2009. LNCS, vol. 5619, pp. 13–22. Springer, Heidelberg (2009)
31. Stickel, C., Scerbakov, A., Kaufmann, T., Ebner, M.: Usability Metrics of Time and Stress - Biological Enhanced Performance Test of a University Wide Learning Management System. In: Holzinger, A. (ed.) 4th Symposium of the Workgroup Human-Computer Interaction and Usability Engineering of the Austrian-Computer-Society, pp. 173–184. Springer, Berlin (2008)
32. Seffah, A., Metzker, E.: The obstacles and myths of usability and software engineering. Communications of the ACM 47(12), 71–76 (2004)
33. Seffah, A., Donyaee, M., Kline, R.B., Padda, H.K.: Usability measurement and metrics: A consolidated model. Software Quality Journal 14(2), 159–178 (2006)
34. Holzinger, A., Searle, G., Kleinberger, T., Seffah, A., Javahery, H.: Investigating Usability Metrics for the Design and Development of Applications for the Elderly. In: Miesenberger, K., Klaus, J., Zagler, W.L., Karshmer, A.I. (eds.) ICCHP 2008. LNCS, vol. 5105, pp. 98–105. Springer, Heidelberg (2008)

35. Bevan, N.: Usability is Quality of Use. In: Anzai, Y., Ogawa, K., Mori, H. (eds.) 6th International Conference on Human Computer Interaction. Elsevier, Amsterdam (1995)
36. Kirakowski, J., Corbett, M.: SUMI: The Software Usability Measurement Inventory. British Journal of Educational Technology 24(3), 210–212 (1993)
37. Brooke, J.: SUS: A "quick and dirty" usability scale. In: Jordan, P.W., Thomas, B., Weerdmeester, B.A., McClelland, A.L. (eds.) Usability Evaluation in Industry. Taylor & Francis, Abington (1996)
38. Raskin, J.: The Humane Interface: New Directions for Designing Interactive Systems. Addison-Wesley-Longman, Boston (2000)
39. Harbich, S., Auer, S.: Rater bias: The influence of hedonic quality on usability questionnaires. In: Costabile, M.F., Paternó, F. (eds.) INTERACT 2005. LNCS, vol. 3585, pp. 1129–1133. Springer, Heidelberg (2005)
40. Smith, L.A., Turner, E.: Using Camtasia to develop and enhance online learning: tutorial presentation. Journal of Computing Sciences in Colleges 22(5), 121–122 (2007)

Accessibility of Educational Software:
A Problem Still to Be Solved

Giovanni Paolo Caruso and Lucia Ferlino

Istituto Tecnologie Didattiche - Consiglio Nazionale delle Ricerche, Genova
{caruso,ferlino}@itd.cnr.it

Abstract. In recent years the issue of accessibility of digital resources has been increasingly studied by the world of research, training, associations and law-makers. If educational software is built without keeping in mind the principles of Design for all, might be considered a new obstacle to learning and an occasion to highlight the limits and not the potential of disabled people. Starting from this, we have carried out a survey among more than four thousand (italian and foreign) educational softwares available on our Educational Software Documentation Service. The result - as one could predict - shows that there are very few software products that can be used for educational purposes which completely satisfy the main accessibility criteria.

Keywords: E-inclusion, Software, Accessibility, Usability, Open Source.

1   Introduction

Some time ago, we wrote: "The accessibility[1] of Information Technology is a concrete problem which can drastically reduce the learning possibilities of certain categories of students; this is reflected in educational practice also due to the fact that nowadays teachers are to be aware of this matter and bear it in mind when choosing the software to be used in class. [...] So if, on one hand, accessibility is a highly relevant topic for teachers who are requested, on an institutional level, to make correct operational choices, on the other hand it is a sensitive matter for software developers too, who are formally obliged to follow some fundamental rules to guarantee the accessibility of their products."[3][Bocconi et al., 2006]. Based on these considerations, we carried out a survey among more than four thousand educational softwares available on our Educational Software

---

[1] Definition of Accessibility from the glossary of Italian law no. 4/2004 "Accessibility is the ability of information technology, in the forms and limits allowed for by technological know-how, to supply services and give usable information, without discrimination, also to those who, because of their disability, need assistive technology or special configuration".

A. Holzinger and K. Miesenberger (Eds.): USAB 2009, LNCS 5889, pp. 193–208, 2009.
© Springer-Verlag Berlin Heidelberg 2009

Documentation Service.[2] The result, predictably, showed that there are very few software products that can be used for educational purposes which completely satisfy the main accessibility criteria. This conclusion spurred us to ask ourselves various questions, for which we found replies by making a detailed analysis of the data in our possession. Our curiosity drove us to examine, in particular, if there were noticeable differences between commercial software and free[3] and open source[4] software, given that the latter, by its very nature can be easily modified, if this is necessary. But before setting out the results of our survey and the considerations involved, we believe it is useful to make a brief digression into the topic of accessibility and to explain the context in which our analysis took place.

2   Accessibility: A Recent Awareness

In recent years the issue of accessibility of digital resources has been increasingly studied by the world of research, training, associations and law-makers.[5] "The Information Society is rapidly becoming an essential part of economic, educational and social life [...]. For this reason, disabled people's access to products and services based on The Information Society is a highly important matter, in order to allow and ease their integration into society", as maintained in the European Action Plan eEurope. The topic is treated in the disabled people's Universal Rights Convention, which even in its preface recognises "the importance of accessibility in physical, social, economic and cultural environments as well as health, education, information and communication, in order to allow disabled people to fully enjoy human rights and fundamental freedoms." [5] [Gubbels, Kemppainen, 2002] Universal Access is now considered a fundamental objective for most developed countries[6][Klironomos et al., 2006] to meet in the near

---

[2] As from 1999 in agreement with the Ministry of Education, it is an "outsourced service regarding documentation and advice on Educational Software" (http://sd2.itd.cnr.it) with 2 main objectives:
   - Allowing teachers access to objective information on the availability, features, and practicalities of software products which can be used in education.
   - Helping teachers to develop operative skills as regards the use of educational software, so that they are better informed to choose products and to plan educational programmes based on the use of software.

[3] From Wikipedia: Free software is software released with a licence which allows anyone to use it and its study, change and redistribution is encouraged. Because of its features it contrasts with proprietary software and is different from the concept of open source, being focused on the user's freedom and not only on the opening of the source code.

[4] From Wikipedia: In IT, open source indicates a software whose authors (more precisely the rights holders) allow and in fact encourage its free study and modification by other independent programmers. This is done by applying special use licences.

[5] Even though since the 70's specific indications had been included in a law paragraph (Section 508 of the American 1973 "Workforce Rehabilitation Act").

future, and this concept refers to almost all aspects of social life, including education [4][Bocker et al., 2005]. In this context the role of Assistive Technologies (AT's) in synergy with Communication and Information technologies, appears decisive in guaranteeing disabled people access to computer equipment. There have been many efforts made on an international level (WCAG and WAI, e-inclusion actions within eEurope, Law no. 4/2004[6] in Italy) in order to make websites accessible; in many countries some special Guidelines have been drawn up to show how to render information and material available on Internet accessible. In Italy Law no. 4/2004 was issued, which contains a detailed description of the requirements that web sites (Enclosure A of the law 22 requirements) and off the shelf products (Enclosure D of the law 11 requirements) must possess in order to be considered accessible (see Table 1). The law indicates for each requirement the specific references to Section 508 (in force in USA) and to WCAG 1.0 (which is an international standard), thus matching the existing international trends.

Table 1. Summary of the 11 requirements of Law 4/2004

Requirement	Short description
1	Accessible from the keyboard
2	Compatible with the operative system's accessibility features
3	Reading of interface objects by the AT's
4	Meaning of graphic symbols
5	Means of presenting text content
6	Presence of visual or textual equivalents in correspondence with audio items
7	Non uniqueness of the information/communication channel
8	Preservation of the display settings defined by the user
9	Flashing items featured
10	Recognition and operation within focus
11	Accessibility of documentation

In particular, article 5 of this law (Accessibility of educational and training tools) is directed to schools:

1. The present law's provisions are to be applied also to educational and training material used in schools of every rank and level.

2. The agreements drawn up between the Education, University and Research Ministries and editorial associations for suppliers of school libraries always provide for supply of copies of fundamental educational materials in digital format, which are accessible to disabled pupils and assistant teachers, as far as budget constraints allow for. During 2006, the Ministry of Education launched the project New Technologies and Disability, constructed around 7 actions, one of which the 3 "Accessibility of Educational software", following law no. 4/2004,

---

[6] Law no. 2/2004, converted into decree 8/2005, shows, in line with international standards, the Instructions to encourage the access of Disabled people to IT material.

was entrusted to the Institute of Educational Technologies (ITD)[7] of the National Research Council (CNR) in Genoa. On this occasion, the ITD designed a system for evaluating the compliance of software, on a technical level, with each of the 11 requirements of enclosure D of law no.4/2004. The appraisal also produced a concise verdict consisting of 5 levels (accessibility level) for each of the four types of disability examined (physical disability, deafness, partial sight, blindness). The aim[8] was to supply useful information to teachers when choosing software to be used with the whole class, including a disabled pupil, by means of the Educational Software Documentation Service Website. Finally on 30th April 2008, in Italy, a Decree was published which dictates the technical rules regulating accessibility to educational and training tools for disabled pupils (GU n. 136 dated 12-6-2008). In particular, enclosure B sets forth the guidelines for educational software accessibility for disabled pupils. This enclosure shows a series of factors to be considered when designing educational software, whilst complying with the 11 accessibility requirements defined in enclosure D of law 4/2004. Now all the necessary elements in order to create accessible products have been supplied, this means that the road has been marked out, all we now need to do is follow it.

3   Accessible Educational Software: Why Must It Be Made So?

If it is built without keeping in mind the principles of "Design for all"[9], educational software might be considered a new obstacle to learning and an occasion to highlight the limits and not the potential of disabled people[3][Bocconi et al., 2006].

Let's consider in detail, with the help of some examples, what kind of accessibility problems educational software may present.

If in a class where a deaf pupil is present, software is employed which uses in its interface only an audio channel, over and above the visual channel (pictures) without a textual format, a barrier to reaching educational goals is created and at the same time discrimination between deaf users and the other users too. In this case, the use of technology instead of helping learning, highlights the limits relative to a deficit.

If in a class there is a partially sighted student who uses assistive technology such as a magnifier, which allows him to see only a part of the screen magnified

---

[7] http://www.itd.cnr.it

[8] Action 3 also had another 2 objectives closely linked between them:

- Make aware and inform schools about problems linked to accessibility in educational and management software used the various school activities.

- Encourage innovation by schools as regards accessible documents and learning units. The results can be found on the project website: http://asd.itd.cnr.it/

[9] "Design for all" assumes that human beings are not all equal and thus when we imagine, we design, we create anything, we must think of the needs of everyone who will use it. Further details are available on-line:
http://www.pubbliaccesso.gov.it/biblioteca/documentazione/

at a time, the teacher must pay attention to the choice of programs which require having vision as a whole to reach educational goals, in order to avoid limiting the chances of their use. An activity such as completing a puzzle which requires manual skills (as well logical and visual/spatial skills) cannot be executed in a traditional way by people who are physically handicapped in their upper limbs. Technology aids us, making available various electronic puzzles, which may even be the only the only chance to play and the only chance to carry out an activity which is useful for cognitive development. But instead, if there are cognitive problems, even "simple" software such as puzzles can create new obstacles. They may show a complex interface, difficult to manage, requiring a hard cognitive effort from the student to organise his thoughts in order to be able to find his way around a large number of pieces with very similar sizes and shapes. Furthermore, having to place a piece using only the mouse and not a touch screen could cause further problems.

The situations mentioned above are aimed to allow consideration of the problems a teacher may have to face or bear in mind when choosing software. A software in order to be used without discrimination must be accessible and usable by all. It must be compatible with assistive technologies which help some "categories" of disabled people, workable using the keyboard and not only the mouse, allow good legibility of the information contained on the screen, and it must use various information/communication channels when interacting with the user. These principles correspond with the four macro-categories which gave rise to the 11 requirements of Law no.4/2004[3][Bocconi et al, 2006].

4 Accessibility: From Theory to Practice

Among the tasks entrusted to ITD as part of Action 3, as previously mentioned, it was requested to evaluate the accessibility of educational software catalogued and present on the Educational Software Documentation Service website, with the aim of activating an information service (for documentation and guidance) on accessibility (regarding disabled people) of educational software with respect to law no. 4/2004 and its means of usage. This activity was divided into two stages, which brought about the creation of an evaluation form which completes the documentation already present:

- Regarding accessibility, showing in detail the features of the software products based on the rules provided for by law 4/2004.

- Regarding the usability of software products in different situations of disability. This form, more closely connected to the educational employment of the software, is intended to directly record the accessibility features of the various software products, based on tests carried out with disabled users, with specific reference to a school context and different types of disability.

"Usability is defined by the International Organisation for Standardisation, as the effectiveness, efficiency and satisfaction with which certain users reach certain goals in certain contexts. In practice, it defines the degree of ease and satisfaction with which human-tool interaction takes place. The term does not refer to an intrinsic feature of the tool, but rather to the interaction process between classes of users, the product and its purpose"[10].

The development of a documentation form for usability of educational software and its means of evaluation was entrusted by ITD to the National Work Group of the Electronic and Computerised aid centres (GLIC in Italian)[11].

This effort was included, in a specific way, in the Educational Software Documentation Service. The evaluation activity provided for usability analysis (accessibility practically tested) on 70 software products and was based on survey methods which included appraisal of each educational software considering its possible input and output devices, following a detailed list of tests which analyse how the software works in its main features. Each of these tests was then related to six types of disability (physical, cognitive-mental retardation, partial sight, blindness, deafness, specific learning disorder).

The two appraisals complement each other: the one regarding accessibility is technical and follows law 4/2004, and the one about usability chooses to examine the theme from the user's point of view and following his needs linked to the specific details of possible operations. Together they offer different points of view, which could enrich law 4/2004 with further content and constitute a base for drawing up guidelines for developers and producers of educational software,[1][Besio, Ferlino, 2007,[2] Besio et al. 2008].

4.1 Accessibility Evaluation

An ITD research group, using its own expertise, performed the activity of evaluating the accessibility of educational software. Such activity featured:

- Building up of an evaluation grid based on Law 4/2004's requirements;
- Choosing and analysing around 300 softwares from the accessibility point of view, following specific criteria;
- Issuing of the relative accessibility forms, containing the results
- Input (with amendment of the form and search engine) of new information into the database, in order complete that already present.

The evaluation grid was created by a working group made up not only of ITD researchers, but also experts in the field, teachers and disabled people, using a co-operative knowledge building method, developed with meetings in person and on-line discussions within a discussion list created for this occasion; every member of the group thus made available his own expertise, to finally create to a product that all can share.

The grid contains:

- specific questions to check compliance with each of the 11 requirements;
- practical suggestions for appraisal;
- comparative references to Section 508 of the U.S. Rehabilitation Act[12];
- indication of the field where the requirement is applicable.

---

[10] Definition taken from Wikipedia.
[11] http://www.centriausili.it
[12] See note 5.

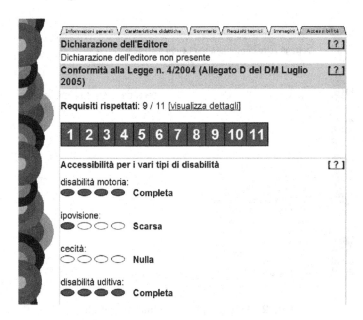

Fig. 1. Example of an information page regarding the accessibility of a particular product, from the Educational Software Documentation Service

This grid was given to an evaluation group who analysed the chosen software, carrying out every test prescribed. If the outcome of the test was uncertain, the researcher contacted another researcher, in order to compare and decide together. The activity was co-ordinated with the aim of monitoring the whole process, but also to verify and validate its own products.

Parallel to this, thanks to the co-operation of a work group (made up of experts with various qualifications: teachers, researchers, therapists, technicians) a form regarding the accessibility of educational software was drawn up, which can be easily understood by everyone, to be made available in the Educational Software Documentation Service database (Fig. 1).

In the evaluation grid, five levels/degrees of accessibility were specified: Complete, Good, Partial, Poor, Nil. Such levels were obtained using an automatic procedure in our IT system for evaluation, which, considering the input from testers (through the grid created) was able to give the correct importance (weight) to each item analysed (for every requirement) with regard to the chosen disability (Fig. 2).

Compliance with each requirement was tested by examining the software and analysing the features of its interface and interactivity compared to the requirements prescribed by the law. For example, let's consider requirement 1 which reads: "The functions provided by the user interface must be able to be activated by keyboard commands too, when a description of this function or the result of its implementation can be supplied". In this case the interface was analysed and the accessibility of the command system (menus, tools, browsing) and the work page was evaluated, by means of specific questions present in the evaluation grid such as:

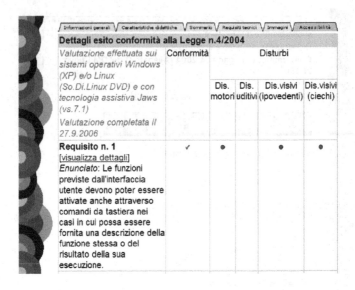

Fig. 2. An example of evaluation details

- Menu bars: can they be reached, activated, browsed using the keyboard?
- Tool bars: can they be reached, activated, browsed using the keyboard? (e.g. Tab, Pag., cursor arrow keys)
- Scroll bars: can they be reached, activated, browsed using the keyboard?

Are all items in the work page reachable and usable in the correct sequence and is it possible to work with them or inside them from the keyboard, in all possible or typical actions of the software? (To be checked especially that the following actions can be performed from the keyboard: access to text input fields, "tabulation" in a logical and sequential order, movement of objects, selection operations such as for text for example)

Can pop-up windows be managed from the keyboard? (open, close, move around inside the windows)?

Every test outcome affected the overall result in percentage terms and in a different proportion according to the type of disability it was related to. In this particular case, keyboard use options were given great importance for the accessibility of blind people and the physically handicapped, but little importance for the accessibility of the hard of hearing.

The final result regarding compliance with the 11 requirements prescribed by the law was given by the system which interpreted the input supplied by the testers, "weighing" it correctly. From a percentage value of 100 (= full compliance), scores arising from "non compliance" were subtracted. Compliance is "Complete" when the percentage is between 80 and 100, "Good" with a percentage between 60 and 80, "Incomplete" between 40 and 60, "Poor" between 20 and 40, "Nil" if less than 20.

During evaluation, apart from accessibility factors, cases were also considered where the software offers some paths which cannot be followed by someone with a particular disability. For example a software which includes comprehension of the spoken word (foreign language) cannot be performed/enjoyed by the hard of hearing. In order to comply with the law, whatever is presented through audio, must use other channels, such as writing, but this evidently conflicts with the activity's objectives. In these cases however, non accessibility does not influence the overall evaluation result.

To keep account of these cases, it was decided to input them in the evaluation grid and display them graphically using parameter CO meaning that the software's educational objectives are in conflict with law no. 4/2004's requirements.

4.2 Evaluation Results

For the test, 313 educational softwares were selected out of the over four thousand present in the Educational Software Documentation Service.

The evaluation result only regard accessibility (compliance with law 4/2004) and not software usability. The choice took account of various factors, among these were requests which arrived at the Consultation Service (Educational Software Library). In particular, products with the following qualities were considered:

- widespread in schools (known and suggested by teachers)
- used to experiment in inclusion courses[13]
- contain different scholastic levels
- for different subject areas
- for different operative systems
- commercial (156) but also free and open source (157)

The appraisal helped us find out what we really expected (bearing in mind that most of the sw analysed were published before the law) which is that an extremely small fraction (9 out of 313) of software products, usable for educational purposes, actually comply completely with the accessibility criteria prescribed by the law.[3][Bocconi et al., 2006].

Here below we present some considerations made after processing the data involved:

In the graph in figure 3, each column represents the number of evaluations which fulfil the exact number of requirements shown on the axis. It can be seen, for example, that only 9 software tests show a result of compliance to all 11 legal requirements and so are completely accessible. The highest value (75) regards a law compliance of 6 requirements out of 11; this means that, at best, the softwares examined are only partially accessible.

But what are the requirements fulfilled most often? Are any requirements more essential than others? Are any of them in some way unimportant? Which kinds of disabilities are penalised the most by inadequate compliance? And, last

---

[13] See note 8 regarding Action 3 objectives.

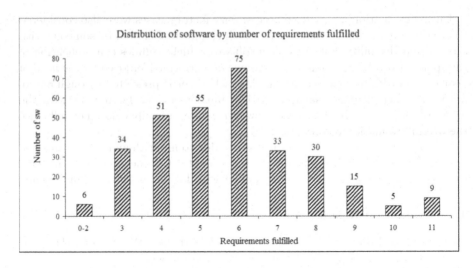

Fig. 3. Distribution of software by number of requirements fulfilled

of all, is there a noticeable difference between open source and non open source products?

Let's consider one aspect in particular "open source and non open source" products, comparing them in every graph. The reason we choose this topic is that, in a parallel way to the current activity, we are also involved with an open source research project for education. Since open source is, due to its very nature, easily changed and improved, thanks to the community which is created around the software, understanding and highlighting the sw accessibility level seemed to be very useful and constructive.

In the graph in figure 4[14], for the first time, we have compared the evaluation results of open source and non open source software. The first column shows the evaluation result for open source softwares which fulfil the number of requirements shown on the axis (related to the total third column and to the "non-open" sw result in the second column); for example 13 open source evaluations and 21 non open source (total 34) have, as a result, compliance to the law of 3 requirements out of 11.

From reading the graph it is evident that open source software, overall, has greater compliance than non-open software. This can be seen in the data regarding the number of evaluations which give a result of 6 to 11 requirements fulfilled.

In the graph in figure 5 we have shown the number of evaluations/software that comply with the single legal requirements. For example, 99 softwares comply with requirement 1, of which 57 open source and 42 non open source.

---

[14] The insignificant number of evaluations which fulfilled from 0 to 2 requirements has not been considered.

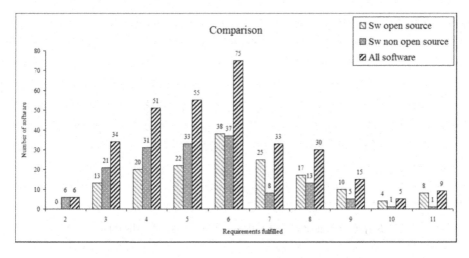

Fig. 4. Comparison of the number of requirements fulfilled, between open source and non open source software

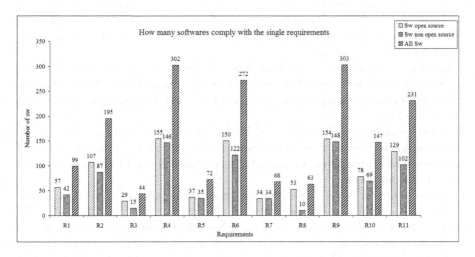

Fig. 5. Number of evaluations/softwares which comply with the single requirements of the law

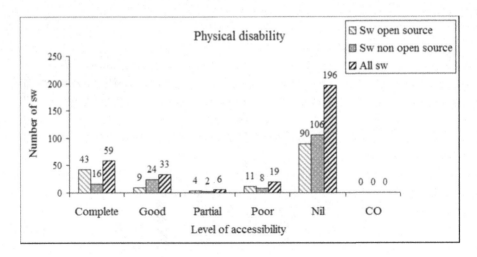

Fig. 6. Level of accessibility for the physically disabled

The requirements most complied with are, in order, no. 9 (flashing light features), no. 4 (meaning of graphic symbols), no. 6 (presence of visual or textual equivalents with sound items) and no. 11 (Accessibility of documents).

In the graphs that follow we have analysed how many softwares (open and non open source) are accessible to the physically handicapped, the deaf, the partially sighted and the blind, and to what extent.

In the graph in figure 6 we analysed how many softwares (open, non open) are accessible for the physically handicapped and to what extent. For example, out of 59 softwares which were given a Complete, accessibility level, 43 were open source and 16 non open source.

In the graph in figure 7 we analysed how many softwares (open, and non open) are accessible for the deaf and to what extent. For example out of 216 softwares which were given a Complete, accessibility level, 131 were open source and 85 non open source.

In the graph in figure 8 we analysed how many softwares (open, and non open) are accessible for the partially sighted and to what extent. For example, out of 12 softwares which were given a Complete, accessibility level, 11 were open source and 1 non open source.

In the graph in figure 9 we analysed how many softwares (open, and non open) are accessible for the blind and to what extent. For example, out of 11 softwares which were given a Complete, accessibility level, 9 were open source e 2 non open source.

Another result worth commenting about is the one regarding accessibility "Nil".

The number of softwares with accessibility level "Nil" is higher in the physically handicapped than in those with sight impairment (divided into the blind and the partially sighted).

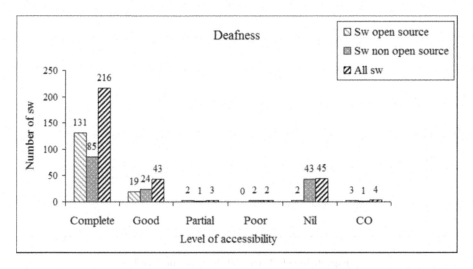

Fig. 7. Level of accessibility for the hard of hearing

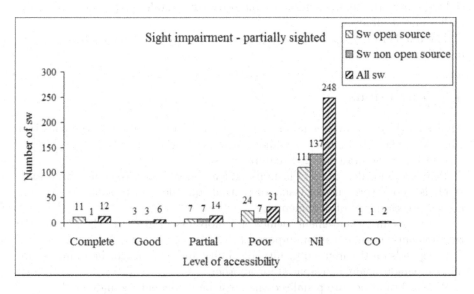

Fig. 8. Level of accessibility for the partially sighted

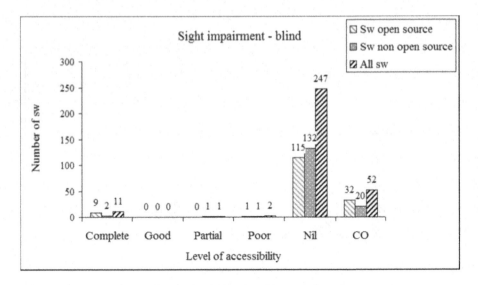

Fig. 9. Level of accessibility for the blind

The almost identical number (respectively 247 and 246) in the categories of "the blind" and "partially sighted" can in fact be reduced for the blind due to the number of softwares which show conflict with their educational aims. This can bring us to say that the most penalised category belongs to the partially sighted where the number of accessible softwares (totally or partially) is really rather low at all levels.

The number of Open Source softwares is lower than non open software for all disabilities.

5   Conclusions

Analysing the data we have in our hands, we have tried to reply to the questions which we have asked ourselves while treating this subject.

Which are the most fulfilled requirements?

They are, in order, no. 9 (Flashing light features), no. 4 (meaning of graphic symbols), no. 6 (presence of visual or textual equivalents with sound items) and no. 11 (Accessibility of documents).

Are there any requirements which are more essential than others? Are any requirements in some way 'unimportant'?

It depends on the user's difficulty/disability and what might be unimportant for one person might be essential for another.

Which disabilities are penalised the most be inadequate compliance?

Above all sight impairment, blindness especially, and, after that partial sight then physical disability. Hearing difficulties are not particularly affected by this problem.

Finally, is there a noticeable difference between open source and non open source products?

There is a difference, that open source software, overall, has greater compliance than non open sw (see the graph in figure 4).

Open source software, as we have seen, due to the fact it can be shared more easily, can be a real training ground for software developers and users who have their own limits. It can provide a valuable occasion for direct exchange between 'builders' and testers, which will maybe open a new age based on 'on demand' bringing with it noble ethical principles. What maybe today is still a hope, may, with everyone's efforts, soon become reality and a model which can be transferred to commercial software.

Digital learning resources, in fact, if they are not planned around the principles of "Design for all", can create new barriers to those who don't have the physical abilities or the cognitive skills necessary to perform the activities expected. Instead of being a tool which encourages and makes acquiring knowledge and skills, and developing abilities, easier, it risks taking on a discriminatory role.

Rules and regulations regarding design have been issued, but whoever creates these tools needs a renewed awareness of the problems that may be encountered by people who live in a condition of "special normality"[7][Ianes, 2006].

In recent years, the idea of software to be used by all people, including the disabled, has been slowly replacing the concept of "special" software, "for the disabled". This is the road which needs to be followed, even though there is still a long way to go.

Our reflections stem from an analysis based on a selection of italian and foreign educational software and on a grid as an evaluation tool which matches the major international trends. For this reason, even though the reflections refer to the italian context, these could be, unpretentionsly, proposed as a stimulus to a more international arena of practitioners in this field and in particular to both developers and users of educational software.

References

1. Besio, S., Ferlino, L.: Accessibility of Educational Software: from the Technical to the User's Point of View. In: Eizmendi, G., Azkoitia, J.M., Craddock, G. (eds.) Challenges for Assistive Technology - AAATE 2007, Proceedings of AAATE 2007 9th European Conference for the Advancement of Assistive Technology in Europe, San Sebastian (Spain), Octobre 3-5, vol. 20, pp. 844–849 (2007) ISBN 978-1-58603-791-8
2. Besio, S., Laudanna, E., Potenza, F., Ferlino, L., Occhionero, F.: Accessibility of educational software: from evaluation to design guidelines. In: Miesenberger, K., Klaus, J., Zagler, W.L., Karshmer, A.I., et al. (eds.) ICCHP 2008. LNCS, vol. 5105, pp. 518–525. Springer, Heidelberg (2008)
3. Bocconi, S., Dini, S., Ferlino, L., Ott, M.: Le nuove barriere tecnologiche: a proposito di accessibilità del Software Didattico, TD Tecnologie Didattiche 39/2006
4. Bocker, M., Cremers, A., Mellors, W.: From Accessibility Standards to Accessible Products: a Best-Practice Example from ETSI Usability Standards in Universal Access in HCI. Exploring New Dimensions of Diversity 8 (2005)

5. Gubbels, A., Kemppainen, E.: A Review of Legislation Relevant to Accessibility in Europe, eEurope 2002 Action Plan, Final draft (November 15, 2002)
6. Klironomos, I., Antona, M., Basdekis, I., Stephanidis, C.: EDeAN Secretariat for 2005, White Paper: Promoting Design for All and e-Accessibility in Europe Universal Access in the Information Society. International Journal 5(1) (June 2006)
7. Ianes, D.: La Speciale normalità. Strategie di integrazione e inclusione per le disabilità e i Bisogni Educativi. Speciali. Erickson (2006)

Accessibility-by-Design: A Framework for Delivery-Context-Aware Personalised Media Content Re-purposing

Atta Badii, David Fuschi, Ali Khan, and Adedayo Adetoye

Intelligent Media Systems and Services Research Centre, School of Systems Engineering,
University of Reading, Whiteknights Campus,
RG6 6AH Reading, United Kingdom
{atta.badii}@reading.ac.uk

Abstract. This paper describes a framework architecture for the automated re-purposing and efficient delivery of multimedia content stored in CMSs. It deploys specifically designed templates as well as adaptation rules based on a hierarchy of profiles to accommodate user, device and network requirements invoked as constraints in the adaptation process. The user profile provides information in accordance with the opt-in principle, while the device and network profiles provide the operational constraints such as for example resolution and bandwidth limitations. The profiles hierarchy ensures that the adaptation privileges the users' preferences. As part of the adaptation, we took into account the support for users' special needs, and therefore adopted a template-based approach that could simplify the adaptation process integrating accessibility-by-design in the template.

Keywords: Digital Item Adaptation, Media Content, Personalisation, Re-purposing, Delivery-Context, Accessibility-by-Design, Transcoding.

1 Introduction

The introduction of Sony's Walkman revolutionised the way music is consumed. Since then a growing number of mobile players have emerged to allow multimedia consumption wherever and whenever desired.

Nowadays the technology trend in mobile phones and personal digital assistants (PDA) provides the same degrees of freedom in communication and content access as the first Walkman did with regards to music; still the availability of the right media content in the present internet-enabled world with huge multimedia content[1] represents a major challenge.

The term multimedia has been known to a wide audience since the 1960s thanks to Bob Goldstein who used it to promote the opening of his show *"LightWorks at L'Oursin"* Southampton, Long Island [2]. Only in the 1990s has this term taken the current connotation (i.e. a multiplicity of media encompassing text, still images, animations, videos, audios and interactive applications). This occurred when the first

---

[1] BrightPlanet estimated about 550 billion documents stored on the Web already in 2000.

A. Holzinger and K. Miesenberger (Eds.): USAB 2009, LNCS 5889, pp. 209–226, 2009.

CD-ROM equipped PCs were launched on the market stressing their ability to provide access to video, audio, images and interactive applications. Yet in most cases multimedia content is at most audio-visual while tactile/force-feedback is usually limited, if available at all, to virtual reality applications or to support some special need (e.g. Braille). Additionally, in most cases multimedia content is designed according to a *"what you see is what you get"* (WYSIWYG) paradigm and any accessibility considerations are taken into account at the very last stage. The education domain taken as a whole, and public services are better supported as far as accessibility is concerned (mostly due to the recent enforcement related to Section 508 [75] and the corresponding EU regulation [16]), yet this is still inadequate as a basis for accessibility assurance. For example, motion pictures with educational content appeared as early as 1943 and in 1973 Robert Heyman introduced the term *"edutainment"* while producing documentaries for the National Geographic Society [59]. Such products originally designed for fruition in cinemas, have progressively migrated to other distribution media such as video-tapes, CD/DVDs and more recently on-line (see the BBC iPlayers) becoming an integral part of available multimedia; yet their provision of features to support differently-enabled users, e.g. subtitling techniques, is fragmentary and anyhow inadequate.

Telecom operators are seeking content owners who could provide them either *"off-the-shelf"* or *"premium"* content traffic that would thus be a source of more profit through the deployment of their infrastructure. Furthermore, current technological evolution combined with a growing demand for more specialised and personalised services is fostering the birth of new businesses where the provision of personalised, contextualised and varied content is a must. This requires firstly that the device manufacturers should support the consumption of a wide range of content on their devices, and secondly that the content owners should provide suitable content for the consumer mobile devices, and, thirdly but above all, that distributors must bridge the wide gap between content production and its fruition on the myriads of mobile devices used by the consumer. From the content production point of view, the producer has to consider aspects such as the physical limitations of the device, its capabilities and supported standards, as well as the channels through which the consumer can access the content. The diversity of the channels and the myriad of available devices, standards and capabilities make the matching of the content to devices an arduous task. Content producers and providers typically choose to produce a limited number of content versions, relying on the distributor to adapt and match the content to various consumer devices. Distributors, on their side, tend to make the content available in the most commonly supported formats and rely on the consumer to pick a suitable one. Thus one of the most significant challenges, as far as content for mobiles is concerned, is to seamlessly match and adapt content to the specific device, taking into account its attributes; as accomplished through the work reported in this paper.

2 Page Formats and Templates

Each reputed content producer has, over time, developed a well-defined house style (branding) based on a well-studied combination of page layout, colours, type-fonts, styles, etc. and all this is usually reflected in defined/adopted templates (both for off- and on-line content). In some cases the same producer may have different product lines, each with a well-defined image reflecting the expectations of the targeted consumers. It is common, for example, to have products targeted for consumption by children made colourful, with large fonts and plenty of drawings and those for scholars characterised by relatively dull colours, and densely packed fonts [8,35,36,42]. Yet there are also types of content and formats that are generically acceptable to a wide audience. This is actually the segment that is addressed in this paper, as it is best suited to automatic composition and adaptation.

Our objectives included the enhancement of both the content production process, and the accessibility of the derived content, particularly in the re-purposing of content stored in databases or content management systems (CMS). We associated with each content component a functional role. As a result of the analysis performed, we could characterise typical content as holding: a *title*, a *sub-title* (if needed), a *body* text (re-size-able and scrollable in the display area), some *multimedia* (with related controls when needed), some *navigation control* (if needed to allow content browsing) potentially comprising (or associated with) *additional controls* (to allow overall content management) plus a *footer* usually holding copyright information.

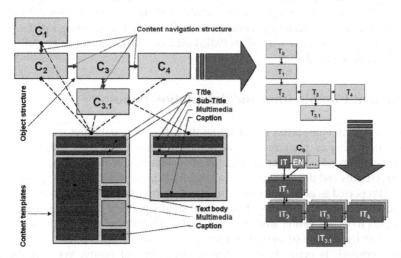

Fig. 1. Generic content structure *(left)*, functional and structural template-based multi-language content *(right)*. Templates have to be manually produced and can then be used in the adaptation process as part of the parameters set.

Original content has been analysed, segmented and labelled according to the criteria above in order to be able to define a set of functional templates as well as a set of navigation templates. This enabled the content to be easily managed, re-combined and adapted according to the required objective as per the user's request and user's preferences as well as device and network characteristics.

It was concluded, that it is possible to automatically decompose existing content, and identify, classify and label its components. However, the production of a content template is part of a creative process that requires the human-factor as the source of qualitative value adding, aesthetic or other goal-oriented, judgement that cannot be replaced by automation. Furthermore, traditionally, publishers would deal with multi-language content through co-editions leading to objects differing in language and format but not in overall layout. This problem has also been addressed in our context via templating. The functional templates, used to give form to content components, represent the first level of presentation; while structural templates allowing access to resources depending on the selected language represent the second level.

The automated production/adaptation process would then logically structure the newly adapted content through invoking a cascade of templates, the first being functional, the second navigation related, the third a layout definition and the last one the language management template. Additionally, the process was refined so as to be able to optimise content for a specific purpose taking into account a combination of factors ranging from harmonising the format of embedded media to a specified reference optimal format, up to template replacement or insertion of additional resources (such as alternate text) for enhancing accessibility.

A template-based approach is already possible in some cases and to a certain extent with tools such as Adobe Director, Dreamweaver, ColdFusion, Flash or Breeze [1,43] when used in combination with a content management system (CMS). However, the challenge we faced was to be able to fully automate the fetching of multi-language, multi-media content from legacy CMS setups, and their adaptation for delivery to a different device either retaining a consistent look-and-feel or adopting a different one. To this end we dealt only with (X)HTML-based or SMIL content to be delivered to PC, PDAs and smart-phones.

3   Content Combination and Adaptation Issues

There are several approaches to managing the different possibilities derived from the combination of user preferences and delivery/device constraints [43,39,40,67,73]. The process depends on either differentiated content production or selection based on user preferences and device capabilities (usually expressed via sets of keywords often collected/reported as attributes of specific fields in profiles). Publishers often prefer to have device-dependent versions of content to simply perform preference-related adaptation, thus most adaptation work is completed at production level and the user simply has to select the desired (if available) format.

This approach is certainly more time-consuming and costly, yet it is the most common. Device-specific content is prepared and stored in a structure reflecting device dependencies; this latter stage is for easing the user's access to the desired content (e.g. via HPPT, WAP, etc.) with minimal latency as users will be accessing the content on a *"pay per use"* basis having signed a specific contract comprising a quality of service agreement (QoS). It is worth mentioning that, following this approach, the content available is usually a subset of the overall available one. An alternative solution often adopted is based on adaptation via two-step filtering. In this case both user preferences and device dependencies are invoked as keywords for performing a two-step consecutive filtering. The ideal would be to have a single step for filtering and adaptation leading to ready-to-use content directly from the original.

A key principle of accessibility is designing content layouts and applications that are flexible to meet the idiosyncratic needs of different users, their preferences, and situations i.e. the delivery context [78,81]. What follows is a set of basic recommendations for content and layout design that can be directly derived from literature [8,13,26,29,35,36,41,42,50,60,75,78,79,80,81,82] and will ensure high quality (as well as accessible) results.

- Content should be presented with appropriate balance in the relative prominence of its components, respecting rules related to Areas of Interest (AoI)
- Each content element must be consistent with the others and as a whole
- Content should be properly indexed and designed to be understandable and accessible
- The language used should be plain
- Explanation of technical/specific terms should be provided via glossary or notes
- Translation of foreign words should be available either as subtitling or by content transcription
- Navigation should be logical and available in text form (for text to speech readers)
- Any foreseen synchronised content should work correctly under all working conditions
- Media characteristics (format, quality, resolution, compression, colour space, etc.) should be selected according to usage
- Rendering standard should be user-selectable and players needed for fruition should be available for installation along with related supportive information if needed
- The user should be able to select GUI effects, while interactive content components (buttons, etc) must be: 1) easy to use, 2) fully reliable and resilient, 3) compatible with target platforms and 4) compatible with distribution network servers if responses are required.

Premium content is typically developed ad hoc for the expected specific target device-based media item delivery. This is simply to allow fine-tuned optimisation; consequently porting to other delivery platforms would often need to be manually performed. This is necessary so as to retain the same level of quality in the finishing of the adapted version as in the original and, as far as accessibility is concerned, if this is not already taken into account in the design, it would lead to difficulties. Our work has led us to conclude that for a large portion of available multimedia content, content structuring and templating allows much easier and more effective adaptation even when taking into account accessibility constraints.

The most frequent change between a PC-based and a PDA-based content rendering is the screen orientation. Unless the PDA is able to automatically flip the screen (presently this feature is supported only in a limited number of devices such as the iPhone and a few others), such a transformation has to be applied prior to delivery. Additionally, PDAs often have lower computational power, smaller displays with lower resolution and colour space, and smaller fonts which often expose anti-aliasing effects more noticeably. Thus a page which has been designed for delivery through a PC screen may often have to undergo a substantial set of changes, for it to be best

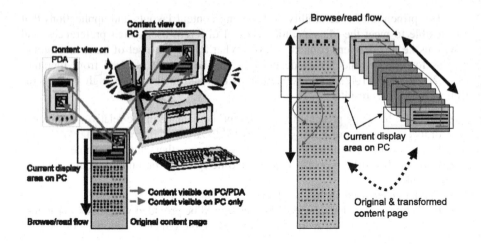

Fig. 2. a) Page changes due to device and b) navigation changes in adaptation

presented on a PDA screen. Content is very likely to be shrunk with substantial changes in area, size and location of page components. Furthermore, it may be necessary to split one page into several. In this case, links between portions of the same page (anchors) are turned into links between pages (URLs). This process, if performed manually, is long, time consuming and potentially error prone as it could lead to programming problems such as "dead links", whereas if it is performed automatically it may be quicker and less error-prone once tested (although it requires quite a complex environment). In more detail this can be achieved thanks to sets of purposely-defined rules.

Given that our primary work context was related to applications in tourism and cultural heritage ("edutainment"), we have taken into account two kinds of possible templates: one that could be defined as static (XHTML and HTML); the other that could be defined as dynamic because of the possible transitions and dynamic effects to be deployed (for SMIL-based objects). Both template sets have been defined and are based on the same rationale exposed so far, thus following a well-specified functional approach. In terms of layout we have basically identified two main template formats, which primarily differ in the basic kind of presented content and in their distribution. Additionally, all these templates could include audio support (in terms of both spoken text and background music).

The first template best fits to content that mainly comprises a balanced mix of text and images (e.g. life of an author, a masterpiece, or a period and its masterpieces, authors, craftsmen, performers, artists, etc.). This has a basic structure consisting of a title, an image area and a text area plus a set of functional and navigational controls located at the bottom of the page. The image (video or animation) could also be linked to additional pages; similarly the text could hold hyperlinks to other content or objects depending on the authors' taste and available content.

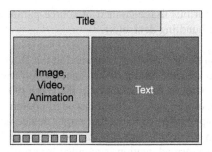 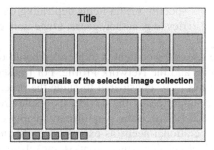

Fig. 3. a) Simple page template and b) "gallery" style template

The second template best fits a gallery of objects that could either represent masterpieces, the authors, craftsmen, performers, artists, etc. of a certain period or artistic movement, etc., thus providing a visually oriented approach to a collection of content. Also in this template there is a title, a collection of image thumbnails (each corresponding to a link to another object) plus a set of functional and navigational controls located at the bottom of the page.

Both templates can be used to generate different objects via rules as well as be adapted to special needs by means of transformations (e.g. addition of alternate text for images and the linearisation of the gallery into a list).

4   The Adaptation Process

The seventh part of ISO/IEC 21000 (MPEG- 21) [28] specifies tools for the adaptation of Digital Items. More specifically, it proposes a set of normalised tools describing the usage environment of a digital item to command the design of the adaptation tools. In order to fulfil these dynamic media adaptation requirements, we have envisaged the requirements for five different kinds of profile elements derived from MPEG-21 DIA [28], which when deployed in combination enable enhanced personalised services. These profiles can be broadly categorised as follows:

1. *User Profiles*: This profile type represents the salient personal information about the user and his preferences, e.g. presentation preferences, auditory or visual impairment, etc. (completed on an opt-in basis).
2. *Device Profiles*: This profile represents the salient information about the user's device(s) including both hardware and software specific information, e.g. codecs, formats, I/O, etc. (retrievable from the manufacturer sources).
3. *Network Profiles*: This profile represents the salient information about the distribution channel that the service provider must use for the delivery of the content, e.g. QoS-related elements, bandwidth, error rate, security, etc.
4. *Context Profiles*: This profile represents the salient delivery context information about the user and his usage environment.
5. *Business User Profiles*: This profile is the Distributor's or Prosumer's (producer-consumer) profile to support B2B media transaction scenarios, e.g. licences acquired, licensing terms preferences generally or particularised to

specific media items depending on various usage-context or source parametrics (e.g. author, genre, usage-zones, bundling deal, etc.).

The requested content is transcoded based on the information contained in the Device Profile and the Network Profile. For transcoding, the user's device-specific information has to be considered to guide the processing of the content (e.g. the types of codecs supported by the device, its display resolution, etc.). The transcoded content is adapted to match the play-display quality capabilities of the actual target device and its operational needs as expressed in the device profile and constrained by the other available profiles (user, context, etc). Unnecessary adaptation is avoided by prioritising constraints resulting from profiles (i.e. if there are several possible solutions at device level, but the network allows only one of the possible solutions due to its bandwidth limitations, then the other candidate solutions are automatically dropped, etc.). Once the adaptation has been achieved, the new content can be sent to the end-user with the related usage licence. Thus individualised media selection and adaptation follows the explicit needs and preferences of the particular user.

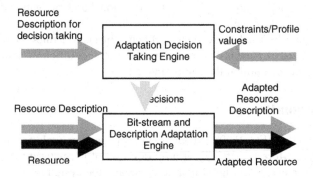

Fig. 4. Constituents of the Adaptation Engine, their relations, inputs and outputs

The profile processing Decision Engine adjusts the user interface or configuration of the learning environment, locates needed resources and adapts the resources to match them to the needs and preferences of the user. Optimal accessibility requires optimal transcoding which needs as input both the parameters of the source data as well as the characteristics set out in the profiles of the user and his/her natural environment, the network and the user client device to which it is to be delivered.

In our case, the Adaptation Engine input spaces takes in an object (set of constituent resources), together with a set of resource descriptions and constraints i.e. profile values. The adaptation process performs necessary activities to arrive at adapted constituent resources (collectively an adapted object) and the adapted resources descriptions. The input sets and output sets of the DIA Decision Engine can be further characterised as

$$X = f \text{ (resource descriptor values, UP, NP, DP)} \qquad (1)$$

Where *UP* is User Profile, *NP* is Network Profile, *DP* is Device Profile and *X* is the target set of adaptation-actionable (*aa*) sub-sets of the respective profile values; as follows:

$$X = (aa\text{-}UP, aa\text{-}NP, aa\text{-}DP) \tag{2}$$

Essentially the adaptation decision-making needs to identify the intersection of all the relevant constraint sets by identifying those elements of the UP, DP and NP that have to be the decision drivers, i.e. logically the prevailing criteria in deciding the value of each aspect of the way the content has to be rendered on the target screen. This amounts to an attempt to find the intersection of four sets namely Resource Description, UP, DP, NP, plus the presentation template (for compound SMIL objects).

We consider the problem of extracting an adaptation strategy from the client profiles for optimal and contextualised content adaptation and propose a technique for its automation. In a typical scenario, we are presented with a digital resource which must be adapted to a target that must conform to a set of profile specifications. These specifications can be considered as constraints guiding the adaptation process. Hence, the systematic selection of a solution space of feasible adaptations is amenable to the well-established artificial intelligence technique of constraint satisfaction [14,62]. Thus the problem can be viewed as a general Constraint Satisfaction Problem (CSP), which provides us with generic tools to automate the discovery of solution spaces.

4.1 Constraints Modelling Illustration

Suppose an un-cropped image is to be displayed on a mobile phone screen with size *l* × *w* (measured in inches). This device can display images at different resolutions *r* taken from the set $\{r_1,...,r_n\}$ in pixels per inch (assuming that the horizontal and vertical resolutions are the same) and supports several image formats such as JPEG, GIF, BMP; data connectivity modes over WIFI, Satellite, GPRS are also supported. This information is gathered from the device profile. Furthermore, depending on the network used, the cost to the user could vary depending on the variable tariffs of network service providers based on the available bandwidth and duration of data transfer. Let us assume that a goal might be to minimise delivery time and consumer cost for this service with minimal compromise on image quality by choosing an optimal network and image format combination. This may also involve the selection of an image format with efficient compression capability to minimise the size of the image to be transferred across the network. All such factors that affect any media delivery operation are constraints bearing down on the solution space. As such these constraints shape the selection of an appropriate media adaptation strategy for optimal delivery.

In this particular example, the necessary parameters to our constraint satisfaction problem include the target screen dimensions (*l* × *w*), the device resolution *r* in $\{r_1, ..., r_n\}$, the image format *f* in *{JPEG, BMP, GIF, ...}*, the network type *n* *{WIFI, Satellite, GPRS, ...}* as may be supported by the target device. We can begin by considering the file size (*s*) of the target adapted image; this needs to be calculated. In this context, for simplicity, we assume that there is a constant, k_f, associated with each image format *f* describing the compression capability of that format; that is, a factor which translates the number of pixels to be encoded to a file size in the target format. Hence, we compute the file size of the image (under any format *f*) as follows:

$$s_f = l \times w \times r^2 \times k_f. \tag{3}$$

Since the network service providers charge by download size, we need to compute the duration of the image download, as well as, the size of the image to be sent over the network. Thus we need to compute the duration (d_n) that it takes to send the target adapted file over the network n. For simplicity, we assume that this duration is a linear function of the file size; calculated as:

$$d_n = (d'_n \times s) / b_n, \tag{4}$$

Where d'_n is the network-related data transfer overheads for sending a file of size s over a network n and b_n is the associated data-rate (that is, "*bandwidth*") of the network. The parameters d'_n and b_n are derived or extracted from the profile of network. Finally, let us assume that the cost c_n of transferring a file of size s within a duration d_n over network n is computed as:

$$c_n = c'_n \times s \times d_n, \tag{5}$$

where c'_n is some pricing factor for the network n.

In this example, we are just interested in checking what combination of parameters are possible as candidate adaptation strategies, on the basis of just the constraint satisfaction parameters given above but in practice additional constraints could be included depending on the requirements for personalisation of a media delivery instance for a particular customer. As highlighted earlier, the goal might be to minimise or maximise the parameters identified above for cost efficiency or quality of service purposes. Thus additional constraints could be included and this would be supported by our framework.

The script shown below is a Constraints Model for the example presented earlier; for which as can be seen below, various constants have been assigned values and domains have been defined and assigned to the various model parameters. This illustrates the flexibility of the framework and the declarative nature of the solution.

```
typedef DIM[1:10]; l, w : DIM;
bandwidth[1:10, 20:30]; size [1:50]; resolution[1:10];
data_rate[3:5, 20]; cost[100:500];
size = l * w * resolution * resolution * 1;
data_rate * bandwidth = 3 * size;
cost = 3*size*data_rate;
Solution:
No.  ({l, w, bandw, size, resolution, cost, data_rate})
1.        {1, 1, 25, 25, 5, 225, 3}
....... .
72. {5, 3, 9, 15, 1, 225, 5}
```

4.2 Constraints Resolution Engine

We have developed a powerful constraint solving system for decision-making in the adaptation process. This engine deploys Gecode [21] in the process of solving the constraint satisfaction problem. The key aspect of this is a modelling language, which we have developed for defining domains and expressing constraints in the system. The key idea is that parameters in our adaptation strategy such as user preferences, device profiles and possible target adaptations of a resource can be used in the development of a Constraints Model which is passed to the Constraints Satisfaction Engine in a fairly high-level language. This model is automatically solved by invoking Gecode and the solutions, if any, form the basis of our decision for a particular resource adaptation strategy.

The Constraint Resolution Engine performs semi-symbolic computation, based on a model written in a very flexible and expressive modelling language to find the set of solutions to a constraint problem. The result is a solution object which can be queried for possible solutions to be used in the adaptation stage. This interface to the engine can accept modelling data from arbitrary input streams such as files, URLs and so on.

The sub-symbolic analysis uses a model specification written in a fairly high-level modelling language that we have developed. This model is semantically analysed to check whether it conforms to the grammar of the modelling language. Accordingly, the Gecode object representations representing the problem are generated to be consequently resolved. The model Lexical and Grammar Analysers are based respectively on GNU Flex and Bison.

The Media Adaptation Engine comprises of various scripts, each with the assigned role of dealing with a specific media type. They invoke the relevant transcoding algorithms for adaptation of the constituent resources of the media object that is to be transcoded (e.g. text, image, video, audio); and in this way deploy the adaptation strategy provided by the Constraint Solving Engine to arrive at an adapted object as output.

The Media Adaptation Engine adapts media types namely image, video, audio and text as well as SMIL. For all these media types, the Media Adaptation Decision Engine incorporates the general media-type-independent component of the adaptation rules as well as the media-type-specific component of the adaptation rules.

In the case of video and image resources, some adaptation features that can be deployed as the Decision Engine processes include: **1)** Acquisition and analysis of the user's preferences regarding image brightness, saturation and contrast, in addition to the user's information regarding visual impairments (if any), as well as the resource information, **2)** Adaptation of the resource for optimal presentation on the target device, **3)** Screen size – re-sizing the image if necessary, **4)** Visual impairments – as may be accommodated in the adaptation process, **5)** Device capability – colour capability, image display capability as per specifications of the target delivery device etc.

In the case of Audio resources, these steps include **i)** Resource transmission information acquisition e.g., sampling frequency, bit rate, number of channels etc, **ii)** Acquisition of the user's preferences and terminal capabilities to ascertain optimal audio adaptation parametric values, e.g. adapting stereo content to mono if the target device can only support mono, **iii)** Changing the audio sampling rate, bit rate, and the number of channels.

For the Text resource, the following steps are taken: **a)** Resource Information Acquisition, **b)** Converting to a format compatible with the receiving terminal (if not already conformant), **c)** Converting text resources to image using ImageMagick [25] or MikTeX [44].

SMIL resources in the object require necessary regional and positional adaptation. The Media Adaptation Engine carries out such modifications by **I)** Adapting the region, text, image and video features, e.g. re-sizing, re-positioning and re-synching, the constituent elements as necessary to ensure that the overall compound media object is composed adaptively for best play-display presentation to match the target delivery context, i.e. to suit the preferences and limitations of the user, device, network, etc., **II)** Adapting text clickable area size and position, **III)** Adapting image clickable area size and position, etc. The Media Adaptation Engine also determines if device and network limitations in relation to the overall size of the object would have adverse effects on the Quality of Service (QoS), and whether a given adaptation strategy would be feasible for actual delivery given network limitations.

This Media Decision Engine for Dynamic Digital Item Adaptation (DIA) has been tested with various compound objects using device profiles for mobile devices such as Samsung i320, Motorola Z3 and imate JASJAR. Some results are shown below:

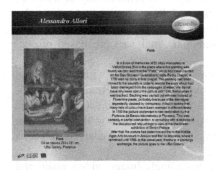
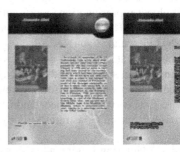

Fig. 5. a) Original Page, b) Object adapted for Motorola Z3 with text to image conversion using MikTeX, c) Object adapted for Motorola Z3 with text to image conversion using ImageMagick

5   Some Application Scenarios

As already mentioned, we had some specific scenarios to deal with in the experimentation of the devised, solution, namely a general one related to tourism and a more specific one related to cultural heritage related education.

5.1   A Tourism Related Scenario

Visitors to a museum, or an archaeological site, are equipped with wireless enabled PDA, the movement of which are tracked inside the location. Whenever the user reaches specific locations, content is pushed to the PDA via WiFi. In this case the delivered content depends on the combination of what is available at the specific location, as well as on the choices and characteristics of the user (based on the user's profile).

5.2   An Educational Scenario

Pupils are equipped with wireless and RFID-enabled PDA within a museum where objects have been tagged with RFID. In addition to what was presented in the tourism scenario above, this education scenario offers the possibility of interaction with "tagged" objects. By deploying the RFID reader and specific software, the user's PDA enables a simple interaction with the environment through tagged objects. Additionally, the user has some special tagged objects that can be used to control the navigation and application management (login, search, print, store, provide-details, seek, locate, etc.). Whenever the user reaches a location, the list of available related content is pushed to the PDA. The user can decide which object to access. Presented objects at this point are basic objects; nevertheless they have links to drilldowns and additional information that is easily accessible with the above-mentioned interface methodology.

6 The Accessibility Paradox

In the past, there have been several attempts to produce *"encyclopaedic content"* that would strive to fully cover what is known on either a specific domain or encompassing several domains (e.g. the works of Aristotle, Ptolemy, Averroes, Avicenna, or the *Naturalis Historia* by Pliny the Elder, the *Encyclopédie, ou dictionnaire raisonné des sciences, des arts et des metiers* by Diderot, etc.), but at present this is neither possible nor envisaged. Yet the digitally connected world aspires to make accessible the complete collection and to be easily and fully accessible.

Actually here lays a paradox: the quantity and quality of fully and freely accessible knowledge whilst being directly proportional to the number of people who can pay for it, is indeed inversely proportional to the number of people who could access it.

This is somehow similar to the accessibility paradox currently being faced in e-Government where disadvantaged and socially marginalised people, who depend on public services most of all, are also among the least likely to have access to computers [19]. The current spectacular growth in tools and methods available to access digital content could either provide a solution or further exacerbate such a digital divide depending on the availability of carefully designed ICT services and specifically targeted initiatives.

7 Conclusions

According to the European Commission report "Innovation in Europe's regions, promoting innovation among practitioners and policy-makers" dated 2006, it will be necessary to exploit also *"mobile phones, digital TV, on-line kiosks and other delivery channels, simply because broadband internet connections are unlikely ever to cover the whole population"*. Additionally, *"delivered, services will need to be useful, easy to use, and backed up by good support for both users and providers. To avoid reinventing the wheel, there is a great need to share solutions and best practices, and software should be based on standards, open specifications and open interfaces wherever possible"*.

This implies that in terms of content, it is important to be able to recognise and highlight content value (in terms of completeness, readability, understandability, trackability), so as to be able to select what to provide to a particular audience in adherence to standards, intellectual property (IP) protection and remuneration, on any needed or required delivery media.

In terms of user acceptance, it is necessary to take into account content suitability and acceptability to the individual users' needs as well as appeal and appropriateness. In this way some users may be persuaded to access media content for free when needed either for educational needs or as part of the right of inclusion in an equal opportunity information society; and, some users may pay for certain content and thus remunerate the producer and therefore contribute to a free media market as well as encourage media creativity.

To support such a digital economy, e.g. more specifically through facilitating viable re-purposing of available content collections, specific solutions for media adaptation have to be designed, tested and validated. Our research work has proven that, in certain contexts and given the availability of certain information, the deployment of a template-based and dynamic digital item adaptation approach makes all this viable in a (semi) automated fashion; thus accommodating the selection of media delivery formats as suited to the user's preferences and operational transmission-play-display constraints of the media delivery context. Furthermore, the proposed solution allows an easier management of content storage increasing the scope for persistence, searchability, trace-ability compatibility and adherence to standards.

Acknowledgment

The authors would like to thank the EC IST FP6 for the partial funding of the AXMEDIS project, and all AXMEDIS project Partners including the Expert User Group and all affiliated members for their support and encouragement.

References

1. Adobe products and Solutions, http://www.adobe.com/ (last accessed: 02/05/2007)
2. Albarino, R.: Goldstein's LightWorks at Southhampton, Variety 213(12) (August 10, 1966)
3. AXMEDIS Framework for All, http://www.axmedis.org/tiki/index.php
4. AXMEDIS web site, http://www.axmedis.org/ (last accessed: 02/05/2007)
5. Badii, A., Sailor, M., Nair, R.R.: Profiling Management for Personalised Multimedia Delivery On-Demand within the AXMEDIS Framework. In: Proceedings of AXMEDIS 2006 Conference, December 2006. University of Leeds, UK (2006)
6. Badii, A.: Context, Context, Wherefore Art Thou? C-Assuring shared sense-making and meta-scaffolding for Collaborative Creative Communities Doing Society with IS. In: Proc.UKAIS-AIS (2000)
7. Badii, A., Hoffman, M., Heider, J.: MobiPETS-GRID context-aware mobile service provisioning framework deploying enhanced Personalisation, Privacy and Security Technologies (.PETS). To appear at the 1st IEEE international conference on Communication Systems Software and Middleware (COMSWARE), New Dehli (2006)
8. Baird, R.N., McDonald, D., Pittman, R.H., Turnbull, A.: The Graphics of Communication: Methods, Media, and Technology, 6th edn. Harcourt Brace Jovanovich (1993)

9. Bo, G., Vaccaro, R., Lorenzon, A.: iTutor: Mobile/Wearable Technologies and Adaptive Multi-modal Interaction for supporting Information Management and Training in Industrial Environments. In: IFAWC 2nd International Forum on Applied Wearable Computing (2005)
10. Bugelski, B.: The Psychology of Learning Applied to Teaching, 2nd edn. Bobbs-Merrill, Indianapolis (1971)
11. Canny, J.: Collaborative filtering with privacy via factor analysis. In: Proc. 25th Int. ACM SIGIR Conference Information Retrieval (2002)
12. Da Bormida, G., Bo, G., Lefrere, P., Taylor, J.: An Open Abstract Framework for Modeling Interoperability of Mobile Learning Services. In: WSMAI 2003, pp. 9–16 (2003)
13. DCMI Type Vocabulary, http://dublincore.org/documents/dcmi-type-vocabulary/ (last accessed: 02/05/2007)
14. Dechter, R.: Constraint Processing. Morgan Kaufmann, San Francisco (2003)
15. Developing the multimedia mobile market, The Netsize Guide 2004 Edn. (2004), http://www.netsize.com/
16. Directive 2001/29/EC (2001), http://eur-lex.europa.eu/LexUriServ/LexUriServ.do?uri=CELEX:32001L0029:EN:HTML
17. Druckman, D., Bjork, R.: In the Mind's Eye. National Academy Press, Washington (1991)
18. Druckman, D., Swets, J.: Enhancing Human Performance. National Academy Press, Washington (1988)
19. European Commission, Directorate-General for Enterprise and Industry, Innovation in Europe's regions, promoting innovation among practitioners and policy-makers, in euroabstracts A review of European innovation and enterprise, vol. 44 (June 2006)
20. Fischer, F., Bruhn, J., Grasel, C., Mandl, H.: Fostering collaborative knowledge construction with visualization tools, Learning and Instruction 12, 213–232 (2002)
21. Gecode. Generic Constraint Development Environment, http://www.gecode.org
22. Gough, J.: MicroWorlds as a Learning Environment: Years 5 - 7: Tools Versus Thinking. In: Symp. on Contemporary Approaches to Research in Mathematics, Science, Healthand Environmental Education, Deakin University, December 2-3 (1996)
23. Hilgard, E.R., Bower, G.H.: Theories of Learning, 4th edn. Prentice-Hall, Englewood Cliffs (1975)
24. Hoyles, C., Healy, L., Sutherland, R.: Patterns of Discussion between Pupil Pairs in Computer and non-Computer Environments. Journal of Computer Assisted Learning 7, 210–228 (1991)
25. ImageMagick, http://www.imagemagick.org/script/index.php
26. Internet Media Types, http://www.iana.org/assignments/media-types/ (last accessed: 02/05/2007)
27. Ishii, H., Ullmer, B.: Tangible Bits: Towards Seamless Interfaces between People, Bits and Atoms. In: Proceedings of the SIGCHI conference on Human factors in computing systems, Atlanta, Georgia, USA, pp. 234–241 (1997)
28. ISO MPEG-21, Part 7 - Digital Item Adaptation, ISO/IEC JTC1/SC29/WG11/N5231 (October 2002)
29. ISO639 Language specifications, http://www.loc.gov/standards/iso639-2/ (last accessed: 02/05/2007)
30. Ng, K., Ong, B., Neagle, R., Ebinger, P., Schmucker, M., Bruno, I., Nesi, P.: AXMEDIS Framework for Programme and Publication and On- Demand Production. In: Proc. AXMEDIS 2005 (2005)

31. Swearingen, K., Rashmi, S.: Interaction Design for Recommender Systems. In: Designing Interactive Systems 2002. ACM, New York (2002)
32. Kearsley, G.: Explorations in Learning & Instruction: The Theory Into Practice Database TIP Version 2.6 (May 2006), http://tip.psychology.org/index.html
33. Ng, K., Badii, A., Sailor, M., Ong, B., Neagle, R., Quested, G.: Programme and Publication Tools Integration with workflow-enabled communication and process control. In: Proceedings of AXMEDIS 2006 Conference, Leeds, UK (December 2006)
34. Klausmeier, H.J., Goodwin, W.: Learning and Human Abilities, 4th edn. Harper & Row, New York (1975)
35. Knight, C., Glaser, J.: Effective Visual Communication for Graphic Designers (Creating Hierachies with Type, Image and Colour). RotoVision SA (2003)
36. Kristof, R., Satran, A.: Interactivity by Design: Creating and Communicating with New Media. Adobe Press (1995)
37. Lee, E., Kang, J., Choi, J., Yang, J.: Topic-Specific Web Content Adaptation to Mobile Devices. In: IEEE/WIC/ACM International Conference on Web Intelligence, pp. 845–848 (2006)
38. Lefrancois, G.R.: Theories of Human Learning (Kro's Report), 3rd edn. Brooks/Cole, CA (1995)
39. Lemlouma, T., Layada, N.: Content Adaptation and Generation Principles for Heterogeneous Clients, http://www.w3.org/2002/07/DIAT/posn/inria/DIAT-PositionPaper.html (last accessed: 02/05/2007)
40. Lemlouma, T., Layaida, N.: Context-aware adaptation for mobile devices. In: Mobile Data Management, Proceedings, pp. 106–111 (2004)
41. Lloyd, R.: Three Approaches to Multilingual Content Management - Using a Content Management System (CMS). KM World (Special Supplement) (2002)
42. Lynch, P.J., Horton, S.: Web Style Guide, 2nd edn. Yale University Centre for Advanced Instructional Media's, http://www.webstyleguide.com/index.html (last accessed: 02/05/2007)
43. Matsuyama, K., Saito, N.: Two-Phased XML Content Adaptation for Appropriate Handling of User Context. In: Internet and Multimedia Systems and Applications - 2005 Proceeding (2005)
44. MikTeX, http://miktex.org/
45. MPEG-21 DIA, http://www.chiariglione.org/mpeg/tutorials/technologies/mp21-dia/index.htm
46. Mukherjee, D., Kuo, G., Hsiang, S., Liu, S., Said, A.: Format-Independent Scalable BitStream Adaptation Using MPEG-21 DIA. In: International Conference on Image Processing 2004. IEEE, Los Alamitos (2004) 0-7803-8554-3/04 02004
47. Mukherjee, D.: MPEG-21 DIA: Objectives and Concepts, HP Labs. Lecture slides as part of ECE 289J - Multimedia Networking at UC Davis taught by Prof. Mihaela van der Schaar (2004)
48. Nichols, S.: Physical ergonomics of virtual environment use. In: Handbook of Virtual Environments: Design, Implementation, and Applications, pp. 999–1026. LEA, Hillsdale (2002)
49. Norman, D., Draper, S.: User Centered System Design. LEA Hillsdale (1986)
50. OCLC. OCLC Bibliographic Formats and Standards, http://www.oclc.org/bibformats/en/0xx/098.shtm (last accessed: 02/05/2007)
51. OKI - Open Knowledge Initiative, Specs, http://www.okiproject.org/specs/

52. Bellini, P., Bruno, I., Nesi, P.A.: Distributed Environment for Automatic Multimedia Content Production based on GRID. In: Proc. AXMEDIS 2005 (2005)
53. Papert, S.: Mindstorms. Basic Books, New York (1980)
54. Papert, S.: The Children's Machine: Rethinking School in the Age of the Computer. Basic Books, New York (1993)
55. Pemberton, D., Rodden, T., Procter, R.: Groupmark: A WWW recommender system combining collaborative and information filtering. In: Proc. 6th ERCIM Workshop on User-Interfaces for All, ERCIM, October 2000, vol. (12), p. 13 (2000)
56. Dechter, R.: Constraint Processing. Morgan Kaufmann, San Francisco (2003)
57. Reigeluth, C.M.: Instructional Design Theories and Models. Lawrence Erlbaum, Hillsdale (1983)
58. Resource Description Framework, http://www.w3.org/RDF/ (last accessed April 2006)
59. Rey-López, M., Fernández-Vilas, A., Díaz-Redondo, R.P.: A Model for Personalized Learning Through IDTV. In: Wade, V.P., Ashman, H., Smyth, B. (eds.) AH 2006. LNCS, vol. 4018, pp. 457–461. Springer, Heidelberg (2006)
60. RFC3066 Language specifications, http://www.ietf.org/rfc/rfc3066.txt (last accessed: 02/05/2007)
61. Richey, R.: The Theoretical and Conceptual Basis of Instructional Theory. Kogan Page, London (1986)
62. Rossi, F., van Beek, P., Walsh, T.: The Handbook of Constraint Programming. Elsevier, Amsterdam (2006)
63. Sahakian, W.: Learning: Systems, Models, and Theories, 2nd edn. Rand McNally, Chicago (1976)
64. Shen, J., Sun, P., Zhang, J., Song, S.: iMMS: Interactive multimedia messaging service. IBM Journal of Research and Development 48(5/6) (2004)
65. Slavin, R.E.: Research on cooperative learning and achievement: What we know, what we need to know. Contemporary Educational Psychology 21(1), 43–69 (1996)
66. Snelbecker, G.: Learning Theory, Instructional Theory, and Psychoeducational Design. McGraw-Hill, NY (1974)
67. Sofokleous, A.A., Angelides, M.C., Schizas, C.N.: Multimedia Content Adaptation: Operation Selection in the MPEG-21 Framework. In: Internet and Multimedia Systems, and Applications - 2005 Proceeding (2005)
68. Soloway, E., Guzdial, M., Hay, K.: Learner-Centered Design: The Challenge for HCI in the 21st Century. Interactions 1(2), 36–48 (1994)
69. Soloway, E., Scala, N., Jackson, S.L., Klein, J., Quintana, C., Reed, J., Spitulnik, J., Stratford, S.J., Studer, S., Eng, J.: Learning theory in practice: case studies of learner centered design. In: Proceedings of CHI 1996, pp. 189–196. ACM Press, New York (1996)
70. Tanner, S., Deegan, M.: Exploring Charging Models for Digital Cultural Heritage. In: HEDS 2002 (2002), http://heds.herts.ac.uk/mellon/charging_models.html
71. The AXMEDIS, Consortium, http://www.axmedis.org/ (last accessed April 2006)
72. The Mobile Is Open For Business, The Netsize Guide 2005 Edn. (2005), http://www.netsize.com/
73. Tong, M.W., Yang, Z.K., Liu, Q.T., Liu, X.N.: A Novel Content Adaptation Model under E-learning Environment. In: 36th ASEE/IEEE Frontiers in Education Conference - 2006 Proceeding (2006)
74. Travers, R.M.: Essentials of Learning, 5th edn. Macmillan, NY (1982)

75. U.S. General Services Administration's Office of Governmentwide Policy, Section 508, http://www.section508.gov/index.cfm (last accessed: 02/05/2007)
76. UAProf Schema and Information, http://www.openmobilealliance.org/
77. Kieling, W., Balke, W.T., Wagner, M.: Personalized Content Syndication in a Preference World. In: Proc. EnCKompass, Eindhoven (2001)
78. W3C Accessibility Initiative, http://www.w3.org/WAI/ (last accessed: 02/05/2007)
79. W3C CC/PP Information Page, http://www.w3.org/Mobile/CCPP (last accessed April 2006)
80. W3C Guidelines for language tags, http://www.w3.org/International/articles/language-tags/ (last accessed: 02/05/2007)
81. W3C Web Content Accessibility Guidelines 1.0, http://www.w3c.org/TR/WCAG10/ (last accessed: 02/05/2007)
82. W3C. Synchronized Multimedia, http://www.w3.org/AudioVideo/ (last accessed: 02/05/2007)
83. WIPO, World Intellectual Property Organization, http://www.wipo.int/portal/index.html.en
84. Lum, W.Y., Lau, F.C.M.: A Context-Aware Decision Engine for Content Adaptation. IEEE, University of Hong Kong (2002)

Generating Dialogues from the Description of Structured Data

Luděk Bártek

Faculty of Informatics, Masaryk University
Botanická 68a, 602 00 Brno
Czech Republic
bar@fi.muni.cz

Abstract. Generating dialogues from the description of structured data is a part of the WebGen system for generating web-based presentations by means of dialogue. Although the system allows the user to create the most common presentations types, such as personal presentations or blogs, the user may need to add a new presentation type. To add a new presentation type the user must specify the content and structure of the presentation descriptor using the XML Schema, the dialogue interface used to collect requested information and finally the layout of the resulting pages. This paper discusses limitations on the XML Schema structure allowing us to generate dialogue interfaces automatically from the presentation descriptor and basic principles and algorithms used during the transformation. In addition, this paper includes some illustrative examples of the data, corresponding XML Schema, XSL Transformation, resulting VoiceXML document and experiments used to evaluate the user satisfaction with generated dialogues.

1 Introduction

There exists a large number of visually oriented authoring tools for creating web presentations like Microsoft Expression Web [1], Mozilla Composer [2], OpenCMS [3], Wiki [4,5], etc. These tools are however not very suitable for some type of users such as not experienced ones or some handicapped users, especially print impaired and visually impaired.

The WebGen system [6] offers the possibility to create common types of web presentations, such as personal pages, product presentations and blogs by means of a dialogue. The paper describes methods used to add a support for a new presentation type into the WebGen system.

2 Algorithms and Principles

The entire process of generating a dialogue interface from the data description is based on a transformation of the XML Schema [7,8], describing the presentation content and structure, into VoiceXML [9] documents [10] used to implement a dialogue interface. The process proceeds in the following steps:

A. Holzinger and K. Miesenberger (Eds.): USAB 2009, LNCS 5889, pp. 227–235, 2009.
© Springer-Verlag Berlin Heidelberg 2009

1. Description of the content of the presentation – the user has to supply an XML Schema describing the structure of the data included in the presentation of the particular type. To create the XML Schema, the user may use some supporting visually oriented tools like NetBeans IDE [11] or XML Mind [12]. To enhance the accessibility of the process to non-experienced and visually impaired users, there is a plan to develop a dialogue application supporting the XML Schema creation.
2. The generation of a dialogue interface for a particular presentation type – this process utilizes a set of XSL Transformations [13] used to transform the schema into the corresponding VoiceXML documents and speech recognition grammars [14].

3 Requirements on the Presentation Description

To be able to generate a dialogue interface from a presentation description [15], the description must contain the following information:

- Description of all slots to be filled – a prompt for a user describing the slot semantic, prompts to be used when there is either no input from the user or the input is incorrect, etc.
- Information needed to generate speech recognition grammars for input slots – the grammar is either generated from the specification of the particular XML element type in the case of user-defined types otherwise a grammar corresponding to the particular predefined type is used.

To be able to utilize the XSL Transformation, the structure of the descriptor must start with the XML Schema element with the attribute name assigned to the value *page*. The content of the element is a complex type describing the structure of the presentation descriptor. The next limitation implied by the XSL Transformation is that types of all elements must be specified within the corresponding element declaration. The type specification can use either the attribute type in the case of elements of the predefined XML Schema type or a child element in the case of a user-defined type.

3.1 Information Describing the Slots

The XML Schema is used to describe the structure of the XML document as well as the types of all elements included in the document. The XML elements definitions are transformed into the corresponding VoiceXML fields. To generate the prompts required by VoiceXML fields, the user can:

1. Add a description for every element in the form of XML Schema annotation [7] – the annotation is specified by the user during the process of a description specification.
2. Create a description from available information – it requires the descriptive names of the input slots. And because the names are identifiers, they can not contains white spaces. This limitation can be eliminated using the Java-like mixed-case syntax [16] of identifiers for example.

While the acquisition of the description is more user-friendly than annotations, the annotations are supported, because they are more expressive.

3.2 Information Used to Generate Speech Recognition Grammars

The speech recognition grammars are used to limit the set of possible input values of the corresponding slot. They are described using the SRGS standard [14] and correspond to the XML Schema element types.

There is a problem with transforming the basic XML Schema types like the string, integer and decimal for example, because the SRGS grammar expects that all possible values are explicitly specified. There are two approaches solving this problem:

1. Use of the GARBAGE SRGS rule [14] – the analysis of the rule is implementation-specific, therefore its usage is platform dependent. This rule can be utilized when using the OptimTalk platform [18] for example.

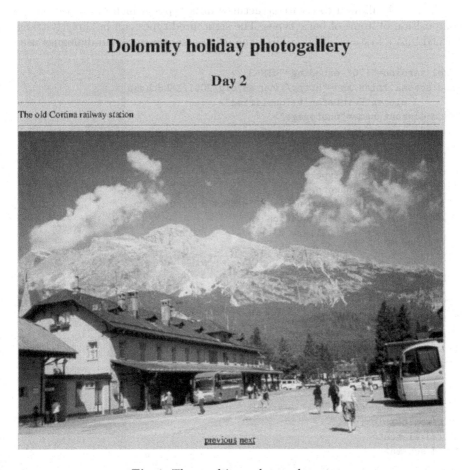

Fig. 1. The resulting web page layout

2. Avoiding the problem using rules for spelling the values – this solution is not very user-friendly. The advantage of the method is that it is supported by most of the VoiceXML platforms. The spelling can be used for a DTMF input using the Multi-Tap method [17] as well.

The XML Schema offers user-defined atomic types as well. The user-defined types are based on:

  – a restriction of a basic type – either pattern-restriction or range-restriction of the basic type;
  – an enumeration of possible values.

Transformation of the restriction types can be done either by the spelling rule described in the previous paragraph or by a transcription of the restriction rules into the form of an SRGS grammar.

The other kind of user-defined basic types is enumeration. The corresponding SRGS grammar is a list of all possible values.

The user is allowed to create structured data types, which are based on the composition of items of basic types. The structured types can be directly transformed into a system-initiative dialogue using a sequence of sub-dialogues used

```
<?xml version="1.0" encoding="UTF-8"?>
<xsd:schema xmlns:xsd="http://www.w3.org/2001/XMLSchema"
          elementFormDefault="qualified">
  <xsd:element name="photopage">
    <xsd:complexType>
      <xsd:sequence>
        <xsd:element name="heading">
         <xsd:complexType>
            <xsd:sequence>
              <xsd:element name="h1" type="xsd:string">
                <xsd:annotation>
                    Gallery title
                </xsd:annotation>
              </xsd:element>
                  ...
            </xsd:sequence>
         </xsd:element>
         <xsd:element name="photo">
            ...
         </xsd:element>
         <xsd:element name="navigation">
            ...
         </xsd:element>
      </xsd:sequence>
    </xsd:complexType>
  </xsd:element>
</xsd:schema>
```

Fig. 2. XML Schema of the generated page

to acquire values of all parts of the structured type. When the mixed initiative dialogue is used the corresponding grammar can be built by deriving the rules from the unrecognized responses using data acquired by the system-initiative correcting dialogue. To extract the rules from the unrecognized answers the pattern matching [19] can be utilized [20].

The fragment of the XML Schema used to generate a dialogue for the acquisition of data included in the page in Fig. 1. is shown in Fig. 2.

4   Generating Dialogue Interfaces from the Data Description

To generate a system-initiative VoiceXML dialogue from an XML Schema the following recursive algorithm is used:

1. For all elements included in the root element, generate the corresponding dialogues as follows:
   (a) When the type of the element is a simple type, either user-defined or predefined, generate directly corresponding input field. To generate the prompt and the grammar of the input field use the methods described in the previous section.
   (b) When the type of element is complex, process all included elements using step 1.

The fragment of the XSL Transformation corresponding to the XML schema shown in Fig. 2. is shown in Fig. 3. The corresponding part of the generated dialogue is shown in Fig. 4.

The XML Schema offers several types of element cardinality next. The previous text dealt with elements with cardinality one. The other possibilities remaining are:

1. Optional elements – they need not appear in the resulting structure.
2. Elements with cardinality more than one.

To solve the issue of the optional parts two different methods has been proposed:

1. Every optional part has assigned a simple yes/no question to find whether the information should be included or not.
2. Ask the user for the optional data and allow him to exclude the data in this step.

There is an issue how long the system should wait to assume that the user did not enter any data when the second method is used. This time is user specific and therefore the first solution was selected to resolve the problem.

To solve the problem with cardinality two or more the following algorithm can be used:

```
<?xml version="1.0" encoding="UTF-8"?>
<xsl:stylesheet xmlns:xsl="http://www.w3.org/1999/XSL/Transform"
                version="1.0"
                ...
                extension-element-prefixes="">
    <xsl:output method="xml" indent="yes"/>
    <xsl:template match="/xsd:schema">
        <vxml xmlns="http://www.w3.org/2001/vxml" version="2.0">
            <xsl:element name="form" >
                <xsl:attribute name="id">
                    <xsl:value-of select="./xsd:element/@@name"/>
                </xsl:attribute>
                <xsl:apply-templates/>
            </xsl:element>
        </vxml>
    </xsl:template>
        ...
    <xsl:template match="xsd:element">
        <xsl:element name="field">
          <xsl:attribute name="name">
            ...
          </xsl:attribute>
            ...
          <xsl:element name="prompt">
              <xsl:value-of select="xsd:annotation/xsd:documentation"/>
          </xsl:element>
          <xsl:element name="grammar">
              <xsl:attribute name="src">
                  <xsl:value-of select="substring(./@@type,5)/>
              </xsl:attribute>
          </xsl:element>
            ...
        </xsl:element>
    </xsl:template>
</xsl:stylesheet>
```

Fig. 3. Example of the XSL Transformation

1. An auxiliary variable with array of values of the selected type is created.
   When particular information is filled the value is added into the array and
   the dialogue field is cleared. The dialogue proceed until either the user wants
   to stop or the maximal cardinality is reached. To find if the user is supposed
   to add new value the methods described in the algorithm for optional parts
   can be used.
2. The second possibility is to repeat the corresponding subdialogue including
   the submitting of the acquired data to the server until user wants to stop.
   This solution needs a support on the side of the server therefore the first
   option is used.

```
<?xml version="1.0" encoding="UTF-8"?>
<vxml xmlns="http://www.w3.org/2001/vxml" version="2.0">
  <form id="photopage">
    <field name="h1">
      <prompt>Gallery title</prompt>
      <grammar src="string" root="string"/>
    </field>
    <field name="h2">
      <prompt>Photo set name</prompt>
      <grammar src="string" root="string"/>
    </field>
      ...
    <field name="next">
      <prompt>Address of the next page in the gallery</prompt>
      <grammar src="anyURI" root="anyURI"/>
    </field>
      ...
  </form>
</vxml>
```

Fig. 4. Example of the generated VoiceXML dialogue

5 Experimental Results

The objective of the experiment was to test a user satisfaction with the generated dialogues.

To test the user satisfaction two sets of dialogues has been created. The first one has included the dialogues generated as described in the paper. The second set of dialogues has been created manually.

The task for the user was to perform and to evaluate the dialogue. The user did not know which kind of the dialogue is used. To evaluate the dialogue the following criteria were used:

1. Number of steps of the dialogue - to get this information the dialogues were slightly modified to count and submit the total number of steps used in the dialogue.
2. Dialogue success - answers were yes or no.
3. The user satisfaction with the dialogue - scale is 0 - unsatisfied, 1 - partially satisfied, 2 - satisfied. In the case of evaluation either 0 or 1 the user may write his recommendations.
4. How natural the dialogue seemed to the user - possible answers were 0 - terrible, 1 - it was obvious I do not communicate with a human, 2 - not sure if the dialogue partner is either a computer or a human, 3 - it seems almost like an interaction with a human, 4 - a human-to-human communication. When the evaluation was worse then 4, the user may fill his recommendation how to improve the dialogue.

The results of the experiment are shown in the table on Fig. 5.

Dialogue	Mean number of dialogue turns	Relative number of successful dialogue	Mean user satisfaction	Mean dialogue naturalness
Created by developer one address	9	100%	1	3
Created by developer two addresses	14	100%	2	2.5
Generated one address	8.5	100%	1.5	2
Generated two addresses	15	100%	2	1.5

Fig. 5. Results of the experiment

The conclusion of the experiment is that the created dialogue seems to be slightly more natural to the users as expected. The evaluation of the other criteria is similar for both sets of dialogues.

The only recommendation from the users was to improve the grammar for recognition of numbers. To keep the grammar simple and small the numbers has to be spelled. The users would like to enter the numbers in a standard form (sixty five instead of six five for example).

6   Conclusions and Future Work

The paper describes the basic principles of generating dialogue interfaces from descriptors of structured data. Illustrative examples of the page layout, corresponding XML Schema, XSL Transformation and VoiceXML dialogue are presented as well. The experiment has proved that the generated dialogue interface is comparable to the developer created one.

Our next efforts will focus on the design and implementation of a dialogue interface used to acquire a descriptor for a custom presentation. The succeeding tasks involve improving the dialogue strategy as well as the implementation of methods used to generate the grammars utilized by the mixed-initiative dialogue strategy.

Acknowledgement

The author is grateful to James Thomas for proofreading a draft of the paper and the students and staff of the Support Center for Students with Special Needs of Masaryk University for their advice, support and collaboration. This work is supported by the Grant Agency of Czech Republic under the Grant 201/07/0881.

References

1. Microsoft Expresion, http://www.microsoft.com/Expression/
2. The SeaMonkey Project, http://www.seamonkey-project.org
3. OpenCMS, the Open Source Content Management System/CMS, http://www.opencms.org/

4. MediaWiki, http://www.mediawiki.org/
5. TikiWiki – CMS/Groupware, http://www.tikiwiki.org/
6. Kopeček, I., Bártek, L.: Web Pages for Blind People — Generating Web-Based Presentations by means of Dialogue. In: Miesenberger, K., Klaus, J., Zagler, W.L., Karshmer, A.I. (eds.) ICCHP 2006. LNCS, vol. 4061, pp. 114–119. Springer, Heidelberg (2006)
7. W3C XML Schema, http://www.w3.org/XML/Schema
8. Gullbransen, D.: Using XML Schema: special edn. Que, Indianapolis (2002)
9. McGlashan, S., Burnett, D.C., Carter, J., Danielsen, P., Ferrans, J., Hunt, A., Lucas, B., Porter, B., Rehor, K., Tryphonas, S.: Voice Extensible Markup Language (VoiceXML) Version 2.0, http://www.w3.org/TR/2004/REC-voicexml20-20040316/
10. Annamalai, N., Gupta, G., Prabhakaran, B.: Accessing Documents via Audio: An Extensible Transcoder for HTML to VoiceXML Conversion. In: Miesenberger, K., Klaus, J., Zagler, W.L., Burger, D. (eds.) ICCHP 2004. LNCS, vol. 3118, pp. 339–346. Springer, Heidelberg (2004)
11. NetBeans IDE, http://www.netbeans.org/
12. XMLmind XML Editor, http://www.xmlmind.com/xmleditor
13. Clark, J.: XSL Transformations (XSLT), http://www.w3.org/TR/xslt
14. Hunt, A., McGlashan, S.: Speech Recognition Grammar Specification Version 1.0, http://www.w3.org/TR/speech-grammar/
15. González-Ferreras, C., Cardeñoso-Payo, V.: Building Voice Applications from Web Content. In: Sojka, P., Kopeček, I., Pala, K. (eds.) TSD 2004. LNCS (LNAI), vol. 3206, pp. 587–594. Springer, Heidelberg (2004)
16. Code Conventions for the Java™ Programming Language, http://java.sun.com/docs/codeconv/html/CodeConvTOC.doc.html
17. Schumacher Jr., R.M.: Phone-based interfaces: research and guidelines. In: Proceedings of HFS, 36th Annual Meeting, p. 1051 (1992)
18. OptimSys, http://www.optimsys.cz/
19. Aoe, J.: Computer algorithms: string pattern matching strategies. IEEE Computer Society Press, Los Alamitos (1994)
20. Bártek, L.: Generating the dialogue interfaces (in czech), PhD. thesis, Masaryk University, Brno (2005)

Book4All: A Tool to Make an e-Book More Accessible to Students with Vision/Visual-Impairments

Antonello Calabrò, Elia Contini, and Barbara Leporini

ISTI - CNR
Via G. Moruzzi, 1 – 56124 Pisa, Italy
{antonello.calabro,elia.contini,barbara.leporini}@isti.cnr.it

Abstract. Empowering people who are blind or otherwise visually impaired includes ensuring that products and electronic materials incorporate a broad range of accessibility features and work well with screen readers and other assistive technology devices. This is particularly important for students with vision impairments. Unfortunately, authors and publishers often do not include specific criteria when preparing the contents. Consequently, e-books can be inadequate for blind and low vision users, especially for students. In this paper we describe a semi-automatic tool developed to support operators who adapt e-documents for visually impaired students. The proposed tool can be used to convert a PDF e-book into a more suitable accessible and usable format readable on desktop computer or on mobile devices.

Keywords: e-book, e-document, accessibility, accessible publishing, semi-automatic support, DAISY.

1 Introduction

Accessing information as well as reading educational materials has always been a challenge for people unable to read printed material. Electronic materials are gaining more and more importance in daily life for everybody [9], especially for people with vision impairments. As technology advances and more books move from hard-copy print to electronic formats, people with print disabilities will have a great opportunity to enjoy access to books on an equal basis with those who can read print. This is particularly important for blind students (e.g. [4] and [8]).

To assure this is the case, associated mechanisms for guaranteeing accessibility as well as usability for all are required. Furthermore, in several countries, specific accessibility laws have been approved, which require publishers to provide electronically accessible versions of school textbooks. Nevertheless, students with disabilities in mainstream classrooms do not always have access to the same learning tools as their classmates. For example, students with visual impairments rely on alternative-format books (such as large or Braille print or audio versions).

Unfortunately, the time-consuming process of turning books or other materials into Braille, audiotape, or large-print editions means that visually impaired students often start the school year without their textbooks. Thus, while the other students receive

A. Holzinger and K. Miesenberger (Eds.): USAB 2009, LNCS 5889, pp. 236–248, 2009.
© Springer-Verlag Berlin Heidelberg 2009

complete printed books, vision-impaired students receive their study material chapter by chapter with the risk that it does not arrive in time for them to keep up with the learning schedule. Moreover, visual learning tools are often totally unsuitable for blind students. This means that a special adapting process to make them accessible to students with vision impairments can be labour intensive. As a consequence, students must rely on teachers or classmates, who have to try to describe visual content as best they can. This situation can limit the educational opportunities of blind students.

We use the term e-document for contents (text, figures etc.) that is stored in electronic format. Thus, an e-document can be a simple text, a more complex document, with title, paragraphs and subparagraphs, or an electronic book organized into chapters and sections. In other words, all these considerations and the solutions we propose are relevant to a general e-document as well as to more highly structured e-books. Starting with these considerations, in the following we use the terms e-document and e-book synonymously.

The format of a large of e-documents available to visually impaired people can be fairly simple and easy to modify to provide accessibility, as is often the case for story books. However, scientific e-documents for example may contain complicated explanations, graphs, tables and formulae. In this case it is more difficult to create accessible and usable texts, since a complex network of alternative explanations and other complementary descriptions need to be included in the electronic format.

Overall, our work is aimed at addressing the accessibility and usability issues in electronic publishing. Specifically, it aims to develop technical and methodological solutions to the main barriers to creating cultural/scientific e-documents that can be accessed and used able by disabled users. In addition this work is intended to provide recommendations for the creation of accessible e-documents as well as support for converting inaccessible e-documents to an accessible format.

In this paper, first we introduce the main issues related to e-book user experience by considering both end-users – i.e. blind students – and adapting-center operators. Next, we describe our approach by showing how it has been developed. For this purpose, we describe the solution applied to two e-documents available on line.

2 Related Work

In order to overcome limitations for those people who cannot meet their information needs from standard printed material, electronic documents can represent a very appropriate solution. In this direction several attempts have been made to develop specialised formats, especially for people with a visual impairment. One of these is a by-product of the Daisy consortium (Digital Accessible Information SYstem), which is working on producing a standard for talking books characterized by navigational information to better move through the document (http://www.DAISY.org). With this system, hybrid books can be made available in the DAISY format, ranging from audio-only, to full text and audio, to text-only [3]. In November 2008, a new version of guidelines for DAISY standard 3.0 has been published [7]. These Guidelines provide information on the correct usage and application of DAISY XML (the DTBook XML element set) in the creation of DAISY publications. Another major change in the DAISY 3 Structure Guidelines is the inclusion of information about NIMAS

(National Instructional Materials Accessibility Standard) mark-up [16]. NIMAS is the required electronic format in the U.S. for textbook publishers which produce K-12 textbooks.

Other studies on this topic include the work of Sun et al. [17], who designed e-Book browsers that aid users in perceiving and understanding the important conceptual structures of a book, and hence improve their comprehension of the book content. A number of authors have proposed ad-hoc solutions for visually-impaired people. Adjouadi et al. [1] introduced a new automatic book reader for blind people. Their objective is the design of a fully integrated system that is relatively fast, but inexpensive and effective with a high reading accuracy. Scientific contents present additional difficulties in reading through a screen reader. Kanahori et al. [14] proposed an integrated system for scientific documents including mathematical formulae with speech output interface. "ChattyInfty" is a system composed of a recognizer, editor and speech interface for scientific documents, including PDF documents. The system tries to recognise the content from the PDF as it was a page image and provides the interpreted content through a simple and customizable interface. Using this system, visually impaired people can read printed scientific documents with speech output.

In our study we prefer to propose solutions to design, develop or adapt accessible and usable e-books, which can be read with traditional tools (e.g. adobe reader, Web browser) in order to obtain more general solutions, with the greatest benefits for all. In this sense, we consider solutions aimed at converting and adapting e-documents in order to make them more usable for blind people.

The large amount of information available today can be potentially accessed in real time through intranet or internet. This has increased the need for syntactic and semantic characterization of documents and for tools that allow their effective access and exploitation on the Net as well as their annotation to adapt and personalize them on the base of users' characteristics and diversities. In [2] the authors propose a system aimed at improving e-document editing, annotating, and at exploiting the description of the logical structure of the document itself to squeeze the information about the document content. In [5] an approach for automatically generating an e-textbook on the Web for a user specified topic hierarchy is described. That approach consists of generating an e-book on the Web starting with a topic indicated by the user. Users can then browse through the descriptive pages like a book. Hence, e-books are increasingly providing new ways to obtain and study information. In [11] the problem related to tagged PDF is faced by using an XML-based structure. The tool implemented is an Acrobat Plugin, which means that it can be used in conjunction with Acrobat products. Conversely our methodology is aimed at developing a semi-automatic support to adapt a single format to various ones by taking into account specific user requirements.

3   The e-Book User Experience (UX)

In order to understand the main issues related to the interaction with an e-book, let us first consider the user experience when handling an e-book itself. Two different perspectives can be identified:

- The end-user viewpoint;
- The adapting-center viewpoint.

As end-users we consider blind people and in particular students who need to use books for educational purposes. The adapting-center viewpoint is provided by the operator who has to manage the content to make it accessible.

3.1 End-Users' Viewpoint

Even though school books are available in a digital format such as TXT, XHTML or PDF, this fact alone is not enough to guarantee accessibility and usability features to support the studying process. Students should be able to read books not exclusively in a sequential way, as with story books: they should be able to move quickly through the content as well as to take notes and to mark interesting parts. In short, blind students should have the same opportunities to interact with an e-book as a sighted student has with the paper format.

Currently available e-books do not enable students t perform this kind of task, because the contents are not well structured, images do not have textual descriptions, data tables do not have text explanation, and it is difficult to mark parts or take notes. Consequently, these issues increase the learning effort and the cognitive load by the students as well. In fact, when the students need to revise specific parts, they have to read the contents in sequential way or try to find the required text by searching for a certain string or sentence. This is not practical when studying, because the students can lose focus while searching for the text. More details of blind people's experiences with e-documents can be found in [6] and [13]. In order to enhance the learning process, the contents should not only be accessible, but also – and equally importantly – usable [15]. This means that appropriate mechanisms and adequate descriptions need to be available in the e-book.

3.2 Adapting-Center Viewpoint

Nowadays, a serious problem is the slow and expensive production of e-books that are both accessible and for all, including people who have to interact with assistive technologies (e.g. a screen reader). To obtain a concrete accessible and usable e-book, the contents and the structure have to conform to appropriate procedure and rules. The e-book content is adapted by a person - called an operator -. Carrying out those actions manually is time-consuming and requires a lot of actions by the operators.

The main reasons for this limitation can be summarized as follows:

- lack of clear guidelines that help authors/publishers to build a really accessible and usable e-book;
- lack of tools able to support the entire conversion process;
- lack of a standard intermediate format that makes it possible abstract data book content and that is not limited to final distribution formats such as PDF, XHTML, HTML5, DAISY 3.0 and Braille;
- Lack of consideration by publishers of blind and visually impaired student needs.

The work carried out is mainly focused on producing accessible versions of the textbooks received by the publishers possibly in electronic format. Simplifying the work of the adaptors in translating contents into a more adequate version that can be easily used via a screen reader would be an important contribution to rectify this limitation.

4 Our Approach

In order to solve problems related to e-book UX we propose a very practical approach with the following components:

- A set of guidelines that allows users and adapting-centers to obtain an excellent e-book UX;
- Semi-automatic tools to speed up the process of e-book conversion and adaptation (ad-hoc PDF viewer and Book4All);
- A very powerful and flexible Intermediate Book Format (IBF) to manage contents of e-books and provides a solid base to generate accessible and usable final formats.
    Currently we provide a simple way to generate XHTML 1.0 Strict or DAISY 3.0 e-book.

The solution proposed in this work is an evolution of our previous case study [6]. Based on our previous experience, we are proposing a new and updated methodology. In particular, we selected two documents available on line ([9] [18]) in order to show how our approach can be applied to practical cases.

4.1 Guidelines

The generation of accessible and usable e-books is closely linked to a well structured content: each element within a book must be marked with the right tag and each complex element such as images and tables must be described using an alternative description.
    When generating the e-book UI to be provided to the blind students, we consider five main guidelines:

1. Titles and subtitles (i.e. sections and subsections) must be marked with the appropriate tags. If titles are tagged it is possible to automatically generate the content index and to provide a basic and non-sequential navigation structure;
2. Paragraph and elements within paragraph (e.g. links, abbreviations and so on) must be marked. If paragraphs are tagged then it is possible to easily search the content of e-book, take notes and create bookmarks;
3. images must be tagged and each image must have an appropriate textual description that clearly explains the information provided;
4. tables must be tagged and each table must have an appropriate textual description that clearly explains the structure of table (e.g. Table has two columns) and the data contained in it (e.g. The first column contains users' names and the second one email);

5. Unordered and ordered lists must be tagged to improve navigation between items and to better identify each list (e.g. by using screen reader special command, the user is able to skip from one list to another).

4.2 Semi-automatic Tools

Our approach also includes two tools aimed at supporting adapting-centers to accelerate the conversion and adaptation process. Based on the consideration that book editors mainly provide e-book in PDF format, we consider this format as the source version. Consequently, our solution is based on a process that takes a PDF document as input file and provides an accessible and usable final electronic format as output, following various semi-automatic manipulations (the intervention of an operator is necessary).

4.2.1 PDF Viewer

In our case study, the first tool we created was an ad-hoc PDF Viewer that allows operators to gather useful data on the PDF source. This is necessary to obtain as much correct information as possible from the source version in order to facilitate the operators in manipulating the content to be adapted. As a consequence, an important assumption we made is about the presence of the operator in the conversion process. This means that (as described below) the more input information provided to the manipulation tool before starting the conversion process, the better the obtained results are. From this prospective, the user (i.e. the operator) could be asked to input some information on the PDF source document. The main goal of our proposed PDF Viewer is to provide styles and formats features as well as select and copy parts from the entire content. For example, the PDF Viewer obtains information on the fonts such as name and size of the selected content.

In addition, with this supporting tool it is possible to manage PDF with multiple column layout. The selection of text in a multiple column layout PDF is a problem recently considered also by Apple Inc, which used artificial intelligence and implemented it in the new version of the Preview tool[1]. Our ad-hoc PDF Viewer provides a simpler and more detailed solution than the one proposed by Apple. And in fact, our tool also provides information about the selected text.

Figure 1 shows an example of multi-column text extraction with Ad-Hoc PDFViewer; in the popup window we have information about font face and size.

4.2.2 BOOK4All

The information gathered about fonts is passed to the second tool "Book4All" which uses such information to extract text and images from the PDF source. Extracting information from a PDF document is a critical issue to be implemented. Similarly to our approach, in [12] a possible method developed to obtain text and images from a PDF file by analyzing the layout structure is proposed. Book4All reconstructs the

---

[1] Apple Preview Tool,
http://www.apple.com/macosx/refinements/enhancements-refinements.html#preview

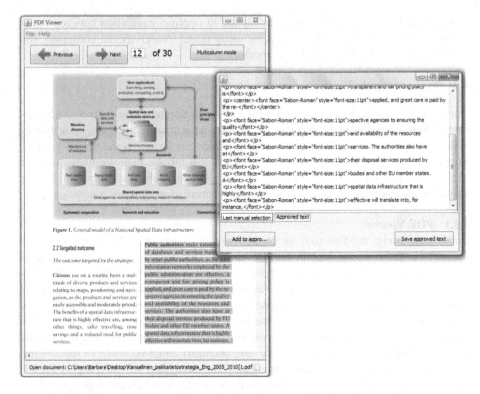

Fig. 1. Ad-hoc PDF Viewer. Text extraction from a multi-column layout document.

semantic structure of the e-book by analyzing the extracted data and saves the result in the Intermediate Book Format (IBF) (see 4.3). Each element is tagged according to the guidelines described above (see 4.1). After this step, it is possible to edit contents, add images and table descriptions and finally to export the result in one of the final supported formats (i.e. XHTML 1.0 or DAISY 3.0).

4.3 Intermediate Book Format (IBF)

The key issue of our solution is the Intermediate Book Format (IBF) that enables the user to tag elements of the e-book in an easy way. Overall, this XML-based format is designed to abstract the content of e-book and make such content independent from the final e-book format provided to the final users, the students.

IBF is a XML based language with an easy syntax that provides a tag for each element usually contained within a school textbook. At the current time, we can provide support only for simple text books: the work to obtain support for scientific books, such as mathematics, chemistry or physics, is in progress.

The following example shows a fragment of IBF code:

```
<page number="1">

<headingLevel1>Chapter title</headingLevel1>

<paragraph>Lorem ipsum dolor sit amet, consectetur
adipiscing elit. Quisque non felis sed augue aliquam
eleifend nec ac lectus. Donec tempus, quam vitae
euismod ullamcorper, nisi nisl malesuada nulla, <em-
phatyzed>a adipiscing nunc dolor et
nunc</emphatyzed>. Nullam eleifend, arcu sed
ullamcorper mollis, justo velit dapibus leo, sed
fringilla nisi arcu vel nulla. <strong>Sed euismod
dapibus tortor ac bibendum</strong>.

    </paragraph>

    <headingLevel2>Paragraph Title</headingLevel2>

    <list type="ordered">

      <listItem>Item 1</listItem>

      <listItem>Item 2</listItem>

      <listItem>

          <list type="unordered">

              <listItem>

                  <paragraph>Lorem ipsum dolor sit amet,
consectetur adipiscing elit. Phasellus a vestibulum
justo. <image source="image.png" width="88" height="33"
description="image description" />

                  </paragraph>

              </listItem>

          </list>

      </listItem>

    </list>

</page>
```

4.4 A Typical Workflow

Based on our procedure, a typical workflow would be the following:

1. The Editor provides a PDF school textbook ;
2. The operator uses ad-hoc PDF Viewer to gather information about fonts and make the content linear in case of multiple column layout (see 4.2);
3. The operator uses Book4All to extract text and images and automatically mark all text elements (title, paragraph and so on) with the right tag, by using the fonts information gathered by ad-hoc PDF Viewer

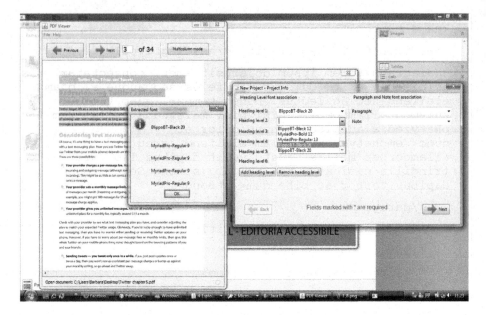

Fig. 2. Association of a font with structure elements with ad-hoc PDF Viewer aid

4. After the tagging step, the operator adds descriptions to images, corrects possible extraction and tagging mistakes (using particular reviews lists), and reconstructs the table manually;
5. At this point, the obtained IBF file is ready to be exported in one of the final formats;
6. The final format can be provided to students.

5 Architecture

As mentioned above our solution is composed of two main tools: an ad-hoc PDF Viewer and Book4All based on the IBF API 1.0 (Stone Eater).

The IBF API 1.0 is the core of our architecture and it is completely GUI independent. Fig. 3. shows the main infrastructure based on our solution. This means that developers can create both Desktop GUIs and web applications.

The main research work was concentrated on the Book4All tool. In this paragraph we discuss its architecture, what issues occurred and which solutions we proposed during the design and the implementation phases.

The Book4All tool is divided into four main components:

1. Extractor;
2. Tagging Engine;
3. IBF Editor;
4. Exporter.

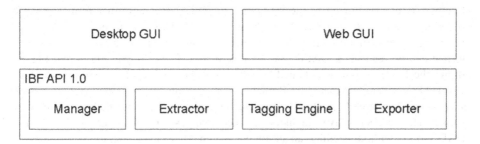

Fig. 3. IBF API 1.0 infrastructure

5.1 Extractor

The Extractor is the component of the tool that extracts text and images. The extracted text contains raw information about fonts (size and face). The extracted images are stored in a directory related to each page. A heuristic engine tries to relocate the images within the pages. The heuristic algorithm is based on the knowledge that in the raw text there are groups of blank lines instead of images. The number of blank lines is proportional to the image size. Using these data, the heuristic engine identifies the image position by computing the consecutive blank lines.

5.2 Tagging Engine

The Tagging engine marks the extracted raw text using the operator input. The operator associates tags with font size and face. Using the ad-hoc PDF viewer, the operator inspects the PDF to gather information about font, by simply selecting the interesting text. The viewer then returns font face and size.

The Tagging Engine marks all text elements with IBF tags and using the operator input, and tries to reconstruct ordered and unordered lists by using a heuristic. The Tagging Engine output is valid IBF, which is ready to be adapted and extended by the operator.

5.3 IBF Editor

Book4All provides a powerful IBF editor that simplifies:

- Heading level editing;
- Paragraph editing;
- Addition and editing of image descriptions;
- Table reconstruction;
- Lists optimization and insertion;
- Note handling and editing.

5.4 Exporter

The Exporter is the element that exports IBF file into final format such as XHTML 1.0 Strict or DAISY 3.0, by mainly using XSLT transformations. The flexibility of the

Exporter is closely linked to the flexibility of XSLT: the new final format can be added by simply adding a new XSL Transformation. The final format XHTML 1.0 can be read through a common browser and a screen reader like Jaws[2]. The DAISY format can be read via a DAISY SW or HW reader. For example, Fig. 4 and Fig. 5 shows the DAISY content obtained by extracting the book [18] by using Book4All. The DAISY version extracted by Book4All can be transferred to the symbian-based smartphone Nokia N95. A DAISY multimedia player[3] can be installed on the mobile phone. The DAISY player includes a voice synthesizer, which reads the XML-DAISY book without needing an additional screen reader loaded on the smartphone.

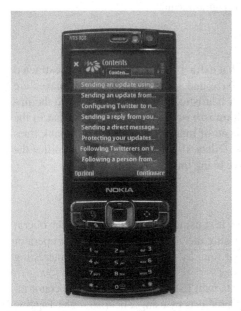

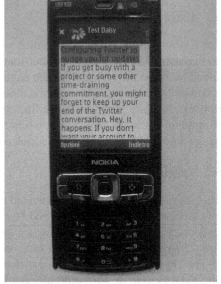

Fig. 4. Exporting in DAISY 3.0. Reading book index using a mobile screen reader

Fig. 5. Exporting in DAISY 3.0. Reading book content using a mobile screen reader

6   Conclusions and Future Work

As described in this paper, the existing manual process for conversion and adaptation of e-documents to an accessible and usable version for students with visual impairments is time consuming due to the numerous manipulations carried out manually by operators. With our approach several tasks can be performed in as semi-automatic

---

[2] Jaws for Windows,
http://www.freedomscientific.com/products/fs/jaws-product-page.asp
[3] Daisy player for Nokia N95 8 GB,
http://codefactory.es/descargas/family_3/product_16/version_57/MobileDaisyPlayer_S60_3_0_v_2_2_3.zip

way which makes the process easier and in addition saves time. . The proposed tool is able to convert the source PDF document into more accessible DAISY and X/HTML versions. In this perspective, the proposed tool is also appropriate for preparing X/HTML documents to be published on the Web based on a PDF version. This can be useful for Public Administration that cannot rely on experts in developing accessible Web pages. Moreover, the tool could be also valuable for additional purposes, such as for generating a variety output versions (e.g. Braille or audio formats). In short, from a single source version it is easy to obtain various accessible outputs. Future work will concern the development of features and components aimed to simplify the editing tasks as well as a Web-based usage in a collaborative way. For this purpose, tools like Microsoft Word and OpenOffice.org Writer plug-ins; a web application for conversion, adaptation, collaboration and sharing will be consider.

Acknowledgements

This project is supported by the Italian Department of the Education.

References

1. Adjouadi, M., Ruiz, E., Wang, L.: Automated Book Reader for Persons with Blindness. In: Miesenberger, K., Klaus, J., Zagler, W.L., Karshmer, A.I. (eds.) ICCHP 2006. LNCS, vol. 4061, pp. 1094–1101. Springer, Heidelberg (2006)
2. Bottoni, P., Ferri, F., Grifoni, P., Marcante, A., Mussio, P., Padula, M., Reggiori, A.: E-Document management in situated interactivity: the WIL approach. Universal Access in the Information Society 8(3), 137–153 (2009)
3. Brzoza, P., Spinczyk, D.: Multimedia Browser for Internet Online Daisy Books. In: Miesenberger, K., Klaus, J., Zagler, W.L., Karshmer, A.I. (eds.) ICCHP 2006. LNCS, vol. 4061, pp. 1087–1093. Springer, Heidelberg (2006)
4. Burgstahler, S.: Universal Design of Distance Learning. Information Technology and Disabilities (2002),
   http://www.rit.edu/~easi/itd/itdv08n1/burgstahler.htm
5. Chen, G., Li, Q., Jia, W.: Automatically Generating an E-textbook on the Web. World Wide Web 8(4), 377–394 (2005)
6. Contini, E., Leporini, B., Paternò, F.: A Semi-automatic Support to Adapt E-Documents in an Accessible and Usable Format for Vision Impaired Users. In: Miesenberger, K., Klaus, J., Zagler, W.L., Karshmer, A.I. (eds.) ICCHP 2008. LNCS, vol. 5105, pp. 242–249. Springer, Heidelberg (2008)
7. DAISY/NISO Standard, Structure Guidelines (2008),
   http://www.DAISY.org/z3986/structure/
8. Edmonds, C.: Providing access to students with disabilities in online distance education: Legal and technical concerns for higher education. American Journal of Distance Education 18(1) (2004)
9. Finnish Government Information Society, Ministry of Agriculture and Forestry,
   http://www.mmm.fi/attachments/maanmittausjapaikkatiedot/5g7g
   69SqF/Kansallinen_paikkatietostrategia_Eng_2005_2010%5B1.pdf

10. Gil-Rodríguez, E.P., Planella-Ribera, J.: Educational Uses of the e-Book: An Experience in a Virtual University Context. In: Holzinger, A. (ed.) USAB 2008. LNCS, vol. 5298, pp. 55–62. Springer, Heidelberg (2008)
11. Hardy, M.R.B., Brailsford, D.F., Thomas, P.T.: Creating structured PDF files using XML templates. In: Proc. of the 2004 ACM symposium DocEng 2004 (2004)
12. Hassan, T.: Object-Level Document Analysis of PDF Files. In: Proc. Of ACM Symposium DocEng 2009, Munich, Germany (2009)
13. Hersh, M., Leporini, B.: Making Conference CDs Accessible: A Practical Example. In: Miesenberger, K., Klaus, J., Zagler, W.L., Karshmer, A.I. (eds.) ICCHP 2008. LNCS, vol. 5105, pp. 326–333. Springer, Heidelberg (2008)
14. Kanahori, T., Suzuki, M.: Scientific PDF Document Reader with Simple Interface for Visually Impaired People. In: Miesenberger, K., Klaus, J., Zagler, W.L., Karshmer, A.I. (eds.) ICCHP 2006. LNCS, vol. 4061, pp. 48–52. Springer, Heidelberg (2006)
15. Leporini, B., Paternò, F.: Increasing Usability when Interacting through Screen Readers. Universal Access in the Information Society 3(1), 57–70 (2004); Guidelines, Standards, Methods and Processes for Software Accessibility
16. NIMAS, National Instructional Materials Accessibility Standard, http://nimas.cast.org/about/nimas
17. Sun, Y., Harper, D.J., Watt, S.N.K.: Design of an e-book user interface and visualizations to support reading for comprehension. In: Proc. of the 27th Annual International ACM SIGIR Conference on Research and Development in Information Retrieval, pp. 510–511 (2004)
18. Twitter Tips, Tricks, and Tweets - Paul McFedries. Pdf twitter, http://mcfedries.com/cs/content/TwitterTTT.aspx

Enhancing Accessibility of Web Content for the Print-Impaired and Blind People

Aimilios Chalamandaris[1,2], Spyros Raptis[1,2], Pirros Tsiakoulis[1,2], and Sotiris Karabetsos[1,2]

[1] Institute for Language and Speech Processing – Athena Research Center
[2] Innoetics ltd, Knowledge and Mutlimodal Interaction Technologies
Artemidos 6 and Epidavrou, 15125 Athens, Greece
{achalam,spy,ptsiak,sotoskar}@ilsp.gr,
{aimilios,sraptis,ptsiak,sotoskar}@innoetics.com

Abstract. Blind people and in general print-impaired people are often restricted to use their own computers, enhanced most often with expensive, screen reading programs, in order to access the web, and in a form that every screen reading program allows to. In this paper we present *SpellCast Navi*, a tool that is intended for people with visual impairments, which attempts to combine advantages from both customized and generic web enhancement tools. It consists of a generically designed engine and a set of case-specific filters. It can run on a typical web browser and computer, without the need of installing any additional application locally. It acquires and parses the content of web pages, converts bi-lingual text into synthetic speech using high quality speech synthesizer, and supports a set of common functionalities such as navigation through hotkeys, audible navigation lists and more. By using a post-hoc approach based on a-priori information of the website's layout, the audible presentation and navigation through the website is more intuitive a more efficient than with a typical screen reading application. *SpellCast Navi* poses no requirements on web pages and introduces no overhead to the design and development of a website, as it functions as a hosted proxy service.

Keywords: Web accessibility, Speech synthesis, Print-Impairment, Screen Reader.

1 Introduction

This paper presents *SpellCast Navi*, a web based tool that can serve as a web-reader used by blind and print-impaired individuals. Currently, the typical aids for blind computer users, as far as computer usage is concerned, are software programs called screen readers, and they are responsible for converting visual information of the computer screen into speech, providing at the same time the necessary shortcut keys for navigating through programs and screens. These programs, more often, are expensive because of their complexity and the relative small market they are addressing, posing a significant obstacle to the blind computer users to acquire one, through private means.

Similarly to the screen readers, which address mainly blind people as their main target group, there are other applications and tools that aim to simply enhance visual

A. Holzinger and K. Miesenberger (Eds.): USAB 2009, LNCS 5889, pp. 249–263, 2009.

interfaces with aural and spatial information, in order to accommodate cases such as of dyslexia or illiteracy. These programs typically enhance visual features of the interface and often incorporate text to speech synthesizers for producing aural interfacing to the content. These applications are also most of the times commercial, with costs that vary from few Euros to a few hundreds Euros, depending on the complexity of the functions they provide.

In this paper we present a hybrid approach for providing an efficient and generic aid to print-impaired people, which actually can be customized and be adapted according to personal needs, with different settings and preferences for users of different impairments, such as blindness, limited vision, or dyslexia. Additionally to these target groups, one can also include people with temporary inability to read textual content, like for instance while driving a car, or people who face difficulties in reading in a specific language, like for example immigrants.

In the following section of this paper a brief overview of available web accessibility technologies is given, along with a classification of the different approaches met in the industrial and research field of web accessibility software. The *SpellCast Navi* system is described in section 3, with enhanced details when necessary, about its design, operation and the functionalities it offers. Finally, a discussion of a pilot evaluation phase of the systems and of the future plans for further developing the systems are given in the final paragraphs of the paper, in order to provide a more complete idea of the described system and its roadmap for evolution.

2   Web Accessibility Technologies and Tools

The World Wide Web's increasing importance and penetration into daily activities makes the need for its accessibility more imperative than ever. Information repositories, communication means and interactive services, based on the internet, are some of the most active development areas today [1].

As true universal access and inclusive design are now becoming critical requirements, efforts to design and implement browsing helpers encounter a typical dilemma: generality versus specialty. A general web enhancement tool (such as a screen reader or a text browser) is able to deal with virtually any web page based on uniform, systematic and widely applicable interaction patterns. On the other hand, a custom tool tailored and adapted to the specifics of a website will perform better and more efficiently, since by being able to exploit available a-priori information of the site's structure, it can convey information more coherently to the user, while at the same time it can cope more efficiently with different types of impairments, by adjusting its features and its functionalities. Moreover, it will be able to support richer and more accurate interaction patterns than in the case of a typical screen reading program. The choice of the appropriate tool is strongly linked with the intended application and the required use cases.

Web accessibility means access to the World Wide Web by everyone, regardless of the type of the disability [2]. The following discussion in this section is confined mainly to the case of web accessibility technology for visually impaired people and it provides a general idea of the status of the web accessibility currently.

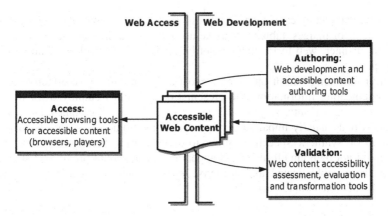

Fig. 1. The main parts involved in web accessibility: The content, the authoring tools, and the browsing tools

Web accessibility evolves around content [3]. Content needs to possess a set of attributes, which ensure the completeness of the information it is intended to convey to the user. This is directly related to the way content is presented, i.e. the content access, and significantly affects the way it is produced, that is content authoring and development.

There has been a lot of research and work in the field of web accessibility and in closely linked fields; fields drawing from, or contributing to it. A special reference is due to the W3C Web Accessibility Initiative [4], and especially to its Web Content Accessibility Guidelines [5], the Voice Browser Activity [6], and the Alternative Web Browsing considerations.

2.1 Accessible Content

As already mentioned, web accessibility evolves around web content. Obviously, the major role of the web content is to capture and convey information to the user. Content presentation is of a separate concern, involving creating views and projections of the content to specific representational patterns in order to provide ease or additional spatial information. Much of the content accessibility relies in assuring that no questionable assumptions are hard-wired in the content concerning the way, means and techniques that will be used to present it.

Accessible web content, namely web content desired to be accessible via screen reading programs, possesses a set of attributes that ensure sufficient consistency and presentational independence (often calling for redundancy) of the information it is intended to provide. In practice, content accessibility suggests conformance to a set of requirements that assure an "accessible format". A widely acceptable specification of such a format is provided by W3C's Web Content Accessibility Guidelines. The primary goal of the W3C's Web Content Accessibility Guidelines is to promote content accessibility and to set the common ground for consistent behavior of aid-tools, such as of screen readers. These guidelines are summarized as a list of organized and prioritized checkpoints that web pages need to be verified against, along with suggested techniques for adopting them.

Some typical examples of specific aspects covered by the WCAG document are alternative text for images, tables that make no sense when their elements are read in a sequential manner, web forms that cannot be navigated into with a meaningful order and so on.

With vision being one of the richest, most appealing and most effective channels for communicating information, the presentational patterns employed for delivering web content, significantly rely on images, charts, tables and graphics. However, the sole means that visually impaired persons often have to access such information are aids based on synthetic speech. In order to avoid marginalizing such users, content itself should not be bound to its visual appearance, and should provide what is necessary for these sophisticated and attractive page layouts to significantly reduce to meaningful audible counterparts.

2.2   Content Authoring

Accessible web content calls for content authoring tools that can produce such content as well as tools that can assess, evaluate, and transform web content into an "accessible format".

Content authoring and development tools for accessible content have evolved significantly in the recent years; however they are out of this paper's scope and therefore they will not be covered. Detailed information on the technologies and tools can be found through the W3C website.

2.3   Content Presentation and Access

Software used to access web content is usually referred to as user agent. Obviously, accessible user agents that can make web content truly available to all users are the terminus. These tools, unless they incorporate a-priori information about the layout of the site they are asked to process, they simply convey the textual information of the content with limited spatial and prioritized information. What however is necessary is to employ efficient content presentation schemes, tailored to the special needs of their users, enhancing the content perception and understanding. Moreover, these tools need to implement appropriate user interaction patterns so that the users can effectively interact with the content and navigate through it.

User agents include desktop graphical browsers, text browsers, voice browsers, mobile phones, multimedia players, and so on. Assistive software technologies used in conjunction with browsers such as screen readers, screen magnifiers, and voice recognition software, are also of concern. Some of the most relevant user agent technologies for the case of visually impaired people are shortly discussed in the following paragraphs.

2.3.1   Alternative Browsing
Text browsers offer an alternative to graphical user interface browsers. They can be used in combination with standard screen readers to render content through synthesized speech. Lynx is a typical example of a text browser.

Voice browsers allow the people to interact via spoken commands and synthetic speech and navigate through the web, with alternative means than the typical mouse or keyboard. They offer the promise of allowing everyone to access web-based services from any phone, making it practical to access the web anytime and anywhere, whether at home, on the move, or at work. Work in the field of voice browsers is closely related to people with visual impairments since voice is used as a replacement of the vision to convey the necessary information, very similarly to accessing the web through the phone.

The term *alternative browsing* refers to all approaches, including the ones mentioned above, and which deviate from the typical browser setting, providing specific support for specific types of disabilities.

2.3.2 Content Transformations

There are several different operations that need to be carried out in order to convert a web page into an audible form. Some of the operations, most relative to this discussion are the web page adaptation, restructuring and, finally, rendition of it into synthetic speech.

2.3.2.1 Adaptation. The adaptation of the web page to the user profile (personalization), involves the alteration of the page's format to fit the user needs and preferences. It includes special processing and transformations that may be necessary to the page so that it becomes more accessible to a specific user.

For example, increasing the contrast or the font size for people with low vision, serializing page contents for blind people so that they are read more efficiently by a screen reader, enlarging the active page elements to facilitate their access by motor-impaired people and so on, are only a few of the adaptation processes that need to be carried out.

Adaptation can take place locally in the user's (client) computer, e.g. as in the case of the AVANTI web browser [7], or through a proxy server that intervenes between the web server that provides the content and the user's computer e.g. as in the case of WebFACE [8] and WebAnywhere [9].

2.3.2.2 Restructuring of the Web Page and Custom Interactivity. Restructuring of the web page involves determining the role of the web page elements and element groups, and provide the user with a more efficient manner to access them.

The role of an element is not only related to the type of the element (e.g. an edit box in a web form or a side link), but also its intended use in the site. Examples of elements, with specific semantics in a site, are the global navigation menus and sub-menus in websites, elements that are systematically used throughout a site, and which have a specific purpose, specific formats that signify section breaks or special types of transitions to other pages or sites, and so on.

It is worth noting that although website templates significantly differ in their aesthetics and their spatial layout, they do share a lot of common structural properties. Global site navigation menus, option bars, and copyright notices appear in the vast majority of the sites. Such usable and efficient website design patterns have been widely adopted and people not only have they become very familiar with them, but also they actually try to identify such structures in every new website they visit, as a fist step of familiarization with the website.

An important property of some of these elements is the fact that they appear in every page of the site providing a tree log of the website. This property assigns to them a more global characteristic, that is, as website's functional elements rather than web page elements. Reading these elements to the user in each page rarely makes sense and it would probably tire the user. Computer users are somehow familiarized with and aware of the website's layout, and they have always in mind that these elements exist in the website and they can follow them anytime they want; however they do not pay attention to them in every web page of the website they visit. Similarly, print-impaired people should not be provided with the same information on every page they visit, but simply they should be notified about their existence only at their request and not in every page they navigate to.

Identification and proper handling of elements with specific roles in a website can provide the means for supporting custom enhanced interaction patterns, which can significantly improve the usability of a website and the quality of the interaction with the user. The navigation through the website is more efficient and less tiring for the print-impaired user. However, this can only be accomplished with a priori information about the design of the specific website.

2.3.2.3 Speech Rendering. Speech has become a mainstream technology in the computers field. Speech synthesis (text-to-speech, TtS) [10] is particularly relative to visually impaired people, since it can be one of the most effective substitutes for vision. Text-to-Speech systems are now widely available for many different languages and are supported even at the level of the operating system as, for example, in the case of Microsoft Speech API for Windows, while their performance has significantly improved during the last few years mainly due to the adoption of statistical methods [11].

In the context of accessibility tools and as far as the location of the software is concerned, a TtS component could be available:

- Locally as part of the operating system, an accessibility tool (as a screen reader) or the web browser itself, like for instance is IBM's Home Page Reader [12]. This does not pose any overhead in the web connection bandwidth, since speech rendering takes place locally, by only consuming local computational resources. However, in this case, the software requires to be downloaded and installed, including regular updates.
- Remotely as a service provided by a speech server like *SpellCast Navi*, ReadSpeaker [13], Talklets [14]. In this case there is no need to install locally a Text-to-Speech software, with the trade-off of higher requirements on the connection for audio files transfer (higher internet bandwidth).

Although in the recent years the local version of TtS software was preferable due to speed limitations as far as the internet connections were concerned, currently they provide a better architectural scheme overall, since they can be maintained more easily and efficiently and they can offer service to the user immediately, to a wider set of devices, without the need of any software installation.

2.4 Existing Systems

A brief overview of the mostly used approaches for the speech-enhanced web access is provided in Figure 2 below. Some features of each category are given below.

- *Category 1*. In this category the most simple and common settings for speech-enhanced web access are included. A normal web browser such as Internet Explorer, Firefox, Safari etc., has the role of accessing and retrieving the web content, while a separate tool such as a screen reader, like for instance JAWS [15], a desktop accessibility tool, like for instance Apple VoiceOver [16], or a web browser plug-in (e.g. FireVox [17]) are responsible for rendering the visited web pages through synthetic speech. In this case, the browser is responsible for performing any necessary adaptations to the web content to meet user needs and preferences. In this category, no restructuring or custom interactivity can be supported since there is no way to exploit a-priori website information.
- *Category 2*. A slightly different approach is that of an entirely custom browser. The new browser is responsible for all the tasks: accessing and retrieving the web content, adapting it to user needs and preferences, and rendering it to speech. A typical example of a custom browser with adaptation and speech capabilities is IBM's Home Page Reader. Additionally, it provides support for other media types such as Adobe PDF and Macromedia Flash content. Normally, this approach does not support web page restructuring. However, special versions of these tools have been deployed in order to provide enhanced support for specific websites, as for the case of the American Association of People with Disabilities (AAPD) website. Other selected sites which demonstrate specific features are also supported (e.g. the sites of Adobe, Macromedia and W3C).
- *Category 3*. In this case, the adaptation of a web page to meet user needs and preferences is performed by a remote server. That server keeps the user profiles and intervenes between the web content provider (web server) and the user agent (client computer). WebFACE is an example of this approach. Speech rendering can be performed either by a screen reader or a desktop accessibility tool (as in Category 1), or by using a custom web browser (as in Category 2). Restructuring and custom enhanced interactivity are not addressed in this approach.
- *Category 4*. In this case, speech rendering is undertaken by a remote "speech server". A normal web browser is used and a synthesized spoken version of the web page is produced and transferred by the speech server on demand, e.g. when the user presses a designated hotkey. The ReadSpeaker system and SpellCast basic are typical examples of this approach. The advantage of this approach is that the users do not need to install any software component locally at their computers while at the same it is cross-browser and cross-platform available. Restructuring and custom enhanced interactivity are not addressed in this approach either and audio files are provided as an independent stream of media.
- *Category 5*. A more recent approach is when a user obtains a speech-based connection with the web content through a proxy server. The SpeechHTML [18] system and WebAnywhere are examples of this approach as well as our approach, *SpellCast Navi*. The reconstruction of the content into distinct elements and its prioritization is also performed in this approach, based on the use of a-priori information

of the website's structure. This approach is the most recent one since it is based on technologies and infrastructures that only recently have shown significant levels of maturity and robustness.

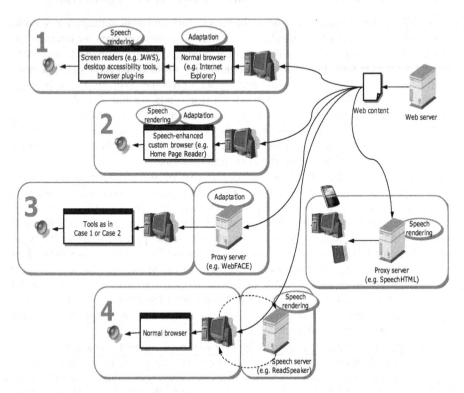

Fig. 2. Overview of different approaches for the speech-enhanced web access

3 The SpellCast Navi System

SpellCast Navi is a tool developed at innoetics ltd, a spin-off company of the Institute for Language and Speech Processing of Research Center Athena, in collaboration with ILSP and it is based on an entirely different approach compared to its predecessor WebSpeech [19].

It is intended to be an accessibility enhancement tool that not only enhances websites via synthetic speech, but it also provides support for page restructuring and enhanced interactivity. It is designed to be a cross-platform and cross-browser application and it operates without the need of any software installation on local computers.

The design of this approach aimed to fulfill a three-fold goal:

1. To provide the functionality of a screen reader for accessing web sites without the need of installing one locally.
2. To provide service in a cross-platform and cross-browser manner, and run on different devices.

3. To offer advanced functionalities and advanced interactivity with the user, depending on the user's preferences and based on a priori information about the website.

By doing so, our approach seems to cover efficiently some of the most important issues concerning the web accessibility and the print-impaired people, while at the same time it constitutes a free, easy to use aid, with intuitive interface for all people. It offers high availability for everyone with advanced functionalities, while, maybe most importantly, it is freely available for all end-users.

3.1 Functional Description

SpellCast's main concern is not only to make web content accessible through synthesized speech, but also to offer more efficient presentation and interaction patterns and facilitate the browsing process by providing a more intuitive and comprehensive aural interface.

The requirements when listening to the content of a webpage are significantly different than those when reading it from the screen or a printout. Our methodology adopts a more natural approach for reading a web page than when using a typical screen reading application, and it consists of two stages: (i) the first one focuses on conveying higher level information such as the title of the page and the distinct elements on the page, such as menus, links etc, and (ii) the second one focuses on reading exhaustively the contents of each section. This permits a quick browsing of the content's structure of the webpage, followed by a detailed reading of the section the user selects. This approach simulates more efficiently the way a non-impaired person would skim a new web page before starting reading it thoroughly.

The most intuitive paradigm for how a web page should be read is when a person is asked to read a webpage aloud to another person, trying to provide, as efficiently as possible, and any information that is implied in the web page. The role of a content mediator is not just to lookup for some specific information for the user, but rather to mediate the user's access to the web content. A typical "session" would include three different steps:

1. Initially to provide a general outlook of the webpage by identifying the title of the webpage and by providing once, only at the beginning of the session or at user's request, the information and the necessary help about the use of the service and about the options given to the him at any time by the service (i.e. menu lists, links lists, shortcut keys etc).
2. The provided service initiates to read aloud all textual web-content, providing also information about different items that are included in the web page, such as images, tables etc. The prioritization of the content elements is performed through a pre-programmed internal service filter that identifies different page elements based on a-priori information fused by the service provider.
3. At any time during the session, the user is given the choice to navigate through restructured audible lists of the page's menus, the page's links and the page's identified distinct textual items. By doing so, the navigation through the website via this enhanced interface, simulates better the way a non-impaired person would be able to do so in the website, rather than with a simple screen reader. In other words, the visually impaired person can navigate, in a non serialized manner

through the website, without the need to go through potentially unnecessary information that would tire him or make the session less efficient.

In order to illustrate and clarify the processes of the service, a specific example site will be used, namely the website of the Secretariat General of Communication-Secretariat General of Information of Greece (http://www.minpress.gr), of which the website's entry page is shown in Figure 3.

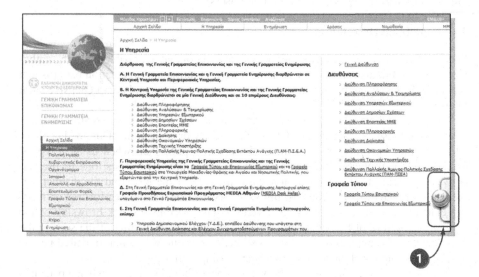

Fig. 3. The example of the website of the Secretariat General of Communication-Secretariat General of Information of Greece (Greek ministry of press)

In the first page and at the beginning of the session the user is notified both visually (for the non-blind people) and aurally, that the website is supported by the *Spell-Cast Navi* service and it can be activated through a combination of hotkeys.

Should the user chooses to activate the service, the user is then given the most essential information about the website, such as the webpage's title, and possible shortcut key combinations for help, menu and link items lists, and navigation inside the webpage elements, such as paragraphs, phrases or tables.

This process is designed to be carried out only once at each user session, via the use of cookies technology. After the first time, the user can listen to this information again at his request, by pressing a hotkey.

Once the process of reading aloud the webpage has started, additional helping tools like highlighting of the current phrase and/or word, and the increased size and contrast of the current cursor position, also provide extra visual aids for people with other print-impairments than blindness, such as dyslexia, limited eyesight, or even illiteracy issues. As it is depicted in figure 4, although the page includes menu items and links that are consistent throughout the website, and they are not read aloud on every page the user visits, but the user can activate any of these menus and browse through them,

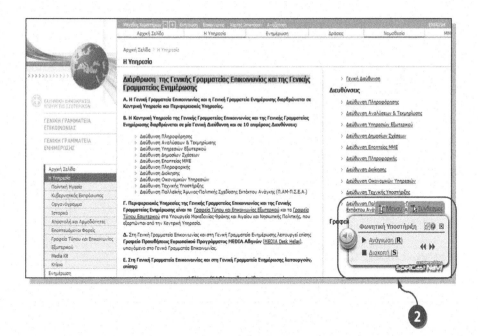

Fig. 4. The example of the website of the Secretariat General of Communication-Secretariat General of Information of Greece (Greek ministry of press). Reading aloud of a webpage.

at his request. This technique improves significantly the interactivity of the user with the website and makes navigation in it more efficient, less time consuming and effortless. One has to note here though that the above information, i.e. of what is a menu and what is the main content item on a website, is fused manually in the service by making through a scripting language especially designed for this service. Although this seems to be one of the drawbacks of this approach, it is only performed once during the adaptation of the service to the specific website, ensuring a more consistent and efficient web reading session for the user.

It remains at the user's request, at any time during his navigation through the website, to stop or restart the audio, jump to next or previous elements, browse in menu items and link items lists and follow one of them by simply selecting one with the arrow keys and the enter button on his keyboard. By doing so the visually-impaired user is gaining quickly an intuitive structure of the website, similar to the one a non-impaired user shapes when viewing the website on a computer screen, without the need for the repetitive pronunciation of items that are present on all web pages of the site.

3.2 Design and Deployment

As already mentioned, the developed system is designed as a web application for speech enhancing websites and for navigating in them, without the need of any software

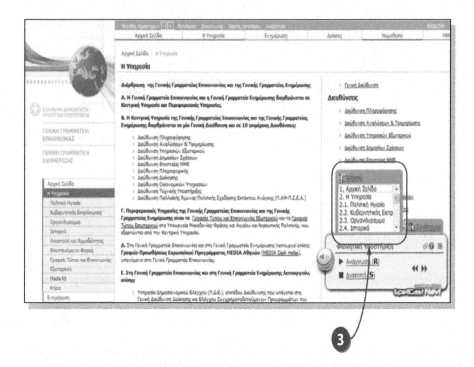

Fig. 5. The example of the website of the Secretariat General of Communication-Secretariat General of Information of Greece (Greek ministry of press). Menu items aural list.

installation on user's local computer. It is entirely developed on a client-side Javascript language, with main concern given to cross-browser and cross-platform capabilities.

The system traverses the DOM of each webpage of a specific website and through a post-hoc approach, based on a-priori information about the website's spatial structure, it re-structures its elements, and via a text to speech rendition, it provides the user with a simplified and intuitive aural representation of the webpage.

In order to be able to identify the roles of page elements and to provide enhanced interactivity, the system requires a priori knowledge of a website. These are encapsulated into site-specific filters; each one of them contains all the necessary specific information for a website along with specific interactivity patterns when necessary.

The system consists of two different components: (i) the client-side Javascript engine which is responsible for the interaction of the system with the user and for the support of the navigation through the website, and (ii) the server side component which is responsible for audio generation, caching and transformation proxy for the web pages. The proposed architecture makes the task of maintenance easier and it ensures high availability and quality levels of the service.

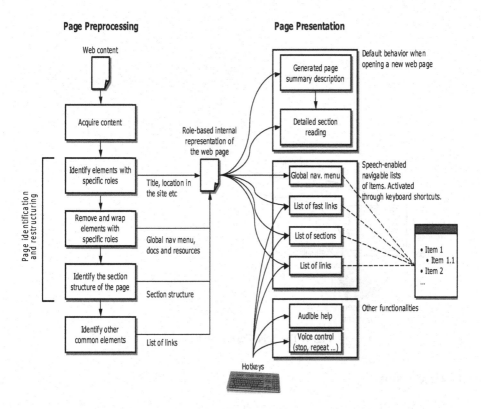

Fig. 6. The processing steps and presentation patterns in SpellCast

The text-to-speech component is incorporated on server-side with additional components such as website specific pronunciation lexica, and a sophisticated production and caching schema of the audio files, for every website's content, ensures high availability and low latency. The latter provides better resources management with improved scalability.

One should note at this point that our system poses no requirements on a website and introduces no overhead to its design and development or functioning processes. Based on its engine + filter approach, it can deal with any website without any modifications in its engine.

For every supported website, there is simply the need to develop a customized filter, which for consistently designed sites (for example sites that are backed by a content management system) it can be a mater of a few days. One of the main advantages of this target-specific approach, as far as the web content is concerned, is that it allows to any web content, even to content that does not conform to the accessibility guidelines, to become accessible through different devices and systems.

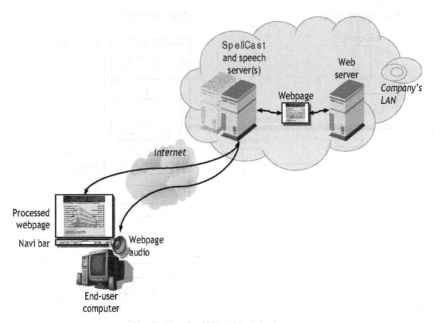

Fig. 7. The *SpellCast Navi* deployment

4 Discussion

SpellCast Navi has already been deployed onto several large websites, mainly of the Greek public sector, and it provides an important tool for rendering vast web content accessible to end users through a web application that can work the majority of computers and web-enabled devices.

Pilot evaluation tests have shown that it offers advanced usability and improved web accessibility compared to typical screen readers and large scale evaluation tests and experiments are currently being carried out. Future improvements have been planned for the development and evolution of the system, such as customizable visual aids for different types and levels of visual impairments, and support for more web elements such as different file types and so on.

In summary, *SpellCast Navi* lies in between a generic and a specialized accessibility tool trying to combine advantages from both categories. Its engine + filter design allows it to support individual websites and to efficiently compensate for any deviations from the recommendations and standards for accessible web design. Common browsing tasks such as following links, navigating back and forth, listening to the page content again, navigating to site menus, obtaining audible help etc., are supported through hotkeys and it provides enhanced aided web navigation.

Relying on site-specific filters to appropriately identify and restructure the web content, it achieves a natural way of conveying the information to the user, by trying to simulate the way one would use to read aloud a website to another person and help him navigate through its pages. It extends beyond the limits of a desktop accessibility enhancement tool and its approach can be also used as a basis for implementing voice browsing where users can interact with web pages through devices as simply as with the telephone.

References

1. Savidis, A., Stephanidis, C.: Unified User Interface Design: Designing Universally Accessible Interactions. International Journal of Interacting with Computers 16(2), 243–270 (2004)
2. Coyne, K.P., Nielsen, J.: Beyond alt text: Making the web easy to use for users with disabilities. Design Guidelines for Websites and Intranets Based on Usability Studies with People Using Assistive Technology (2001)
3. Bigham, J., Cavender, A.C., Brudvik, J.T., Wobbrock, J.O., Ladner, R.: WebinSitu: A comparative analysis of blind and sighted browsing behavior. In: Proc. of the 9th Intl. Conf. on Computers and Accessibility, ASSETS 2007 (2007)
4. W3C links on alternative web browsing,
   http://www.w3.org/WAI/References/Browsing
5. W3C Voice Browser Activity, http://www.w3.org/Voice/
6. W3C Web Content Accessibility Guidelines, http://www.w3.org/TR/WAI-WEBCONTENT/
7. Stephanidis, C., Paramythis, A., Karagiannidis, C., Savidis, A.: Supporting Interface Adaptation in the AVANTI Web Browser. In: 3rd ERCIM Workshop on User Interfaces for All, Obernai, France, November 3-4 (1997)
8. WebFACE from FORTH, http://www.ics.forth.gr
9. Bigham, J.P., Prince, C.M., Ladner, R.E.: Webanywhere: A Screen Reader On-the-Go. In: Proc. of the Intl. Cross-Disciplinary Conf. on Web Accessibility, W4A (2008)
10. Black, A., Taylor, P., Caley, R.: The Festival Speech Synthesis System (1998),
    http://festvox.org/festival
11. Hunt, A., Black, A.: Unit selection in a concatenative speech synthesis system using a large speech database. In: Proceedings of ICASSP 1996, Atlanta, Georgia, vol. 1, pp. 373–376 (1996)
12. Home Page Reader from IBM,
    http://www-306.ibm.com/able/solution_offerings/hpr.html
13. ReadSpeaker VoiceCorp Website, http://www.voice-corp.com/
14. Talkets Technologies, http://www.textic.com/
15. JAWS from Freedom Scientific, http://www.freedomscientific.com
16. Apple Accessibility VoiceOver,
    http://www.apple.com/macosx/accessibility/
17. Chen, C.: Fire vox: A screen reader firefox extension (2006),
    http://firevox.clcworld.net/
18. SpeechHTML from Vocalis, http://www.vocalis.com
19. Raptis, S., Spais, I., Tsiakoulis, P.: A Tool for Enhancing Web Accessibility: Synthetic Speech and Content Restructuring. In: Proc. HCII 2005: 11th International Conference on Human-Computer Interaction, Las Vegas, Nevada, USA, July 22-27 (2005)

Towards the Era of Mixed Reality:
Accessibility Meets Three Waves of HCI

Per Olof Hedvall

Certec, Dept. of Design Sciences
Lund University
P.O. Box 118
SE-221 00 LUND
Sweden
+46 46 222 40 94
per-olof.hedvall@certec.lth.se

Abstract. Today, the underlying theoretical and methodological foundations as well as implementations in the field of accessibility are largely based on plans, metrics and heuristics. There is an obvious tension between these norms and those of the overall spirit of the times, which leans heavily towards improvisations, diversity, and ever-changing affordances. The parallel evolution of human computer interaction (HCI) has been characterized as three waves, each building on the previous one, resulting in an in-depth understanding of the interwoven activity of humans and non-humans (artifacts). Now when facing the era of mixed reality, accessibility can gain considerably from HCI's, usability's and interaction design's bodies of knowledge.

Keywords: Accessibility, Usability, HCI, Interaction design, Mixed Reality, Situated action, Activity theory, Norms.

1 Introduction

As Manuel Castells [1] has pointed out, only the technologies that the surrounding culture is open to can spread. There are, however, not only cultures but subcultures, one of which is accessibility with its own issues and development; HCI, on the other hand, is based on a different context and has a different development.

It is possible to distinguish three waves in the development of HCI [2]. The first was characterized by what is large-scaled, rule-based and pre-planned; the second focused on single individuals, who stand-alone with different conditions; and the third on different individuals in a state of many-to-many-communication. The accessibility field has not progressed through these three phases and is still based on the large-scale, predictability and rule management. This explorative paper deals with these differences and their background – and how the accessibility field can and should be inspired by HCI/usability development and benefit from it.

Despite the ever so distinguishing symbols (cf. Fig. 1) and diagnoses, people with disabilities are first and foremost human beings (cf. "people first" [4]) and increasingly integrated in their environment. They are, however, being challenged when the

A. Holzinger and K. Miesenberger (Eds.): USAB 2009, LNCS 5889, pp. 264–278, 2009.

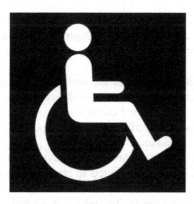

Fig. 1. Rehabilitation International's well-known symbol of access, which was adopted in 1969 [3]

current norms in the accessibility field are not in phase with the norms in society. The field of disability studies, which is more focused on a social and ideological level, is doing better. But the experienced accessibility – as it is for the acting individual in her social context – is about actual implementations. It is currently based on a view of technology and of human beings that was more relevant 25 years ago than it is today. The accessibility area could gain considerably from a closer relationship to the HCI waves over the last decades, not least of all now when approaching the era of mixed reality.

2   Wave 1 of HCI and Its Relation to Accessibility

The starting point of HCI is often connected to Doug Engelbart's famous demonstration called *The Mother of All Demos* where, among other inventions, he showed the first computer mouse [5]. Another important breakthrough came in 1981 with the first what-you-see-is-what-you-get interface of the Xerox STAR computer. The first HCI wave was highly influenced by information processing psychology and ergonomic approaches such as human factors, with the design largely depending on rules, guidelines and other formal methods [2]. These later resulted in criticism that the human users and their real life were excluded instead of being an influential part of the process [6].

Accessibility usually refers to how people with activity limitations can access the physical world or content on the Internet, mainly web pages. The accessibility area started its expansion during the second part of the 20th century. For many reasons, the area has never been particularly variable or open to change: it has been collectively rooted and often tied to infrastructure, legislation and economic structures. Its experts have often had medical or social backgrounds. The target of the results has often been society at large rather than individuals. It may also have played a role that very few researchers with disabilities have been active and affected the accessibility area.

When a certain accessibility level has been negotiated all the way into political decisions and then implemented, this has been the result of such a great effort that it in itself then becomes preservative. In that sense, the accessibility area interacted better with the continuous and relatively slow development during the authoritarian era than with the current one, which is characterized by empowerment, dynamic diversity and individual demands.

Value-wise, accessibility is related to the individual – as in the UN *Convention of the Rights of Persons with Disabilities*, where the concept of accessibility is defined as "the physical, social, economic and cultural environment, to health and education and to information and communication, in enabling persons with disabilities to fully enjoy all human rights and fundamental freedoms" [7]. But in reality, the individual's individuality and improvisational wishes have always been outside the main scope of the accessibility field, which is better suited to streamline how to respond to various human factors than different human actors. This is also reflected in how the field approaches the Internet. Web accessibility relies on several components, one of them being the *Web Content Accessibility Guidelines* [8].

The European initiative entitled *Design for All* [9], aims to support architects and designers in their work with new buildings or new products by doing the aftermath of accessibility issues beforehand. It is based on strategies for equal access to society by using plans, guidelines and heuristics. Among others, the work with *design for all* is based on the following two principles:

1. That which is good for people with impairments is often good for everyone else.
2. Accessibility can largely be established by thinking ahead, which means that the preconditions for accessibility can already be created on the drawing board.

The concept *design for all* has counterparts in other concepts such as the American *universal design* and the British *inclusive design* [10]. The work on accessible design is based on following principles and guidelines for how products should be designed to be used by as many as possible. See, for example, Connell et al. [11]. These are necessarily general, not situated in actions and not connected to an experienced accessibility, which more fully expresses environmentally-relative accessibility.

To some extent, it may be problematic to use concepts such as *universal* or *for all* and to see *design for all* as a desirable ideal. In his article, "Is There Design-for-All?", Harper argues that a *design for one* is needed as a counterweight to the impossible-to-achieve-practice perspective *for all* [12]. Anderberg [13] sees a need to nuance the term *design for all* and proposes the complementary concept *design for me* as a way to focus on the individual and the situated aspects of accessibility. Harper and Anderberg both discuss their individual design perspectives in relation to the field of computers and the Internet (Fig. 2).

To sum up the first two sections, the current view of accessibility as a predefined characteristic represents a structuralistic approach to accessibility that turns the individual into an un-situated passive robot without desires or idiosyncratic whims [15]. However, what determines if an individual can manage in a given situation can just as easily be a broomstick that happens to be available, as well as something specially designed and placed there to be accessible. This in itself is not an argument against *design for all* – the pre-defined is necessary – but the scope needs to be expanded to also capture the dynamics affecting accessibility for empowered individuals.

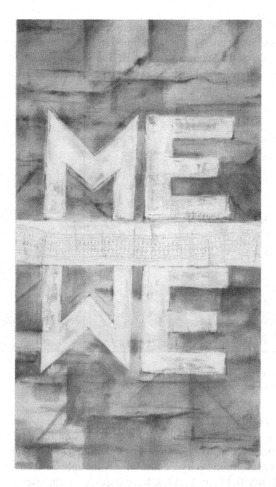

Fig. 2. The perspectives *design for all* and *design for me* do not need to be contradictory. Instead, ME and WE can be seen as each other's reflections and preconditions. Illustration by Mattias Christenson [14] after a text by Bodil Jönsson.

3   Wave 2 and 3 for HCI – But Not for Accessibility

The growing criticism that the human users and their real lives were excluded instead of being an influential part of the process [6] led to the second wave of HCI. One of its obvious starting points was the groundbreaking paper, "From Human Factors to Human Actors", by Bannon [16]. Some examples of second wave HCI are *situated action* [17], *participatory design* [18] and increased interest in activity as described in *activity theory* [19].

In her keynote paper at NordiCHI 2006, Susanne Bødker [2] described the third wave of HCI as a consequence of the ever-increasing penetration of computers around us, at work, at home and following us from context to context. She writes: "Pervasive technologies, augmented reality, small interfaces, tangible interfaces, etc., seem to be changing the nature of human-computer interaction in ways that we don't quite understand" [2:2]. Bødker argues for a Scandinavian approach where the user-sensitive theories and methods of the second wave of HCI are applied to gain understanding of the entangled and technology dense everyday lives in a third wave of HCI as well (Fig. 3).

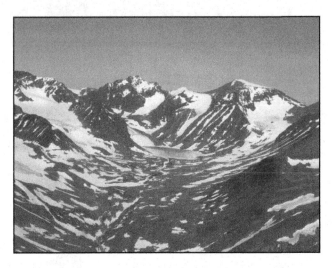

Fig. 3. Today, high up in the mountains far north in Scandinavia, there is also excellent cell phone coverage. Photo by Bodil Jönsson.

The development that Bødker [2] describes also has consequences for accessibility, not only regarding computers and accessibility, but in an increasing extent to larger and larger domains of our lives, where combinations of humans and non-humans continuously influence the activity conditions. Although Jönsson et al., active in the disability/accessibility field for decades, have focused on the user's needs, wishes and dreams [20], there is no doubt that HCI, usability and interaction design as a whole have come further than the field of accessibility in describing and understanding the experienced consequences of the ever changing area of information technology.

The fields of HCI and usability are interwoven. Advancements in the usability field in the last ten years have progressed as follows:

1. Originally, ISO 9241-11 [21] defined usability as: "...the extent to which a product can be used by specified users to achieve specific goals with effectiveness, efficiency and satisfaction in a specified context of use."
2. ISO FDIS 9241-171 [22] defines accessibility as: "...usability of a product, service, environment or facility by people with the widest range of capabilities."
3. The new draft ISO standard ISO/IEC CD 25010.2 [23] proposes a more comprehensive breakdown of *quality in use* into *usability in use* (covered by ISO 9241-11), *flexibility in use* (which is a measure of the extent to which a product is usable in all potential contexts of use, including accessibility) and *safety* (which is concerned with minimizing undesirable consequences) [24].

4. Since 2008, however, there has also been a *user experience (UX) standard*, ISO CD 9241-210 [25], defining user experience as: "...all aspects of the user's experience when interacting with the product, service, environment and facility."

This UX standard exposes the absence of a corresponding standard for *accessibility experience* (AX). The absence can be seen as a sign of the lag in development of the concept *accessibility* compared to that of *usability*, and a need for a renewal of the accessibility field to allow for the empowered and experiencing user, and an activity-relative accessibility rather than an absolute one.

4   A Complement: Activity–Tied and Experienced Accessibility

Categorizations are often followed by descriptions that can turn into assumed causal relations. Words control thought, thought controls words and we tend to realize our thoughts [26]. A well-established thought is that people with disabilities have "special needs" and that accessibility is meant to accommodate those needs with special solutions. But what really are these needs and how do they differ from the needs of non-disabled people [20]? In fact, it is not the needs that are different or special, but the human conditions that manifest themselves when the individual wants to do something.

In all of the existing accessibility standards, accessibility is viewed as a phenomenon that can be achieved by planning ahead, not for the affected individuals, but for thought models of individuals and contexts. In the moment of action, however, the only accessibility that matters is that which is individually experienced and activity-tied. Laboratory experiments, guidelines or blueprints can only partially predict this, and there are no contextually valid properties before or beyond participation in a specific activity. An individual is subjected to the current contextual circumstances and conditions and has to manage with the actual level of accessibility – however satisfying or discriminating this may be.

According to the sociologist Lucy Suchman [17], people rely on their abilities and experiences to handle different situations in the here and now. She has introduced the term *situated action* as a way of understanding how people act and how they relate to their planning. Situated action represents a view where every chain of events depends on the current material and social circumstances. According to Suchman, the term encompasses all action and all planning (Fig. 4).

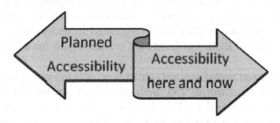

Fig. 4. There is a tension between the plans and how accessibility is actually experienced in the action. Illustration by the author.

Those who care about and depend on accessibility have good reasons to consider that actions are situated in the past, the present and the future. The planned accessibility covers only parts of the experienced accessibility in action. There is a need to broaden the understanding of accessibility to include not only what can be planned using guidelines, heuristics and logistics, but to increase the focus on situated and activity-tied accessibility. A previous plan may be ever so good, but it is not until the action in the here and now that accessibility is realized. In that sense, accessibility is tied to a specific activity in a particular situation, where both other humans and artifacts take part.

Accessibility today is under-theorized and lacks methodological sensitivity to the particular conditions for access and participation in concrete activities. The field has yet to account for several of the characteristics of and impacts on individually experienced and activity-tied accessibility.

5 Reframing Accessibility in the Era of Mixed Reality

The information technology (IT) area and its focus on non-physical materials [27] has stimulated those working with accessibility and IT to discuss the design of active and adaptive technologies that change for the user's varying conditions [28, 29]. What is desirable in the IT field is not that the possibilities are the same for all, but rather that they may be different for everyone. In the IT age, afforded uniqueness caters to equality.

In 2001, Gregor and Newell introduced the concept of *design for dynamic diversities* [30] as an approach for the design of information technology for older people. They pointed out that the user is not a static average person that does not change over time. As people age, they may lose physical and cognitive functions. The products they rely on in daily life must therefore be able to meet them based on their functional level here and now [30, 31].

HCI has shifted focus over the decades from the relationship between man and computer, such as the design of user interfaces, to an increasing concentration on the total experience, including aesthetic, ergonomic, narrative and other dimensions [32]. Current interaction design [33-35] includes knowledge from all the previous HCI areas. As humans and technology become more and more entangled so do the potential for their intertwined activity. This yields a mixture of the real and virtual elements that together form what is called *mixed reality* (Fig. 5) [36, 37]. In recent years, several related fields such as ubiquitous computing, tangible interaction, augmented reality, augmented virtuality, pervasive computing, enactive computing and so on, have emerged. In this article, they are all squeezed in under mixed reality as an umbrella term, but each of them has traits that are important for a future elaboration of accessibility.

Now with the mixed reality era well on its way, it is important that the accessibility field draws inspiration, theories and methodologies from HCI in its broadest sense, rather than from the physical world only. One of the many reasons is that it is more evident than ever that not only the interactive parts but all the artifacts in our surroundings exert an active influence on us. To design for many different opportunities and to be systematically open to the unexpected can be a way to avoid costly and

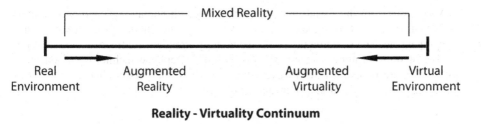

Reality - Virtuality Continuum

Fig. 5. The Reality-Virtuality Continuum by Milgram et al. [36]

stigmatizing special solutions for specific groups of people. Design for rich opportunities and redundancy increases people's degrees of freedom and allows for improvisation and whims while decreasing the likelihood that someone is suddenly caught standing there with no possibility at all. Donald Schön [38] is one of those who described the importance of having access to a repertoire of solutions, strategies and procedures. In meeting different situations, these provide opportunities to see the similarities and differences from previous experiences and can thus help to move forward.

On the whole, technology changes the conditions for humanity at the same time as individual products influence the individual person, and the accessibility as well. The combination of an active view of people and an active view of technology, like that in Actor Network Theory (ANT) [39-42], influences humanity and technology in many ways, large and small.

Over the last ten years or so, new technologies have taken their place in our daily lives. Internet, the cellular phone and the PC are now commonplace for the vast majority of people in the West. Technology affects individuals and their lifestyles. The cellular phone has led to greater freedom, Internet to new ways to search for information and e-mail to other ways to stay in touch, while the computer in itself is an everyday tool for not only written language but also for lots of pictures and sound, including computer games and all the media. Overall, it has meant that we now have many more contacts with many more individuals in many more ways, rendering a multitude of perspectives and possibilities (Fig. 6).

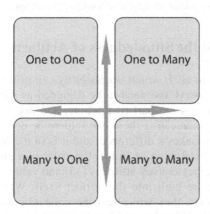

Fig. 6. The lower right corner has never before been available. Now it represents one of the most attractive possibilities of the information technology. Illustration by the author.

ANT focuses on the social processes involving both humans (H) and non-humans (NH) that are related to one another in similar ways, like nodes in a network. On a comprehensive level, humanity and technology mutually influence one another (means of transportation, energy systems, cellular telephone technology, food technology). There is also a level of everyday life where the person chooses and influences her artifacts, which in turn influence her (Fig. 7).

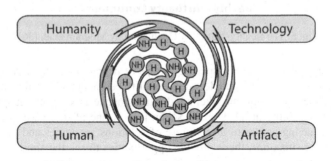

Fig. 7. Never before have humans been involved with so many people and so much technology at the same time [9]. Illustration by the author.

When a human utilizes an aid – an artifact – this activity does not occur in isolation. On the contrary, humans and artifacts are interwoven, together determining the terms for accessibility. Their activity interplays with both humanity and technology, both developing and changing in anticipation of the future. Being dependent on an artifact also means being dependent on this artifact's relation to everything else. Thus, the field of accessibility ought to be based on a view of the human being *together* with her technology, just as most of HCI, usability and interaction design are today.

Technology in itself boosts or poses challenges that can support, spur on, hinder or delay a given plan. Affordance [43, 44] can change dynamically in the moment and based on the current situation, alter the opportunities that the technology offers. Viewed through ANT eyes, the future challenges and opportunities are not static but depend on a dynamic environment where affordance changes.

6   Accessibility and the Situatedness of Artifacts

Another insight gained in HCI, which accessibility can profit from, is that artifacts always are parts of a context and need to be designed as such. Technology development and new prototypes are part of a whole, and dissociating them from that when evaluating or communicating them can seldom be done successfully. It is the effect on the whole that makes a difference, and it is in the whole that research can be conducted. When looked upon as influential parts of a greater picture, artifacts are not neutral. Instead, they convey attitudes [13] and values because of the knowledge and meaning that are built into the artifact itself. When the artifacts are included in various contexts, they will affect the collective meaning of the context. The artifact's potential is defined in and by the current situation's horizon of possible actions. This means that researchers, developers and others must be involved in people's everyday lives and in their activities, because this is where the artifact's further potential can be captured.

Vygotsky's [45, 46] discussion of how knowledge and meaning are being co-created, for example during a normal conversation, can also be applied to technology. Series of mock-ups, user trials, small breakdowns and corrections have a different profile than a technology built on component refinements and a determinist linear approach (Fig. 8). Instead, technology is, at every point in time, seen as the resulting expression of the implemented meaning, as far as this has reached [15]. Most (in my opinion all) technology developments would benefit from being thought of and described as the non-linear processes they actually are.

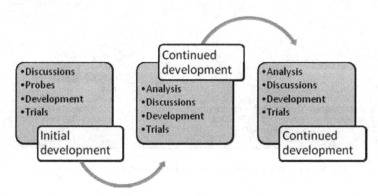

Fig. 8. An iterative design process can open the way up for richer initiative and participation, thus enhancing the shared implemented meaning. Illustration by the author.

In the initial development of a given technology, the designer and the users rarely share the same picture of the meaning the artifact should provide. Nor do they see the same meaning in the finished product. But the chances that the artifact actually can play a useworthy [47] and positive role increase considerably if the affected person's perspective is part of the knowledge and meaning that is built into the artifact.

A look at current participatory design (PD) methods reveals that they rely on text or speech to a large extent. This is not surprising at all, since PD arose in a workplace context [18]. Ong [48] describes technological aspects of written language. But how do you cater to a dialogue when written or spoken language is not an option? In situations with inherent asymmetries, due to disabilities or age differences for instance, the notion of technologies as intermediaries can facilitate communication that hardly could be achieved by relying on written or oral modalities [20, 49, 50].

7 Artifacts for Mutual Information and Inspiration

In the mixed reality era, the object of methodical inquiry becomes part of a mixture consisting of humans and non-humans entangled in a network (Fig. 7). This requires and offers new and complementary techniques other than today's. When information and actions are distributed across networks, it is not enough to focus solely on the human actors; there is also a need to turn to the ever-increasing number of non-humans that are part of the studied context. With such an approach, the systematic introduction of new artifacts also can serve as a method for mutual information and inspiration.

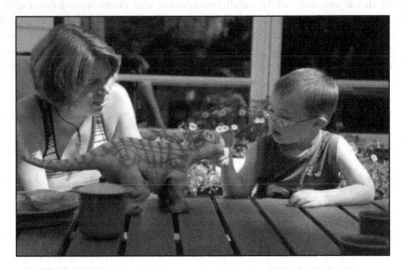

Fig. 9. A mother and her son play with Pleo™. Photo by the author.

It is a matter of artifacts being physically here among us. We can gather around them and interact with them – they are an integral part of a situation in which the living communication between mother and son, here illustrated, can be afforded structure, direction and other significance for those involved. This is based on the simultaneous focus on the artifact as one in the context, such as the robot dinosaur Pleo™ in Fig. 9.

If spoken or written language is insufficient, technology can often offer other means of communication. It is possible both to ask and to receive answers via artifacts, as soon as the acting individual has a chance to do something with them. One quick way of getting started is to develop mock-ups at an early stage, models or sketches that definitely are not good enough to function as prototypes and that can lack much of the functionality, but that still have the weight, the size and some functions available that resemble those of the intended product [15].

By presenting these to the user, it is possible to get feedback in action at an early stage. The designer consciously or unconsciously has a strong inner image of the future results, and it is this early image that will be realized, unaffected by the surrounding world if the surrounding world is not given a chance to provide input. Trial implementations, in the form of mock-ups without any demands whatsoever on precision, can make a huge difference. It is only an advantage if the user does other things than those intended with the mock-ups, or even rejects them. Artifacts can be big and small, hard and soft, compliant and reluctant, meet expectations and act mischievously. Surprises like that spur on thoughts that contribute to the continued development process.

8 To Sum Up: Time for Accessibility 2.0?

While the framework and applications of HCI, usability and interaction design have developed continuously and long since reached their "2.0" level, the considerations, elaborations and applications of accessibility have proceeded noticeably slower. The relative delay of accessibility has its reasons as well as its consequences. It takes years of initiating, norm confrontations, lobbying and realization before a certain level of accessibility is reached. In itself, it then plays a conservative role – nothing steers a development as ruthlessly as an implemented infrastructure, and when HCI, usability and interaction design have reached their 2.0 level, accessibility is only in its 1.2.

As explored above, the era of mixed reality has several characteristics that can substantially add value to the field of accessibility, both in terms of new methodologies regarding inquiry and participation and in the form of a richer, warmer and more flexible accessibility that bends to fit the individual's dreams wishes, needs and even idiosyncratic whims and pure improvisation. This shift has dynamic effects, not only in technology (where an active network-embedded technology obtains a different and stronger position) but also on the human side. A person who becomes accustomed to opportunities being within reach, and being able to manage with the help of them, is influenced by her experience to have the expectation that she will manage the next time. These expectations concern both herself and her human and technical environment.

Let us return to *The Rise of the Network Society* [1] and Manuel Castells' clear statement that no new technology can be established unless the culture and its thought climate allow for it. There is, however, a follow up to this statement: when a technology is finally established, especially a technology in the societal sector, it can be very robust and almost aggressive in its efforts to block further development. The evolution of HCI and usability have not by themselves led to a comparative evolution of accessibility – the accessibility area is its own subculture and relies heavily on a slow development of rules and laws. This results in a tension regarding the ever-accelerating evolutions of attitudes and norms. There is an enhanced and challenging need for a thought climate that allows and urges design thinking on social concerns, that disclaims instrumentalistic disability attitudes and that strengthens improvisation (both individually and socially) to benefit the lived life.

These situated and individually oriented characteristics of our times can and will change the materiality of everyday life, with or without disabilities. A society that actually listens to its people necessitates an accessibility that can be adjusted to fit the individual. In the mixed reality era, it is the combinatoric sum of human and technological affordances that together determine the conditions for action in the here and now. If the combined environment wants the individual's success and adapts accordingly, it can offer an optimal potential in the moment of action. In the future, this also ought to be reflected in how metrics, heuristics and generalizations are utilized to facilitate access, and the ways it is designed.

It is about time to roll out the next wave of accessibility, version 2.0.

Acknowledgements

The author gratefully acknowledge Bodil Jönsson, professor at Certec, Department of Design Sciences, Lund University, Sweden, for her continuous inspiration, critical questioning and constructive feedback, and Eileen Deaner, international coordinator at Certec, for translation services and comments on the text.

References

1. Castells, M.: The Rise of the Network Society. Blackwell, Malden (1996)
2. Bødker, S.: When second wave HCI meets third wave challenges. In: Proceedings of the 4th Nordic conference on Human-computer interaction: changing roles, pp. 1–8. ACM, Oslo (2006)
3. Rehabilitation International, http://www.riglobal.org/about/index.html
4. People First movement, http://www.people1.org/about_us_history.htm
5. Doug Engelbart's, Demo (1968),
   http://sloan.stanford.edu/MouseSite/1968Demo.html
6. Kuutti, K.: Activity theory as a potential framework for human-computer interaction research. In: Nardi, B. (ed.) Context and Consciousness: Activity Theory and Human Computer Interaction, pp. 17–44. MIT Press, Cambridge (1995)
7. UN.: Convention on the Rights of Persons with Disabilities,
   http://www.un.org/disabilities/default.asp?navid=12&pid=150
8. W3.: Web Content Accessibility Guidelines 2.0,
   http://www.w3.org/WAI/intro/wcag.php
9. EIDD.: The EIDD Stockholm Declaration,
   http://www.designforalleurope.org/Design-for-All/
   EIDD-Documents/Stockholm-Declaration
10. Klironomos, I., Antona, M., Basdekis, I., Stephanidis, C.: White Paper: promoting Design for All and e-Accessibility in Europe. Universal Access in the Information Society 5(1), 105–119 (2006)
11. Connell, B.R., Jones, M., Mace, R., Mueller, J., Mullick, A., Ostroff, E., Sanford, J., Steinfeld, E., Story, M., Vanderheiden, G.: The Principles of Universal Design (Version 2.0 -4/1/97) (1997),
    http://www.design.ncsu.edu/cud/about_ud/udprinciples.htm
12. Harper, S.: Is there design-for-all? Universal Access in the Information Society 6, 111–113 (2007)
13. Anderberg, P.: FACE – Disabled People, Technology and Internet. Certec, LTH, Lund (2006)
14. Christenson, M.: Bildrör, B4PRESS, Gothenburg (2008)
15. Hedvall, P.O.: Situerad Design för alla – till improvisationen lov (Situated Design for All – In Praise of Improvisation). Licentiate thesis. Certec, LTH, Lund (2007)
16. Bannon, L.: From human factors to human actors: the role of psychology and human-computer interaction studies in system design. In: Greenbaum, J., Kyng, M. (eds.) Design at work: cooperative design of computer systems table of contents, pp. 25–44. Lawrence Erlbaum Associates, New Jersey (1991)
17. Suchman, L.: Human and Machine Reconfigurations: Plans and Situated Actions, 2nd edn. Cambridge University Press, Cambridge (2006)
18. Ehn, P.: Work-Oriented Design of Computer Artifacts. Lawrence Erlbaum Associates, New Jersey (1988)
19. Kaptelinin, V., Nardi, B.A.: Acting with Technology: Activity Theory and Interaction Design. MIT Press, Cambridge (2006)
20. Jönsson, B. (ed.): Design Side by Side. Studentlitteratur, Lund (2006)

21. ISO 9241-11, Ergonomic requirements for office work with visual display terminals (VDTs) – Part 11: Guidance on usability. International Organization for Standardization, Geneva (1998)
22. ISO CD 9241-210, Ergonomics of human-system interaction – Part 210: Human-centred design process for interactive systems. International Organization for Standardization, Geneva (2008)
23. ISO FDIS 9241-171, Ergonomics of human-system interaction – Part 171: Guidance on software accessibility. International Organization for Standardization, Geneva (2008)
24. Bevan, N.: Classifying and Selecting UX and Usability Measures. In: Law, E.L.-C., Bevan, N., Christou, G., Springett, M., Lárusdóttir, M. (eds.) Proceedings of the international workshop on meaningful measures: Valid useful user experience measurement (VUUM), pp. 13–18. Institute of Research in Informatics of Toulouse, Toulouse (2008)
25. ISO/IEC CD 25010.2, Software engineering – Software product Quality Requirements and Evaluation (SQuaRE) – Quality model. International Organization for Standardization, Geneva (2008)
26. Jönsson, B., Rehman, K.: Den obändiga söklusten. Brombergs, Stockholm (2000)
27. Löwgren, J., Stolterman, E.: Thoughtful interaction design: a design perspective on information technology. MIT Press, Cambridge (2005)
28. Savidis, A., Antona, M., Stephanidis, C.: A decision-making specification language for verifiable user-interface adaptation logic. International Journal of Software Engineering and Knowledge Engineering 15(6), 1063–1094 (2005)
29. Darzentas, J.S., Miesenberger, K.: Design for All in Information Technology: A Universal Concern. In: Andersen, K.V., Debenham, J., Wagner, R. (eds.) DEXA 2005. LNCS, vol. 3588, pp. 406–420. Springer, Heidelberg (2005)
30. Gregor, P., Newell, A.F.: Other impairments and rehabilitation technologies: Designing for dynamic diversity: making accessible interfaces for older people. In: Proceedings of the 2001 EC/NSF workshop on Universal accessibility of ubiquitous computing: providing for the elderly WUAUC 2001, pp. 90–92 (2001)
31. Heller, R., Jorge, J., Guedj, R.: Workshop report: EC/NSF workshop on universal accessibility of ubiquitous computing: providing for the elderly event report. In: Proceedings of the 2001 EC/NSF workshop on Universal accessibility of ubiquitous computing: providing for the elderly WUAUC 2001, pp. 1–10 (2001)
32. Hochheiser, H., Lazar, J.: HCI - and Societal Issues: A Framework for Engagement. International Journal of Human-Computer Interaction 23(3), 339–374 (2007)
33. Löwgren, J.: From HCI to interaction design. In: Chen, Q. (ed.) Human-computer interaction: Issues and challenges, pp. 29–43. Idea Group Pub., Hershey (2001)
34. Shedroff, N.: Experience design 1. New Riders Pub., Indianapolis (2001)
35. Preece, J., Rogers, Y., Sharp, H.: Interaction Design: beyond human-computer interaction, 2nd edn. J. Wiley & Sons, New York (2007)
36. Milgram, P., Takemura, H., Utsumi, A., Kishino, F.: Augmented Reality: A Class of Displays on the Reality-Virtuality Continuum. In: SPIE. Telemanipulator and Telepresence Technologies, vol. 2351, pp. 282–292 (1994)
37. Behringer, R., Christian, J., Holzinger, A., Wilkinson, S.: Some Usability Issues of Augmented and Mixed Reality for e-Health Applications in the Medical Domain. In: Holzinger, A. (ed.) USAB 2007. LNCS, vol. 4799, pp. 255–266. Springer, Heidelberg (2007)
38. Schön, D.A.: The Reflective Practitioner – how professionals think in action. Ashgate Publishing, UK (1983/1991)

39. Latour, B.: Technology is society made durable. In: Law, J. (ed.) A Sociology of monsters: Essays on Power, Technology, and Domination. Sociological Review Monograph, vol. 38, pp. 103–131. Routledge, London (1991)
40. Latour, B.: Pandora's Hope: Essays on the Reality of Science Studies. Harvard University Press, Cambridge (1999)
41. Latour, B.: Reassembling the Social: An Introduction to Actor-Network-Theory. Oxford University Press, Oxford (2005)
42. Akrich, M.: The de-scription of technical objects. In: Bijker, W., Law, J. (eds.) Shaping technology, building society: Studies in sociotechnical change, pp. 205–224. MIT Press, Cambridge (1992)
43. Gibson, J.J.: The ecological approach to visual perception. Lawrence Erlbaum Associates, New Jersey (1986)
44. Norman, D.A.: The psychology of everyday things. Basic Books, New York (1988)
45. Vygotsky, L.S.: Mind in Society: Development of Higher Psychological Processes. Harvard University Press, Cambridge (1978)
46. Vygotsky, L.S.: Thought and Language. MIT Press, Cambridge (1986)
47. Eftring, H.: The useworthiness of robots for people with physical disabilities. Certec, LTH, Lund (1999)
48. Ong, W.J.: Orality and Literacy: The Technologizing of the Word. Methuen young books, London (1982)
49. Jönsson, B., Philipson, L., Svensk, A.: Certec.: Vad vi lärt oss av Isaac; What Isaac taught us. Certec, LTH, Lund (1998)
50. Jönsson, B.: Enabling communication: pictures as language. In: MacLachlan, M., Gallagher, P. (eds.) Enabling technologies: body image and body function. Churchill Livingstone, New York (2004)

Investigating Agile User-Centered Design in Practice: A Grounded Theory Perspective*

Zahid Hussain[1], Wolfgang Slany[1], and Andreas Holzinger[2]

[1] Institute for Software Technology, Graz University of Technology, Austria
zhussain@ist.tugraz.at, slany@ist.tugraz.at
[2] Institute of Information Systems and Computer Media,
Graz University of Technology, Austria
a.holzinger@tugraz.at

Abstract. This paper investigates how the integration of agile methods and User-Centered Design (UCD) is carried out in practice. For this study, we have applied grounded theory as a suitable qualitative approach to determine what is happening in actual practice. The data was collected by semi-structured interviews with professionals who have already worked with an integrated agile UCD methodology. Further data was collected by observing these professionals in their working context, and by studying their documents, where possible. The emerging themes that the study found show that there is an increasing realization of the importance of usability in software development among agile team members. The requirements are emerging; and both low and high fidelity prototypes based usability tests are highly used in agile teams. There is an appreciation of each other's work from both UCD professionals and developers and both sides can learn from each other.

Keywords: Agile Methods, Extreme Programming, Scrum, Usability, User-Centered Design, Grounded Theory, Interviews.

1   Introduction

The adoption of agile software development methods is growing in the industry. However, in their development lifecycles, these methods still lack the realization of the importance of usability and usable user interfaces. Holzinger [1] draws attention to the need for an awareness of various usability techniques by software practitioners that should be applied according to the nature of a project. Both the agile methods and user-centered design methodologies have many similarities: both methodologies focus on delivering value, both focus on customers/users, and their iterative nature and continuous testing are the key

* The research herein is partially conducted within the competence network Softnet Austria (www.soft-net.at) and funded by the Austrian Federal Ministry of Economics (bm:wa), the province of Styria, the Steirische Wirtschaftsförderungsgesellschaft mbH. (SFG), and the city of Vienna in terms of the center for innovation and technology (ZIT).

A. Holzinger and K. Miesenberger (Eds.): USAB 2009, LNCS 5889, pp. 279–289, 2009.

similarities for integrating them easily [2]. However, there has not been much investigation regarding how these two methodologies are actually practiced in industry; and how to successfully integrate HCI/usability techniques into agile methods is an area worthy of exploration.

In this paper, we report our findings, the emerging themes of our qualitative research conducted using grounded theory [3]. The data was collected by semi-structured interviews with professionals who have already worked with an integrated agile UCD methodology. Further data was collected by observing these professionals in their working context, and studying their documents- the various artefacts produced during their work, where possible. All the interviews were conducted by the first author. We also confirm some of the previously identified themes by Ferreira et al. and Fox et al. [4][5][6].

The next section describes related literature studies. Section 3 provides details about the research method and participants' profiles. Section 4 describes the results – the emerging themes along with quotes from the participants. Section 5 concludes the paper with future work.

2 Related Literature Studies

There have been studies present in the literature that report about the various aspects and efforts for the integration of agile methods and usability/user-centered design. Patton [7] reports about how to combine interaction design into his agile process and emphasized the participation of all stakeholders into the design process. His team was responsible for the UCD practices as there was no dedicated UCD professional[1] present in the team. In his recent article, Patton [8] describes the twelve best practices for adding user experience (UX) work to agile development. Chamberlain et al. [9] propose a framework for integrating UCD into agile methods by presenting similarities between two methodologies. McInerney and Maurer [10] interviewed three UCD professionals for integrating UCD within agile methods and their report was positive. Holzinger et al. [11] presented the idea of extreme usability by integrating XP and usability engineering which then, they implemented into software engineering education. At her company, Miller [12] reports her experience where both interaction designers and developers were working in parallel tracks coordinating their work smoothly. Meszaros and Aston [13] describe how they introduced paper prototype based usability testing into agile process. Memmel et al. describe the benefits of including usability engineering into agile development, "When usability engineering becomes part of agile software engineering, this helps to reduce the risk of running into wrong design decisions by asking real end users about their needs and activities" [14]. Sy [15] reports the parallel tracks used at her company by both UCD professionals and developers to integrate UCD with agile methods. At every iteration cycle, the coordination between UCD professionals and developers was smoothly done so that UCD professionals were always one cycle ahead, in order

---

[1] We use the term UCD professional equivalent to usability engineer, interaction designer, UI designer, user experience designer, etc.

to be able to gather requirements and design for the next cycles while testing the previous cycle's work. Ferreira et al. [4][5] have investigated four projects in four different countries for the integration of UI design and agile methods. They have used the grounded theory qualitative method for their study where they have conducted semi-structured interviews from the two members of each project, one who concentrated on UCD and one who concentrated on programming. Some themes that emerged from their data are: there is an advantage in doing up-front interaction design; do most of up-front design; much of interaction design consists of studying clients and users; interaction design learns from implementation by developers; cost and time are constraints; both usability testing and development affect each other; and agile leads to changing the relationship of UCD professionals and developers. Using the same grounded theory qualitative approach, Fox et al. [6] also investigated the integration of UCD with agile methods. They conducted semi-structured interviews from ten participants, one member from each team, in North America and Europe where the majority of the participants were UCD professionals and only few were developers. They describe three approaches taken by the participants to achieve the integration and term these approaches as generalist, specialist, and hybrid approach. In the generalist approach, there is no UCD professional present in a team but this role is performed by a developer interested in usability/UCD. In the specialist approach, one UCD professional is present in the team; whereby in the hybrid approach, a team member has both formal UCD training and also has experience in software development. Brown et al. [16] report that they use various artefacts, such as stories, sketches, and lists between UCD professionals and developer in their agile process. Ungar [17] reports the advantages of introducing a Design Studio, a collaborative workshop, into the agile UCD process. "The design studio is a rapid process that allows designers, developers and stakeholders to collaborate and explore design alternatives. Participants grow their skills by exchanging viewpoints with their peers and openly discussing the strengths and weaknesses of their work. The design is enriched and strengthened from the feedback" [17]. In their work, Wolkerstorfer et al. [18] and Hussain et al. [2], [19] report on the integration of various HCI techniques, e.g., field studies, usability tests, paper prototypes, usability expert evaluations, etc., into their agile process. In their case study Federoff et al. describe the struggle of UX teams when transitioning to agile development [20]. Recently, Miller and Sy [21] discussed issues regarding agile user experience.

With a few exceptions, many studies are anecdotal, albeit providing important information how the UCD is integrated with agile methods at various levels and at various levels of efforts. Studying the various aspects of the integration of agile methods and usability/UCD is an area worth to explore for developing usable and quality software products. Our research is aimed at enhancing this knowledge base to identify new themes, and supporting and confirming the existing empirical evidence by using qualitative approach of grounded theory.

3   Method

Besides technical focus, software development is mainly a human activity carried out by team members, so a qualitative approach is needed to study this human behavior, as with qualitative approach, researcher is forced to delve into the problem's complexity thus achieving richer and more informative results [22]. As we wanted to study how the integration of agile methods and user-centered design is carried out in practice, which and how team members are integrating and using usability/UCD techniques into agile methods, we chose to use grounded theory qualitative research method [3]. The grounded theory method is used to discover theory from data [23] - mostly from the 'voices' and 'experience' of the practitioners [24], i.e., interviews but also from other forms of data, such as observations and documents; and its application to human behavior is well-known [24]. Grounded theory is "useful for discovering behavioral patterns that shape social processes as people interact together in groups" [23]. It is used to generate a mid-level substantial theory that is directly derived from the data rather than verifying prior hypotheses [23]. Coleman and O'Connor [24] describe the analytical process of grounded theory, "The analytical process involves coding strategies: the process of breaking down interviews, observations, and other forms of appropriate data, into distinct units of meaning, which are labelled to generate concepts. These concepts are initially clustered into descriptive categories. They are then re-evaluated for their interrelationships and, through a series of analytical steps, are gradually subsumed into higher-order categories, or one underlying core category, which suggests an emergent theory." Basically for social sciences and specifically in nursing, grounded theory has also been applied in information systems, software engineering as well as in agile software development [25][24][26][4][5][27][6][28].

Since the initial discovery of grounded theory by Glaser and Strauss [3], there are now at least three versions of grounded theory [23] but we employed the Strauss and Corbin approach [29] and [30], because they argue that "the researcher's personal or professional experience is supportive of theory building and contributes to theoretical sensitivity, the ability to understand the data's important elements and how they contribute to theory" [24]. We have the experience of both as professionals as well as researchers in the study area, i.e., agile usability/UCD; and are already familiar with the literature, thus this knowledge supports theoretical sensitivity. Another reason for selecting the version of Strauss and Corbin is that "they favour setting the research question in advance of commencing a grounded theory study, rather than it being allowed to emerge at the coding phase as advocated by Glaser" [24]. We also set a few questions in advance: How the integration of agile methods and user-centered design is carried out in practice? Which HCI techniques are being used in agile methods? How the role of UCD professional is carried out in agile teams? Besides finding new themes, we also wanted to confirm the studies of Ferreira et al. [4][5] and Fox et al. [6].

Grounded theory consists of a set of established procedures and guidelines for the systematic collection and analysis of qualitative data [26]; of which the constant comparison method is the heart of grounded theory [23], where data and concepts are constantly compared to each other during collecting and analyzing the data, to ensure that an integrative theory is developed, which is grounded in the raw data [26]. In theoretical sampling, the sampling is continuously selected based on emerging categories and concepts [3]. So the interview questions are being changed according to these emerging categories as well as "the researcher may decide to interview certain types of individual or seek out other sources of data" [24]. We developed an initial interview protocol with the help from literature and from our own experience. Initially, we conducted a pilot interview with a project manager who is also a certified scrum master and works in a software developing company on a project about social networking and is employing scrum agile method. We then adjusted our interview protocol by getting feedback from his interview and it was slightly but continuously modified as the interviews were conducted and data was gathered. For the analysis, we used Atlas TI software tool, which is suitable for grounded theory analysis. In grounded theory analysis, the first step is open coding, where codes or labels are allocated to data obtained from interview transcripts and from other sources, if any [24]. The purpose is to identify important concepts in the data and then categorize it [6]. During our open coding analysis, codes were allotted to data, which were then constantly compared to subsequent data. At the end of open coding, initial concepts and categories are identified, which are then used in axial coding to make relationships among categories and their sub-categories, and identifying core category/categories. We compared initial categories with subsequent categories and made relationships among them in the form of categories and subcategories. Finally, in selective coding, core categories are used to find themes or high-level concepts that emerge from the data [6]; and that explain how the participants are carrying out their work and solving their problems. Another ongoing technique in grounded theory is memoing which is "the ongoing process of making notes and ideas and questions that occur to the analyst during the process of data collection and analysis" [31]. These memos play an important role in identifying ideas or hypotheses and generating the themes or high-level concepts [24]. We continuously wrote memos during the interviews and during the analysis of the data, which helped us in generating the themes during all phases of the analysis and those emerging themes are described in the results section.

3.1 Participants

We denote the participants as P1, P2, P3, P4, and P5. Based in Austria, P1 is a usability expert who provides consultancy to both agile and non agile projects ranging from banking sector to transport to typical web based applications whose durations vary from 6 months to 3 years. He also delivers lecture at a local university. He works with the companies whom either do not have expert UCD professionals or have certain knowledge of usability but they do not have resources to manage it, so they have to buy resources. Depending upon the projects, sometimes he is the only UCD professional and sometimes his two other colleagues also work as UCD professionals in the projects. In one of the companies that is employing the XP process, he works as a UCD professional, so according to Fox et al. he is performing the role of specialist [6].

Based in Austria, P2 is a developer who also has an interest in usability so he is performing the role of generalist [6]. He works in a team with 3 team members: one project manager and two developers. They use a combination of XP and Scrum and modified their practices according to their context. The web based product is for sales people to optimize their sale process.

P3 is based in Finland, and works in a large mobile phone company. He is a program manager and works on multiple projects using scrum. They develop mobile phones and telecom applications and also configuration tools for internal use. After failure on a project using the traditional waterfall process, he switched to agile methods and now he is continuously working on different projects by employing scrum. In one of the projects, the team size is about 6 people, one person as tester, 3 to 4 developers, and a UCD professional; so the role of specialist is being carried out in this team [6].

P4 is based in Germany and is an agile coach, a consultant and a certified scrum master. Mostly, he has been working as a project manager consultant with telecom sector and has been developing and leading teams for mobile phone applications. In one of the agile projects where he is working as a coach and project manager using scrum, there are 8 members who all are developers as well as having good background in usability as according to [P4], *"In that team, most of the people are actually coming from user interface design for mobile phones, so they almost all have a feel of what is a good UI because they saw many of those... They already have quite a lot experience of developing UI and some of them are developing these types of things something like 14 years but, one even 15 years, even before working in agile process. Usability was a part of our job description since quite long time... The general concepts about usability are discussed together by the whole team including management; and the low level usability, so what happens when the user presses a button, how for example scrolling goes, those are mostly decided by the engineers themselves."* The role of UCD professional in this case is carried out differently as all are both developers as well as having good experience in UI design, nevertheless, we would call this type of role a hybrid approach, as described by Fox et al. [6].

Based in Austria, P5 is a developer and project manager who has also experience in usability. He works on products which are used in hospitals for the medical staff and he also develops software for clinical research. They are using an agile process, which has been adapted to their context where many agile practices have been taken from pragmatic programming, scrum, and XP. The team consists of 3 to 4 persons, among them one is a usability engineer who is not present in the team all the time but is accessible on demand. He is contacted for the formal usability tests, otherwise mostly the usability tests, i.e., low and high fidelity tests and thinking aloud tests are conducted by P5. Here again, the role of UCD professional is carried out differently as both the role of specialist as well as generalist is present in this project. So again, this is a new situation for the role of UCD professional compared to that described by Fox et al. [6].

4 Results

This section describes some of the main themes and concepts that emerged after the analysis of the data. The relevant passages from the interview participants are also presented.

Among agile team members, there is an increasing realization of the importance of usability in software development, whereas agile methods also provide advantages to usability/UCD for its integration.

[P1] *"This is also an indicator for me that it is good to use agile developments because then you have shorter cycles and then you have the possibility to integrate in the next cycle. If you use conventional project processes, you don't have the possibility, for example for half a year, to integrate. So agile development is good in that the usability results can be easily integrated in its short cycles and end users become more satisfied."*

[P2] *" We have no usability engineers, but I have interest in usability... Usability fixes can be done because of agile development we always have a working software so it is easy to find usability changes which then can be fixed according to the priority."*

[P3] *"The usability guy has value for the project... He thinks how the process and one sitting proceeds; so which functions are more used, which should be more easily available, which is used, which is the harder way to access, how to jump in from one component to other, and that kinds of issues. He has better vision and intuition what is better and what is not."*

[P4] *"Usability testing and taking care of UI into agile process, it is beneficial...The usability tests and evaluating UI with users bring lot of feedback to be fixed, so it was easy for us to fix those usability results into small iterations of agile process."*

[P5] *"Being both a developer and having interest, experience in usability is a plus point. If your product is usable, the user acceptance is far better than if it is only functional but unusable... Usability is always a main feature of the software, so the good usability is really important."*

Almost all the participants mentioned that integrating usability/UCD into agile process has enhanced the quality and the usability of the product and increased the satisfaction of the users. Some also pointed out that this integration has added value to their team and the process.

[P1] *"We also have some numbers showing about the company that they compared page usage with user sessions and it doubled their usage and this was because of our usability work."*

[P2] *"Yes, we have good experience with that and customers, who are both customers and end users, are happy about that; they give us good feedback; they get what they want; and so we don't have bad experience about that."*

[P3] *"Yea, well, on this case I say, it's quite good proof because we tried on traditional way and it crashed and burned and nothing got. It was totally unusable, and this [using usability into agile process] we got... also the short iterations are good or the customer doesn't forget what he has asked for. Because in first case, they had changed their minds over the half year period, so that's why it wasn't any more what they expected and wanted. So now in agile, we can show the customer what he asks for immediately... The integration of usability techniques into agile method has added value to our team and the process. I definitely would like to use more."*

[P4] *"As the product is new and not yet public so we don't have real external users but it has increased the satisfaction of the internal users... Usability testing and taking care of UI into agile process, it is beneficial."*

[P5] *"Of course, yes."*

Almost all the participants mentioned that they do some up-front design to understand users, their goals, and the project vision; and the requirements are emerging. This result is consistent with other studies [4][5][6].

[P2] *"For the initial vision of the project we do paper prototyping with the customers [who are also end users] to understand their goals; and then we are getting continuously requirements from the customers during every cycle."*

[P3] *'Initially, we [as a team] did prototyping with end users, we discussed it with them and said this is what you are and on which you are comfortable and then on demo when we went through and we sat after wards and asked does it work for you? How are your feelings? ....The requirements are gathered for about one sprint. The usability guy takes feedback from the team members, from customers and user representatives, and shows them and asks them how they feel it; and of course there is feedback that this design works very well and this does not work and then it as taken as a requirement for the next sprint and so then it is fixed.'"*

[P4] *"The requirements are emerging and they are not fixed up front. As the product is completely new, so the customer had no clear requirements, he just provided few requirements and the majority of the requirements are generated internally by us [the team and the internal users at the company]; and there were few requirements also generated by technology. So the customer just had the vision of the product, a generic vision and we are putting meat into it [the features]. There was informal feedback got from outside but no formal feedback because they wanted to keep their product secret...Initially, paper prototype was something used in brainstorming and even in product manifest period and were shown internally. So in visionary meetings we used drawing boards, and also simulated them using NetBeans with GUI designer with the screen shots and how you move."*

[P5] *" The requirements are always emerging. The customer has only the vision. So only 20% to 30% requirements are already fixed and the rest are emerging. So the html mockup is the first version we implement and evaluate them to the customer to get more requirements."*

There is an appreciation of each other's work from both UCD professionals and developers and both sides learn from each other. This result is also consistent with [4][5][18][19].

[P1] *"Because of different understanding, from developer perspective from us-ability perspectives, we are presenting the results in the form of workshop; so we try to invite developers and the other team members to discuss and to ask ques-tions, because this is more efficient. During the discussion a developer pointed out technical, legal and security issues. And this was also an information for us; so we said ok we have to consider it in future."*

[P3] *"Of course we have to consider how it is difficult to implement. So we have the conversation that what is possible at technical level and in this way the usability guy also got feedback from the developers. For example, the usability guy is presenting something and saying this is good and then when it is tested for example, in a testing environment and then it came out that it's response time is too long and on paper it looks good but it is not usable."*

Both low and high fidelity prototype based usability tests are frequently con-ducted in the agile teams of these participants. The forms of prototypes vary and include paper prototypes, screenshots, powerpoint presentations, html mockups, etc. This result is also consistent with [13] and [19]. Holzinger [32] describes the advantages and disadvantages of both low and high fidelity prototypes during their application in the development of a virtual medical campus interface. Us-ability tests on working software were also conducted by some of the participants. Other HCI techniques that were mentioned by the participants and sometimes also conducted are heuristic evaluations and thinking aloud. Fixing the usability feedback results by developers in an iteration cycle depends upon how big the usability change is. If it is big then it is implemented in the next iteration cycle, otherwise it is fixed in the same iteration cycle.

5 Conclusion

This paper investigated how the integration of agile methods and user-centered design is carried out in practice using grounded theory. The emerging themes that the study found show that, among agile team members, there is an increas-ing realization of the importance of usability in software development; whereby agile methods also provide advantages to usability/UCD for its integration. The participants also mentioned that integrating usability/UCD into agile process has enhanced the quality and the usability of the product and increased the satisfaction of the users. Some also pointed out that this integration has added value to their team and the process.

Some up-front design is carried out to understand users, their goals, and the project vision. The requirements are emerging. The usability changes are fixed in the same iteration cycle or in the next iteration cycle depending upon how big they are. Both low and high fidelity prototypes based usability tests are highly used in agile teams. There is an appreciation of each other's work from both UCD professionals and developers and both sides can learn from each other. Almost all the results are consistent with the existing studies present in the literature. We also confirmed some of the previously identified themes by Ferreira et al. and Fox et al. [4][5][6].

It should be noted that the sample data set of five participants for grounded theory research is small which may be the limitation of the study but we plan to conduct more interviews from various participants working on different projects to verify and extend the results found during the current study. The current qualifying core category is "the realization of the importance of usability in software development", which will be verified by conducting further interviews and collecting various forms of data.

References

1. Holzinger, A.: Usability Engineering for Software Developers. Communications of the ACM 48(1), 71–74 (2005)
2. Hussain, Z., Lechner, M., Milchrahm, H., Shahzad, S., Slany, W., Umgeher, M., Wolkerstorfer, P.: Agile User-Centered Design Applied to a Mobile Multimedia Streaming Application. In: Holzinger, A. (ed.) USAB 2008. LNCS, vol. 5298, pp. 313–330. Springer, Heidelberg (2008)
3. Glaser, B.G., Strauss, A.L.: The Discovery of Grounded Theory: Strategies for Qualitative Research. Aldine (1967)
4. Ferreira, J., Noble, J., Biddle, R.: Agile development iterations and UI design. In: Agile 2007, pp. 50–58. IEEE Computer Society, Los Alamitos (2007)
5. Ferreira, J., Noble, J., Biddle, R.: Up-front interaction design in agile development. In: Concas, G., Damiani, E., Scotto, M., Succi, G. (eds.) XP 2007. LNCS, vol. 4536, pp. 9–16. Springer, Heidelberg (2007)
6. Fox, D., Sillito, J., Maurer, F.: Agile methods and User-Centered design: How these two methodologies are being successfully integrated in industry. In: AGILE 2008, pp. 63–72 (2008)
7. Patton, J.: Hitting the target: adding interaction design to agile software development. In: OOPSLA 2002 Practitioners Reports, Seattle, Washington. ACM, New York (2002)
8. Patton, J.: Twelve emerging best practices for adding UX work to agile development (June 2008),
   http://www.agileproductdesign.com/blog/
   emerging_best_agile_ux_practice.html
9. Chamberlain, S., Sharp, H., Maiden, N.: Towards a framework for integrating agile development and user-centred design. In: Abrahamsson, P., Marchesi, M., Succi, G. (eds.) XP 2006. LNCS, vol. 4044, pp. 143–153. Springer, Heidelberg (2006)
10. McInerney, P., Maurer, F.: UCD in agile projects: dream team or odd couple? Interactions 12(6), 19–23 (2005)
11. Holzinger, A., Errath, M., Searle, G., Thurnher, B., Slany, W.: From extreme programming and usability engineering to extreme usability in software engineering education (XP+UE→XU). In: COMPSAC 2005: Proceedings of the 29th Annual International Computer Software and Applications Conference (COMPSAC 2005), Washington, DC, USA, vol. 2, pp. 169–172. IEEE Computer Society, Los Alamitos (2005)
12. Miller, L.: Case study of customer input for a successful product. In: Agile Conference, pp. 225–234 (2005)
13. Meszaros, G., Aston, J.: Adding usability testing to an agile project. In: Agile Conference 2006 (2006)

14. Memmel, T., Reiterer, H., Holzinger, A.: Agile methods and visual specification in software development: A chance to ensure universal access. In: Stephanidis, C. (ed.) HCI 2007. LNCS, vol. 4554, pp. 453–462. Springer, Heidelberg (2007)
15. Sy, D.: Adapting usability investigations for agile user-centered design. Journal of Usability Studies 2(3), 112–132 (2007)
16. Brown, J., Lindgaard, G., Biddle, R.: Stories, sketches, and lists: Developers and interaction designers interacting through artefacts. In: AGILE 2008. Conference, pp. 39–50 (2008)
17. Ungar, J.: The design studio: Interface design for agile teams. In: AGILE 2008. Conference, pp. 519–524 (2008)
18. Wolkerstorfer, P., Tscheligi, M., Sefelin, R., Milchrahm, H., Hussain, Z., Lechner, M., Shahzad, S.: Probing an agile usability process. In: CHI 2008: human factors in computing systems, pp. 2151–2158. ACM, New York (2008)
19. Hussain, Z., Milchrahm, H., Shahzad, S., Slany, W., Tscheligi, M., Wolkerstorfer, P.: Integration of extreme programming and user-centered design: Lessons learned. In: Abrahamsson, P., Marchesi, M., Maurer, F. (eds.) XP 2009. LNBIP, vol. 31, pp. 174–179. Springer, Heidelberg (1975)
20. Federoff, M., Courage, C., Villamor, C.: Agile success: A user experience case study. In: UPA 2009 International Conference, Usability Professional's Association (2009)
21. Miller, L., Sy, D.: Agile user experience SIG. In: Proceedings of the 27th international conference extended abstracts on Human factors in computing systems CHI, Boston, MA, USA, pp. 2751–2754. ACM, New York (2009)
22. Seaman, C.B.: Qualitative methods in empirical studies of software engineering. IEEE Trans. Softw. Eng. 25(4), 557–572 (1999)
23. Adolph, S., Hall, W., Kruchten, P.: A methodological leg to stand on: lessons learned using grounded theory to study software development. In: CASCON 2008: Proceedings of the 2008 conference of the center for advanced studies on collaborative research, pp. 166–178 (2008)
24. Coleman, G., O'Connor, R.: Using grounded theory to understand software process improvement: A study of irish software product companies. Information and Software Technology 49(6), 654–667 (2007)
25. Hansen, B.H., Kautz, K.: Grounded theory applied - studying information systems development methodologies in practice. In: HICSS 2005: Proceedings of the Proceedings of the 38th Annual Hawaii International Conference on System Sciences. IEEE Computer Society, Los Alamitos (2005)
26. Whitworth, E., Biddle, R.: The social nature of agile teams. In: Proceedings of the AGILE 2007, pp. 26–36. IEEE Computer Society, Los Alamitos (2007)
27. Cao, L., Ramesh, B.: Agile requirements engineering practices: An empirical study. IEEE Software 25(1), 60–67 (2008)
28. Hoda, R., Noble, J., Marshall, S.: Negotiating contracts for agile projects: A practical perspective. In: Abrahamsson, P., Marchesi, M., Maurer, F. (eds.) XP 2009. LNBIP, vol. 31, pp. 186–191. Springer, Heidelberg (2009)
29. Strauss, A., Corbin, J.M.: Basics of Qualitative Research: Techniques and Procedures for Developing Grounded Theory, 1st edn. Springer, Heidelberg (1990)
30. Strauss, A., Corbin, J.M.: Basics of Qualitative Research: Techniques and Procedures for Developing Grounded Theory, 2nd edn. Springer, Heidelberg (1998)
31. Schreiber, R.S.: The 'how to' of grounded theory: avoiding the pitfalls. In: Schreiber, R.S., Stern, P.N. (eds.) Using Grounded Theory in Nursing. Springer, Berlin (2001)
32. Holzinger, A.: Rapid prototyping for a virtual medical campus interface. IEEE Software 21(1), 92–99 (2004)

A Bridge to Web Accessibility from the Usability Heuristics

Lourdes Moreno, Paloma Martínez, and Belén Ruiz-Mezcua

Computer Science Department, Universidad Carlos III de Madrid
Avda. Universidad 30, 28911 Leganés, Madrid, Spain
{lmoreno,pmf,bruiz}@inf.uc3m.es

Abstract. There is not a clear distinction between accessibility and usability for all. This work shows the overlap between usability and accessibility proposing a bridge from the usability heuristics to WCAG 2.0 guidelines. The mapping between some usability and accessibility concepts can be a useful resource to know what aspects of accessibility were collected when the usability is taken into account.

Keywords: web accessibility, usability, Heuristic Evaluation.

1 Introduction

The relationship between accessibility and usability generates discussion due to an unclear distinction between them [1], [2]. Some things are clearly accessibility issues, some are obviously usability; and others are in an area where accessibility and usability overlap. There is not a clear distinction between accessibility for people with disabilities and general usability for all.

Accessibility has a technical component and a user interface component. Accessibility of user interfaces can be approached through a usability field. International Organization for Standardization (ISO) 9241-11 defines usability as the "extent to which a product can be used by specified users to achieve specified goals effectively, efficiency and with satisfaction in a specified context of use." [3] Accessibility focuses on including people with disabilities as the "specified users" and a wide range of situations [4], including assistive technologies (ATs), as the "specified context of use".

In a simpler way, usability means designing a user interface that is effective, efficient, and satisfying. Accessibility makes sure the user interface is designed to be effective, efficient, and satisfying for more people—especially people with disabilities, in more situations—including with ATs.

One way to start looking at the distinction between the two is to categorize interface problems: the usability problems equally impact all users, regardless of ability; that is, a person with a disability is not disadvantaged to a greater extent by usability issues than a person without a disability, whilst the accessibility problems decrease access to a product by people with disabilities. When a person with a disability is at a disadvantage related to a person without a disability then it is an accessibility issue.

A. Holzinger and K. Miesenberger (Eds.): USAB 2009, LNCS 5889, pp. 290–300, 2009.

Apart from this, the distinction is further blurred by the fact that features for people with disabilities benefit people without disabilities because of situational limitations (limitations from circumstances such as environment or device) and additionally accessibility increases general usability.

Another point that confuses the distinction is usable accessibility, that is, how usable are accessibility solutions. If a website uses images for navigation and there's no alt text, the site is clearly not accessible, one might say that the site is technically accessible because there is alt text. However, the alt text is so bad that the usability of the site is awful for anyone who relies on alt text. When designing products, it's rarely useful to differentiate between usability and accessibility. However, there are times when such a distinction is important, such as when looking at discrimination against people with disabilities and when defining specific accessibility standards. In some usability test reporting it may be important to distinguish between accessibility and usability problems [5].

Another perspective to consider is the accessibility and usability in the context of a development process. Beside compliance issues at the level of implementation of accessibility standards as WCAG [6], we must guarantee the user satisfaction and usability. In this line, to follow the standard ISO 13407 (Human-centred design processes for interactive systems) [7] is a solution framework, with the use of usability techniques in the web development process [8]. Usability must be considered before prototyping takes place. When usability inspection, or testing, is first carried out at the end of the design cycle, changes to the interface can be costly and difficult to implement, which in turn leads to usability recommendations. Thus, user interface design should more properly be called user interface development [9].

In section two works about Web Accessibility standardization are outlined. Section three describes the overlap between usability and accessibility and provides a bridge from concepts of usability to WCAG 2.0 Success Criteria. The last section includes some conclusions.

2 Web Accessibility Standardization. The Web Content Accessibility Guidelines 2.0 (WCAG 2.0)

In web accessibility standardization, the W3C must be highlighted along with the Web Accessibility Initiative (WAI) [10]. WAI includes documentation of suggestions on how to use the guidelines in the developments. The Web Content Accessibility Guidelines (WCAG) [6] is one of the most important components, and it is considered to be the official standard in the European Union. These guidelines appear in the majority of legislation worldwide. There are other laws such as Section 508 [11] in the United States. In Spain there is also a standard [12], but all of them are similar to those established by WCAG 1.0 [13].

However, the WCAG do not cover all situations; a study [14] investigated the accessibility of Web sites concluding the need to extend WCAG because, in some cases, pages that did pass that WCAG test were inaccessible in another way and almost certainly would have failed usability test and the resources could be inaccessible.

Over the years, two different versions of the WCAG, the WCAG 1.0 and the WCAG 2.0, have been published as W3C Recommendations, with the latter having come into official existence in December 2008. The publication of the WCAG 2.0 became necessary to accommodate not only HTML and CSS, but also scripting and non W3C Web technologies such as RIAs. WCAG 2.0 incorporate techniques of the Accessible Rich Internet Applications (WAI-ARIA) specification for RIA technologies.

In this work the new version WCAG 2.0 [15] has been followed. The WCAG 2.0 is built on four basic principles of accessibility: perceivable, operable, understandable and robust. Within these principles, there are guidelines that contain Success Criteria. Each Success Criteria has one of three defined Levels of Conformance (A, AA, AAA). Regarding the fulfillment of these success Criteria, a Web site can have an A, AA, or AAA level of conformance. The priority levels are designed to indicate a Web site's level of accessibility, with A being the lowest and AAA being the highest.

3   Correspondence between Usability Principles and WCAG 2.0

In the field of human-computer interaction (HCI), one of the most common informal and popular inspection-based methods for evaluating usability is the Heuristic Evaluation (HE) as described originally by Nielsen and Molich [16] and later refined by Nielsen [17]. The HE is seen as an economical alternative to empirical usability tests involving actual users. HE involves having a small set of evaluators examine the interface and judge its compliance with recognized usability principles (the "heuristics"), the group of evaluators apply heuristics during their independent review of a system. The evaluators explore the system, considering each heuristic in turn in an effort to identify potential usability issues. They are most valuable as an early evaluation technique on a first prototype in an effort to identify the major usability problems.

HE method continues to be considered somewhat of a standard in the HCI industry, although many evaluators have found that Nielsen's original list does not always meet their specific needs. As a result, several modifications of Nielsen's heuristics have been developed over the years in an effort to improve their interpretation, reliability, and adequacy for new technologies.

In this work, the criteria of HE method have been used with the approach of "Site Usability Heuristics for the Web" of Keith Instone [18], based on Nielsen [19]. It is a solid reference with other heuristics based on it and it can be adapted to a current project due to the fact that it consists of generic usability principles that can be matched with current criteria.

A study has been made to find relationships between concepts of accessibility and a very generic usability. We must emphasize that it was not considered the usable accessibility or usability in contexts of use with accessibility barriers, since in this case the conceptual overlap is misleading, as is the usual case to consider providing an alternative text to images (WCAG 2.0 success criteria 1.1.1) as usability criteria.

To show the overlap between usability and accessibility issues, Table 1 introduces a correspondence between the criteria of usability heuristics by Nielsen in web environments and the WCAG 2.0 Guidelines.

Then, to provide a brief explanation of each heuristic criterion, the related WCAG 2.0 Success Criteria are described. They are denoted by their levels of conformance in parentheses next to the WCAG 2.0 techniques applied in each case.

Table 1. Overlap between usability heuristics and WCAG 2.0 guidelines

Usability Heuristics	WCAG 2.0 Success Criteria
Visibility of system status	2.4.2 / 2.4.3/ 2.4.4/ 2.4.6/ 2.4.8/ 2.4.9/ 2.4.10
Match between system and the real world	3.1.2 / 3.1.3/ 3.1.4/ 3.1.5/ 3.1.6/ 3.2.3
User control and freedom	1.4.2/ 1.4.4/ 1.4.8/ 2.2.1/ 2.2.2/ 2.2.4
Consistency and standards	3.2.3/ 3.2.4
Error prevention	3.3.1/ 3.3.2/ 3.3.4/ 3.3.6
Recognition rather than recall	1.3.1/ 2.4.2/ 2.4.6/ 2.4.10
Flexibility and efficiency of use	2.4.1/ 2.4.3
Aesthetic and minimalist design	
Help users recognize, diagnose and recover from errors	3.3.3
Help and documentation	3.3.5

3.1 Visibility of System Status

The system should always keep users informed about what is going on, through appropriate feedback within reasonable time. Probably the two most important things that users need to know at your site are "Where am I?" and "Where can I go next?"

Make sure each page is branded and that you indicate which section it belongs to. Links to other pages should be clearly marked. Since users could be jumping to any part of your site from somewhere else, you need to include this status on every page. One of the biggest problems for users when browsing the network is the disorientation

WCAG 2.0 Success Criteria correspondence:

The WCAG 2.0 Guideline 2.4 said: "Navigable: Provide ways to help users navigate, find content, and determine where they are". Different criteria are specified:

Related to documents:

✓ 2.4.2 (A)/G88 (Providing descriptive titles for Web pages) y H25 (Providing a title using the title element), ARIA 1 (Using Accessible Rich Internet Application described by property to provide a descriptive, programmatically determined label).

✓ 2.4.6 (AA)/G130 (Providing descriptive headings), G131(Providing descriptive labels).

✓ 2.4.10(AAA)/G141 (Organizing a page using headings)

Concerning the target link:

✓ 2.4.3 (A)/G59 (Placing the interactive elements in an order that follows sequences and relationships within the content), H4 (Creating a logical tab order through links, form controls, and objects), C27(Making the DOM order match the visual order) y SCR26(Inserting dynamic content into the DOM immediately following its trigger element), SCR27(Reordering page sections using the DOM).

✓ 2.4.4 (A)/ G91 (Providing link text that describes the purpose of a link), G53 (Identifying the purpose of a link using link text combined with the text of the enclosing sentence), ARIA 1 (Using ARIA described by property to provide a descriptive, programmatically determined label).

✓ 2.4.9(AAA)/G91 (Providing link text that describes the purpose of a link), C7 (Using CSS to hide a portion of the link text).

✓ 2.4.8 (AAA)/ G63 (Providing a site map), G65 (Providing a breadcrumb trail), G128 (Indicating current location within navigation bars), G127 (Identifying a Web page's relationship to a larger collection of Web pages) con H59 (Using the link element and navigation tools).

3.2 Match between System and the Real World

The system should speak the users' language, with words, phrases and concepts familiar to the user, rather than system-oriented terms. Follow real-world conventions, making information appear in a natural and logical order.

On the Web, you have to be aware that users will probably be coming from diverse backgrounds, so figuring out their "language" can be a challenge. ". Different criteria are specified:

WCAG 2.0 Success Criteria correspondence:

The related guideline 3.1 specifies: "Readable: Make text content readable and understandable". We must use a language that is familiar to the user, with simple phrases and concepts. In fact, the WCAG 2.0 guidelines provide how to fix this mismatch between the "conventions of the real world" and the system. The guidelines through techniques indicate that there is a need to offer a mechanism for users to identify what content is unusual or technical words in another language, problems with reading ability, etc, and to provide help about how to access this additional content to understand.

✓ 3.1.2 (AA)/ H58 (Using language attributes to identify changes in the human language).

✓ 3.1.3 (AAA)/ G55 (Linking to definitions), G112 (Using inline definitions), G62 (Providing a glossary).

✓ 3.1.4 (AAA)/ G102 (Providing the expansion or explanation of an abbreviation), G97 (Providing the abbreviation immediately following the expanded form), H60 (Using the link element to link to a glossary), G55 (Linking to definitions), H28 (Providing definitions for abbreviations by using the abbr and acronym HTML elements).

✓ 3.1.5 (AAA)/ G86 (Providing a text summary that requires reading ability less advanced than the upper secondary education level), G103 (Providing visual illustrations, pictures, and symbols to help explain ideas, events, and processes), G79 (Providing a spoken version of the text).

✓ 3.1.6 (AAA)/G120 (Providing the pronunciation immediately following the word), G121 (Linking to pronunciations), G62 (Providing a glossary).

✓ 3.2.3 (AA)/ G61 (Presenting repeated components in the same relative order each time they appear).

3.3 User Control and Freedom

Many of the "emergency exits" are provided by the browser, but there is still plenty of room on your site to support user control and freedom. Or, there are many ways authors can take away user control that is built into the Web. A "home" button on every page is a simple way to let users feel in control of your site.

Be careful when forcing users into certain fonts, colors, screen widths or browser versions. And watch out for some of those "advanced technologies": usually user control is not added until the technology has matured. One example is animated GIFs. Until browsers let users stop and restart the animations, they can do more harm than good.

WCAG 2.0 Success Criteria correspondence:

The related guideline 2.2 establishes: "Enough Time: Provide users enough time to read and use content". It includes different success criteria that indicate characteristics associated and offering the user control in the interaction with web content. The success criteria 1.4.2 is related too, and said: "Audio Control: If any audio on a Web page plays automatically for more than 3 seconds, either a mechanism is available to pause or stop the audio, or a mechanism is available to control audio volume independently from the overall system volume level". Finally, the Success criteria 1.4.4 and 1.4.8 in relation to CSS implementation ensure the freedom of the user to change the text size, color etc.

Different criteria are specified:

✓ 1.4.2 (A) / G170 (Providing a control near the beginning of the Web page that turns off sounds that play automatically), G171 (Playing sounds only on user request).

✓ 1.4.4 (AA)/ C28 (Specifying the size of text containers using em units), G178 (Providing controls on the Web page that allow users to incrementally change the size of all text on the page up to 200 percent).

✓ 1.4.8 (AAA)/ G148 (Not specifying background color, not specifying text color, and not using technology features that change those defaults), H87 (Not interfering with the user agent's reflow of text as the viewing window is narrowed), G175 (Providing a multi color selection tool on the page for foreground and background colors), C20 (Using relative measurements to set column widths so that lines can average 80 characters or less when the browser is resized), G188 (Providing a button on the page to increase line spaces and paragraph spaces).

✓ 2.2.1 (A)/ G198 (Providing a way for the user to turn the time limit off), SCR16 (Providing a script that warns the user a time limit is about to expire), SCR1 (Allowing the user to extend the default time limit).

✓ 2.2.2(A)/ G4 (Allowing the content to be paused and restarted from where it was paused), G186 (Using a control in the Web page that stops moving, blinking, or auto-updating content), G191 (Providing a link, button, or other mechanism that reloads the page without any blinking content).

✓ 2.2.4 (AAA)/ G75 (Providing a mechanism to postpone any updating of content), G76 (Providing a mechanism to request an update of the content instead of updating automatically).

It would be also related criteria such as 2.3.1 and 2.3.2 which provide restrictions on the use of animated images. In the WCAG 2.0 documentation warns that "since any content that does not meet this success criterion can interfere with a user's ability to use the whole page, all content on the Web page (whether it is used to meet other success criteria or not) must meet this success criterion".

3.4 Consistency and Standards

Users should not have to wonder whether different words, situations, or actions mean the same thing. The site must maintain a consistent structure of content, styles and conventions. The use of style sheets (CSS) helps maintain a graphical design consistency of the site.

Conventions should ensure the labeling of links with the same criteria and the links have to be identified in the same way throughout the website.

In relation to the standards there is a clear overlap with web accessibility and conformance with the WCAG, which includes an implementation of all recommendations of the W3C on Web technologies ((X) HTML, CSS, XML, SMIL, etc..) to ensure compatibility.

WCAG 2.0 Success Criteria correspondence:

The related guideline 3.2 said "Predictable: Make Web pages appear and operate in predictable ways", and more specifically the success criteria 3.2.3: "Consistent Navigation: Navigational mechanisms that are repeated on multiple Web pages within a set of Web pages occur in the same relative order each time they are repeated, unless a change is initiated by the user". Besides, the success criterion 3.2.4 is considered, that is, "Consistent Identification: Components that have the same functionality within a set of Web pages are identified consistently".

Different criteria are specified:

- ✓ 3.2.3 (AA)/ G61 (Presenting repeated components in the same relative order each time they appear).
- ✓ 3.2.4 (AA)/ H44 (Using label elements to associate text labels with form controls (HTML)), H65 (Using the title attribute to identify form controls when the label element cannot be used (HTML)).

3.5 Error Prevention

Even better than good error messages is a careful design which prevents a problem from occurring in the first place, must ensure that instructions are clear to the data entry forms providing mechanisms for identifying required fields.

WCAG 2.0 Success Criteria correspondence:

The guideline 3.3 said "Input Assistance: Help users avoid and correct mistakes", it is related and their success criteria are:

- ✓ 3.3.1 (A)/ G83 (Providing text descriptions to identify required fields that were not completed), SCR18 (Providing client-side validation and alert (Scripting)), G85 (Providing a text description when user input falls outside the required format or values), G84 (Providing a text description when the user provides information that is not in the list of allowed values).
- ✓ 3.3.2 (A) / G131 (Providing descriptive labels AND G89|G83).

✓ 3.3.4 (AA) y 3.3.6 (AAA) / G98 (Providing the ability for the user to review and correct answers before submitting, G155 (Providing a checkbox in addition to a submit button), G99 (Providing the ability to recover deleted information) and G155 (Providing a checkbox in addition to a submit button).

3.6 Recognition Rather Than Recall

Make objects, actions, and options visible. The user should not have to remember information from one part of the dialogue to another. Instructions for use of the system should be visible or easily retrievable whenever appropriate.

For the Web, this heuristic is closely related to system status. If users can recognize where they are by looking at the current page, without having to recall their path from the home page, they are less likely to get lost. Good labels and descriptive links are also crucial for recognition.

For the Web, this heuristic is closely related to system status. If users can recognize where they are by looking at the current page, without having to recall their path from the home page, they are less likely to get lost.

Good labels and descriptive links are also crucial for recognition. Therefore the success criteria to "Visibility of system status" heuristic is also considered.

WCAG 2.0 Success Criteria correspondence:

Among the guidelines considered: success criteria 1.3.1, the success criteria 2.4.10 that said "Section Headings: Section headings are used to organize the content". Others related criteria are: the 2.4.2 ("Page Titled: Web pages have titles that describe topic or purpose") which indicates that the pages should have title. This approach does not require unique page titles but descriptive and usable ones as success criteria 2.4.6 establishes "Headings and Labels: Headings and labels describe topic or purpose".

The related success criteria are:

✓ 1.3.1 (A)/ H42 (Using h1-h6 to identify headings), ARIA 1 (Using ARIA described by property to provide a descriptive, programmatically determined label).
✓ 2.4.2 (A)/G88 (ARIA 4(Using ARIA to programmatically identify form fields as required).Providing descriptive titles for Web pages) y H25 (Providing a title using the title element), ARIA 1 (Using ARIA described by property to provide a descriptive, programmatically determined label).
✓ 2.4.6 (AA)/G130 (Providing descriptive headings), G131 (Providing descriptive labels).
✓ 2.4.10(AAA)/G141 (Organizing a page using headings).

3.7 Flexibility and Efficiency of Use

Accelerators – unseen by the novice user – may often speed up the interaction for the expert user such that the system can cater to both inexperienced and experienced users. Allow users to tailor frequent actions.

When users do become experts of the program, they may want to speed up some task with shortcuts. This does not mean to change the interface such that tasks can be done quickly but non-intuitively. The principle here suggests that the program should cater to both the inexperienced and the experienced users.

WCAG 2.0 Success Criteria correspondence:

Advanced users could prefer not to move their hands from the keyboard to the mouse and make use of the keyboard shortcuts to speed up the process. In this point the *WCAG 2.0* criteria about keyboard shortcuts are considered. There are Additional Techniques (Advisory) for 2.4.1 that said: Providing keyboard access to important links and form controls (future link), Providing skip links to enhance page navigation (future link), Providing access keys (future link) and Using accessibility supported technologies which allow structured navigation by user agents and ATs (future link).

The related success criteria are:

✓ 2.4.1(A)/G1 (Adding a link at the top of each page that goes directly to the main content area), G123 (Adding a link at the beginning of a block of repeated content to go to the end of the block), G124 (Adding links at the top of the page to each area of the content), H69 (Providing heading elements at the beginning of each section of content), H50 (Using structural elements to group links).

Following the 2.4.3 criteria if a Web page can be navigated sequentially and the navigation sequences affect meaning or operation, focusable components receive focus in an order that preserves meaning and operability this applies to the element with control type included in a form.

✓ 2.4.3 (A)/G59 (Placing the interactive elements in an order that follows sequences and relationships within the content), H4 (Creating a logical tab order through links, form controls, and objects), C27 (Making the DOM order match the visual order) y SCR26 (Inserting dynamic content into the Document Object Model immediately following its trigger element), SCR27 (Reordering page sections using the Document Object Model).

The WCAG 2.0 Principle 4: "Robust – Content must be robust enough that it can be interpreted reliably by a wide variety of user agents, including assistive technologies" is related too because to provide Flexibility and efficiency of use it is necessary to maximize compatibility with user agents and ATs.

3.8 Aesthetic and Minimalist Design

Dialogues should not contain information which is irrelevant or rarely needed. Every extra unit of information in a dialogue competes with the relevant units of information and diminishes their relative visibility.

Extraneous information on a page is a distraction and a slow-down. Make rarely needed information accessible via a link so that the details are there when needed but do not interfere much with the more relevant content.

WCAG 2.0 Success Criteria correspondence:

In this case, the next guidelines and success criteria are not directly concerned but if there is some dependence guidelines, the WCAG 2.0 pursue the goal of simplicity, for a better understanding of the user.

3.9 Help Users Recognize, Diagnose and Recover from Errors

Error messages should be expressed in plain language (no codes), precisely indicate the problem, and constructively suggest a solution.

Errors will happen, despite all your efforts to prevent them. Every error message should offer a solution (or a link to a solution) on the error page.

WCAG 2.0 Success Criteria correspondence:

The criterion 3.3.3 said "Error Suggestion: If an input error is automatically detected and suggestions for correction are known, then the suggestions are provided to the user, unless it would jeopardize the security or purpose of the content".

✓ 3.3.3 (AA)/ G83 (Providing text descriptions to identify required fields that were not completed), SCR18 (Providing client-side validation and alert (Scripting)), G85 (Providing a text description when user input falls outside the required format or values), G84 (Providing a text description when the user provides information that is not in the list of allowed values).

3.10 Help and Documentation

Even though it is better if the system can be used without documentation, it may be necessary to provide support and help documentation. Any information should be easy to search, focused on the user's task, list concrete steps to be carried out, and not be too large.

Some of the more basic sites will not need much documentation, if any. But as soon as you try any complicated tasks, you will need some help for those tasks.

For the Web, the key is to not just slap up some help pages, but to integrate the documentation into your site. There should be links from your main sections into specific help and vice versa. Help could even be fully integrated into each page so that users never feel like assistance is too far away.

WCAG 2.0 Success Criteria correspondence:

The criterion directly related to is:

✓ 3.3.5 (AAA) / G71 (Providing a help link on every Web page), G89 (Providing expected data format and example).

4 Conclusions

The mappings among some usability and accessibility criteria have been introduced in this work. This correspondence provides a resource to help professionals to include usability in their Web projects, in such a way that they know what aspects of accessibility were collected.

Thus, for each criterion of usability heuristics the guidelines of the WCAG 2.0 with their associated techniques are provided together with useful resources to use at design, implementation and evaluation activities. This work is an additional resource to evaluate the accessibility closely to usability, because the evaluation will be complete only by testing with real users.

Acknowledgments. This research work has been supported by the Spanish Ministry of Education under the project BRAVO (TIN2007-67407-C03-01) and by The Spanish Centre of Captioning and Audio Description (see http://www.cesya.es).

References

1. Petrie, H., Kheir, O.: The relationship between accessibility and usability of websites. In: Proceedings of the SIGCHI Conference on Human Factors in Computing Systems, CHI 2007, San Jose, California, USA, April 28 - May 03. ACM, New York (2007), http://doi.acm.org/10.1145/1240624.1240688
2. Pühretmair, F., Miesenberger, K.: Making Sense of Accessibility in IT Design - Usable Accessibility vs. Accessible Usability. In: DEXA Workshops 2005, pp. 861–865 (2005)
3. International Organization for Standardization ISO 9241-11. Ergonomic Requirements for Office Work with Visual Display Terminals, Part 11: Guidance on Usability (1998)
4. Miesenberger, K., Ossmann, R., Archambault, D., Searle, G., Holzinger, A.: More Than Just a Game: Accessibility in Computer Games. In: Holzinger, A. (ed.) USAB 2008. LNCS, vol. 5298, pp. 247–260. Springer, Heidelberg (2008)
5. Henry, S.L.: Just Ask: Integrating Accessibility Throughout Design. ET\Lawton, Madison, WI (2007), http://www.uiAccess.com/justask/
6. Web Content Accessibility Guidelines (WCAG), http://www.w3.org/WAI/intro/wcag.php
7. International Organization for Standardization ISO 13407 International Standard, ISO 13407. Human-centred design processes for interactive systems (1999)
8. Moreno, L., Martínez, P., Ruiz, B.: Inclusive Usability Techniques in Requirements Analysis of Accessible Web Applications. In: Weske, M., Hacid, M.-S., Godart, C. (eds.) WISE Workshops 2007. LNCS, vol. 4832, pp. 423–428. Springer, Heidelberg (2007)
9. Holzinger, A.: Usability Engineering for Software Developers. Communications of the ACM 48(1), 71–74 (2005)
10. W3C, Web Accessibility Initiative (WAI), http://www.w3.org/WAI/
11. United States Laws, Overview of the Rehabilitation Act of 1973 (Sections 504 and 508) (1998), http://www.webaim.org/articles/laws/usa/rehab.php
12. AENOR, Spanish technical standards. Standard UNE 139803:2004: Requirements for WebPages accessibility, http://www.aenor.es
13. Chisholm, W., Vanderheiden, G., Jacobs, I. (eds.): W3C, WAI, Web Content Accessibility Guidelines 1.0, W3C Recommendation 5-May-(1999), http://www.w3.org/TR/WAI-WEBCONTENT/
14. DDC report The Web Access and Inclusion for Disabled People (2004), http://www.drc.gov.uk/publicationsandreports/2.pdf
15. Caldwell, B., Cooper, M., Guarino Reid, L., Vanderheiden, G. (eds.): W3C, WAI, Web Content Accessibility Guidelines (WCAG) 2.0, W3C Recommendation (December 11, 2008), http://www.w3.org/TR/WCAG20/
16. Nielsen, J., Molich, R.: Heuristic evaluation of user interfaces. Paper presented at the ACM CHI 1990 Conference on Human Factors in Computing Systems, Seattle, WA (1990)
17. Nielsen, J.: Heuristic evaluation. In: Nielsen, J., Mack, R.L. (eds.) Usability Inspection Methods. John Wiley & Sons, Inc., New York (1994)
18. In stone, K.: Site usability heuristics for the Web (1997), http://instone.org/heuristics
19. Nielsen, J.: Ten usability heuristics, http://www.useit.com/papers/heuristic/heuristic_list.html

E-Inclusion in Public Transport: The Role of Self-efficacy

Günther Schreder, Karin Siebenhandl, and Eva Mayr

Danube University Krems, Department for Knowledge and Communication Management,
Research Center KnowComm, Dr.-Karl-Dorrek-Straße 30,
3500 Krems, Austria
{Günther.Schreder,Karin.Siebenhandl,Eva.Mayr}@donau-uni.ac.at

Abstract. Many subgroups in today's society are not skilled in using novel technologies. Even everyday technologies pose a barrier to technically non-skilled people and – if they fail to use them – exclude them from important parts of daily life. In this paper we discuss the relevance of self-efficacy for the use of one specific kind of everyday technology: the ticket vending machine. Results from observations and interviews within the research project InnoMat are presented to answer the question how self-efficacy influences the ticket buying behavior and show that this motivational factor leads to an active avoidance of ticket machines. Negative experiences seem to be one of the strongest influences, which indicate that the group of technically non-skilled users should be given special attention when developing a new generation of ticket vending machines.

Keywords: e-Inclusion, self-efficacy, digital divide, ticket vending machine, public transport, usability, accessibility.

1 Motivation

Some social groups are disadvantaged by novel technologies either in using or having access to them or in resources and skills needed to effectively participate in the digital society. This phenomenon is referred to as the digital divide. Problems not only include potential limitations in gathering information e. g. from the internet, but also difficulties due to the increasing need to use digital devices in everyday life. Bank opening hours are shortened as ATMs sprout; in public transport, ticket counters are substituted by ticket vending machines. While it might still be easy to maintain a normal life without using a personal computer or participating in newly created forms of communication (like virtual communities, blogs and so on), being unable to withdraw money or to buy a ticket for public transport is a severe restriction.

The InnoMat research project[1] sought to develop a design framework for a new generation of ticket machines in order to best meet the needs of different user groups.

---

[1] The InnoMat project was funded by the Austrian Federal Ministry for Transport, Innovation and Technology's "Ways2go" (Innovation and Technology for Evolving Mobility Needs) research programme. In a project managed by ÖBB Personenverkehr AG, the Danube University Krems (Department for Knowledge and Communication Management), Plot EDV-Planungs- und Handels Ges.m.b.H. and AlliedPanels Entwicklungs- und Produktions GmbH developed the framework for a new generation of ticket vending machines.

A. Holzinger and K. Miesenberger (Eds.): USAB 2009, LNCS 5889, pp. 301–311, 2009.

The aim of the project can be characterized as a contribution to e-inclusion by "design for all": with regard to groups who often face barriers in using public transport systems in everyday life the target group was defined with senior citizens, people with limited affinity for technology and disabled people.

The first step was to identify the special needs and requirements of the target group in using public transport systems based on the insights from relevant literature. Specific needs of disabled persons are mostly connected to questions of accessibility, such as the existence of voice-output for visually impaired persons or the optimal height of hardware elements to allow wheelchair users the access to the machine. A similar approach can be found concerning the group of senior citizens who are often seen as persons with reduced physical and mental abilities due to their age. Relevant design aspects therefore include the contrast of screens, the size of (virtual) buttons and text, the speed of required input and so on.

As important as these factors may be, older people (but not only them) are likely to face further problems that are not identified as easily: Research into ticket queues at 12 major stations in Great Britain supports this assumption. Among those who could have bought their ticket from a machine the decision to purchase at the counter was driven by a lack of confidence in using the machine as well as a lack of confidence in the ability to select a ticket [1].

ÖBB's (Austrian Rail) sales statistics indicate that elderly people use ticket machines less frequently than other groups [2]: 63 % of senior citizens purchase tickets from a ticket machine, while 31 % opt to go to a ticket counter. ÖBB passengers under the age of 26 use ticket machines almost exclusively (91 %), while holders of regular travel cards ("Vorteilscard") or family travel cards use ticket machines relatively frequently (69-74 %).

To identify possible reasons for avoidance of ticket machines the role of the users´ confidence in their abilities to successfully buy a ticket at the vending machines will be investigated. Insights into this aspect of the digital divide should allow creating a new generation of ticket vending machines which should not only be easy to use without much experience with novel technology, but also reduce subjective fears associated with potential failure to use them.

A tendency to avoid novel technologies and a lack of technological knowledge can build barriers that effect mobility and lifestyle. This certainly holds true for elderly people and other socio-economic groups disadvantaged by the digital divide as they especially rely on public transport [3].

2 Theory

From the mid-90s on studies showed that age, gender, ethnicity, social status, education and income are the major socio-economic indicators for the societal gap that exists in the usage of digital technologies. While the discussion of the digital divide was focused on the access to the internet and the necessary hardware, strategies of inclusion showed that users´ lack of know-how seems to contribute to the emergence of the digital divide as well. It is argued that a rather poor usability of novel technologies combined with few or completely missing experiences with digital technologies in school or workplace as well as a lack of support by social networks lead to a reduced chance of acquiring adequate skills [4].

The question of so-called technological literacy [5], which includes the ability to use not only computers and consumer electronics products but also everyday items like cash and ticket machines, becomes more relevant among older generations. People born before 1939, for example, did not have any opportunity to learn how to use digital technologies at school or in the workplace [6].

In addition to senior citizens, some other groups are also disadvantaged by the so-called "secondary digital divide" that emerges due to reduced technological literacy [7]: people with lower levels of education and members of ethnic minorities number relatively frequently among those with little experience of technology. Gender, income level and occupation are also seen as predictors of a lower level of technological literacy [8], [9].

Furthering opportunities for learning and skill acquisition might seem invaluable; still a remarkable part of the population is actively avoiding the use of computers and the internet. In the representative German Online Nonusers Survey [10] 234 (54%) of the 501 nonusers stated that they did not want to connect to the Internet. A variety of reasons are listed in Figure 1. It should be noted that only half of the nonusers (47%) rejected private computer use partly due to financial limits, whereas the more numerous answers pointed at a lack of interest or need or a general dislike. Van Dijk and Hacker [4] see these results as an argument for not neglecting motivational factors contributing to the digital usage gap.

According to Eastin and LaRose [11] social cognitive theory offers an alternative to the socio-economic explanations normally used when discussing the digital divide. "Self-efficacy is a person's belief in her capabilities to organize and execute the courses of action required to produce given attainments". [12] People with lower self-efficacy display less motivation to engage in a task than do those with higher self-efficacy. A correlation between learning to use computers and self-efficacy was demonstrated by Karavidas, Lim and Katsikas [13], indicating that computer self-efficacy also depends on the subjective feeling of having made progress during training.

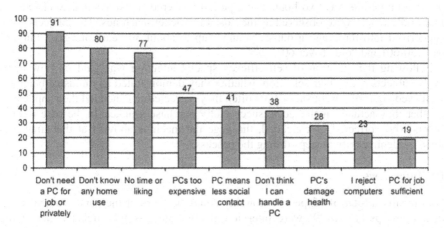

Fig. 1. Reasons for not using the internet [10]

In [8] "computer self-efficacy" was an important predictor for the use of technical devices, while being influenced by "computer anxiety" as a mediator. For persons with a low level of self-efficacy the probability of using the technology was generally reduced. Additionally, persons with a high level of computer anxiety had less experience with computers and the internet and used these technologies for a smaller number of different activities. The combination of both resulted in an active avoidance of technological devices. As senior citizens are frequent among the described group, the authors stressed the importance to use technology that allows senior citizens to experience success so that they are able to build up confidence in their abilities.

Following these ideas the focus of this study is to answer some research questions closely related to self-efficacy: Do the users´ or non-users´ beliefs to be able to successfully buy the ticket show any relevancy concerning the purchase process? Are any negative experiences connected to buying tickets at the machine? Furthermore the research team sought to identify those elements of the current ticket machines that have the strongest effects on users' perception of their ability to cope with them.

3 Methods

With the aim of learning from users' actual experiences, the project team decided to observe the usage and specifics of the machines currently being used at Austrian railway stations. Interviews gave additional information and helped to identify particular problems and elements that currently hinder use.

3.1 Observations

The main aim of the observations was to identify those people who had problems in using the ticket machines. The observations took place at two different railway stations, one in Baden (Austria), one at a major station in Vienna (Südbahnhof). The observation period was two hours each, periods covered weekdays and weekends. A total of 50 people were observed as they used the ticket machines. The subjects were categorized into three age groups: "young" (up to about 30 years of age), "middle-age" (30-60) and "old" (over 60).

Following the question of self-efficacy special attention was paid on how decisively subjects made their selection, whether they demonstrated any unusual behavior or showed signs of nervousness, how often they corrected or cancelled their input, and whether they actually managed to successfully purchase a ticket. In the case of customers who corrected or cancelled, the page the machine showed at that time was noted to identify critical steps during the process.

3.2 Interviews

Additionally a total of 65 people (roughly equal numbers of men and women) from all age groups (15 to 89) were interviewed after purchasing a ticket either at the ticket counter or from a machine. They were asked about their experiences in using ticket vending machines and problems they had encountered so far. The interviews took place on two weekdays at the railway station in Baden (Austria) and on a Friday and a Saturday at the Südbahnhof in Vienna. To identify their level of affinity for technology, the subjects were also asked about their use of mobile phones, computers, cash machines and the internet.

3.3 Log File Analysis

A sales data log file analysis was additionally carried out to support the observations and interviews. Internal logs of an ÖBB ticket machine at Vienna Südbahnhof for the time between 06:24 and 10:56 a.m. on 14 October 2008 were analyzed.

4 Results

The 50 people observed were split fairly evenly across both genders (45 % men, 55 % women). One third of these people were classed as "uncertain" by two observers (inter rater agreement: 100%). In contrast to other passengers, they did not make a clear and direct selection or seemed to be not sure whether to use the machines and how to do so. As displayed in Figure 2, the number of young people (i.e. estimated to be under the age of 30) in the group of "uncertain" users was very low (only four out of a total of 17), while about half of the middle-aged and elder customers were rated as "uncertain".

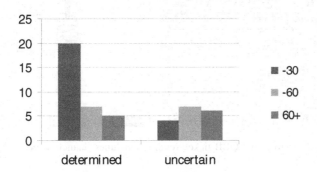

Fig. 2. Number of determined and uncertain customers in the three different age groups

Almost 70 % of the customers rated as uncertain had to cancel the purchase process and start again at least once, while nearly two thirds ultimately gave up and left the machine without purchasing a ticket (Figure 3). This means that the chance for successfully operating the machine can be predicted to a very high degree during the first few seconds after a person approached the machine!

We also observed some distinctive patterns of behaviour among members of this group. They repeatedly watched other customers using the machines and frequently received assistance from their companions or other customers, e.g. those using the adjacent machine. Also typically, this group spent a lot of time looking at the machines from a distance and approached it hesitantly; some members of this group cancelled the purchase process and went away from the machine, only to return a short time later and try again. We also observed that they spent a particularly long time studying both the launch screen (Figure 4, *left*) and the options screen (Figure 4, *right*).

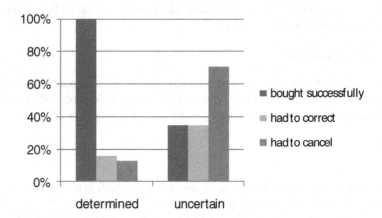

Fig. 3. Percentage of determined and uncertain customers who bought successfully, had to correct their input at least once and had to cancel

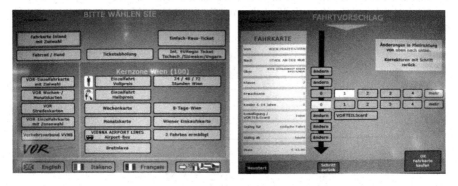

Fig. 4. Screen shots from the ÖBB ticket vending machines: launch screen (*left*) and options screen (*right*)

Our analysis of the sales data log files indicated that this is a fairly common pattern of behaviour. Of the 144 purchase processes started during this period, 61 were cancelled before completion: 54 % at the launch screen and 20 % at the options screen.

The observations suggest strong evidence for the role of uncertainty, but it remains unclear, whether actual thoughts corresponding to a low self-efficacy are responsible for this behaviour. Therefore, the results were complemented by interviews with users and non-users of ticket vending machines.

Similar to the observations most customers interviewed had little problems buying their tickets from the ticket machine. Of the 65 persons interviewed only 5 have never used the ticket machines and one person did not even know they existed at all. Nevertheless 78% of those persons who had at least once used a ticket machine reported problems or difficulties to understand some aspects of the purchasing process. The most common negative experiences were problems in operating machines, such as pressing the wrong keys or buying the wrong ticket, difficulties in understanding the complexity of the system, and having the impression that the machines are not always working properly. Problems with payment, such as credit cards being not accepted or wrong amounts of change were reported as well though less frequently (see Figure 5).

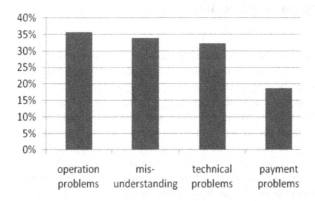

Fig. 5. Percentage of experienced problems reported by customers

Different age groups clearly had different problems with the machines. While older passengers with little technical experience reported problems in actually operating the machines, such problems were rare among younger interviewees: the group of passengers under the age of 19 reported no problems of this kind at all.

For more information on the role of technological literacy, interviewees were asked how frequently they used the ticket vending machine and also other everyday technologies (ATM, mobile phone, computer, internet). The results showed that seldom use of other everyday technologies is correlated to buying a ticket at the machine less often (Rho=.21, p<.05, N=64).

Qualitative analysis of the interviews showed that about two thirds of the customers who experienced operating problems or misunderstanding seemed to attribute this failure externally, which means they actually spoke of usability problems, referring to an inflexible system or an overloaded screen. The remaining third interpreted their failures as a result of their know-how and some of them even expressed to be helpless in the face of the machine (C17:"It just didn't work. Each time I tried I got something different."). Not surprisingly, all of these customers were prone to avoid the ticket machines, two persons stated to never use the machine again after one bad experience with it (C5:"I once tried to buy one, but I was completely confused and got a wrong ticket.").

Negative experiences were often combined with an expression of uncertainty: some people mentioned their fear of inadvertently buying the wrong ticket (M15: "One of my friends even once bought a ticket for a dog instead of a normal ticket!") or paying more out of ignorance (C28: "If you ask me, the counter's better, because someone there tells you what's what. If you buy a ticket from a machine, you might pay twice as much as you had to!"). This is complemented by a conviction that they would not be able to buy a ticket from a machine without help (C21: "Nobody showed me what to do, and I don't know what I am doing. If I knew how it worked, I would try it myself."). It should be mentioned, that even some of those people who used the ticket machines regularly said that they had only learned to use them with the help of other passengers (M19: "*I sometimes help people who don't use the trains so often. I also found the machines difficult to use at first.*")

5 Discussion and Conclusions

Our observations and interviews showed that "typical accessibility problems" like letter size, contrast or button size did not occur even with elder people. In contrast, most people were able to use the machine without any problems. But to ensure eInclusion it seems to be important to focus on the problems of those who did not succeed. For these people our studies revealed a number of serious barriers to the use of the ticket machines, above all among older and middle-aged passengers.

Especially in these age groups some customers had little confidence in their ability to successfully buy a ticket at the machine: Often they approached it only carefully and sometimes even had to cancel their purchase process. When asked why they avoid the machines, they referred to bad experiences, doubt in their own abilities, and distrust with respect to the technology. These are clear indicators of low self-efficacy in the context of using everyday technologies. A similar result was found in Great Britain [1], where elderly did use the ticket machine only seldom and did confide less in their own abilities.

When developing a new layout of a ticket vending machine, it will be important to ensure that people with low technological self-efficacy are given the feeling that they can buy a ticket easily and without the help of others. A relative easy and intuitive step is to avoid computer terminology and to use everyday language instead (e.g., yes instead of ok).

Additionally it is necessary that the purchase process in some way resembles their cognitive scripts of this process. While a salesman at the ticket counter can easily adjust the sales process to the customers' diverse cognitive scripts, the ticket machine is not as flexible. It only meets one possible cognitive script – the programmer's. This poses a barrier to people whose cognitive scripts are not addressed. To meet their needs as well, the ticket machine's interface could be split up into two modes: A fast purchase mode and a step-by-step-mode that leads customers through the purchase process and poses only one question after the other.

A considerable number of users were clearly already daunted by the multiple options offered on the launch screen which may have caused problems because of the rather unstructured, large amount of options it provides. The problem gets worse for users who are not familiar with the fare systems of Austrian Rail and the local transport services that sell their products on the same machines. The relevant fare and discount options have to be entered before some products can be selected. As initial steps, the choice of options could be better structured and a clearer visual demarcation between higher level menu elements could be introduced. Furthermore, special knowledge of the fare system should not be necessary to buy a ticket. Therefore it would also be worth considering which of these factors could be calculated automatically in the background without the need for user input.

Design examples gathered from systems currently in use in other countries provide some clues to a more user-friendly graphic design: the French ticket machines show that it is possible to reduce the number of options on the launch screen while maintaining a maximum of possible interactions (buying and exchanging tickets for national and international journeys, printing tickets bought online, see Figure 6).

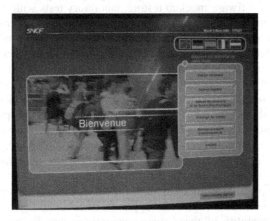

Fig. 6. Start screen of the French ticket machines by SNCF

A further barrier was encountered on the screen offering a so-called suggested route that can be partly modified by the user. An increased number of users cancelled the process on this screen, indicating that they either felt overwhelmed by the information they were asked to provide or did not succeed in changing the information in the way they wanted. The Austrian system displays the choices made by customers as a virtual ticket in the left part of the screen. To make changes, it is necessary to start at the top and to proceed in only one direction (see Figure 4, right). It could be observed that some people tried to make changes by touching the left, virtual ticket area. In the Netherlands, this problem does not exist as the buttons also serve as information about the choices already made and changes are possible in any order (see Figure 7). A demonstration of the system is available at http://www.ns.nl.

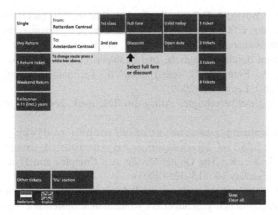

Fig. 7. Options screen of the Netherland's ticket machines by NS

In further development phases of the new generation of ticket machines, an iterative usability engineering approach is planned: To support the user-driven design methods, hard- and software mockup testing, laboratory tests with scenario machines and (partial) working systems will be conducted with multiple users to ensure a barrier free and easy to use prototype. This prototype will be evaluated in laboratory experiments and field observations including users with high and low self-efficacy.

The suggested improvements in the design and the usability of ticket vending machines will not only help people with low technological literacy, but also ease the purchase process for all customers. In addition to the improvement of the design, further measures should be taken to facilitate the access for people with low self-efficacy, as the results by Karavidas et al. [13] suggest: at-home-trainings, local support, information leaflets and advertisements can reach also those, who might even avoid the railway station. An easy-to-use system will not only facilitate access to public transport systems for people with low technological affinity, but could be a chance to develop positive attitudes towards digital technology in general.

Many projects and ideas follow the approach of accessibility in order to support and promote the mobility of these socio-economic groups by providing accessible computer-based technologies and information services. Certainly the physical barriers to access will be eliminated, but barriers like limited acceptance and limited affinity for technology still remain. In addition, failing to use everyday technology can decrease their feeling of mastery for technology in general. However, if everyday technologies enable mastery and the user gains a feeling of success, self-efficacy can be increased in the long run and might also reduce the perceived barriers with other kinds of media. Thereby, easy-to-use everyday technologies can contribute to the inclusion of technically non-skilled people in the eSociety. The project Innomat provides an example how a neglected factor, the users' self-efficacy, can be taken into account and can improve the design beyond existing approaches.

References

1. Passenger Focus: Buying a Ticket at the Station; Research on Ticket Machine Use; Technical report, London (2008), http://www.passengerfocus.org.uk [26.01.09]
2. Schreder, G., Siebenhandl, K., Mayr, E., Smuc, M.: Hindernis Fahrkartenautomat? Höhere Mobilitätschancen durch zugängliche und benutzerfreundliche Fahrkartenautomaten. In: von Hellberg, P., Kempter, G. (eds.) uDayVII. Technologienutzung ohne Barrieren, pp. 105–114. Pabst, Lengerich (2009)
3. ÉGALITÉ, Ein gleichberechtigter Alltag im Telematik gestützten Verkehrsgeschehen. Wien (2006),
   https://forschung.boku.ac.at/fis/suchen.projekt_
   uebersicht?sprache_in=de&menue_id_in=300&id_in=5863 [26.01.09]
4. Van Dijk, J., Hacker, K.: The Digital Divide as a Complex and Dynamic Phenomenon. The Information Society 19, 315–326 (2003)
5. Funiok, R.: Ich fange erst gar nicht an, mich damit zu beschäftigen - Schwierigkeiten und Wünsche älterer Menschen gegenüber der Kommunikationstechnik – eine generationsspezifische Fallstudie. Literatur- und Forschungsreport Weiterbildung 42, 63–72 (1998)
6. Weymann, A., Sackmann, R.: Technikgenerationen. Literatur- und Forschungsreport Weiterbildung 42, 23–35 (1998)

7. Hargittai, E.: Second-Level Digital Divide: Differences in People's Online Skills. First Monday 7(4), 1–20 (2002)
8. Czaja, S.J., Charness, N., Fisk, A.D., Hertzog, C., Nair, S.N., Rogers, W.A., Sharit, J.: Factors Predicting the Use of Technology: Findings From the Center for Research and Education on Aging and Technology Enhancement (CREATE). Psychol. Aging 21, 333–352 (2006)
9. Doh, M.: Ältere Onliner in Deutschland - Entwicklung und Prädiktoren der Internetdiffusion. IT-basierte Produkte und Dienste für ältere Menschen – Nutzeranforderungen und Techniktrends, 43–64 (2005)
10. ARD/ZDF-Arbeitsgruppe Multimedia. ARD/ZDF Online Studie 1999. Media Perspektiven 8, 388–409 (1999)
11. Eastin, M.S., LaRose, R.: Internet Self-Efficacy and the Psychology of the Digital Divide. JCMC 6 (2000)
12. Bandura, A.: Self-Efficacy: The Exercise of Control. Freeman, New York (1997)
13. Karavidas, M., Lim, N.K., Katsikas, S.L.: The effects of computers on older adult users. Computers in Human Behavior 21, 697–711 (2005)

Smart Home Technologies: Insights into Generation-Specific Acceptance Motives

Sylvia Gaul and Martina Ziefle

Human Technology Centre (HumTec),
RWTH Aachen University,
Theaterplatz 14,
52056 Aachen, Germany
{Gaul,Ziefle}@humtec.rwth-aachen.de

Abstract. In this research we examine the generation specific acceptance motives of eHealth technologies in order to assess the likelihood of success for these new technologies. 280 participants (14 - 92 years of age) volunteered to participate in a survey, in which using motives and barriers toward smart home technologies were explored. The scenario envisaged was the use of a medical stent implemented into the body, which monitors automatically the health status and which is able to remotely communicate with the doctor. Participants were asked to evaluate the pros and cons of the usage of this technology, their acceptance motives and potential utilization barriers. In order to understand the complex nature of acceptance, personal variables (age, technical expertise, health status), individual's cognitive concepts toward ageing as well as perceived usefulness were related. Outcomes show that trust, believe in the reliability of technology, privacy and security as well as intimacy facets are essential for acceptance and should be considered in order to proactively design a successful rollout of smart home technologies.

Keywords: Aging, technology acceptance, smart home technology, perceived usefulness, TAM, medical technology.

1 Introduction

The profound demographic change in many countries of the world imposes considerable challenges on modern societies. Due to increased life expectancy, improved medial health care, and reduced fertility rates, increasingly old and frail people will need medical care in the near future, e.g. [1] [2] [3]. At the same time, considerable bottlenecks arise from the fact that increasingly fewer people are present which may take over the nursing and decreasing supply shortfalls of societal health insurance funds [2].

In order to master the requirements of an aging society, technological innovations in information and communication technologies as well as medical engineering technologies come into fore, which offer novel or improved medical diagnosis, therapy, treatments and rehabilitation possibilities. Technologies in this context are subsumed

A. Holzinger and K. Miesenberger (Eds.): USAB 2009, LNCS 5889, pp. 312–332, 2009.

under different terms, as e.g. electronic health systems (ehealth), smart health, ambient assisted living (AAL), or personal health care systems, e.g. [4] [5] [6]. Technological innovations in this sector are fast developing. Yet, the spectrum of technical applications in the eHealth sector available covers a broad variety of developments, reaching from internal technologies (implants for monitoring bio signals, so called medical stents or chips) over devices integrated into clothes (tissue engineering) up to healthcare robots, which continuously monitor the health status by wireless technologies and support older people to keep up safe and independent living at home (e.g., [7] [8] [9] [2]).

However, recent experience shows that it is not predominately the technical barrier, which hampers a successful rollout and a broad responsiveness of users. Rather, far-reaching acceptance barriers are prevalent which represent serious obstacles to technical solutions, which are so badly needed [10] [11]. One major reason for this reluctant acceptance and a still negative evaluation might be due to the fact that current developments in this sector are predominately focusing on technical feasibility, inspired by technical disciplines, in combination with medical and computer science knowledge, while the "human factor" in these systems is fairly under developed. Of course, the technical aspect and the concentration on feasibility, signal power and compatibility with other systems is a sine qua non for smart technologies [7], which must be the primary goal of technical design in the first round. However, at least at the current maturity of technical solutions, the human perspective should be incorporated into technical designs as soon as possible. This is especially important for the older user group, which is not basically disinclined to the usage of technology in general [12], but has specific demands, needs and requirements and put strong emphasis on usability and acceptance issues [13] [14] [15] [16]. Thus, we need to understand seniors' needs and wants, and their specific using motives as well as acceptance barriers. This problem space was addressed in the present study. We examined users of a broad age range and collected their acceptance ratings and barriers towards smart health technologies.

1.1 Technology Acceptance

Looking back, it is evident that peoples' acceptance of technology is predominating the public discourse and the scientific discussion in times of technological cycles in which new technologies are penetrating into personal and working environments. In the 1980ies and 1990ies, alongside with the ubiquitous introduction of personal computers, there was a boom of research dealing with technology acceptance [17] [18] [19]. As technology cycles are increasingly faster, technology acceptance continued to be a key research issue. Technology acceptance deals with the approval, favourable reception and ongoing use of newly introduced devices and systems and explores the relation of end-users using motives, cognitive and affective attitudes toward the respective technology and the technological impact assessment. The huge majority of technology acceptance studies dealt with the impact of information technologies in the working context and addressed the young and healthy adult as a major user group of information and communication technologies (e.g.). It was found that the perceived ease of using a system and the perceived usefulness are the key components of technology acceptance (e.g. [20] [17] [18]). However, with the increasing diversity of users, the diversity of technical systems (visible vs. invisible, local vs. distributed) and using contexts (fun and entertainment, medical, office, mobility) end-users are confronted with, more aspects are relevant for understanding users acceptance – beyond the ease of using a system and the perceived usefulness. Especially, user characteristics (economic status, culture, gender, age, experience, and the voluntariness of system usage) had been added to the original model and considered in the comprehensive UTAUT-model [21].

To date, a few studies were concerned with acceptance of medical and ehealth technologies from the human perspective [22] [23] [3] [24] [25] [26]. Outcomes show that it is highly questionable that acceptance for medical technologies can be fully understood on the base of the prevailing knowledge of technology acceptance drivers so far. Rather, technology acceptance for the medical technology sector seems to be still more complex than it is for other technical systems, out of different reasons. A first argument in this context is that eHealth technologies are predominately addressing the seniors, which are increasingly prone to diseases with increasing age. Ageing, dependency and illness are – still - negatively connotated in our societies and, thus, carry a stigmatizing potential, which could impact the acceptance of medical technology. A second argument refers to the fact that many technologies incorporated in smart homes (walls, furniture or clothes) do overstep personal intimacy limits and therefore could be bothered by justifiable worries about privacy, intimacy and loss of control. Third, it should be considered that the status of health and resulting feelings of independency or dependency on technology also could impact the willingness to accept ehealth applications. Finally, and this is of specific interest, the acceptance of medical technology might also be influenced by age, and the generational perspective. As aging is a key factor in this context, the next section will detail the aging impact on acceptance of medical technologies.

1.2   The Aging Impact for the Use of Technology

In the last decades, an increasing number of studies had been concerned with the interacting of older users with different technologies, as e.g. Internet and web applications (e.g. [27]), computers (e.g. [28] [29]) and mobile small screen devices (e.g. [20] [30] [31] [32] [33] [34]). Outcomes show that older adult face enormous difficulties when interacting with modern technology. Though, it had been also demonstrated that a human-centred design of devices' interfaces might considerably reduce, if not compensate, the aging handicap and enable older adults to efficiently handle modern technical devices (e.g. [31] [32]).

With respect to older adults' acceptance, considerably less and less unequivocal knowledge is prevalent. On the one hand, older users' hesitant approach towards new technical devices in general is well known (e.g., [20] [30] [11] [14]), and older adults' hesitant acceptance towards ehealth technology in particular (e.g., [23] [34] [11]). A possible source of older adults' lower acceptance is their lower computer knowledge [35], and a completely different understanding of how technology works. Older adults were often educated in times where technical devices were far less complex and, therefore, are often not experienced with the handling of current technology models. In addition, the olds' lower levels of self-confidence when using technology might be a serious obstacle for accepting a technology [20] [36] [33] [16]. On the other hand, there are studies which reveal that older adults show high interest in modern technologies (e.g. [12] [33]), but they are much more critical regarding the social compatibility of technology, the usefulness and the fair balance between costs and benefits of the respective technology [14] [15]. Also, older adults have a much more exclusive claim for usable technical designs compared to younger technology users [20] [30] [11] [37].

Especially for the evaluation of acceptance of ehealth technologies, age and technology generation is assumed to play a prominent part. For young and technology-experienced adults (about 20-30 years of age), which are not personally touched by the application of medical technologies in the near future, medical technology could represent attractive and appropriate technological solutions for societal problems. The middle-aged adults (about 45-60 years of age) could adopt another attitude. As they have the duty to care for their older parents, ehealth technologies could guarantee the well-being of their parents. Also, modern medical technologies could help save them costs (e.g. for nursing homes) and could spare them family caring duties. Finally, from the perspective of the over 70+ years olds, still different and controversial aspects could impact the degree of acceptance of medical technologies. One the one hand, medical technologies could allow them to feel safe in the privacy of one's home and to stay independently from the help of others. On the other hand, feelings of being permanently controlled in combination with low trust in technology could provoke ambivalent feelings towards medical technologies.

1.3 Questions Addressed and Working Model

The main goal of this research was to analyze the contribution of age and technical generation to the motivation patterns for the intention to use an implanted stent if necessary. In order to differentiate the different technology generations, we rely on a model of technology generation [38], in which three technology generations and age groups, respectively, are distinguished: the *early-technical generation* (65+), the *household revolution generation* (49+), and the *computer generation* (26+). As the mentioned research stems from 1989, there was a need to categorize still younger participants accordingly. To this end, the *GameBoy generation* was established, comprising an age range from 14-25 years of age.

The goal was to determine technology acceptance for medical technology in each generation and to identify the impact of potential generation specific barriers (con's) and using motives (pro's) on the intention to use the respective technology. In order to consider the generation related user factors, we examined the health status of participants and their experience with technical devices.

According to the model, the following hypotheses were specified:

H1:   Generations differ in their ageing concepts.
H2:   Generations differ in their intention to use the medical device.
H3:   Age concepts are affecting the pros and cons for usage of medical technology.
H4:   The barriers and using motives directly influence the using intention.
H5:   Technical experience is related to barriers and using motives within generations.
H6:   Generations differ within reported using motives and barriers in relation to the reported intention to use medical technology.
H7:   No specific hypotheses for gender effects were on hand (dashed line in Figure 1), and were therefore not considered in this paper.

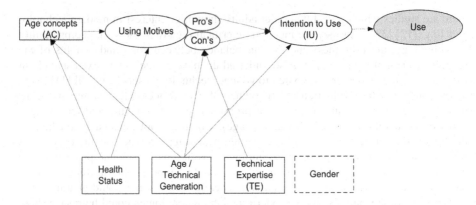

Fig. 1. Research Model comprising variables selection in our study. Independent variables are given in quadratic, dependent variable in round boxes.

2   Method

We assume that acceptance of (smart) medical technology is a rather complex phenomenon. In order to learn which components might be decisive for the forming of technology acceptance toward medical technology, we used an investigative and explorative approach. In order to examine a large number of participants and to consider the diversity within the older age group, the questionnaire-method in combination with a scenario technique was chosen as empirical approach.

Participants were introduced into a medical scenario: "Imagine that in the year 2025 a vast majority of people in our societies are 65 years and older. Many of these people will be frail and therefore reliant on medical care. Due to shortcomings in the caring sector (economic bottlenecks and a decreasing number of nursing staff) it is a basic question how older people can live independently at home, and have access to medical services. Yet, there are already mature technical developments, which enable continuous medical care at home. One example for these developments is a so-called medical stent, an electronic miniature chip, which can be implemented in a blood vessel inside the body. This device is able to monitor bio signals continuously and unobtrusively (e.g. blood pressure, blood quality). The device communicates bio signals automatically to the doctor/medical staff and contacts the emergency ambulance if necessary." Participants were instructed to envisage the use of such a device and to evaluate, if it may be helpful for them, to state if they would accept technologies like these and to report the most important pros and cons regarding the usefulness of these technologies. In order to ensure peoples' understanding of the scenario and its consequences the described scenario was tested in a sub sampling before the main data collection began.

2.1   Variables

Independent variables: Independent variable is the age of participants. As age can only be taken as an indicator of other critical variables, which might be carried by age and which influence the attitude towards medical technology and the acceptance of it, we classified participants according to their technology generation [38] and, in addition, assessed mediating factors as the technical expertise and individual health status.

Dependent Variables: Dependent variables were the perceived usefulness of the medical technology and the intention to use the medical device if necessary. Participants were instructed to envisage the use of this device and to evaluate the pro's and con's regarding its usefulness and their willingness to use it. Items were formulated from the perspective of participants (first person), in order to enhance understandability by the very olds. Items were to be confirmed or denied on a four-point Likert-Scale from 1 (totally disagree) to 4 (totally agree). Usefulness and intention to use were formulated as pros and cons.

The potential using motives (pro's) focused on potential

-*pragmatic* reasons ("the usage of the device reduces the duty to constantly visit the doctor")

-*control* reasons ("I prefer using the device in order to have continuous feedback about my health status").

The potential barriers (con's) focused on

-*dependency* reasons ("I do not trust the reliability of the device")

-*privacy* reasons ("I fear that others could come to know about my health status").

In order to collect potential individual annotations, the questionnaire offered at some places the possibility, to note personal remarks if necessary.

2.2 The Questionnaire

Overall, the questionnaire was arranged in different sections. First socio-demographic variables were assessed, followed by the items to individual aging concepts. Then the scenario was introduced to which the questions regarding the intention to use, using motives and utilization barriers were related to. In the following, dimensions and items are described in detail.

Aging Concepts (AC)

For the assessment of aging concepts, the following questions had to be answered:

Table 1. Items for Ageing Concepts (1 = totally disagree to 4 = totally agree)

When I am aged
I want to live independently from others
I do not want to burden s.o. with the care for me
I would accept to rely on technical support
I plan to move into a nursing home
I would accept to rely on mobile nursing services
I plan to move into my children's homes

Intention to Use (IU)

Participants were given the following answers regarding their intention to use the technology, if necessary.

Table 2. Items for the Intention to Use (1 = totally disagree to 4 = totally agree)

Using the medical device... (implanted chip)
... would increase my life contentment and satisfaction
... allows a sensible medical care
Can you imagine to use the device to...
... live longer independently at home?
... facilitate your living conditions?

Pro's and Con's

Using motives and barriers were assessed through the following questions:

Table 3. Items for the pros (using motives) (1 = totally disagree to 4 = totally agree). "Under which conditions would you use the medical stent?".

I would use the implemented medical device
... in order to save caring costs
... in order to escape from the indignity of being cared
... in order to keep independency
... because it reliefs me from worries about life-menacing situations
... because this medical device is unobtrusive without attracting public attention
... because it reliefs me from the duty to constantly visit the doctor

No, I would be reluctant to use the implemented medical device
...because I fear that the device is not reliable
...because others would come to know about my health status
...because I do not want to feel stigmatized as old and sick
...because the implemented device could shift and get out of place inside my body
...because I dislike the idea of a contaminant and foreign particle inside my body

Technical Expertise (TE)

Technical experience might also be connected to acceptance outcomes. However, technical experience is a broad construct and is not limited to the experience with information and communication technologies, especially not in the older generation. Therefore, we assessed technical experience in a broad context (Table 4).

Table 4. Items for Technical Expertise (1 = totally disagree to 4 = totally agree)

Which of the following actions apply to you
I can assemble a prefabricated object (e.g. furniture) from pieces by myself
I can hang up a picture on the wall by myself
If something breaks I usually seek to repair it by myself
I easily handle a mobile phone and use it regularly
I easily handle a computer and use it regularly

2.3 Reliability and Validity of Scales

In order to assure a high measuring quality, reliability and validity of items were analyzed prior to testing. The reliability of the (latent construct) scales *Intention to Use* (IU) and *Technical Experience* (TE) was assessed by scale reliability analysis. Table 5 shows the outcomes.

Table 5. Factor analysis of the scales IU and TE. Bold values indicate items' loadings on correct latent construct.

	Factor loadings	
	IU	TE
Intention to Use: Using the medical device…		
…would increase my life contentment and satisfaction	**.925**	.133
…allows a sensible medical care	**.853**	.183
Can you imagine to use the device to…		
…live independently at home?	**.900**	-.033
…facilitate your living conditions?	**.912**	.117
Technical expertise		
I can assemble a prefabricated object (e.g. furniture) from pieces by myself	.111	**.820**
I can hang up a picture on the wall by myself	.108	**.756**
If something breaks I usually seek to repair it by myself	.100	**.726**
I easily handle a mobile phone and use it regularly	-.044	**.722**
I easily handle a computer and use it regularly	.146	**.720**

Cronbach's Alpha values for IU reached .93, .80 for TE, suggesting high reliability. Convergent and discriminant validity were examined using principal factor analysis with varimax rotation. The rotated factor matrix in Table 6 suggested convergent validity within scales (loadings greater than .70) and discriminant validity across scales (cross-loadings less than .20).

2.4 Participants

A total of 280 respondents participated, with an age range between 14 and 92 years of age (M = 46.7). Participants were recruited through the social network of authors and came from a broad range of professions. All participants volunteered to take part and showed a very high and personal interest in the topic, what can be taken from - for questionnaire studies - high response rates of about 80%. Participants were not gratified for their efforts. The sample was allocated to four technology generation groups, according to the theory of technology generations by Sackmann and Weymann, 1998.

-*Early-technical generation* - Group: 71 participants (42% men, 58% women), between 65 and 92 years of age (M=75.4, SD=6.2).

-*Household revolution generation* - Group: 72 participants (47% men, 53% women), with an age between 49 and 64 years of age of M=54.1 years (SD=3.8).

-*Computer generation* - Group: 75 participants (45% men, 55% women), with an age between 26 and 48 years of age of M=33.8 years (SD=8.1).

-*GameBoy generation* - Group: 64 participants (53% men; 47% women), with an age between 14 and 25 years of age of M= 21.4 years (SD=3).

Participants' health status and the experience with the usage of medical technology were assessed (Table 6).

Table 6. Health status and experience with medicine-technical aids. Given is the absolute number of participants, which suffer from a chronic disease and which use medical devices (the total number of participants in the respective generation is given in brackets).

Group	"I suffer from a chronic disease"		"I use a medical technical device (e.g. blood pressure device, hearing aid, heart pacemaker)."	
	N (N all)	%	N (N all)	%
1 Early-technical generation	34 (71)	47.9	39 (71)	54.9
2 Household revolution	23 (72)	31.9	9 (72)	12.5
3 Computer generation	11 (75)	14.7	3 (75)	4.0
4 GameBoy generation	4 (64)	6.3	2 (64)	3.1

As shown in table 6, the number of persons suffering from a chronic disease rises with increasing age ($r = .3.8$; $p < 0.05$) and also the need of using medical technology ($r = .48$; $p < 0.05$). Though, in all generation groups there were participants, which indicated to suffer from a chronic disease and which reported to use medical technical devices, respectively.

3 Results

Results were analysed by ANOVA - procedures (differences between generation groups) and bivariate correlation analyses (Pearson, Spearman as well as nominal correlation procedures) to assess the interrelation between factors and variables. ANOVA - procedures were carried out which are sufficiently robust regarding varying numbers of participants in different groups.

The result section is structured as follows. First, the findings regarding aging concepts, the intention to use the medical technology and the using motives and utilization barriers in the different technology generations are reported. If necessary, the quantitative findings are underpinned with qualitative findings (personal remarks and free answers of participants). The section closes with the research model in which the relations between factors and variables are complemented.

3.1 Aging Concepts in the Different Technology Generations

H1 states differences in the generations' aging concepts. In order test this hypothesis multivariate tests with technical generations as between factor was conducted. The analysis revealed a significant main effect for generations ($F(18,738)= 2.68$; $p<0.01$). Descriptive outcomes are illustrated in Figure 2.

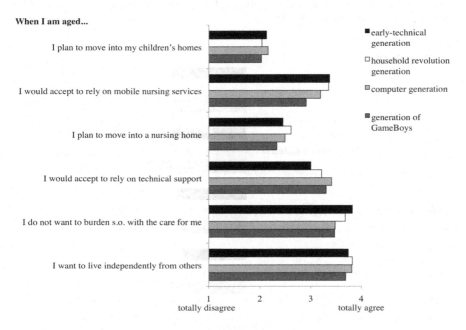

Fig. 2. Aging concepts of the different technology generations

For the early-technical generation it is most important that they do not want to burden s.o. with the care for them ($M = 3.8$ out of four maximal points; $SD = .49$). In contrast, acceptance for technical support is less pronounced (but not refused) in this generation ($M = 3$; $SD = .91$) compared to the computer generation ($M = 3.41$; $SD = .74$). The possibility of relying on mobile nursing services is more confirmed by the early technical and the household revolution generation compared to both younger generations. Beyond the differences between generations, it is though insightful to look at the non-differences. All generations prefer to live independently from others when they are aged. Also, none of the generations really envisaged the possibility to move into their children's homes.

3.2 Intention to Use

First, the four items of the intention to use were analyzed and for further analysis a total mean was calculated for each generation. It was hypothesized (H2) that generations differ in their intention to use the medical stent if necessary, as they might have a very different technical model, knowledge and a different attitude towards technology.

Multivariate analysis reveals that intention to use the medical device differs across generations (F(12,688) =2.03; p<0.05). However, it is important to note that all generations have a basic positive disposition to the use a medical stent (Table 7). Altogether, the most decisive reason in all generations *for* using the medical stent is that the device allows a sensible care (M_{total}=2.88; s=0.92). In contrast, the lowest agreement for using the stent is its ability to increase life contentment and satisfaction (M_{total}=2.52; s=0.95). While this was given again in all generations, it was most pronounced for the very olds (early-technical generation) (Fig. 3).

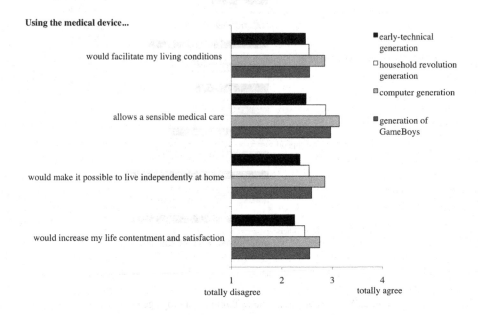

Fig. 3. Intention to use the medical stent in all generations

When focusing on the overall acceptance, the computer generation (average 33 years) turns out to be the group that shows the highest degree of acceptance towards using the medical stent (M = 2.9; SD = 0.78), whereas the early-technical generation (average 75 years) shows the lowest, but still positive, attitude (M = 2.38; SD = .91).

Table 7. Total mean IU for each generation

	Intention to use the medical stent	
	M	SD
early-technical generation (N=69)	2.38	.91
household revolution generation (N=72)	2.59	.82
computer generation (N=74)	2.90	.78
generation of GameBoys (N=64)	2.66	.76

3.3 Barriers and Using Motives

In this section, we report the using motives (Table 8) and barriers (Table 9). Comparing the pro's and con's for using the medical stent in each generation, MANOVA analyses revealed that generations differ in their weighting of reasons for and against usage.

First, the using motives are discussed. It is an interesting finding that - independently of the generation - the unobtrusiveness of the device for avoiding public attention is the less important feature of the device. Within the reasons, which are perceived as

Table 8. Using Motives. Bold values indicate the less important motive in each generation (Standard deviations are given in brackets. Items are abbreviated - for full item text see 2.2).

I would use the medi-cal device...	early-technical (N=67)	household revolution (N=72)	computer (N=73)	GameBoys (N=64)
	M	M	M	M
save caring costs	2.52 (.99)	2.75 (.95)	2.91 (.95)	2.75 (.94)
escape from indignity	2.63 (.99)	2.81 (.87)	3.06 (.81)	2.84 (.86)
keep independency	2.57 (.93)	2.8 (.90)	3.03 (.87)	2.91 (.75)
no worries about life-menacing situations	2.60 (1.1)	2.78 (.95)	2.75 (.95)	2.61 (.92)
unobtrusiveness	**2.30** (1.1)	**2.40** (1.0)	**2.6** (1.0)	**2.45** (.99)
less frequent doctor visits	2.64 (1.1)	2.65 (1.0)	2.97 (.88)	2.55 (.89)

Table 9. Barriers towards using the medical stent - bold values indicate the most important barrier in each generation (Standard deviations are given in brackets. Items are abbreviated -for full item text see 2.2).

I would not use the medical device because I fear...	early-technical (N=67)	household revolution (N=72)	computer (N=73)	GameBoys (N=64)
	M	M	M	M
device is not reliable	**2.58** (.67)	**2.44** (.71)	**2.59** (.80)	**2.6** (.77)
others come to know about my health status	2.37 (.84)	2.29 (.87)	2.11 (.75)	2.18 (.90)
stigmatized	2.17 (.91)	1.96 (.97)	1.95 (.83)	2.05 (.99)
chip could shift	1.98 (.85)	2.08 (.89)	2.14 (.93)	2.34 (.84)
foreign particle inside my body	2.10 (.99)	2.15 (1.0)	2.15 (.99)	2.33 (1.1)

most important, the generations show different ratings. For the early - technical generation, the lower frequency of seeing the doctor, and the escape from the alleged indignity of being cared by others are the most critical factors, which militate in favor of the
usage of the medial stent. In all other generations - the household, the computer and the
GameBoy generation - there are two prominent reasons for using the stent: the escape
from indignity of care and the benefit of keeping independency in older age (Table 8).

Second, the reported barriers are detailed (Table 9). On a first sight, it is noticeable
that the barriers were perceived as less significant (lower values indicate a less crucial
barrier). Independently of the generation, the most important worry is that the device
is not reliable, showing a small trust in technology. The less relevant barrier for not
using the device is the fear of being stigmatized as old and frail.

3.4 Qualitative Insights into Using Motives and Barriers

Any quantification of using motives and barriers in this sensitive field is only a superficial analysis, as long as it is not understood which underlying cognitions or affects
determine the extent of acceptance or rejection of the respective using contexts and
device characteristics. Therefore, participants had been given the possibility to comment on possible reasons in the questionnaire. Overall, participants frequently used
this possibility and showed an enormous commitment to participate in the discussions
about this topic. In the following, some of the comments of participants are detailed
as supplement to the quantified pro's and con's. It allows a fruitful qualitative insight
into possible objections and proposals people have. Here are some examples of what
they wrote.

Arguments, which were given by participants in the category "pro's", reveal first
and foremost the increased mobility and the timely feedback of health status by the
devices as important reasons. This is illustrated by the following original comments.

Mobility:
- "More mobility when I am aged - e.g. when I go on holiday or do not want to stay
  always at home" (female, 21years)
- "to be independent from my flat" (male, 52 years)

Timely feedback of health status:
- "to facilitate diagnostics" (female, 22 years)
- "to simplify conversation with the doctor" (female, 50years)
- "For Sports: to attain more security if my individual limit is reached" (female, 48
  years)

However, some participants reported that they would use this device only under certain circumstances, and that using a chip would be their last alternative when they
have no other opportunities. Interestingly, this conditional acceptance is not age-
specific, but has been reported by participants of all ages.

- "Only, if no family members are nearby" (female, 23 years)
- "Only, if I suffer from a really heavy illness" (male, 64 years)

On the other hand, there are also some significant fears connected to using the implemented device. It is noteworthy that the number of negative comments connected to
fear, reservation towards the usage and the general disliking outnumbered the positive

comments. The primary fear or sorrow referred to feeling of constantly being controlled and even manipulated by technology or others. Also, the fear of physical intolerance reactions inside the body was strongly expressed. This is illustrated in the following quotations.

Control:
   -"Pursuing of my movements by the State" (male, 20 years)
   -"Exactly reconstruction of my activities and emotions with the help of
        physiological values by strangers, doctors or nursing staff" (female, 23 years)
   -"Manipulation!!" (male, 57 years)
Physical Intolerance:
   -"chip could block smaller blood vessels" (male, 21 years)
   -"inflammation as consequences" (male, 75 years)
   -"intolerance" (female, 26 years)
   -"allergic reactions" (female, 33 years)

   But also fear of losing the control in form of having no ability to finally control the device was mentioned several times.

   - "The fact that the device could be controlled from outside and I cannot stop it
        myself" (female, 32 years)

Other fears refer to more fundamental critics touching ethical or normative values. It is astounding that the intrinsic function of medical technology - to save life and to enable older adults to life in dignity at home for a longer time - is also critically evaluated by some participants. This can be demonstrated by the comment of a 58 years old man who refused to use this technology because he fears that the stent would prolonging his lifetime improperly.

   - "if I would use this device, I would not feel human anymore" (female, 52 years)
   - "support life for too long" (male, 58 years)

3.5   Generation Specific Acceptance Patterns

We also hypothesized that the participants' intention to use the medical device depends on the pattern of barriers and using motives, which on their part differ in generations (H6). So far it became clear that generations differ in the weighting of their pro's and con's. Now we examine if these patterns might correlate with the reported intention to use and if we can predict the intention to use by the respective using motives and barriers (stepwise regression analysis).

   In regression analyses, we used the intention to use as dependent variable and those pro's and cons as predictor variables, which turned out to reveal significant generation differences (see 3.3.). The outcomes are reported for each generation, consecutively.

Acceptance Patterns of the Early-technical Generation
In this generation, there were two key factors, which predicted the intention to use for the oldest participant group (average: 75 years of age). Together, the argument that the stent would *save caring costs* and would allow *escaping from the indignity of being cared* explained solid 70% of variance ($F(1,62)=71.93$; $p<0.01$, table 10).

Table 10. Regression analysis for the early-technical generation

Dependent variable: IU				
Predictor	Adj. R^2	β	p	t-Value
Saving caring costs	0.70	0.55	0.00	3.84
Escape from indignity of care		0.31	0.03	2.19

Acceptance Patterns of the Household Revolution Generation
Table 11 shows the regression analysis of the acceptance pattern of the 55-year-old group (household generation). Again, a very clear predictive picture was found, with one main key player *using the stent allows living independently*, which explained 64% of variance after all ($F(1,62)=71.93$; $p<0.01$).

Table 11. Regression analysis for the household revolution generation

Dependent variable: IU				
Predictor	Adj. R^2	β	p	t-Value
Living independently	0.64	0.80	0.00	11.3

Acceptance Patterns of the Computer Generation
In contrast to the early technical and the household generation, the acceptance pattern of the computer generation mean age 33 years does not count on one or two main factors, but relies on four factors to reach a prediction of 66% ($F(4,72)=35.91$; $p<0.01$), possibly hinting at a more diverse acceptance profile (table 12). Among these predictors, the possibility to *save caring costs*, benefit by *escaping from life-menacing situations through technology* and the prevention of the *indignity of being cared* were among the predictors. It is astonishing that the generation, which grew up with digital technology, and the ubiquity of chips, is the one who is reluctant to tolerating a medical chip inside the body and perceives this *as a foreign particle*.

Table 12. Regression analysis for the computer generation

Dependent variable: IU				
Predictor	Adj. R^2	β	p	t-Value
Saving caring costs		0.31	0.00	3.00
Life-menacing situations	0.66	0.22	0.01	2.56
Indignity		0.30	0.00	2.98
Foreign particle		-0.22	0.00	-2.69

Acceptance Patterns of the Generation of GameBoys
Finally, in the gameboy generation (21 years of age), the possibility of *saving costs* by using the chip as well as *to live independently* were prominent predictors of the acceptance pattern in this generation (table 13). Among all generations, unexpectedly, it was the youngest generation, which disliked the possibility that *others could come to know about their health status*. The three items explained 59% of variance ($F(3,63)=31.45$; $p<0.01$).

Table 13. Regression analysis for the generation of GameBoys

Dependent variable: IU				
Predictor	**Adj. R^2**	**β**	**p**	**t-Value**
Saving caring costs		0.37	0.00	3.36
Others come to know about my health status	0.59	-0.35	0.00	-4.12
Living independently		0.30	0.01	2.68

3.6 The Acceptance Model as a First Conclusion of This Work

We started this work by proposing a model, in which single user factors (health status, age and technology generation, technical experience) can be distinguished in their impact on the intention to use the medical stent and acceptance patterns for incorporated medical technology. On the basis of the outcomes these relations between factors can now be furnished. Figure 4 visualizes the overall interrelations for the whole sample, which were outlined in the model. To begin with the impact of age, we now can say that age and technical generation distinctly impacts acceptance, but also the selection of using motives (pro's and con's) as well as the underlying ageing concepts of participants. The most prominent factor within aging concepts is the willingness of participants to rely on technical support when they are aged (H3).

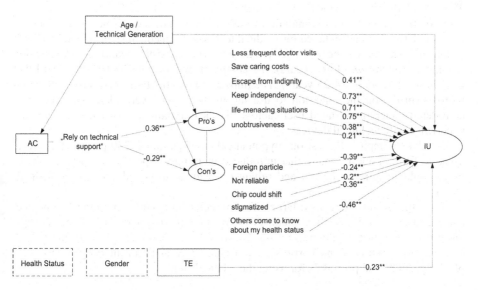

Fig. 4. Research model of acceptance for incorporated medical technology based on the quantitative outcomes

Even independently from generations a strong influence of pro's and con's on the intention to use was confirmed (H4). The pro's turned out to be more strongly related to the intention to use compared to the con's, which showed lower correlation. This finding reflects generation specific acceptance patterns and indicates a greater emphasis on the relevance of the usefulness of technology than of possible barriers, which impede the willingness to use the medical stent. Within the pro's the reasons for *saving caring costs* (.73, Fig. 4), *keeping independency* (.75, Fig. 4) and *escaping from indignity of being cared by others* (.71, Fig. 4) revealed to be the most powerful ones for using the medical stent.

The weakest relations were found for the using condition of unobtrusiveness (.21, Fig. 4) and *the fear that the chip could shift* (-.02, Fig. 4). Unexpectedly, the technical experience of participants was a rather unimportant factor. It relates to the intention to use only by .23 (Fig. 4) and is comparably low correlated to using motives. Thus, we have to assume that the acceptance pattern is not that much influenced by technical experience (H5). It is definitely noteworthy that in none of the analyses the health status did impact participants' acceptance. We had assumed that participants, which have to handle a chronic illness, would be more involved in medical technology, and, as a consequence, show a different intention to use pattern than healthy subjects. This was not the case. Possibly we will have to focus on this outcome in future studies (section 5).

4 Discussion

The aim of the present study was to analyze the contribution of generation specific using motive patterns for the intention to use an implanted stent if necessary. Therefore, we determined acceptance for medical technology (medical stent) in each of four technical generations: the *early-technical generation* (65-92 years), the *household revolution generation* (49-64 years), the *computer generation* (26-48 years), and the *GameBoy generation* (14-25 years). The impact of potential barriers (con's) and using motives (pro's) on the intention to use the medical stent were identified. We also considered generation-related user factors like health status of participants, and the experience with technical devices.

In order to empirically test our hypothetical considerations, 280 participants were asked to fill in a questionnaire that introduced them into a specific scenario in which they should imagine to be old and reliant on medical technical support (a medical stent).

Altogether results confirmed large effect of technical generation on the acceptance and intention to use a medical stent. Also, we identified generation specific acceptance patterns towards intention to use. On top of that, comments of participants on possible using motives and barriers gave a qualitative and fruitful insight into peoples' objections and proposals for using the medical stent.

4.1 Technology Generations and Their Intention to Use the Medical Stent

Overall, all respondents showed a high willingness to use a medical stent, however some of them stressed explicitly that the usage is conditional if there is nothing else left. The fact that they reported several proposals for other pro's and con's beyond the questions to be asked showed great interest and a high involvement in the topic, quite independently of age. They also appreciated that potential end-users of technology are involved in the development process and confirmed the need of a participatory design in this sensitive topic.

The computer generation reported the highest degree of acceptance of the medical stent, followed by the youngest generation (generation of GameBoy) and the household revolution generation. But even the oldest participants (early-technical generation) widely agreed for using the stent though in this generation the variety of acceptance patterns was most pronounced.

These results suggest two main points: First, greater variety within response behavior illustrates the heterogeneity of the older age group and reveals the importance for considering this group as potential users of medical technologies in a special manner. Second, the high degree of acceptance within the computer generation might be a mixture out of a broader general understanding of technology (grown up with digital technologies), and already a higher involvement into the topic compared to the youngest generation (GameBoy). This will be detailed in section 4.3.

4.2 Barriers and Using Motives

Participants' ratings on possible reasons for and against using the medical stent as well as their numerous voluntary proposals for further pro's and con's gave a deeper insight into the topic and suggestions for further factors which should be considered in future research and product development. Basically, all participants reported greater agreement with potential using motives than their hassle with potential barriers. We take this as a confirmation of the current trend to invest in developments of future medical technology, but also as a hint that potential barriers should be taken seriously.

Potential using motives revealed a great difference between the early-technical generation and the other three generations. This generation is the one who are closest to the topic as they will be most likely use these technologies. They not only had the lowest acceptance for the pro's, and at the same time the highest rating on the con's. The main argument for the usage of a medical stent in the very olds is the less frequent visit at the doctor, while the other generations stressed the keeping independency as main acceptance driver.

Across all generation the motive for using the stent to escape the indignity of being cared by others was common. This of course reflects also cultural and societal aging attitudes and public preconceptions.

4.3 Aging Concepts and Generation Specific Acceptance Patterns

The examination of aging concepts revealed a very concise picture of societal trends. People want to be mobile and live independently, they are reluctant to move to the children when they are old and they refuse to move into a nursing home and concede this possibility only, if no other opportunities exist. Also, most respondents want to escape from the indignity of being cared. This picture was found to be universal and did not differ across generations, what could be rather culture-specific and reflect a societal attitude. But people would like to have mobile nursing services which support them living independently at home. Somehow it is an ironic finding that the basic positive attitude towards medical technology could be due to the negative and stigmatizing picture of being old, which is avoided by respondents.

One could have assumed that these very specific aging concepts might be the driver of the positive evaluation of the usefulness of medical technology. However, correlation analyses did not corroborate this assumption. No relation was found between aging concepts and the using motives. On the basis of the present data we cannot explain this finding. Possibly however, yet we have a too small experience with ambient-assisted living technologies (while we all have profound experience and knowledge about family quarrels when caring old parents and negative message about a low quality of nursing homes).

Finally, a last remark is directed to the uniqueness of predictive factors, which turned out to be decisive for acceptance and intention to use. In the two older generations -the early technical generation and the household revolution - one or two factors were decisive (escape from the indignity of being cared, saving costs for care) to reach an explained variance of about 70 %. In the younger generations, more and more diverse factors were needed to reach comparable explained variance levels. Though this must be replicated in future studies, this could be taken as a first hint that the acceptance pattern of older persons is less ambiguous and more palpable in contrast to younger people for which the using situation of a medical device is a rather distant situation.

5   Limitations and Suggestions for Future Research

Future studies will have to investigate to what extent these outcomes may be generalized to specific illnesses or using contexts. A cross-cultural comparison of different societal aging concepts and their relation to acceptance of medical technology could also represent a valuable research topic. Furthermore, gender effects on acceptance of medical technology should be investigated in greater detail. Also, it will have to be found out if the caveats reported by respondents do vanish if people get to know these technologies. Within this context it is also interesting to take a deeper look on the role of technology adaption strategies among each generation. It is assumable that e.g. early-adaptors might be the only one who can imagine to use the technology (which is not yet available) although late adaptors would also use its, but not till they get to know it themselves. Future studies could also address learning style and aspects of life-long learning for deeper insights into the topic.

Finally, a medical device to be implemented in the body is only one form, which might be applicable to enhance mobility with aging. It should be investigated if intelligent clothes or walls or even robots may have another acceptance pattern.

Acknowledgments. Authors would like to thank all participants, but especially the older ones, to patiently fill in the questionnaire and to allow us to gain insights into a sensible topic. Many thanks also to Carola Caesar, Simone Wirtz, and Oliver Sack for their research assistance. This research was supported by the excellence initiative of the German federal and state governments.

References

1. Wittenberg, R., Comas-Herrera, A., Pickard, L., Hancock, R.: Future Demand for Long-Term Care in England. PSSRU Research Summary (2006)
2. Leonhardt, S.: Personal Healthcare Devices. In: Mekherjee, S., et al. (eds.) Malware: Hardware Technology Drivers of Ambient Intelligence, pp. 349–370. Springer, Dordrecht (2005)
3. Weiner, M., Callahan, C.M., Tierney, W.M., Overhage, M., Mamlin, B., Dexter, A.: Using Information Technology To Improve the Health Care of Older Adults. Ann. Intern. Med. 139, 430–436 (2003)
4. Groß, D., Jakobs, E.-M.: E-Health und technisierte Medizin [Ehealth and medical engineering]. LIT, Münster (2007)
5. Jähn, K., Nagel, E.: e-Health. Springer, Berlin (2004)
6. Tan, J.K.H.: Healthcare information systems & informatics: research and practices, Hershey (2008)
7. Warren, S., Craft, R.L.: Designing smart health care technology into the home of the future. Engineering in Medicine and Biology 2, 677 (1999)
8. Starr, P.: Smart technology, stunted policy: developing health information networks. Health Affairs 16(3), 91–105 (1997)
9. Lymberis, A.: Smart wearable systems for personalised health management: current R&D and future challenges Engineering in Medicine and Biology Society. In: Proc. of the 25th Annual International Conference, vol. 4, pp. 3716–3719. IEEE, Los Alamitos (2003)
10. Wirtz, S., Ziefle, M., Jakobs, E.-M.: Autopilot versus hearing aid – domain- and technology type-specific parameters of older people's technology acceptance. In: 9th International Conference on Work With Computer Systems, Beijing, China (2009)
11. Jakobs, E.-M., Lehnen, K., Ziefle, M.: Alter und Technik. Eine Studie zur altersbezogenen Wahrnehmung und Gestaltung von Technik., Aprimus, Germany (2008)
12. Arning, K., Ziefle, M.: What older user expect from mobile devices: An empirical survey. In: Pikaar, R.N., Konigsveld, E.A., Settels, P.J. (eds.) Proceedings of the 16th World Congress on Ergonomics (IEA). Elsevier, Amsterdam (2006)
13. Mynatt, E.D., Melenhorst, A.-S., Fisk, A.-D., Rogers, W.A.: Aware technologies for aging in place: understanding user needs and attitudes. .IEEE Pervasive Computing 20(3) (2004)
14. Melenhorst, A.S., Rogers, W.A., Caylor, E.C.: The use of communication technologies by older adults: Exploring the benefits from an users perspective. In: Proc. of the Human Factors and Ergonomics Society 45th Annual Meeting (2001)
15. Melenhorst, A.-S., Rogers, W.A., Bouwhuis, D.G.: Older adults' motivated choice for technological innovation: Evidence for benefit-driven selectivity. Psychology and Aging 21(1), 190–195 (2006)
16. Zimmer, Z., Chappell, N.L.: Receptivity to new technology among older adults. Disability and Rehabilitation 21(5/6), 222–230 (1999)
17. Davis, F.D.: Perceived Usefulness, Perceived Ease of Use, and User Acceptance of Information Technology. MIS Quarterly 13, 319–337 (1989)
18. Venkatesh, V., Davis, F.D.: A Theoretical Extension of the Technology Acceptance Model: Four Longitudinal Field Studies. Management Science 46, 186–204 (2000)
19. Venkatesh, V., Davis, F.D.: A Model of the Antecedents of Perceived Ease of Use: Development and Test. Decision Sciences 27, 451–481 (1996)
20. Arning, K., Ziefle, M.: Understanding age differences in PDA acceptance and performance. Computers in Human Behavior 23, 2904–2927 (2007)

21. Venkatesh, V., Morris, M.G., Davis, G.B., Davis, F.D.: User acceptance of information technology: Toward a unified view. MIS Quarterly 27, 3 (2003)

22. Arning, K., Ziefle, M.: Different perspectives on technology acceptance: The role of technology type and age. In: USAB 2009, Linz, Austria (submitted, 2009)

23. Ziefle, M.: Age perspectives on the usefulness on e-health applications. In: International Conference on Health Care Systems, Ergonomics, and Patient Safety (HEPS), Straßbourg, France (2008)

24. Meyer, S., Mollenkopf, H.: Home technology, smart homes, and the Aging user. In: Schaie, K.W., Wahl, H.-W., Mollenkopf, H., Oswald, F. (eds.) Aging Independently: Living Arrangements and Mobility. Springer, Heidelberg (2003)

25. Demiris, G., Hensel, B.K., Skubic, M., Rantz, M.: Senior residents' perceived need of and preferences for "smart home" sensor technologies. International Journal of Technology Assessment in Health Care 24, 120–124 (2008)

26. Stronge, A.J., Rogers, W.A., Fisk, A.D.J.: Human factors considerations in implementing telemedicine systems to accommodate older adults. Telemed. Telecare 13, 1–3 (2007)

27. Morrell, R.W., Mayhorn, C.B., Bennet, J.: A Survey of World Wide Web Use in Middle-Aged and Older Adults. Human Factors 42(2), 175–182 (2000)

28. Vicente, K.J., Hayes, B.C., Williges, R.C.: Assaying and isolating individual dfferences in searching a hierarchical files system. Human Facotrs 29, 349–359 (1987)

29. Westerman, S.J.: Individual differences in the use of command line and menu computer interfaces. International Journal of Human Computer Interaction 9, 183–198 (1997)

30. Arning, K., Ziefle, M.: Barriers of Information Access in Small Screen Device Applications: The Relevance of User Characteristics for a Transgenerational Design. In: Stephanidis, C., Pieper, M. (eds.) ERCIM Ws UI4ALL 2006. LNCS, vol. 4397, pp. 117–136. Springer, Heidelberg (2007)

31. Ziefle, M., Bay, S.: How older adults meet cognitive complexity: Aging effects on the usability of different cellular phones. Behaviour and Information Technology 24(5), 375–389 (2005)

32. Ziefle, M., Bay, S.: How to overcome disorientation in mobile phone menus: A comparison of two different types of navigation aids. Human Computer Interaction 21(4), 393–432 (2006)

33. Ziefle, M., Bay, S.: Transgenerational Designs in Mobile Technology. In: Lumsden, J. (ed.) Handbook of Research on User Interface Design and Evaluation for Mobile Technology, pp. 122–140. IGI Global (2008)

34. Ziefle, M., Schroeder, U., Strenk, J., Michel, T.: How young and older users master the use of hyperlinks in small screen devices. In: Proceedings of the SIGCHI conference on Human factors in computing systems 2007, pp. 307–316. ACM, New York (2007)

35. Arning, K., Ziefle, M.: Comparing apples and oranges? Exploring users' acceptance of ICT and eHealth applications. In: International Conference on Health Care Systems, Ergonomics, and Patient Safety, HEPS (2008)

36. Marquie, J.C., Jourdan-Boddaert, L., Huet, N.: Do older adults underestimate their actual computer knowledge? Behaviour and Information Technology 21(4), 273–280 (2002)

37. Noyes, J.M., Sheard, M.C.A.: Designing for older adults - are they a special group? In: Universal Access in HCI: Inclusive Design in the Information Society, pp. 877–881. Lawrence Erlbaum, Mahwah

38. Sackmann, R., Weymann, A.: Die Technisierung des Alltags – Generationen und technische Innovationen [mechanization of daily life- genarations and technical innovations]. Frankfurt: Campus (1994)

User Interaction Design for a Home-Based Telecare System

Spyros Raptis, Pirros Tsiakoulis, Aimilios Chalamandaris, and Sotiris Karabetsos

Institute for Language and Speech Processing – "Athena" Research Center,
Artemidos 6 & Epidavrou, GR-15125, Athens, Greece
{spy,ptsiak,achalam,sotoskar}@ilsp.gr

Abstract. This paper presents the design of the user-interaction component of a home-based telecare system for congestive heart failure patients. It provides a short overview of the overall system and offers details on the different interaction types supported by the system. Interacting with the user occurs either as part of a scheduled procedure or as a consequence of identifying or predicting a potentially hazardous deterioration of the patients' health state. The overall logic of the interaction is structured around event-scenario associations, where a scenario consists of concrete actions to be performed, some of which may involve the patient. A key objective in this type of interaction that it is very simple, intuitive and short, involving common everyday objects and familiar media such as speech.

Keywords: home-based system, speech interface, text-to-speech, smart home, telecare.

1 Introduction

Within the European States the percentage of older people is growing. The population structure of all European countries is changing with a large increase in the proportion of older (65+) and very old (80+) persons. Consequently, the need for caring assistance is increasing and national health services have a responsibility to manage for this need. As the population ages it experiences more chronic health problems. Chronically ill patients account for three quarters of all healthcare expenditures.

The pattern of care is also changing. Current European policy implies transfer of resources to care in the community and informal care to facilitate supporting arrangements. The challenge for Europe will be to provide good-quality care at manageable cost to a growing number of people. Thus, support for informal caring may improve care competence, prolong or extend caring capacity and provide value with respect to care delivery [1].

The increasing cost of providing healthcare services and changing patterns of use of hospital resources (a rise in admissions but a fall in the average length of stay) are powerful forces for shifting the focus of care from the hospital to the home. Moreover,

A. Holzinger and K. Miesenberger (Eds.): USAB 2009, LNCS 5889, pp. 333–344, 2009.
© Springer-Verlag Berlin Heidelberg 2009

there is strong evidence that most people (especially the older ones) prefer to remain at home. One of the key reasons for this is 'independent living'. There is also substantial evidence that healthcare outcomes and quality of life improve when healthcare services are home based [2, 3].

Thus, there is a shift of interest towards enhancing patient independent living and quality of life by providing the means for safe and unobtrusive monitoring and quality care at manageable cost to a growing number of people away from hospitals.

The "Information for Health" document published by the NHS Executive in 1998 [4], recognised that "telecare technology will be used to provide reliable but unobtrusive supervision of vulnerable people who want to sustain an independent life in their own home". The development of telecare and monitoring services is also included in the published national strategic programme for IT in the NHS [5]. The recently completed Australian Coordinated Care Trials identified home telecare as having significant potential for contributing to the management of patients with acute exacerbation of chronic conditions as well as at-risk elderly people living alone at home.

In this direction, there have been numerous efforts to design and develop infrastructures that would enable and support patients with chronic diseases (see for example [6]). Home telecare technologies have been reviewed by several authors [7, 8, 9, 10]. Many of these infrastructures include a home-based component for remote monitoring with integrated medical inference and controlled decision making capabilities. State-of-the-art measurement and data acquisition is employed through communities of devices and artefacts, wireless data transfer and communications, data fusion, medical inference and decision making, and automatic planning and execution of advanced response patterns and interaction scenarios.

Work has been carried out on the user interaction design issues of wearable health monitoring devices (e.g. [11]). However, such systems are quite different in target and scope, since they are tailored towards lightweight portable solutions that are always attached to the patient and can monitor a set of crucial health parameters. They do not fuse multisensory information and they do not need to consider multimodality in the user interaction.

It should be noted that some real and potential problems in the application of telecare and smart homes have been identified [12].

2 The HEARTS System

The HEARTS project (Home-Based Everyday Activities analysis and Response Telecare System) emerged in this context. The aim of the project was to design and develop an adequate infrastructure that, based on information, communications, measurement and monitoring technologies would be able to constantly evaluate the health status of a patient at home and intervene when necessary to avoid deterioration. This involved the development of an integrated home telecare system encompassing devices from different generations available, the investigation of methods of embedding everyday artefacts and smart home technology into this system, enhance available signal processing and data analysis algorithms and finally implement a proof-of-concept system consisting of the relevant sensors, data collection devices, algorithms and networking within a typical home environment.

The project focused on congestive heart failure (CHF) patients. Its scope well exceeding the simple monitoring and plain comparison of measurements to predefined values that could lead to alarms. It also covered the identification of time-varying patterns of important health variables and the prediction of their evolution. The sensitivity and specificity of the system's operation provide the basis for measuring the quality of the performed medical inference and decision-making.

The infrastructure of the HEARTS system comprised of:

- a local *data collection mechanism*, fusing information from multiple diverse sensors, both body-attached and fixed at specific locations at the home environment. These sensors provide not only measurements of important patient health parameters but also information on activities of daily living (ADL)
- a local *data processing system*, that performs some preliminary checking on the obtained data, takes any emergent actions necessary, and forwards the data to the remote server for further processing
- a *remote server* that, based on the collected information, performs preventive medical inference and medical decision making, also taking into consideration the patient's past medical data
- a *local response mechanism* for conveying system feedback to the patient and initiating interaction scenarios when appropriate
- a *remote response mechanism* involving a health service provider to take appropriate measures when deemed necessary.

Minimal daily life disturbance and unobtrusive supervision were very important factors. This relates both to the arrangements required for setting up the system to the patient's home and to the patient participating in the process. Necessary devices and sensors needed to be as transparent to the user as possible and should avoid affecting their mobility. This implies movable wireless low consumption devices (with the exception of the ones that need cannot be to be large or devices that are attached to fixed objects).

The patient's active participation should not be required in the system routine use. However, for tasks where this is inevitable (e.g. during measurements that cannot be done automatically or, periodically, when sensor need to be calibrated) the interaction with the system should be very simple, intuitive and short.

When potentially negative trends are identified in the monitored health variables, the system issues effective pre-alarms or alarms, involving the automatic creation and execution of in-situ responses (such as audible and/or visible feedback through appropriately adapted familiar common devices) and external responses (engaging health service providers and other formal and informal health structures). Interaction scenarios with the user are integrated into the system's operation either as part of a medical data acquisition schedule or as an automatically created system response. These involve a set of (intelligent) communication devices such as visible feedback devices (e.g. a TV set for displaying a message or alert), and audible feedback devices (e.g. a text-to-speech system for voice messages).

3 System Responses

The medical inference and decision making process of the system provide estimates on the patient's health condition, identifying potentially dangerous patterns in the monitored variables based on the patient's personal profile.

To the event of such a potentially dangerous situation being identified, the overall system has to provide appropriate responses the range of which should differ according to the nature of and level of the predicted declination.

Two major response paths can be identified:

- *In situ responses*, i.e. actions taken at the patient's site
- *External responses*, i.e. actions involving the intervention of external health service providers

3.1 In Situ Responses

In situ responses refer to the actions taken at the patient's site, i.e. locally at home. When a declination pattern has been identified, system responses could range from a quite simple to more complex interaction schemes. Such responses ranged from:

- An audible feedback conveyed through to the patients informing them of a potentially dangerous situation
- A voice message being conveyed to the patient providing simple instructions, e.g. informing them that they should take a rest, try to relax, take a medication, etc.
- A voice message prompting the patient to call their attendant physician for further instructions
- A visible feedback conveyed through common house media, such as the television, etc.

Common house communication media provide the main interaction channels used during an in situ response. These devices will need to be appropriately adapted and enhanced with wireless LAN support to serve for these purposes. They offer audio and image.

Audio (sounds and voice) may be conveyed through the patient's stereo or television set. Text-to-speech technology will be employed to synthesise audible messages and prompts. This provides an important advantage over pre-recorded messages since it enables easy customisation, personalisation and maintenance of the message content and alleviates the need for producing recordings of the all required material. Moreover, voice parameters such as rate and pitch can be configured according to each patient's personal preferences.

An important issue that needs to be addressed when designing such interaction schemes, is the location of the patient. Information on which room the patient is currently in is important for the system to route feedback to the appropriate devices, so that the message can reach and be perceived by the patient. Body-attached devices or motion capturing devices can serve for this purpose.

The medication schedule component is an additional function provided by the system. Each patient's medical profile will contain information on the patient's medication program. An in situ response may be produced automatically by the system at appropriate times to remind the patient to take the necessary medication.

3.2 External Responses

When a potentially problematic situation is identified for a patient by the medical inference and decision making module, the system may also trigger alerts directed to the health service provider (in parallel to the in situ responses that may be scheduled) depending on the severity of the situation.

The health service provider will need to respond by taking the necessary actions and intervening, when appropriate, to assist the patient and prevent deterioration.

These actions may range from a telephone call to the subject from a specialist to provide some instructions, to an emergency signal and an ambulance departing to transfer the patient to the hospital.

Of course, the technological and administrative issues related to this framework, including the health service provider signalling and response mechanisms, need to be explicitly defined.

4 Interaction Scenarios

There are certain tasks where the patient's active participation is inevitable, e.g. during measurements that cannot be taken automatically (e.g. systolic, diastolic and mean blood pressure, blood oxygen saturation etc.) or, on a periodic basis, when the sensor will need to be calibrated. In these cases, the interaction with the system should be very simple, intuitive and short.

Scheduled interactions scenarios can be used for different purposes. A regular interaction can be useful for asking simple questions to the patients aiming to evaluate additional aspects of their health (such as their mood, their psychological state etc) and to detect signs or symptoms that are still not evident in the other monitored parameters but which could have predictive value for early identifying an upcoming degradation.

An additional reason for invoking interaction scenarios is the widely recognized significance of patients being aware of their health status, the feeling of active participation in its improvement and the appreciation of the results of the therapy followed.

The aim is to design a module for forming and executing appropriate scenarios. The interaction can be much more immediate and effective if it involves familiar objects and familiar modalities such as speech.

Some of the scenarios that have been foreseen are summarized in Table 1 below:

Table 1. Some examples of possible scenarios involving the user

Scenario	Type[1]
S1. Scheduled daily test. This is actually a variant of the 6-minutes-walk test, that patients carry out daily, usually at morning hours. This test can be used to identify indications that could endanger the patient's health. The test can lead to some preliminary conclusions on how the patient's health evolves.	S
S2. Examining patient's speech. In this scenario the patient's speech is recorded and certain parameters of the signal are analyzed aiming to identify significant deviations from his/her regular speaking patterns. A deviation could, conditionally, be considered as an indication of an impending deterioration.	S
S3. Cardiogram. A cardiogram is an important tool for drawing initial conclusions on the evolution of a patient's health. This scenario is carried out 4 times a day.	S
S4. Basic consultation. Often, it is possible that a patient feels atony, fatigue or dysphoria. The purpose of this scenario is to support to the patient in such cases by providing basic advice and guidance. The scenario is based on a set of questions and answers between the system and the patient through which the system collects information regarding the symptoms and offers suggestions for dealing with the situation such as, for example, taking a rest, taking a medicinal product or contacting the attendant physician or a family member.	U
S5. Medication reminder. Based on stored information regarding the medication schedule of the patient, the system automatically engages into interaction scenarios to ensure that the patients follow their program.	S
S6. Manual alarm. An emergency device, such as an alarm button, can be used to automatically fire an alert for immediate contact with the appropriate recipients, such as the security personnel or a family member, or to raise a (pre-)alarm.	U
S7. Monitored parameter off the limits. Except from the constant and periodic sampling of the patient's monitored health parameters and posting them to the remote server, the local system is also responsible for performing a first check of their values. This check roughly consists of comparing against the personalized limits that have been defined for each patient. A significant deviation from the reference values will activate this scenario.	U

5   The Scenario Execution Module

5.1   Structure and operation

The operation of the interaction scenario execution module is based on *events*. Different situations raise different events. For example, if a monitored parameter of patient is found to be outside its acceptable range, then an event is triggered. The execution module associates every possible event to an *interaction scenario*. As soon as the event is triggered, the module invokes the corresponding scenario step-by-step.

Structuring the execution module on the basis of event-scenario associations, provides an open solution offering flexibility and adjustability to diverse requirements and different needs. New scenarios can be designed and dynamically linked to different events.

Fig. 1 below illustrates the link between measurements, events and scenarios.

[1] Scenario type. Can be "S": Scheduled, or "U": Unscheduled.

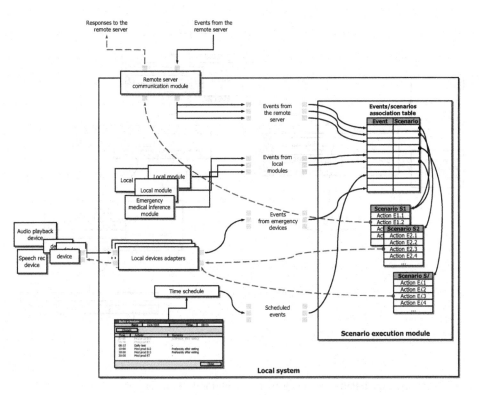

Fig. 1. Measurements, events and scenarios

The basic event categories are shown in the following table.

Table 2. Basic event types

Event Type	Description
Time-scheduled events	Such events are triggered, for example, from the medication scheduler of the system at the times when the patient needs to take a medication. A regular daily test is another example of a time-scheduled event.
Events from local modules	These are events that are triggered from the modules of the local system as, for example, the medical inference module, when significant deviations are observed in the monitored parameters.
Events from the remote server	Such events are triggered from the remote server. This could happen (a) automatically, e.g. in case a problematic situation is identified by the remote medical inference module, or (b) manually, e.g. by the security personnel in response to a pre-alarm.
Events from emergency devices	These events are triggered from specific types of emergency devices, such as emergency buttons, alarms or devices attached to the patient that are able to detect a fall.

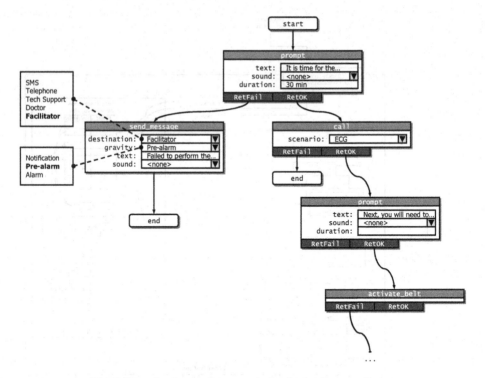

Fig. 2. Part of an interaction scenario for the 6-minutes-walk test

The execution module associates each event to a scenario. Each scenario is composed of a set of *actions* that are executed sequentially, each of which can involve other modules, devices or the patient himself.

In cooperation with the other modules of the local systems, the execution module supports a specific set of possible actions that can be combined to create appropriate responses for any event. Thus, a scenario is basically an action script.

Fig. 2 shows part of an interaction scenario with the respective actions that comprise it. This scenario corresponds to the daily 6-minutes-walk test.

For each action there is a set of associated:

- *arguments*, that specify the different parameters of the action
- *results*, that capture the possible outcomes of the executing the action (success/failure)

Thus, an interaction scenario is actually a script or a "program" written in the language of the system, and every "instruction" corresponds to one of the available commands.

5.2 The Operational Environment

The execution module operates in the background, receiving events from the local system (and, through that, from the remote server too) and executing the corresponding interaction scenarios.

The module interacts with:
1. the *end-user* (the patient) in the course of executing an interaction scenario, for example to remind the patient of a task or to offer information
2. specialized personnel that is responsible for designing and/or configuring the interaction scenarios so that they meet the patient's particular requirements and needs.

Interacting with the End-user. During the execution of certain actions from an interaction scenario, it is necessary to update or to engage the patient. For such interactions, the execution module employs simple patterns involving the equipment of the local system (monitor, speakers, keyboard, mouse etc).

For example, an action that would need to carry a notification message to the patient would display the following window:

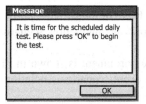

Fig. 3. A message box with an audible notification

This message is also read out loud through synthetic speech and, optionally, accompanied by an audio prompt. If the scenario is required to make sure that the patient gets the message, the synthetic speech (and the audio prompt) would be repeated for a specified number of times or until the patient dismisses the message box by hitting any key on the keyboard. This interaction step, as described above, corresponds to an action of the execution module, the prompt action.

The execution module integrates text-to-speech technology for producing the audio messages and prompts. Synthetic speech presents several advantages over prerecorded messages, since it allows easy adaptation and personalization, and can offer the ability to change the content of the message without the need to manually produce all the new recordings for the necessary prompts. Furthermore, its parameters such as the speech rate and pitch can be adapted to preferences of each patient.

The user has access to the full set of scheduled interaction scenarios, including the ones that relate to the medication schedule. This information is made available through the simple view shown in Fig. 4.

In this figure, the various activities (corresponding to interaction scenarios) are displayed ordered by time. Gray letter font is used to differentiate past activities that have already been performed. In the specific situation displayed in the figure, the current time is 08:13; all activities scheduled for earlier times have already been performed. The next scheduled activity is the daily morning test. The majority of the activities shown in the figure relate to the medication schedule.

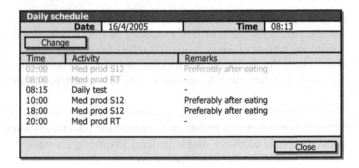

Fig. 4. The list of daily schedule activities

Event-scenario Association Environment. This purpose of this environment is to link possible events to appropriate interaction scenarios and is only addressed to specialized personnel.

The basic interface of the environment is shown in Fig. 5 below. In this view, the user can activate or deactivate event-scenario associations and to define new ones.

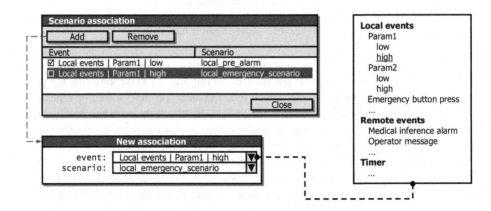

Fig. 5. The event-scenario association environment

Scenario Creation Environment. The execution module offers a basic simplified graphical environment for creating interaction scenarios (scripts), and is addressed to specialized personnel. The approach follows that of a typical simplified programming language.

Starting from an initial state, the user can add commands (selecting from a list of available commands) and configure their arguments. Furthermore, the user can define the execution flow by linking commend results to appropriate following commands.

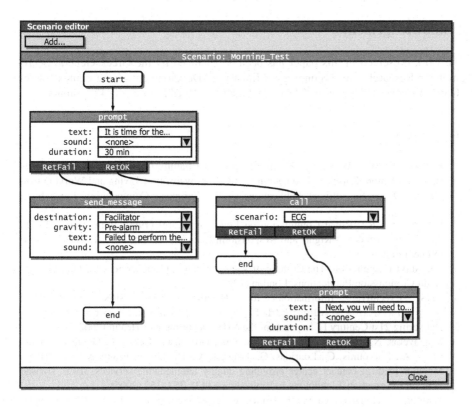

Fig. 6. The scenario editor

6 Conclusions

An overview of the mechanism and the underlying concepts of human-computer interaction for the case of a home-based telecare system has been presented.

The system's operation is designed to be mostly transparent to the patient. However, in certain cases when a potentially hazardous situation is predicted the system intervenes and interacts with the user. The interaction is triggered by events of interest which, in turn, activate interaction scenarios that involve home devices and the user himself. The interaction can be made much more direct, effective and intuitive when it involves common everyday objects such as the TV set, and familiar media such as speech and image. However, depending on the information to be conveyed to the patient, the patient's location within the limits of the house, and other factors, appropriate interaction patterns need to planned and executed. Structuring the execution module on the basis of event-scenario associations, provides an open solution offering flexibility and adjustability to diverse requirements and different needs. New scenarios can be designed and dynamically linked to different events.

Acknowledgements

The work presented in this paper has been co-financed by the Greek General Secretariat for Research and Technology, Ministry of Development in the context of the "Competitiveness" Operational Program under the Third Framework Programme.

References

1. Salvage, A.: Who Will Care? Future Prospects for Family Care of Older People in the European Union, European Foundation for the Improvement of Living and Working Conditions, Office for Official Publications of the European Communities, Luxembourg (1995)
2. Sutherland, S.R.: (Royal Commission on Long-term Care) (1999) With Respect to Old Age: Long-term care—Rights and Responsibilities: A report, Cm 4192-1, The Stationery Office, London
3. UK Audit Commission, The Coming of Age: Improving Care Services for Older People. Audit Commission Publications, London (1997)
4. NHS Executive, Information for Health (1998) ISBN 0-95327190-2, http://www.nhsia.nhs.uk/def/pages/info4health/contents.asp
5. Delivering 21st Century IT Support for the NHS, Department of Health (2002)
6. Maglaveras, N., Chouvarda, I., Koutkias, V.G., Gogou, G., Lekka, I., Goulis, D., Avramidis, A., Karvounis, C., Louridas, G., Balas, E.A.: The citizen health system (CHS): a Modular medical contact center providing quality telemedicine services. IEEE Transactions on Information Technology in Biomedicine 9(3), 353–362 (2005)
7. Kinsella, A.: Home Telecare in the United States. J. Telemed. Telecare 4, 195–200 (1998)
8. Doughty, K., Cameron, K., Garner, P.: Three Generations of Telecare of the Elderly. J. Telemed. Telecare 2, 71–80 (1996)
9. Ruggiero, C., Sacile, R., Giacomini, M.: Home Telecare. J. Telemed. Telecare 5, 11–17 (1999)
10. Stoecke, J.D., Lorch, S.: Why Go See the Doctor? – Care Goes From Office to Home as Technology Divorces Function from Geography. Int. J. Technol. Assess. Health Care 13, 537–546 (1997)
11. Villalba, E., Peinado, I., Arredondo, M.T.: User Interaction Design for a Wearable and IT Based Heart Failure System. In: Jacko, J.A. (ed.) HCI 2007. LNCS, vol. 4551, pp. 1230–1239. Springer, Heidelberg (2007)
12. Celler, B.G., Lovell, N.H., Chan, D.K.Y.: The Potential Impact of Home Telecare on Clinical Practice. The Medical Journal of Australia 171, 518–521 (1999)

A Videophone Prototype System Evaluated by Elderly Users in the Living Lab Schwechat

Johannes Oberzaucher[1], Katharina Werner[1], Harald P. Mairböck[2], Christian Beck[3], Paul Panek[1,3], Walter Hlauschek[1], and Wolfgang L. Zagler[1,3]

[1] CEIT RALTEC, Am Concorde Park 2, 2320 Schwechat, Austria
{j.oberzaucher,k.werner,p.panek,w.hlauschek,w.zagler}@ceit.at
[2] Telekom Austria TA AG Vienna, Austria
harald.mairboeck@telekom.at
[3] fortec – Research Group on Rehabilitation Technology, Vienna Univ. of Technology, Favoritenstrasse 11/029, A-1040 Vienna, Austria
{beck,panek,zagler}@fortec.tuwien.ac.at

Abstract. Elderly people often experience difficulties in using modern Information and Communication Technologies. This paper presents findings of an evaluation and a field test of a touch screen based internet videophone system mounted in a wooden frame in order to provide a non technical appearance. During a 14-day lasting field test in real-life environment the goal was to evaluate if and to what extent the elderly participants would benefit from using such a modern multimodal way of communication. Four prototype systems were installed in four private homes and were tested successfully by six persons. It was found that the elderly users actually benefited from the touchscreen control, the proportionally large-scale GUI and the VoIP-and video-telephone functions. Despite the small scale of the evaluation the gathered data demonstrates the potential this technology might have in daily life in particular for the emerging ambient assisted living (AAL) area.

Keywords: Usability evaluation, elderly, ICT, ubiquitous computing, e-inclusion, VoIP, AAL.

1 Introduction and Aim

Modern convergent Information and Communications Technology solutions, merging telephony, Internet and video applications are often not or only restrictedly applicable for elderly users although elderly people could benefit a lot from using such solutions. [1,10].

As a contribution for overcoming this "digital divide" a research prototype of a new communication platform for elderly people - called the "Interactive Picture Frame" (in German "InterAktives Bild" – IAB) [6,7] - was developed and evaluated. The system is based on the availability of fixed line broadband-access and touch-screen-technology. Whereas it should not be perceived as a technical system, rather as a nice looking piece of furniture [9].

A. Holzinger and K. Miesenberger (Eds.): USAB 2009, LNCS 5889, pp. 345–352, 2009.
© Springer-Verlag Berlin Heidelberg 2009

Potential future users were involved throughout the whole development process and also participated as test-users in a field test in a real-life setting. In order to gather reliable information about the usability of new systems for Human Computer Interaction they should be tested in a real-life setting during a longer period of time [5], what should lead to a better understanding, how the users are interacting with the system. Unlike usability methods like guided interviews, wizard of oz tests or guided user tests, a field test in a real-life setting gives the users the chance to interact with the system in a less influenced way.

The real life evaluation of the video phone prototype was carried out in the so called Living Lab Schwechat for Ambient Assisted Living (AAL) which was established in 2006. Local authorities, social service providers, elderly persons, carers, research entities and companies have started to cooperate closely as full partners in order to invent, discuss, explore, implement, and evaluate innovative technologies to support the independent living of senior citizens. This approach allows focusing on the actual needs of the future users by involving them right from the beginning into the RTD-process [2, 11].

In December 2008 – at the very end of the iterative development and evaluation process in the IAB project – we conducted a field test in a real-life setting. Four IAB-platforms were installed (N=4) in four flats of elderly citizens in Schwechat over a period of 14 days. Whereas the goal was to evaluate if the participants would benefit from using such a modern multimodal way of communication and would not be constrained or intimidated by our system.

2 Usability Evaluation Study

This section briefly describes the participatory design process which was applied for the development of the prototype system. This design process took place together with senior citizens in several iterative steps [6, 7] in the Living Lab Schwechat [2]. The outcome of the design process is the final video phone prototype system which then was used in the field trial described in the main part of this paper.

2.1 Description of the Evaluated System

The „Interactive Picture Frame" (IAB) is used as a video telephone system with a new touchscreen based graphical user interface (GUI). The whole system is "masked" as an ordinary piece of furniture - a picture frame.

In December 2007 15 seniors aged 58 to 86 (average 70 years) took part in two focus group sessions held in the center for senior citizens in the city of Schwechat. They discussed and tested a paper-wood-mockup of the platform and a nonfunctional graphical prototype presented on an Ultra Mobile PC with a touchscreen. Based on the focus group results we developed a first functional prototype, which was capable of conducting VoIP-telephony and conducted a test series with the same senior citizens. A high amount of positive response to the prototype was gained and also a couple of ideas how it could be improved to make it more suitable for elderly people. This included using larger symbols, enhancing the contrast and rearranging some symbols to ensure a more intuitive navigation. Since the first - rapid prototyped - laboratory samples did not include all features, finally we also added the possibility to conduct video calls and tested this redesigned prototype again with 10 senior citizens in August 2008 [6].

The August 2008 prototype consisted of a Paceblade tablet PC (Slimbook P110 Touch and P120 Touch) with a touchscreen and a wooden case, which resembled a picture frame. The size of the touch screen was 25 by 18,5 cm, the overall size of the device including wooden frame was 35 by 29 cm. A small hole in the picture frame made it possible to use the tablet's camera for video telephony and a metal slider was added to cover the camera if the caller did not want to be seen by his/her counterpart.

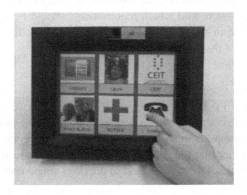

Fig. 1. The final videophone-prototype as it was developed iteratively in the Living Lab. This version was duplicated for use in the field evaluation.

Some modifications of the prototype – as a result of the iterative design process - were necessary to be made in order to ensure that the participants of the field trials can handle the device themselves (e.g. a modified start-up and shut-down procedure or adjustable speakers).

For developing the GUI of the video phone existing framework software was used and modified [4]. This software framework allows the design of multimodal user interfaces focusing on the specific needs and flexibility which is needed in the area of Assistive Technology.

One big difference to an ordinary telephone is that the user can call a close relative or an emergency service just by tipping on the corresponding picture. So the user does not have to remember any speed dial numbers. All the buttons are much larger than they are on an ordinary telephone (the smallest number dial buttons are 4 by 3 cm), so even persons with impaired fine motor dexterity and people with visual impairments can use the device more easily .

2.2 Description of the Field Test

The field test was conducted in December 2008. Four homes in and near Schwechat were equipped with IABs including the necessary fixed line broadband internet connectivity. One month ahead the preparations concerning user-recruitment and test-set-up preparation were started. After two weeks of testing the participants were visited again in order to conduct a final interview about their experiences during the test.

2.3 Recruitment of Users

Most of the participants of the preceding single user tests wanted to take part in the field test as well. As there were only four platforms available it was necessary to select who should participate.

To be able to test all functions of the prototype in a real-life setting as intensively as possible, it seemed to be preferable that the participants knew each other quite well and were used to informal regular communication among each other to ensure that they really would call each other via the videophone system. In order to achieve this, the former participants were told which requirements should be considered as a precondition to participate in the test. Whereupon they discussed and decided on their own who is going to test the system at home.

2.4 Participants

The final test group consisted of six people (N=6) aged between 70 and 82 years, whereas there were two couples and two women who tested the system alone. Two of them regularly use a computer at home, whereas one uses the computer for e-mail and internet actions, the other one for gaming. Four of the users already knew the system and tried it in the period before the field test in previous single user tests.

2.5 Test Preparation and Set Up

Following good practice in user involvement it was very important for us to inform the participants as good as possible about their tasks during the test period, the test itself, the platform and what to do if something would not work as intended or if they were annoyed or constrained by any function of the IAB. This information became part of our informed consent procedure – including a letter of information and a face-to-face meeting - where we explained the above mentioned topics in detail [8]. In addition an easily understandable user manual was designed and we offered the opportunity to get our help 24 hours a day via the emergency-button on the GUI or via a phone-call on a mobile-phone.

Three of the four test sites did not have the possibility to use the internet, so one week before the beginning of the real-life test these apartments were equipped with a broadband connection (aonFlex 2008/04b Telekom Austria, uplink of 340 kbps, downlink of 3500 kbps data rate, measured average values).

It was the participants' decision where to put the videophone platform in their home. The devices were connected wirelessly with the internet to offer the users the possibility to change its location. As it can be seen in Fig. 2 the platforms were almost imperceptible and did not change the flat's appearance negatively. It was also possible to change a "screen-saver" (graphic shown by the system during idle mode), so that a favored picture could be set (e.g. in Fig. 2 on the right picture "Der Kuß" ("The Kiss") from Gustav Klimt, on the left and middle picture an "autumn mood").

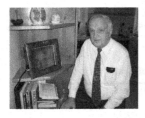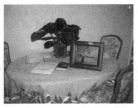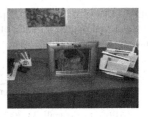

Fig. 2. The participants themselves decided the placement of the devices. They fit pretty well into the different apartments as they rather look like a piece of furniture than a technical device.

2.6 Test Procedure

There was no target given, concerning how often or in what mode (video- or speech-telephony) the users should use the interactive picture frame during these two weeks. For our test-aim and research question it was important, that the users should use the system only if they really wanted to use it. Our intention was to avoid any kind of stress for the elderly people and to minimize the influence on the test setting as far as possible.

During the test-phase the system logged activities that were proceeded with the interactive picture frame. We did not log the called telephone numbers, just the time and length of a call. Beside that we also used an error log to identify periods, where problems occurred.

The seniors themselves helped us in gathering more information by keeping a diary about the amount of calls they conducted, problems that occurred and new ideas that arose when using the device.

At the end of the test period we visited the participants again and carried out a short interview about their experiences with the device.

3 Results

The test in daily life was carried out with 4 video telephony prototype systems in 4 private homes over a period of 14 days involving 6 persons (age between 70 and 82, 2 male, 4 female). During the test three of the four systems were used actively almost every day. Despite the limited duration of the field test overall 114 calls (N=114) were carried out, whereas the video telephony function was used 35 times (N=35). The amount of calls to extern fixed line or mobile telephones was as high as double (N=79).

During the test period the participants were contacted once a week by the researchers. This allowed gathering information about occurring problems but also positive feedback.

After the first supervised single user tests we generally got a very positive feedback about the idea and usability of the IAB. In particular the big push buttons and the good readability of the numbers and control panels - assisted by an optimized contrast, increased dimension of the buttons and unambiguous symbols - as well as the intuitive use were emphasized and commended. This intuitive handling was also approved during the field test, as two elderly people, who have not used the device before, could use the system immediately without further explanation.

Table 1. Usage of the four IAB-platforms during the field test. (Note: Due to some missing log data the actual overall duration of the calls is estimated to be 25-30% higher than documented in the table below).

Platform	Initiated Calls			Duration of a call
IAB01	overall: 37	extern: 25	to IAB: 12	overall: 00:36:38
IAB02	overall: 33	extern: 27	to IAB: 6	overall : 05:09:30
IAB03	overall: 28	extern: 20	to IAB 8	overall : 00:52:27
IAB04	overall: 16	extern: 7	to IAB: 9	overall : 00:15:15
ALL IABs	**overall: 114**	**extern: 79**	**to IAB 35**	**Overall 06:53:50**

The users emphasized as a positive feature, that the IAB worked faster than the familiar telephone system due to the fast dialling process via the picture-buttons.. Comparing the device with their regular fixed line phone the users also pointed out that the feature to correct a wrongly typed number was very helpful. Also, not having to put on glasses for operating the phone was stated to be a big gain in comfort from point of view of the users.

Others told us that even visitors who saw the device were delighted about the possibilities, which arose when having the opportunity to see the counterpart – especially when a relative lives far away and they usually do not see each other very often. One participant who has a lot of friends abroad told us enthusiastically that she could *"reach them faster and in a better quality than with the usual phone"*.

All users also provided the feedback that the system was not considered as a technical system, it was just a part of the furniture and by this they were not averse to the self-contained use.

The seniors were also very comfortable with the manually operated video camera-shutter. By sliding the shutter in front of the camera they felt confident that no picture could be transmitted to anyone. None of the users had the feeling, that someone could get a glimpse of their private home, if they did not want it.

However especially IAB04 was affected by an asynchronism between lips-movement and sound due to insufficient bandwidth, which was caused by a lower internet downlink (measured average 1500 kbps) compared to the other installations.

Another problem on all platforms was that the conversational partner's face sometimes could not be fully seen. This was caused by the fact, that it was not possible to see one's own face on the screen (e.g. with a split-screen) in order to adjust the inclination angle of the IAB device. However this omission of one's own video picture was a decision that was made by the seniors in the course of the participative development process.

Also changes of the location were not accomplished, due to the weight of the prototypes (3,2 kg).

4 Discussion, Conclusion and Outlook

Based on the results of the second single user test in the senior citizen home in Schwechat [7] we had big expectations in the use of the video-telephony during the field test – and those were mainly conformed. However the users used the conventional voice-telephony more than twice (N=79) as much as the video-telephony during the field test (N=35). In a next step it would be of great interest if this proportion would change, if more users would take part in a field test and would have the chance to call more people via a video call.

Although the optimisation of technical problems concerning the video-picture and sound quality was not part of this research project, these problems should be considered in further development projects in this area. It should be commented, that even if the handling of such problems is not part of the project, the incidence of the problems can influence in particular a field test, as especially elderly persons could get the impression, that they would cause the problem by doing something wrong. This could lead to a loss of confidence and in succession to a refusal of acceptance towards the ongoing field test [3]. Linked up with that the topic of a "procreated feeling of a preserved privacy", which was one of our main interests (e.g. the manually operated camera-shutter), has to be considered with a prior ranking during a field-test in that area.

It is also mentionable that concerning the GUI and touchscreen control, this control mode was appreciated across the board. So it was verified that a touchscreen control with a relatively fast adaptable GUI is a very good choice for such purposes. Especially this control-dimension by touch-selection seems to be beneficial in particular for elderly users, if the touchscreen is big enough to display buttons in size like previously mentioned.

Extensive support-services - like we offered - are only possible with a small group of users. So it was approved that it is important to plan and accomplish a field test in a real-life setting for elderly in an iterative way too – a small group of users in a first step and a bigger group in a second.

Despite the small number of users and the limited duration of the real life test the potential of using broadband communication integrated in a device with a non technical appearance could be explored. The findings indicate that similar approaches also might be of value for the emerging ambient assisted living (AAL) research and development area [2].

Acknowledgement

We would like to thank the participants and test users, who helped us developing and evaluating the interactive picture frame for more than a year, the Senior citizen center Schwechat and the "Seniorenbeirat" (seniors' advisory board) of the city of Schwechat for their great support. We also thank fortec research group at TU Vienna for their contributions. The work reported here was funded in part by Telekom Austria TA AG. Ceit Raltec is a non profit research institute owned and partly funded by the municipality of Schwechat.

References

1. ARC Seibersdorf Research. Informations- und Kommunikationstechnologien für Menschen im Alter,
   http://www.lifetool.at/rte/upload/6_Fachforum/
   IKT_studie_2004_Endbericht.pdf [last access: 19/05/2009]
2. Hlauschek, W., Panek, P., Zagler, W.L.: Involvement of elderly citizens as potential end users of assistive technologies in the Living Lab Schwechat. In: PETRA 2009, Corfu. ACM, New York (2009) ISBN 978-1-60558-409-6
3. Isomursu, M., Häikiö, J., Wallin, A., Ailisto, H.: Experiences from a Touch-Based Interaction and Digitally Enhanced Meal-Delivery Service for the Elderly. Advances in Human-Computer Interaction 2008, Article ID 931701 (2008)
4. Software framework package for multimodal user interfaces in assistive technology, fortec, Vienna Univ. of Technology,
   http://www.is.tuwien.ac.at/4/index_en.html [last access: 23/07/2009]
5. Nielsen, J.: Usability Engineering. Academic Press, San Diego (1993)
6. Panek, P., Clerckx, G., Hlauschek, W., Mairböck, H., Zagler, W.L.: Experiences from Developing an Easy-To-Use VoIP Communication Device For and Together with Senior Citizens in the Living Lab Schwechat. In: CD-ROM proceedings IT and Telecom Symposium, Vienna, October 9-10 (2008)
7. Panek, P., Beck, C., Clerckx, G., Edelmayer, G., Haderer, R., Jagos, H., Mairböck, H., Oberzaucher, J., Zagler, W.L.: Partizipative Entwicklung eines intuitiven Kommunikationsgerätes für alte Menschen im Living Lab Schwechat. In: Maier, E., Roux, P. (eds.) Seniorengerechte Schnittstellen zur Technik, pp. 160–167. Pabst Science Publishers (2008)
8. Rauhala, M.: Ethics and Assistive Technology Design for Vulnerable Users: A Case Study. STAKES, Helsinki (2007)
9. Weiser, M.: The Computer for the Twenty-First Century. Scientific American 265(3), 94–104 (1991)
10. Kleinberger, T., Becker, M., Ras, E., Holzinger, A., Müller, P.: Ambient Intelligence in Assisted Living: Enable Elderly People to Handle Future Interfaces. In: Stephanidis, C. (ed.) UAHCI 2007 (Part II). LNCS, vol. 4555, pp. 103–112. Springer, Heidelberg (2007)
11. Schumacher, J., Niitamo, V.-P. (eds.): European Living Labs. A new approach for human centric regional innovation (2008); wvb Berlin, ISBN 978-3-86573-343-6
12. Holzinger, A.: Usability Engineering for Software Developers. Communications of the ACM 48(1), 71–74 (2005)

Avatars@Home

Inter*FACE*ing the Smart Home for Elderly People

Martin M. Morandell[1], Andreas Hochgatterer[1], Bernhard Wöckl[2],
Sandra Dittenberger[2], and Sascha Fagel[3]

[1] AIT Austrian Institute of Technology GmbH, Biomedical Systems
Viktor Kaplan-Strasse 2/1, A-2700 Wiener Neustadt, Austria
{martin.morandell,andreas.hochgatterer}@ait.ac.at
[2] CURE - Center for Usability Research and Engineering
Hauffgasse 3-5, A-1110 Wien, Austria
{woeckl,dittenberger}@cure.at
[3] Berlin Institute of Technology
Strasse des 17. Juni 135
D-10623 Berlin, Germany
sascha.fagel@tu-berlin.de

Abstract. Avatars are a common field of research for interfacing smart homes, especially for elderly people. The present study focuses on the usage of photo-realistic faces with different levels of movements (video, avatar and photo) as components of the graphical user interface (GUI) for Ambient Assisted Living (AAL) environments. Within a usability test, using the "Wizard of Oz" technique, these presentation modes were compared with a text and a voice only interface with users of the target groups: elderly people with ($n_{MCI}=12$) and without ($n_{nMCI}=12$) Mild Cognitive Impairment (MCI). Results show that faces on the GUI were liked by both, elderly with and without cognitive restrictions. However, users' performance on executing tasks did not differ much between the different presentation modes.

Keywords: Avatar, Usability, Elderly, Mild Cognitive Impairment.

1 Introduction

The department "Health and Environment" at the Austrian Institute of Technology (AIT) deals with societal challenges of the aging population. In its sub-group "Biomedical Systems" one research focus lies on strategic research topics referring to Ambient Assisted Living (AAL) solutions and how to adjust supporting technologies to the requirements of elderly people. The shared interests with the Center for Usability Research and Engineering (CURE) on design issues of assistive technologies brought us together to investigate the usage and acceptance of photo realistic avatars deployed in technologies for elderly people. This work is supported by the Department for Language and Communication at the Berlin Institute of Technology which provides experiences and tools for generating photo realistic avatars.

A. Holzinger and K. Miesenberger (Eds.): USAB 2009, LNCS 5889, pp. 353–365, 2009.

1.1 Idea and Background

Feasibility studies on technical aspects of Smart and in particular Assistive Home Environments are available from various sources (i.e. the Gator Tech Smart House [1], the Independent Life Style Assistant [2]), but the requirements for new strategies to make Information and Communication Technology (ICT), and in this case Smart Home Technology, more likely to be used by the elderly population are underestimated and not observed sufficiently.

Many factors play a decisive role for the successful realization of modern technologies. For the group of elderly users criteria such as the way of interaction, usability aspects and even emotional feelings have a crucial effect on the acceptance of devices or services. P. Wu even calls it *a need for an emotional relationship* between the users and their Assistive Technology [3]. Subsequently, users of the target group will reject assistive services and devices if their prospects on usability, accessibility and likability are not delivered, even if the technology has positive effects on safety aspects and prolongs independent living.

Van Berlo [4] emphasizes in the "Design Guidelines on Smart Homes" that the key factor for the acceptance of a smart home and its services is the user interface:

> The user interface is the main component in such systems, upon which the whole systems will be judged. This means that if the interface is confusing and poorly designed, the system will be thought of in the same way. Indeed, it is an extremely complex goal to make such systems appear simple, intuitive and easy to handle for elderly people to achieve a high degree of usability, accessibility and likability. Nonetheless, it is very important to do so.

The major target group within the scope of AAL is the group of older people. For this reason the focus of this study has been put on the identified crucial factor - the user interface - in particular on the output strategies and possible designs of those, using "faces on the interface".

1.2 The Target Group of Elderly People

One of the biggest challenges of the 21st century will be the increasing number of elderly people (and particularly people with age-related cognitive impairments like Mild Cognitive Impairment and Alzheimer's Disease). In 2001, 90.500 elderly people with dementia lived in Austria. If the predicted life expectancy leads to a prolonged duration of the illness, the number of people with dementia will be noticeably higher [5]. By the year 2050 the expected number of people with dementia in Austria will be about 233.800 [6].

Before reaching the status of dementia, many people are diagnosed with Mild Cognitive Impairment.

Mild Cognitive Impairment (MCI) is a general term most commonly defined as a subtle, but measurable memory disorder. A person with MCI experiences more memory problems than expected within the normal aging process, but does not show other symptoms of dementia, such as impaired judgment or reasoning [7]. However, these problems are in general not serious enough to interfere with daily life. Therefore, persons with MCI do not meet criteria for being diagnosed with dementia. The best-studied type of MCI is called *amnestic MCI* and involves a memory problem while nonamnestic MCI does not affect memory [8] [9]. MCI may, but does not have to emerge to dementia. Most commonly, the type of dementia that patients with MCI are at risk to develop is Alzheimer's Disease, but other forms of dementia, such as Vascular Dementia or Frontotemporal Dementia may occur as well [10].

1.3   Avatars and Elderly People

One approach by different AAL-research groups to raise the level of acceptance of assistive technologies is the usage of virtual faces as part of the graphical user interface (GUI). Most research groups focus their work on characters that are not photo-realistic. Some of these approaches in research and more literature can be found in the last year's conference proceedings [11].

At the Austrian Institute of Technology, a pre-study ([12], [13]) dealing with photo realistic avatars applied within GUIs for people with dementia brought promising results. Observations could show that avatars of known faces (formal and informal caregivers) are liked as GUI component by people of the target group and may be used as an *eye catcher* when presenting new information on displays.

Due to the fact that the number of participants within the pre-study was very small, further investigations have been made within the project Avatars@Home.

2   Aim of the Study

The aim of the study is to investigate the suitability of "graphical user interfaces based on photo-realistic avatars" for the interaction of elderly people (with and without Mild Cognitive Impairment) with smart home environments.

To evaluate possible applications of avatars for assistive technologies, a user interface with a photo-realistic avatar and synchronized synthetic speech was compared with similar user interfaces, showing either the same face as video or photo, or the same sequence of synthetic speech in combination with text or as voice only. The aim of the study was to elicit information about the acceptance and likability of avatars within the target group, as well as the influence of the user interface design on task-performance of the user.

3   Study Design

For this study different types of user interface designs have been evaluated with elderly people (with and without Mild Cognitive Impairment). From the initial phase of the project onwards the project team aimed to meet the needs of the target group and provided all information in a way that is easy to understand for all involved persons, in particular the potential test persons. To do so, the main steps were supervised by an expert of gerontology. Furthermore, a "project information folder" and the "informed consent form" were translated following the "easy to read guidelines" by experts of Innovia[1]. The translated versions were validated with persons of the target group before being used in the project.

3.1   Tasks for the Usability Study

For the usability study a test scenario was developed consisting of three kinds of tasks:

Information Tasks: Test subjects were requested to remember information about appointments, news-headlines, weather forecast, etc.
Activity Tasks: Subjects had to perform different activities within the usability lab like: closing a door, watering the flowers, turning off the coffee machine, etc.
Performance Tasks: Step by step the test participants were requested to bring shapes of paper into a certain order.

In total 5 different blocks of tasks were generated, each block consisting of an information, an activity and a performance task. Thus, the task sample consisted of 15 different tasks. The sequence of tasks remained the same for all test subjects. The presentation order was randomized to avoid negative rating effects. Each order of presentation mode was used once for one member of both target groups.

3.2   Selection of Test Persons

The recruiting of potential test persons for the study was performed by a gerontologist using his direct connections to memory clinics, by presenting the project to an Alzheimer affiliation group. In addition, information material was spread via interest groups of elderly people and participants of former usability studies were contacted by mail.

Candidates were requested to get in contact with the responsible person of the usability lab to define an appointment.

The inclusion criteria for the tests were:

- Age: 60 to 75
- Being diagnosed with no (MMSE 28-30) or "amnestic Mild Cognitive Impairment" (MMSE 24-27)
- Fluent German speaking
- Sufficient vision and powers of hearing
- Signed "Informed Consent Form"

Exclusion criteria were

- Being diagnosed with dementia or any other neurodegenerative disease
- People who have any other psychological diagnosis

---

[1] www.innovia.at

- Persons who are dependent on a guardian ("ger.: besachwalterte Personen")
- People with a Vision < 0,2
- People with a hearing loss > 30 dB (when using hearing aids)

3.3   Selection of Faces

Test persons were able to choose one of four different faces for the "personal assistant" which accompanied them during the test series (see fig. 1) The aim was to have young and old, female and male faces. Four persons could be found within the teams of AIT and CURE that agreed to serve as "models" for the study. These persons were not involved in the user trials and thus unknown to the test persons.

Each of these models was videotaped reading the information of the 15 different tasks. The models were requested to read the text in a neutral way, with clear voice, avoiding moveing the head too much. In a next step the recorded videos were cut into short videos for each single task. The generation of the avatars was done by the "Department for Language and Communication" at the Berlin Institute of Technology. They are experienced in creating avatar sequences and synchronizing videos with synthetic speech.

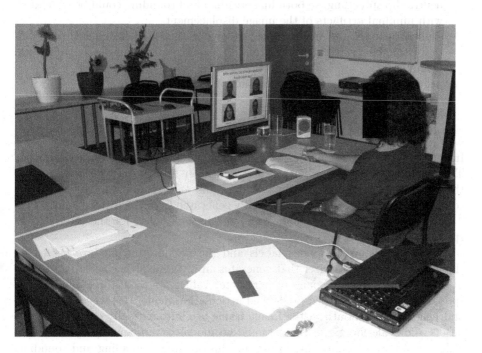

Fig. 1. Setting of the usability lab with a test participant choosing one of the four faces for different personal assistants

3.4   Processing of Videos, Avatars and Synthetic Speech

The audio tracks were extracted from the recorded videos. The audio files were labeled on phoneme level using the analysis and annotation tool *praat* [14]. The result was a phone chain plus phone durations per utterance. Praat was also used to extract the fundamental frequency contour (F0) of the speech signals. Synthetic audio speech was generated by the phone labels, phone durations and the F0 contours where the waveforms were rendered by the mbrola speech synthesizer [15]. One male speaker turned out to speak with relatively high F0. For him the voice de4 was chosen as this voice produces better results at higher F0 than the voices de2 or de6. The voices de3 (female) and de2 (male) were chosen for the other speakers due to subjectively best synthesis quality at the given phonetic descriptions.

The avatars of the speakers were created by the image based visual speech synthesis module of MASSY [16]. This software produces synthetic visual speech by the manipulation of a single image of a speaker. Mouth opening/closing and lip spreading/rounding is simulated by appropriate displacements of parts of the image. The procedure for creating the avatars consisted of three steps. First, one video frame for each of the speakers was selected from the videos. Selection criteria for the image were

- neutral lip spreading: so both lip spreading and rounding could be simulated with minimal artifacts of the image displacement
- slightly open mouth: this provided image data inside of the inner lip contour that could be stretched or compressed according to various degrees of mouth opening
- neutral lip opening: provided visibility of upper and/or lower teeth according to the speaker's characteristics
- open eyes
- absence of motion blur

In the second step a set of feature points was manually marked in each image. These feature points describe the outer and inner lip contour, the upper teeth, the jaw contour from left to right jaw joint, and an area that surrounds the jaw contour. A triangle mesh is automatically generated from the feature points. Fig. 2 shows the marked feature points and the triangle mesh for the elderly male speaker.

In the third step the phone labels and the phone durations are passed to the visual speech synthesizer that generates an image sequence according to the utterance: a sequence of pairs of parameter values for mouth opening and lip spreading is generated by a predefined articulation model [17] where the width and height of the mouth in the image frame are automatically considered (the offsets and scale factors of the articulation model were manually optimized in order to obtain adequate lip closure and lip opening, spreading and rounding magnitude). Image frames for the utterance to be synthesized are generated by displacing the triangle mesh and hence the image pixels that are inside the triangles. Videos are generated from the image sequence at the frame rate of

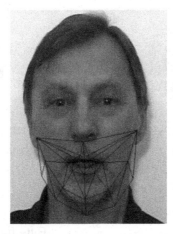

Fig. 2. Triangle mesh of feature points

the original video recordings. The synthetic audio was also used in audio only stimuli (voice- interface) as well as paired with the utterance in orthographic form (text-interface), paired with a still image of the speaker (photo-interface), paired with the synthetic video of the speaker (avatar-interface), and paired with the original video recording (video-interface).

3.5   The Test-Tool

For the "Wizard of Oz' study a test-tool was needed that fulfilled the following criteria:

- provide an easy-to-handle tool for the tests
- being able to allow different sequences of presentation modalities
- being able to handle the different types of multi-media data
- being visually adjustable in an easy way

The test-tool was created using Microsoft PowerPoint 2007 (see Fig. 3). For each of the 4 faces a presentation was generated that showed each task in every presentation mode on a single slide. After each block of tasks (see section 3) a navigation slide was inserted giving the possibility of jumping to the first task of the next block, presented in a certain presentation mode.

3.6   Technical Setting

The test series took place in the laboratories of CURE. All interface conditions were presented on a 19 inch Belinea monitor with a resolution of 1024x768 pixels. The distance between the monitor and the test person was approximately 50 centimeters. The "Wizard of Oz" sat behind the test persons and controlled the test-tool via a Lenovo X61 notebook. Speech was presented with REVEAL stereo loudspeakers. All trials were video recorded.

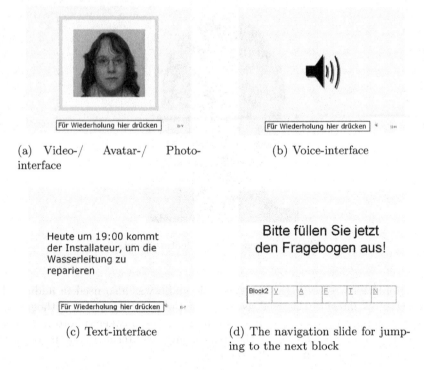

(a) Video-/ Avatar-/ Photo-interface

(b) Voice-interface

(c) Text-interface

(d) The navigation slide for jumping to the next block

Fig. 3. Examples of the test-tool for the younger female face. As the video, avatar and photo interface was based on the same material, the screenshot looks the same.

4   Course of the Test Series

After reading and signing the informed consent form (IC) test persons could select one of the 4 different faces for the virtual assistant. Subsequently the Mild Cognitive Impairment (MCI) screening was conducted with the Mini Mental State Examination (MMSE). Subjects were grouped into MCIs and non MCIs on the basis of the results. The MCI group was defined with a MMSE level between 24-27 points. People with a result higher than 27 points were defined as non MCIs.

Before starting the test series, the test persons were instructed to memorize information and accomplish tasks given by the virtual assistant. If the information or task was not understood the test person had the chance to replay the actual task-instruction, but not more than 3 times (controlled by the "Wizard of Oz"). All 5 different interface settings (video, avatar, photo, text, voice only) in each case with 3 tasks (information, activity, performance) were presented in random order.

After each test block test persons had to fill in an acceptance questionnaire consisting of 4 questions referring to the system. Thereafter, the next test block was started.

After the last block the test persons were asked to rank the likability of the different presentation modes and to answer further questions concerning the presented system.

In the end of the test, the test persons were informed about their result of the MMSE test and where they could get further information on MCI and dementia, if needed. Finally the test persons were reimbursed by an allowance of EUR 30.-.

5   Results of the Study

In total 24 persons participated in the study Avatars@Home, 16 female and 8 male persons. The two groups, test persons with and without MCI, had 12 test persons each.

Table 1. Statistical data

	Test persons with MCI	Test persons without MCI
number	$n_{MCI}=12$	$n_{nMCI}=12$
mean age	M=70.42; SD=6.53	M=65.50; SD=4.48
MMSE	M=26.33; SD=0.89	M=28.67; SD=0.49

Although the participants were grouped into the two groups, for some evaluations they were seen as one group of elderly people.

5.1   Selected Faces

13 of 24 persons selected the younger female virtual assistant followed by the older female (N=4) and male (N=4). The younger male face was only selected by three test persons.

Table 2. Selection of faces

	male	female
younger	3	13
older	4	4

5.2   Presentation Modes

The presentation modes were evaluated in two different steps:

1. Each presentation mode was evaluated right after the test person finished the block of tasks shown in this mode.
2. At the end of the last block the different presentation modes were ranked.

Ranking of the Presentation Modes. 24 users (MCI and non MCI) rated the video-interface best followed by the text-interface. The avatar-interface and the photo-interface are equally in the middle of the 5 point scale. The worst rating got the speech-interface.

Differences between MCI and non MCI users can be seen for the photo and the speech-interface. The photo-interface was more liked by the non MCI than by the MCI users. For the speech-interface it was reverse. MCI users rated the speech-interface worse than the non MCI users.

Table 3. Ranking of the presentation-modes

Group	Video		Avatar		Photo		Text		Voice-only	
	M	SD	M	SD	M	SD	M	SD	M	SD
Both	1.42	0.93	3.33	1.13	3.33	1,27	3.04	1.04	3.88	1.39
MCI	1.42	1.16	3.33	1.23	3.08	1.16	3.00	0.85	4.17	1.27
nMCI	1.42	0.67	3.33	1.07	3.58	1.38	3.08	1.24	3.58	1.51

Acceptance of the Presentation Modes. Overall results of the acceptance analysis show that all modes were rated between very good and good on a 5 point Likert-Scale (very good-very bad) with text-interface rated best (M=1.31; SD=0.72) and speech-interface rated worst (M=1.52; SD=0.91). Video, avatar and photo-interface were rated equally good.

Differences between MCI and non MCI ratings can be seen for the avatar and the photo condition. The avatar-interface is rated worse by users with MCI (M=1.56; SD=0.93) than non MCI users (M=1.36; SD=0.77). For the photo-interface a contrary result can be shown.

Table 4. Acceptance of the presentation-modes

Group	Video		Avatar		Photo		Text		Voice-only	
	M	SD	M	SD	M	SD	M	SD	M	SD
Both	1.46	0.87	1.46	0.81	1.41	0.81	1.31	0.72	1.52	0.91
MCI	1.52	0.91	1.56	0.93	1.30	0.5	1.27	0.5	1.48	0.8
nMCI	1.4	0.86	1.36	0.77	1.52	1.04	1.35	0.9	1.56	0.99

The synthetic voice was the same for all presentation-modes. Being rated after the test series on a 5 point Likert-Scale (very good - very bad) was M=2.75; SD=2.11. Persons with MCI rated the voice worse (M=3.0; SD=2.04) than non MCI users (M=2.5; SD=2.24).

5.3   Performance

In order to investigate the differences between MCI and non MCI users within each presentation mode (video, avatar, photo, text, voice only) Chi-square tests were conducted. Because of the small sample Fisher's exact tests were computed (significant when $p < 0.05$).

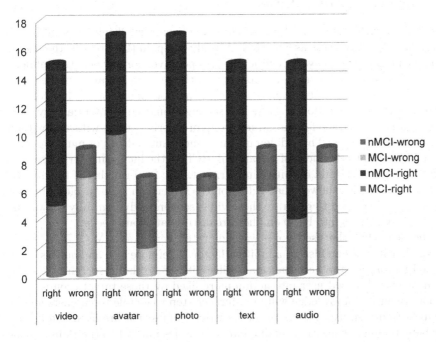

Fig. 4. The graphic shows the number of blocks that were completed without any mistake (right) or at least with one mistake (wrong) per target group and presentation mode

For the video, photo and speech interface the Fisher's exact tests were significant with $p_{Video}=0.045$, $p_{Photo}=0,034$ and $p_{Speech}=0.005$. Non MCI users could solve more tasks within the blocks than MCI users.

In the avatar and text condition the Fisher's exact tests were not significant with $p_{Avatar}=0.185$ and $p_{Text}=0.200$. Non MCI users could not solve more tasks within the blocks than MCI users. Results show that in the avatar and text-interface MCI users performed as good as non MCI users with more solved tasks ($N=10$) than non MCI users ($N=7$) in the avatar-interface (see fig. 4).

5.4   Possible Usage and Personalization

The users rated the likability to use such a system in their home environment on a 5 point Likert-Scale (yes-no) with $M=2.33$; $SD=1.27$. MCI users rated the utilization of the system worse ($M=2.75$; $SD=1.42$) than users without MCI ($M=1.92$; $SD=1.00$), but overall both groups gave positive feedback.

Having the possibility to choose other faces for the virtual assistant, 41.7% of the test users would choose a family member, followed by a "friendly face" with 16.7%.

6   Discussion and Outlook

The different kind of presentation modes did not have as much influence on the task performance of the users as expected. A study in Spain [18] brought the results, that the presence of an avatar neither has any positive, nor any negative influence on recall. The fact, that in the avatar and in the text presentation mode people with MCI performed not significantly worse than people without MCI could be a hint, that a combination of those two settings could be a potential way of designing a user interface for the target group of elderly people, with and without cognitive restrictions. Thus, different kinds and combinations of multi-modality should be put into the focus of research on HCI for the increasing target group of elderly people with mild cognitive impairment. The final ranking of the different presentation modes showed that videos on the screen can raise the acceptance of the system. The need to generate those video sequences dynamically shows, that more investigations into R&D on photo-realistic avatars are needed.

The fact, that the used voice was not rated very good (M=2.75;SD=2.11) shows that its use can also be a limiting factor. Therefore also an analysis on the crucial factors for the acceptance and likability of synthetic speech is essential to make speech based user interaction more liked by those target groups.

The generated knowledge will be a further step to enable researchers and developers to design user interfaces for Assistive Homes that are liked and used by the baby boomer generation coming into ages. Especially when the Baby Boomer generation heads towards 75+, the need for all kinds of assistance will increase. Industrialized countries have the chance to get prepared for this situation by supporting research in all fields dealing with supporting strategies and assistive technologies for elderly people.

If pharmacy and medicine are not able to stop neurodegenerative diseases such as Alzheimer's disease, it might be up to Assistive Technology to provide tools, devices and services which are able to compensate not only cognitive deficits. Even though it is not a pleasant vision, but maybe the day comes when virtual nursing agents have to substitute a weakened family background. For such situations highly efficient and sophisticated tools with adequate user interfaces have to be provided, which are not just accepted but also liked by the user. This can be realized by binding the user emotionally to the system to avoid rejection and attempts to defeat or fool the system. [13]

Acknowledgements

Avatars@Home is funded by the Austrian Research Promotion Agency (FFG) within the benefit program. The authors want to thank all participants of the test series for participating in this study.

References

1. Helal, S., Mann, W.C., El-Zabadani, H., King, J., Kaddoura, Y., Jansen, E.: The Gator Tech Smart House: A Programmable Pervasive Space. IEEE Computer 38(3), 50–60 (2005)

2. Haigh, K.Z., Kiff, L.M., Myers, J., Krichbaum, K.: The Independent LifeStyle Assistant^{TM} (I.L.S.A.): Deployment Lessons Learned. In: AAAI WS on Fielding Applications of AI, San Jose, CA (July 2004)

3. Wu, P., Miller, C.: Results from a Field Study: The Need for an Emotional Relationship between the Elderly and their Assistive Technologies. In: 1st International Conference on Augmented Cognition, Las Vegas (2005)

4. van Berlo, A., et al: Design guidelines on smart homes. A COST 219bis Guidebook (October 1999)

5. Wancata, J., Musalek, M., Alexandrowicz, R., Krautgartnerd, M.: Number of dementia sufferers in Europe between the years 2000 and 2050. European Psychiatry 18, 306–313 (2003)

6. Pfizer Corp Austria GmbH: Praesentation der Studie Alzheimer - Herausforderung für Gesellschaft, Medizin und Pflege (09 2005), http://www.pfizer.co.at/... [200807]

7. Alzheimer Association: Mild cognitive impairment (mci) (2006), http://www.alz.org/national/documents/topicsheet_MCI.pdf [11/03/2008]

8. Alzheimer Association: Mild cognitive impairment, http://www.alz.org/alzheimers_disease_mild_cognitive_impairment.asp [11/03/2008]

9. Mayoclinic: Mild cognitive impairment - mayoclinic.com, http://www.mayoclinic.com/health/mild-cognitive-impairment/DS00553%20 [11/03/2008]

10. Memory, Aging: Ucsf memory and aging center | mild cognitive impairment (mci), http://memory.ucsf.edu/Education/Disease/mci.html [11/03/2008]

11. Morandell, M., Hochgatterer, A., Fagel, S., Wassertheurer, S.: Avatars in assistive homes for the elderly. In: Holzinger, A. (ed.) USAB 2008. LNCS, vol. 5298, pp. 391–402. Springer, Heidelberg (2008)

12. Morandell, M., Fugger, E., Prazak, B.: The Alzheimer Avatar - Caregivers' Faces Used as GUI Component. In: Eizmendi, G., Azkoitia, J.M., Craddock, G. (eds.) Challenges for Assistive Technology AAATE 2007. Assistive Technology Research, vol. 20, pp. 180–184. IOS Press, Amsterdam (2007)

13. Morandell, M.: Day Structuring Assistance for People with Alzheimer's Disease. Master Thesis at the University of Linz, Austria, inaccessible until October 2010 (2007)

14. Boersma, P., Weenink, D.: Praat: doing phonetics by computer (version 5.1.15). [Computer program] (2009), http://www.praat.org/ [30/08/2009]

15. Dutoit, T., Pagel, V., Pierret, N., Bataille, F., der Vrecken, O.V.: The MBROLA project: Towards a Set of High Quality Speech Synthesizers Free of Use for Non Commercial Purposes. In: Proc. ICSLP 1996, Philadelphia, USA (1996)

16. Fagel, S.: Merging methods of speech visualization. ZAS Papers in Linguistics 40, 19–32 (2005)

17. Fagel, S., Clemens, C.: An articulation model for audiovisual speech synthesis - determination, adjustment, evaluation. Speech Communication 44(1-4), 141–154 (2004)

18. Ortiz, A., del Puy Carretero, M., Oyarzun, D., Yanguas, J.J., Buiza, C., Gonzalez, M.F., Etxeberria, I.: Elderly Users in Ambient Intelligence: Does an Avatar Improve the Interaction? In: Stephanidis, C., Pieper, M. (eds.) ERCIM Ws UI4ALL 2006. LNCS, vol. 4397, pp. 99–114. Springer, Heidelberg (2007)

Effects of Aging and Domain Knowledge on Usability in Small Screen Devices for Diabetes Patients

André Calero Valdez[1], Martina Ziefle[1], Andreas Horstmann[2], Daniel Herding[2], and Ulrik Schroeder[2]

[1] Human Technology Centre, Humtec
[2] Computer-supported learning research group, Department of Computer Science
RWTH Aachen University, Germany
calero-valdez@humtec.rwth-aachen.de

Abstract. Technology acceptance has become a key concept for the successful rollout of technical devices. Though the concept is intensively studied for nearly 20 years now, still, many open questions remain. This especially applies to technology acceptance of older users, which are known to be very sensitive to suboptimal interfaces and show considerable reservations towards the usage of new technology. Mobile small screen technology increasingly penetrates health care and medical applications. This study investigates impacts of aging, technology expertise and domain knowledge on user interaction using the example of diabetes. For this purpose user effectiveness and efficiency have been measured on a simulated small screen device and related to user characteristics, showing that age and technology expertise have a big impact on usability of the device. Furthermore, impacts of user characteristics and success during the trial on acceptance of the device were surveyed and analyzed.

Keywords: Usability, Aging, Health care, Performance, Small screen device, Perceived Ease of Use, Perceived Usefulness, Technical experience, Domain knowledge.

1 Introduction

An ever-increasing amount of technical devices with small screens and complex hierarchical menu systems surge into every day life. A simple press of a button on a mobile phone can connect the device to the Internet and add to the unknowing customers bill. Such handling errors on mobile phones are - though bothersome - a mere hassle compared to severe consequences of difficulty in using technical devices in a different context. Small-screen-device penetration in varying medical contexts is soaring for certain diseases. Individual disease related bio-physiological parameters are monitored electronically in order to regulate application of drugs and even enhance connectivity to nursing staff, physicians or family members. Slick usability is becoming the critical factor for acceptance, sustainability and competitive capacity of any mobile technical system, especially in regard of demographic changes, world wide increasing life expectancy and the resulting increase of older users. The share

A. Holzinger and K. Miesenberger (Eds.): USAB 2009, LNCS 5889, pp. 366–386, 2009.

of population over the age of 65 has already reached 20 percent in Germany in 2008 and is expected to swell to a 38 percent level in 2038 [1]. Similar forecasts apply to many western European countries [2]. Usage of electronic devices is also becoming decreasingly voluntary because of either work or everyday life requirements (e.g. [3, 4]). This impact will be even stronger concerning medical appliances of mobile devices. Since the increase of age related illnesses like diabetes accompanies both demographic change and sedentary lifestyle, medical care and age appropriate independent domestic care can only be economically realized through technical solutions (e.g. [5]).

Designing such solutions in a self-explanatory and usable way for heterogeneous user groups has not been realized to date [6, 7, 8]. Device development is still dominantly technical-oriented and criteria of usability and learnability are mostly applied subordinately, if at all [9]. This is directly related to the development of these devices through computer scientists and engineers, and lack of harmonization with psychological and ergonomic knowledge of necessities, capabilities and cognitive structures of the end users.

This paper examines the usability of a small screen device for diabetes patients. In the following, first, the importance of diabetes as a main civilization disease is outlined, followed by the status of knowledge regarding the usability of small screen devices, in combination with the impact of the diverse user group, which is using these devices. The chapter closes with the research questions addressed by a usability experiment.

1.1 Diabetes and Technology

Diabetes mellitus is a metabolism dysfunction, which affects about 8 million people (10% of the population) in Germany alone and for the year 2010 an increase of up to 10 million affected is expected. Diabetes and secondary disorder treatment already covers 20% of Germany's compulsory health insurance funds expenditure. Diabetes alone is expected to cause a hole of 40 billion Euros in Germany's health care budget in 2010 [10].

Diabetes predominantly causes a dysfunction of the blood glucose metabolism and is caused by different phenomena. The body produces either too little insulin or no insulin at all. In some cases the available insulin can no longer be effectively used by the body to regulate blood glucose levels. Generally two types of diabetes are differentiated.

Type-1-Diabetes
Diabetes mellitus type 1 occurs mostly in younger adults between the age of 5 and 50, but can also occur later in life. Type-1-diabetes is an immune mediated disease but causes for its incidence are still unknown. Genetic factor, viral infections and environmental influences are expected to contribute to type-1-diabetes. The immune system of affected patients destroys the pancreas' beta cells, which then no longer produce insulin, causing hyperglycemia. The main symptom of type-1-diabetes is absolute insulin deficiency. Only 8-10% of all diabetes patients are type-1-diabetics [11].

Type-2-Diabetes
Diabetes mellitus type 2 occurs mostly after the 40th year of one's life but increasingly often occurs in children and younger adults today. Main causes for type-2-diabetes are obesity and lack of physical exercise. Typical secondary disorders encompass hypertonia (high blood pressure), micro- and macroangioma (mostly benign tumors) and arteriosclerosis. The main symptom of type-2-diabetes is body cell insulin resistance. This forces the pancreas into an overproduction of insulin (referred to as hyperinsulinism) to prevent hyperglycemia, which further raises insulin resistance in all body cells. This relative insulin deficiency can lead to absolute insulin deficiency when the pancreas' insulin production collapses. About 90% of all diabetes patients are type-2-diabetics [11].

Secondary Disorders
Chronic high blood glucose levels cause long-term damage to the vascular and neural system. Over-frequent exposure to hyperglycemia manifests in diabetic heart disease, retinopathy (eye damage), nephropathy (kidney damage), and diabetic neuropathy (neural damage). These degenerative effects lastly cause blindness, renal failure, amputations and heart failure.

A persisting type-2-diabetes illness may also cause cognitive deficiencies, especially in patients older than 50 years executive functions and the neurocognitive processing speed are affected. Episodic memory, word flow and semantic memory though seem to be unaffected by type-2-diabetes [12].

Another frequent symptom of diabetes is hypoglycemia (insufficient blood glucose level). If a patient's glucose level drops too far (e.g. the patient administers too much insulin) diabetic coma occurs. This constitutes a case of emergency since the patient can no longer help himself and instant application of glucose becomes necessary.

Diabetes Therapy
Goal of any diabetes therapy is a stable and healthy blood glucose level (<135mg/dl postprandial). This can be accomplished by multiple means. Oral anti-diabetic drugs can increase effectiveness of bodily insulin or decrease the rate of intestinal glucose reception. Depending on the severity of the disease, subcutaneous application of insulin is required. Insulin is mostly administered before or after meals, since eating has a big effect on blood glucose level.

Two types of insulin therapy are discerned. Conventional therapy (CT) follows a fixed injection plan and intensive conventional therapy (ICT) requires the patient to measure blood glucose level and inject insulin accordingly. ICT-patients can also be treated with an insulin pump - a device that constantly administers insulin over the day and that offers an interface to increase dosage after meals.

Type-2-diabetes can sometimes be treated by diet and physical exercise alone, since reduction of body weight can in some cases cause full remission [13].

Almost all therapy types require or can at least be assisted with mobile small screen devices, since monitoring, persisting and analyzing of blood glucose levels, insulin dosage and caloric intake increases therapy success, since their correlation and behavior can vary drastically between individuals.

1.2 The Usability Demands in Small Screen Devices

It is a central claim that mobile devices are designed to be in line with users' specificity and diversity. However, the intelligent interface design of mobile devices, which meets the demands and abilities of especially older users, is an extremely sophisticated task. Aging itself represents a highly complex process. Not all users age in the same way, and the onset of aging processes as well as the consequences show considerable differences across humans. Design approaches should therefore take the user-perspective seriously [14, 15, 16, 17]. This includes that adults' behavior with current technical devices is carefully studied and also, that user abilities are identified, which affect the interaction with interactive computing devices.

The miniaturization of small screen devices may also contribute to usability shortcomings. Beyond handling and visibility problems, the restricted screen space allows only little information to be displayed at a time. By this, memory load is increased. In addition, orientation in the menu is complicated, because users do not experience how the menu might be "spatially" structured and how the functions are arranged [6, 7, 18, 19, 20, 21]. In hierarchically structured menus disorientation occurs when complexity is high with respect to the depth and breadth of menu levels [18, 22, 23].

With respect to effects of users' age, the profound changes in sensory, physical, psychomotor and cognitive functioning over the life span are well known (e.g. [24]). These changes may account for older adults' lower performance when using technical devices. Furthermore, due to a different upbringing, older adults often have a lower technical understanding and are less experienced in computer usage. As a result, the majority of older adults possess limited computer knowledge, which may also account for differences in computer-based performance (e.g. [25, 26, 27]). However, it was found that age-related decreases could be compensated by expertise (e.g. [28]). Thus, performance of older adults can be just as good as that of younger adults when they can rely on elaborated domain-specific knowledge.

1.3 Questions Addressed and Logic of Experiment

The present experimental study addresses two basic topics: the impact of aging and domain knowledge of diabetes on task performance on a small screen diabetes living assistant. Therefore participants were selected from different age groups and screened for domain knowledge of diabetes. Additionally, expertise in technology was surveyed.

Although this study was primarily designed exploratory, the following outcomes were expected:

- Younger users, due to aging impacts on both cognitive and perceptual abilities, outperform older users (e.g. [6, 8, 12, 29]).
- Users with higher expertise in technology usage outperform users with lower expertise, due to conceptual transfer of navigation user interfaces (e.g. cell phone navigation) (e.g. [19, 24, 29]
- Users with higher domain knowledge outperform users with lower domain knowledge, due to improved understanding of tasks and higher appreciation of purpose behind functions of the user interface (e.g. a diabetes patient knows about bread unit calculation and its importance) (see [21, 26, 28]).

- Users with type-1-diabetes outperform users with type-2-diabetes, due to the nature of those two illnesses and the coinciding difference in domain knowledge. Type-1-diabetes patients require more frequent and stricter regulation of blood glucose levels as this type of diabetes usually occurs earlier in patients' lives. A good comprehension of the disease is critical for successful long-term treatment. Insulin medication is obligatory for this disease. Type-2-diabetes patients in contrast can be treated in many different ways. Some patients are only medicated with a single daily intake of an oral anti diabetic drug. Real time blood glucose regulation is often not as urgent for therapy success, since patients are mostly too old to experience long-term effects of the illness. Thus comprehension of the disease is not as exigent as in type-1-diabetes.

2 Method

The objective of the study was to understand influence of aging and domain knowledge on task performance on a small screen living assistant for diabetes patients and to gain knowledge of determining factors on navigation performance in small screen touch enabled devices. Since the current study claims to extend the earlier research, efforts were made to keep the method very similar to that used before. In this section the conceptual design and the procedure of the experiment are described.

2.1 Experimental Variables

In our study we considered five independent and five dependent variables. The first independent variable we examined is user age in order to measure influence on both task effectiveness (i.e. the amount of tasks solved correctly) and efficiency (the amount of time required to solve a task). Additionally we analyzed the influence of expertise with medical technology, overall technical expertise and in particular mobile phone navigation expertise on usability (as in EN ISO 9241-11, 1998) of the device. To measure impact of domain knowledge on effectiveness and efficiency knowledge of four key health parameters (blood glucose, HbA_{1c}, blood pressure, body fat percentage) were surveyed and aggregated as an independent variable.

As dependent variables five performances criteria were measured: success rate, total steps, detour steps, total time and time per step. Success rate is measured as the percentage of successfully performed task steps of each task. Effectiveness was not measured as a Boolean variable in order to account for users who were able to solve tasks mostly correct but missed a certain step to solve a task with 100% correctness. These users can still be viewed as effective, as not necessarily all steps are required in order to perform well enough for the device to be useful. Total steps are the amount of program interactions performed for a certain task. A user interaction is an interaction of the user, which changes the state of the program. Pressing on the non-interactive background or missing a button is not included in total steps. Many tasks could be solved in multiple ways allowing users to complete each task in differing amounts of total steps. Detour steps are all program interactions that do not account into solving the task at hand, such as navigation failures, accidently pressed buttons and unnecessary repeated input. Total time is the amount of time the users take to finish all tasks without account for reading time of task descriptions. Time per step is the average amount of time a user takes between to program interactions. A lower value represents a faster navigation pace but not necessarily a better navigation performance. Since total steps, detour steps, total time and time per step are also measured for unsuccessful tasks; data from these dependent variables must always be related to the success rate of the current task.

2.2 Participants

A total of twenty-three adults volunteered to take part in this study. In Figure 1, the age distribution of the sample is depicted. Among those, were seven young adults (2 males, 5 females) with a mean age of 27.4 years (SD = 2.6; range: 25 – 33 years), seven medium aged adults (2 males, 5 females) with a mean age of 51.3 years (SD = 8.3; range: 41 – 59 years) and nine older adults (3 males, 6 females) with a mean age of 67.9 years (SD = 7,8; range: 61 – 87 years). The younger participants were mostly university students of different academic fields (psychology, social science, engineering, medicine). Medium aged and older adults were reached by advertisement in local newspapers and through an exhibition on a local public diabetes convention and covered a broad range of professions and educational levels (e.g. administrative officers, secretaries, teachers, engineers, physicians).

Twelve participants were non-diabetic adults, who were mostly recruited through their social networks (3 males, 9 females, mean age = 44.8; SD = 18.4; range: 25 – 71 years). The eleven diabetic participants (4 males, 7 females; mean age = 56.7; SD = 16.8; range: 26 – 87 years) split up into a group of five participants diagnosed with Type-1-Diabetes (1 male, 4 females; mean age = 43.6; SD = 13.6; range: 26 – 64 years) and 6 participants suffering from Type-2-Diabetes (3 males, 3 females; mean age = 67.7 SD = 10.2; range: 59 – 87 years).

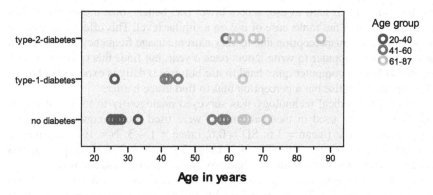

Fig. 1. Age and health status distribution and age group allocation

Regarding the recruitment of older participants a prototypical ideal participant "diabetic but otherwise healthy senior" was aimed at. All medium aged and older adults participating were either active parts of the work force or otherwise mentally fit and not hampered by stronger age-related sensory and psychomotor limitations. All participants were novices to the small-screen device we developed.

In order to relate effects on usage performance to prior experience with modern technology or experience with medical technology, participants were asked about their experience with different nonmedical (mobile phone, computer, GPS navigation, digital camera, microwave oven, alarm clock, gaming console) and medical devices (blood glucose meter, hearing aid, blood pressure meter, heart rate monitor, in-house emergency call). Since the study was performed using a small screen device user experience with mobile phones was surveyed thoroughly as well. Measurement was applied to functions of mobile phones (calling, text messaging, address book, calendar, integrated camera, integrated radio, integrated GPS navigation, internet browser, games, alarm, email). Two types of measurements were applied to three different areas of technology. Perceived Ease of Use (PEU) (see [30, 31, 32]) and Usage Frequency (UF) were aggregated for the three categories of expertise (expertise with technology, expertise with medical technology, expertise with mobile phone menu navigation). Perceived Usefulness (PU) was only measured for mobile phone functions because usefulness in this study was concerned as an attribute of a function of device, rather than of a device it self. In addition to any technical experience, domain knowledge about diabetes was collected for all participants.

Technical expertise was surveyed by measuring the PEU and UF. Both PEU and UF were measured on a Six-Point Likert Scale. PEU was examined with questions like "How easy to use is for you..." (1 = very easy, 2 = easy, 3 = rather easy, 4 = rather hard, 5 = hard, 6 = very hard). UF was similarly examined with questions like "How often do you use a..." (1 = Daily, 2 = 2 - 3 times a week, 3 = once per week, 4 = 1 - 2 times a month, 5 = 1 - 2 times a year, 6 = never). Total expertise is calculated as the square root of the product of the mean of all PEU and the mean of all usage frequency (UF) in order to reflect a value that is also on a Six-Point-Likert scale where 1 reflects a value with highest usage frequency and highest PEU and 6 represent the exact opposite. Intermediary values reflect both PEU and UF, with a tendency to rank equal values of PEU and UF higher than differing values. A person who uses a computer often, but finds it hard to use, scores lower (i.e. better), than a user that uses a computer not as often but ranks ease of use on a similar level. This effect is desired in order to account for misperception due to very extreme usage frequency (e.g. a person that only uses the computer to write letters once a year, but finds this task very easy). A person that finds a computer quite hard to use but uses it daily is expected to have a better computer expertise but a perception bias to find usage harder.

Expertise with medical technology was surveyed analogously to technical expertise. Devices that are used in medical context were used more frequently and perceived as easier to use (mean = 1.6; SD = 0,6; range = 1 – 3; N = 16) compared to normal technology (mean = 4.1, SD = 1.1, range 2 – 6, N = 23). Here, participants who had no experience with medical technology were not taken into account.

Mobile Phone expertise was also surveyed in the same manner (mean = 4.8; SD = 1.1; range = 2 – 6, N = 23) but additionally a total PU was measured (Six-Point Likert scale; 1 = very useful; 2 = useful; 3 = rather useful, 4 = rather not useful, 5 = not useful; 6 = not useful at all) for different functions of the mobile phone.

Domain Knowledge (mean = 4,0; SD = 1.7; range = 2 – 6, N = 23) was surveyed with a Five-point Likert scale ("How well do you know..."). Answers ranged from 1 = "very precise" to 4 = "not at all". Option 5 was labeled with "I don't know" and considers the item at hand to be completely out of the knowledge of the person contrasting to 4, where the person has heard about the measurement, but does not know about his own value for this measurement.

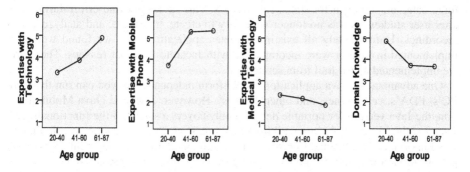

Fig. 2. Means plot of Expertises over age groups

ANOVA-analysis of these four factors regarding to age shows, that technical as well as mobile-phone expertise are both correlated with aging, where expertise with medical technology and domain knowledge are not (Table 1). This is expected since older users should be equally (if not more) prone to using medical technology as younger users. Especially in the case of diabetes domain knowledge should rather depend on the period of time being affected by the illness than on the numerical age.

Table 1. One Way-ANOVA table for mean differences of total technical expertise, total medical technical expertise, mobile phone expertise and domain knowledge regarding differences between the age groups

	SS	MS	df	F	p
Total technical expertise	10.65	5.33	2	6.20	< 0.01
Total mobile phone expertise	12.45	6.22	2	7.38	< 0.01
Total medical technology expertise	0.04	0.02	2	0.17	> 0.05
Domain knowledge	6.67	3.34	2	1.19	> 0.05

Post-hoc Benferroni testing shows that significant differences only exist between young adult users and older adult users for technical expertise (p < 0,01). Medium aged adults are both more experienced than older users and less experienced than younger users, but this difference fails to reach significance level (p < 0,12).

Significant differences in mobile phone expertise only exist between young adult users and both medium (p < 0.05) and older aged users (p < 0.01).

2.3 Development of a Small Screen Device for Diabetes Patients

Our goal is to develop a portable device that supports diabetes patients in their therapy and in their everyday lives. Before dealing with the hardware part of these devices, we wanted to concentrate on the usability of the software. For the user studies, we needed an application that can be run on standard hardware. Another constraint was given by our decision to use the Jacareto capture and replay toolkit (see [33, 34, 35]).

Jacareto can record the user interaction with a Java application, structure the captured data, and export it for statistical analysis. This saves time and effort during and after user studies, as it is no longer necessary to create, transcribe, and analyze video recordings. Unfortunately all existing diabetes applications that we found were not implemented in Java or were incompatible with Jacareto for other reasons. Therefore we implemented a new tool from scratch.

One advantage of Java applications is platform independence: you can run them on PC's, PDA's, cell phones, and other devices[1]. However, Java ME (Java Mobile Edition, the Java version for portable devices) only covers a subset of the functionality of Java Standard Edition. As compatibility with small-screen devices such as cell phones was important to us, we had to meet some constraints during development. For example, we did not use Java 5 language features, and we used the Abstract Window Toolkit (AWT) instead of the more modern Swing. Furthermore we made sure that the user interface could be used without a keyboard, so that it can later be used on a touch screen-enabled mobile device.

Instead of creating a specialized application that is only useful for certain diabetes patients, we decided to include features that are required for the different types of the disease. On the first start, the user has to set up the application by entering his characteristic values (such as drugs that he has to use regularly for his therapy).

The most important feature in everyday use is the so-called diabetes diary (Diabetes-Tagebuch). Every time the patient measures or influences his blood sugar concentration, he is supposed to insert the data into his diary, using a wizard-based input mechanism. For instance, when the patient has measured that his blood sugar is low and has therefore eaten dextrose to raise it onto a normal level, he creates a new entry. He enters the time, the measured blood sugar, and the bread units' equivalent of the ingested dextrose (1 bread unit (BU) = 12 g of carbohydrates). In the wizard, he simply skips values that were not relevant for this entry, such as the bolus insulin. The entered data is then shown in a column of a table. The tabular representation is based on the layout of the paper-made diaries that are in common use in Germany (see fig. 3), and that a large part of our target user group is already familiar with. 61 % of diabetes patients in Germany are using a diary to record their values; 91 % of these are keeping their diaries on paper.

Another application feature that is inspired by a paper template is the health passport, or Gesundheits-Pass. After each quarterly examination, the doctor writes down the results into this booklet. Like the diabetes diary, the values are entered in a table. For example, there are table rows for the HbA_{1c} value, the blood pressure, and the body weight. We were unable to use this table representation in our tool because of screen size constraints. That is why we only show the values of one quarter of a year, while the paper version has columns for four quarters. Besides the actual values of the quarter, we offered the possibility to enter the desirable values that the doctor determined

---

[1] Some of these devices may require a Java Runtime Environment from a third party vendor, such as IBM WebSphere Everyplace Micro Environment for Windows Mobile or Palm for instance.

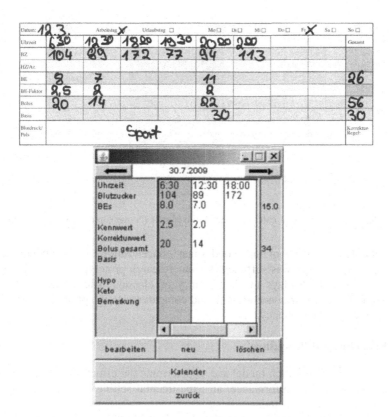

Fig. 3. The paper version of the diary (top) and the diary function of our application (bottom)

during the examinations. We added this feature because the health passport that was in use in 2008 had columns for desirable values. These columns were removed in the 2009 version of the Gesundheits-Pass.

For a successful diabetes therapy, it is important to teach the patients a basic knowledge of the nutrient contents of groceries. Especially patients who inject insulin need to calculate their drug dosage on the basis of the food they consume. Most people use a scale to measure the weight of the food, and then look up the bread units (BU) per gram in a nutrition table. After calculating the product of these values, they enter the result in their diabetes diary. We included an application feature that supports the user in looking up and calculating these values. He can choose a grocery from a predefined list, and then enter a weight or volume. The application then displays the bread units and kilocalories (see fig. 4). The user then repeats these steps with the remaining ingredients of his meal, and copies the resulting BU sum into his diary. To reduce the routine work of choosing the ingredients of regular dishes, the user can save a meal as a favorite, and reuse it later.

There are two features that help the patient to keep track of the progress of his therapy. The first one is the so-called plotter, which shows the course of measured values in a history diagram (see fig. 3). We only implemented a functional diagram

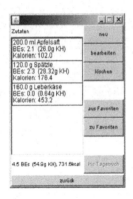 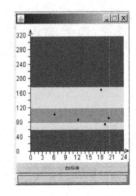 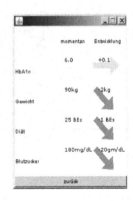

Fig. 4. The bread unit calculator (left), the plotter (center), and the screener (right)

for a one-day overview of the blood sugar concentration. The remaining diagram types are static, which was sufficient for our research prototype. The other feature is called screener. It displays the latest entry of characteristic values such as body weight and blood sugar concentration, and compares it to the previous entry. Colored arrows visualize the tendency.

2.4 Experimental Procedure

In order to test the research model and to determine the effects of domain knowledge and age variables on performance, an experimental setting with a simulated small-screen-device was conducted.

At the outset participants completed a paper-based questionnaire concerning demographical information (age, gender, educational achievement) and information about the familiarity with common technical devices, mobile phone and common medical technology (usage frequency as well the perceived ease of use). The assessing of demographic data was performed paper-based. It was of high importance that this questionnaire was realized prior to the simulation, as performance during the experiment could impact and bias self-assessment and thus expertise ratings.

After completing the survey participants were asked to perform a set of five tasks on the simulated device. Each task regarded a different main function of the device in order to create both a realistically setting and an interaction with various UI elements and uses cases for the device. All medical values that were to be entered into the device were predefined and given to the participant on a paper based task description to create equal preconditions for all participants. Task-information was printed on hardcopy and was available throughout. For all tasks a total time limit of 30 minutes was given implicitly (participants were told that the experiment should last for about 30 minutes). The fastest user completed all 5 tasks in about 6 minutes and all participants finished under 30 minutes.

After completion of the experimental tasks participants were asked to rate the perceived ease of use (PEU) and perceived usefulness (PU) of the used functions in the simulated device to assess the users acceptance of the device.

2.5 Small Screen Device Simulation

The diabetes living assistant was simulated as a software solution one a PC running Windows XP connected to an Iiyama AX3819UT touch screen (15" TFT-display, display resolution 1024x768 pixels). The simulated device spanned over 245x319 pixels (width = 7,27cm; height = 9,47cm) and was displayed in the center of the screen. The rest of the visible screen was covered with an opaque paper cutout to prevent any interaction with the operating system.

Participants were seated on a height-adjustable chair in a comfortable seating position. In order to control viewing conditions, participants were not allowed to choose viewing angle, viewing distance or inclination of the TFT-Monitor. If the participant required any corrective lenses, wearing those was obliged throughout the experiment. Lighting conditions were kept the same by choosing a room with no exterior lighting and a fixed interior lighting system.

2.6 Questionnaires

Perceived ease of use (PEU) and perceived usefulness (PU). Users' technology acceptance was assessed by original items from the Technology Acceptance Model of Davis (TAM [25]). The perceived ease of use (PEU) implies 'the extent to which a person believes that using a particular system would be free of effort', and secondly, the perceived usefulness (PU) which is defined as 'the extent to which a person believes that using a particular system would enhance his or her job performance' [25]. The validity and reliability of TAM items had been proven by several empirical studies (e.g., [30, 31, 32]), and also showed satisfactory values in this study. The 5 presented PEU items had to be judged on a six-point Likert-scale ranging from 1 (very easy) to 6 (very hard). PU items were rated on a six point Likert scale ranging from 1 (very useful) to 6 (not useful at all). Smaller values would reflect a higher acceptance of the device.

Experimental tasks. Five Tasks were to be solved by the participants. In particular users were first asked to setup the "freshly unboxed" device and enter information about their current therapy (i.e. insulin type, dosage and schedule as well as total weekly calories) with given fake values. Secondly users were asked to fill out their health passport in order to complete the setup of the device. After completing the first two tasks participants should enter three blood glucose measurements along with dietary information and insulin dosage for three times of a the given day (morning, noon, afternoon) into the digital diary. Again all values were predefined. The fourth glucose measuring was preceded by a task in which the users had to calculate the bread units of a given meal using the BE-Calculator of the device. This value was then to be used as dietary information in the digital diary for the fourth measurement. The last task required the user to simply view the daily blood glucose graph in the plotter of the device. All tasks were described in natural language but data for all input forms was given numerically.

In the following, examples of two task types are described:

- Example for 'digital diary'-task: *'After finishing configuration of your device, daily blood glucose measurements can be stored in the devices digital diary. Please enter the following measurement into the digital diary. This morning 9:20am:Blood glucose level 123; consumed 3 bread units, no correction of insulin dosage; no basal-insulin dosage; no hypo- or ketoacidosis was measured'*.
- Example for 'BE-Calculator-task: *'You are hungry and want to eat some fish sticks (200grams) and have a glass of apple juice (200ml). Please calculate the bread units for this meal using the BE-Calculator of the device.'*

3   Results

Results of this study were analyzed by one-way ANOVA, bivariate correlations, multivariate analysis of variance and univariate analysis of covariance and linear regression with a level of significance set at 5%.

The result section is designed as follows: first, we assess correlative relations and impact of individual factors (age, health status, domain knowledge, expertise with technology) on users' performance; second, a deeper analysis of aging effects on effectiveness and efficiency is conducted. At last effects of different factors on acceptance of the simulated device is presented.

3.1   Effects of Age, Domain Knowledge and Technical Proficiency on Performance

Relationship between factors and performance. To get a first insight into the data, correlations (Spearman rank analysis) between individual variables and performance measures were carried out (Table 2).

Table 2. Bivariate Correlations between age and user characteristics and performance

	Success Rate	Total steps	Detour Steps	Total Time	Time per step
Age	-0.664**	0.616**	0.472*	0.231	0.693**
Expertise with technology	-0.449*	0.330	0.244	0.476*	0,320
Expertise with medical technology	0.251	-0.266	-0.146	0.101	-0.342
Mobile Phone Expertise	-0.339	0.295	-0.006	0.393	0.301
Health Status	-0.179	0.342	0.181	-0.102	0.421
Domain knowledge	-0.53	-0.167	0.097	0.314	-0.244

$**p < 0.01$, $*p < 0.05$

Correlational analysis shows that only age and expertise with technology show a significant correlation with performance measures. Younger age is highly correlated with better effectiveness (r = -0.664) and efficiency. Younger users need less total steps (r = 0.616), make less navigation errors (r = 0.472) and have a faster navigation pace (r = 0.693). Expertise with technology is mostly correlated with effectiveness (r = -0.449) such that users with better expertise are more effective than users that are more inexperienced. This correlation does only affect one efficiency measurement significantly (i.e. total time r = 0.476), which also shows that higher expertise is related with better performance.

Apparently domain knowledge (r = 0.53) and health status (r = -0.179) seem to have an unexpected adverse effect on effectiveness, but further correlation analysis shows that age is highly correlated with health status, and health status highly correlated with domain knowledge (Table 3).

Table 3. Bivariate Correlations between age, health status and domain knowledge

	Age	Health Status	Domain knowledge
Age	1	0.509*	0.253
Health Status		1	-0.799**
Domain knowledge			1

$$**p < 0.01, *p < 0.05$$

To examine how domain knowledge and health status predict performance, two analyses of covariance (ANCOVA) were conducted using 'domain knowledge' and 'health status' as a covariate. The ANCOVA revealed no significant main effect for domain knowledge (F = 1.817; p > 0.05) with 'domain knowledge' as a covariate. Choosing 'health status' also reveals no significant main effect on effectiveness (F = 1.808, p > 0.05).

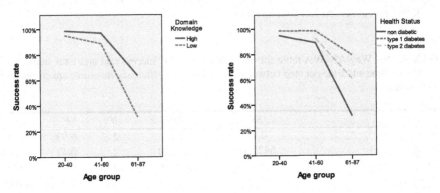

Fig. 5. Means plot: success rate over age group grouped by median split domain knowledge (left); success rate over age grouped by health status (right)

A means plot of effectiveness over age grouped by domain knowledge indicates that domain knowledge might have an effect on effectiveness, even though the significance level was not reached with the data at hand. Similar observations can be made for health status. Means for non-diabetic participants are lower than type 2 diabetes participants, which are lower than means of the type 1 diabetes participants (fig. 5).

3.2 Effects of Age on Navigation Performance

One-way ANOVA-analysis regarding to age group shows significant differences in effectiveness and efficiency between age groups (Table 4 and Fig 6). Since total steps, detour steps and time per step are also measured for tasks, which had not been successfully solved in the time given, correction with success rate has to be performed. Corrected measurements are calculated by division of original measurement by success rate and indicated by "[c]". For instance participants that only completes half of the tasks successfully get a two-fold "penalty" on all efficiency measures. This can lead to overblown values, if very low success rates (e.g. 1%) are reached.

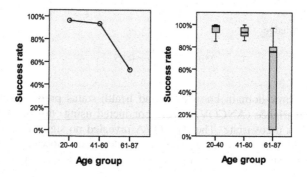

Fig. 6. Means plot of success rate over age group, higher values indicate better effectiveness (left). Box plot of success rate over age (right).

Table 4. One Way-ANOVA table for mean differences of success rate and total steps, detour steps, total time and time per step between age groups. All efficiency measures are corrected by success rate.

	SS	MS	df	F	p
Success rate	0.97	0.48	2	6.93	< 0.01
Total steps [c]	6475.41	3237.71	2	0.47	> 0.05
Detour steps [c]	1951.56	975.78	2	9.01	< 0.01
Total Time [c]	$5.02*10^{12}$	$2.51*10^{12}$	2	2.07	> 0.05
Time per step [c]	$6.89*10^{10}$	$3.45*10^{10}$	2	3.16	> 0.05

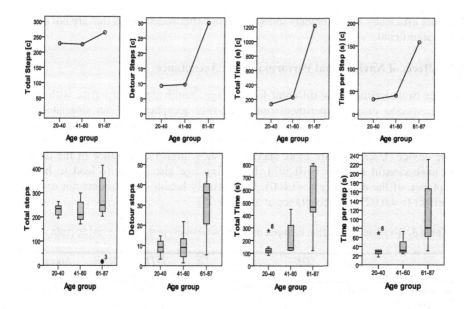

Fig. 7. Means plots of efficiency measurements over age group (top row); from left to right: (1) total steps over age group, (2) detour steps over age group, (3) total time over age group and (4) navigation pace (time per step) over age group; Box plots of efficiency measurements over age group (bottom row)

Comparison of effectiveness shows that younger and medium users performed almost equally, and both outperformed older users. Younger users (Y) averaged a success rate of 96% (SD = 6.2%), similar to medium aged (M) users, who reached 94% (SD = 5.2%), while older users (O) only managed to reach a mean success rate of 53% (SD = 41.1%). The mean of corrected total steps shows almost no difference between age groups ($M_Y = 228.3$, $SD_Y = 25.3$; $M_M = 225.9$, $SD_M = 48.0$; $M_O = 264.3$, $SD_O = 133.8$). Older aged users made more than three times more navigational errors (detour steps: $M_O = 29.9$, $SD_O = 16.1$) during task performance than medium and younger users (detour steps: $M_M = 9.7$; $SD_M = 7.07$; $M_Y = 9.2$; $SD_Y = 4.1$). Older users also required more time to complete all tasks than medium or younger aged users ($M_Y = 136.4s$, $SD_Y = 65.3s$; $M_M = 228.8s$, $SD_M = 139.4s$; $M_O = 1216.5s$, $SD_O = 190.0s$), which also reflects in a slower navigation pace. Older users trigger interactions almost 5 times slower than younger users, who are still almost 30% faster than medium aged users ($M_Y = 32.5s$, $SD_Y = 17.1s$; $M_M = 40.7s$, $SD_M = 18.4s$; $M_O = 157.9s$, $SD_O = 179.1s$).

Post-hoc Bonferroni testing shows that both younger and medium aged adults significantly ($p < 0.05$) outperform older adults in effectiveness (i.e. success rate). Younger and medium aged adults show now significant difference here. Apparently the only efficiency measure that shows significant mean differences is detour steps (corrected by success rate). Post-hoc Bonferroni testing showed similar effects for detour steps between groups as in success rate. Again younger and medium aged users outperform older users ($p < 0.05$), but fail to differ between each other significantly.

All other efficiency measurements show differences betweens means that are not statistically significant.

3.3 Effects of Navigational Performance on Acceptance

In order to understand how different factors (age, health status, expertise with technology, success rate in experiment) influence user acceptance of our simulated device non-parametrical analysis of correlations (Spearman's rho) was conducted (see Table 5). Both age and success rate show a significant correlation with acceptance of the device. Users that are more successful show higher acceptance of the device than unsuccessful users ($r = -0.507$). Increasing age also seems to lead to higher acceptance of the device ($r = -0.460$). Interestingly health status seems not to have any effect ($r = 0.027$) on acceptance at all ($p > 0.05$).

Table 5. Bivariate Correlation between user characteristics, performance and acceptance

	Age	DK	HS	TE	MTE	MBE	Success rate
Acceptance	-0.460*	0.200	0.027	0.276	0.409	0.287	-0.507*

*$p < 0.05$

DK = Domain knowledge, HS = Health status, TE = Expertise with technology, MTE = Expertise with medical technology, MBE = Expertise with mobile phones

To examine how age and success rate affect acceptance, two analyses of covariance (ANCOVA) were conducted using 'age' and 'success rate' as a covariate. The ANCOVA analysis revealed no significant main effect for user age ($F = 3.502$; $p > 0.05$) with 'user age' as a covariate. Choosing 'success rate' as a covariate also reveals no significant main effect on acceptance ($F = 3,378$, $p > 0.05$).

Linear regression though contradicts this finding: both age and success rate explain 65.5% of the variance of acceptance of the simulated device, but success rate is a stronger predictor for acceptance ($\beta = -0.486$, $p < 0.05$) than user age ($\beta = 0.241$, $p > 0.05$). This suggests, that high performance in initial usage of a device might have a high impact on acceptance of a new device.

4   Discussion and Conclusion

The present experimental study was conducted to provide deeper understanding of small-screen-device menu navigation performance in respect to age and domain knowledge in a medical context. A total of twenty-three participants accomplished five tasks designed for a diabetes living assistant. In order to analyze individual factors that may differentially affect user's performance, domain knowledge, expertise with technology, expertise with medical technology, expertise with cell phone navigation and their health status were surveyed and related to performance outcomes.

Basically it could be shown here that small screen devices do have a great potential in monitoring users' disease and therefore should be investigated in greater detail in the near future. The present study was one first step in this direction.

4.1 Impact of User Characteristics on Navigation Performance

The study confirmed the large impact of user characteristics on small-screen-device menu navigation performance. The first influential factor found in the analyses was the user's age. Users technical expertise also showed positive influence on users effectiveness and efficiency. User age in particular stood out to be the best predictor of navigational performance. Especially users that are older than 61 years show drastically inferior navigational performance. They tend to make more navigational errors, require more time between each interaction and are less effective in solving the tasks at hand.

Domain knowledge and health status show no significant influence onto the measured performance criteria, but comparisons of means denote a correlation might exist. Thus, we can assume that the navigational performance is indeed facilitated if users show a high knowledge in both, computer experience and disease-related knowledge. The fact that we could not statistically confirm this on the significance level set is presumably due to the comparably small sample size. Future studies will therefore examine the relationship between the computer and disease-knowledge by enlarging the participant group.

4.2 Potential Applications and Limitations of This Study

The findings underline earlier research regarding usability and aging. Further research is required to prove or increase understanding of influence of domain knowledge or diabetic status on user interaction, since findings of influence of age on performance are being studied. Further analysis of task related problems and identification of required neuropsychological characteristics for different tasks might lead into further input for further research. In this context, the comprehensibility of UI component labeling is of interest, as well as the investigation of the underlying mental model of device usage, which also could have impacted performance. Finally, individuals' coping styles should be incorporated into research scope.

However, the findings as promising as they are, also have to be looked at critically, especially as the participants here represented a kind of best-case scenario, which may not represent the whole group of ill and disease-limited patients.

1. Older non-diabetic users were recruited through social networks and are not representative in regard of total population. A best-case homogeneous user group might have led to skewed findings compared to different populations. Older users were all mentally fit, of relatively high education and mostly all of them had experience with computers.
2. All diabetic participants were highly interested in contributing to advancement of usability of diabetes small-screen-devices and thus highly motivated and to try out our prototype. Real life application cannot assume such perfect preconditions and must perfectly work even when the user is distressed, afraid or even in a case of emergency.
3. The software we used to simulate a living assistant was a prototype. Certain features that are not implemented yet, might have caused user distraction that would not have - or at least to a lesser extend - appeared in a finished retail product. Although this was not observed in the study during user interactions,

perceptual distraction during navigation should be assumed. The UI-components of the device themselves were not all perfectly chosen and will have to be iteratively optimized in the next steps (see [36, 37]).

4. Simulating a small-screen-device on a 15" display is a simplification of the situational context, since holding and handling a real small-screen device requires more cognitive and motor load (coordination of both hands). Therefore all performance measures are probably an overestimation of real life performance especially in regard to using fake values and not real user data. Users might be more concerned about using the device correctly and thus be more disturbed by unexpected behavior in a medical device. This sandbox operation might have led to a more carefree approach. This was reported by two older women (69 and 87 years old) who enjoyed trying out something new without fearing to break a device by accidental mishandling. Both agreed, that trying out the same device at home would have caused earlier abandonment of the device due to lower frustration thresholds. Although the opposite effect could also have occurred (i.e. giving up prematurely in order to not fail in front of a 'supervisor') no participant reported any such feelings after the test trial.

Acknowledgements

This work was funded partly by the RWTH Aachen postgraduate scholarships for students with excellent degrees and partly by the initiative of excellence of the German Federal Ministry of Education and Research.

References

1. Federal Statistical Office Germany: Germany's population until 2050 – 11th coordinated population projection, Wiesbaden (2006), http://www.destatis.de/
2. Siebert, H.: Economic Policy for Aging Societies. Springer, Berlin (2002)
3. Arning, K., Ziefle, M.: Understanding age differences in PDA acceptance and performance. Computers in Human Behaviour 23, 2904–2927 (2007)
4. Arning, K., Ziefle, M.: Barriers of information access in Small-Screen-Device applications: The relevance of user characteristics for a transgenerational design. In: Stephanidis, C., Pieper, M. (eds.) ERCIM Ws UI4ALL 2006. LNCS, vol. 4397, pp. 117–136. Springer, Heidelberg (2007)
5. Leonhardt, S.: Personal Healthcare Devices. In: Mukherjee, S., et al. (eds.) AmIware: Hardware Technology Drivers of Ambient Intelligence, ch. 6.1, pp. 349–370. Springer, Dordrecht (2006)
6. Ziefle, M., Bay, S.: How older adults meet complexity: aging effects on the usability of different mobile phones. Behaviour & Information Technology 24(5), 375–389 (2005)
7. Ziefle, M., Bay, S.: How To Overcome Disorientation in Mobile Phone Menus: A Comparison of Two Different Types of Navigation Aids. Human-Computer Interaction 21, 393–433 (2006)
8. Ziefle, M., Bay, S.: Transgenerational Designs in Mobile Technology. Handbook of Research on User Interface Design and Evaluation for Mobile Technology 1, 122–141 (2008)

9. Holzinger, A., Schaupp, K., Eder-Halbedl, W.: An Investigation on Acceptance of Ubiquitous Devices for the Elderly in a Geriatric Hospital Environment: Using the Example of Person Tracking. In: Miesenberger, K., Klaus, J., Zagler, W.L., Karshmer, A.I. (eds.) ICCHP 2008. LNCS, vol. 5105, pp. 22–29. Springer, Heidelberg (2008)
10. German Diabetes Union: Report on Public Health - Diabetes (2007), http://www.deutsche-diabetes-gesellschaft.de/
11. Tililil, et al.: Guideline of the German Diabetes Association for treatment of Diabetes melliutus type 2, 177 (1998)
12. Yeung, S.E., Fisher, A.L., Dixon, R.A.: Exploring effects of type 2 diabetes on cognitive functioning in older adults. Neuropsychology 23(1), 1–9 (2009)
13. Dixon, et al.: Adjustable Gastric Banding and Conventional Therapy for Type 2 Diabetes. The Journal of the American Medical Association 299(3), 316–323 (2008)
14. Holzinger, A.: Usability Engineering for Software Developers. Communications of the ACM 48(1), 71–74 (2005)
15. Holzinger, A., Searle, G., Kleinberger, T., Seffah, A., Javahery, H.: Investigating Usability Metrics for the Design and Development of Applications for the Elderly. In: Miesenberger, K., Klaus, J., Zagler, W.L., Karshmer, A.I. (eds.) ICCHP 2008. LNCS, vol. 5105, pp. 98–105. Springer, Heidelberg (2008)
16. Nischelwitzer, A., Pintoffl, K., Loss, C., Holzinger, A.: Design and Development of a Mobile Medical Application for the Management of Chronic Diseases: Methods of improved Data Input for Older People. In: Holzinger, A. (ed.) USAB 2007. LNCS, vol. 4799, pp. 119–132. Springer, Heidelberg (2007)
17. Holzinger, A., Searle, G., Nischelwitzer, A.: On some Aspects of Improving Mobile Applications for the Elderly. In: Stephanidis, C. (ed.) HCI 2007. LNCS, vol. 4554, pp. 923–932. Springer, Heidelberg (2007)
18. Lin, D.M.: Age differences in the performance of hypertext perusal. In: Proceedings of the Human Factors and Ergonomics Society 45th Annual Meeting, pp. 211–215. Human Factors Society, Santa Monica (2001)
19. Ziefle, M., Bay, S.: Mental Models of a Cellular Phone Menu. Comparing Older and Younger Novice. In: Brewster, S., Dunlop, M.D. (eds.) Mobile HCI 2004. LNCS, vol. 3160, pp. 25–37. Springer, Heidelberg (2004)
20. Ziefle, M.: Aging and Mobile Displays: Challenges and requirements for age-sensitive electronic information designs. In: Proceedings of the 9th International Conference on Work With Computer Systems, WWCS 2009, Beijing, China (2009)
21. Arning, K., Ziefle, M.: Assessing computer experience in older adults: Development and validation of a computer expertise questionnaire for older adults. Behaviour and Information Technology 27(1), 89–93 (2008)
22. Parush, A., Yuviler-Gavish, T.: Web navigation structures in cellular phones. The depth-breadth trade-off issue. International Journal of Human-Computer Studies 60, 753–770 (2004)
23. Westermann, S.J.: Individual differences in the use of command line and menu computer interfaces. International Journal of Human Computer Interaction 9, 183–198 (1995)
24. Craik, F.I., Salthouse, T.A.: Handbook of Aging and Cognition. Lawrence Erlbaum, Hillsdale (1992)
25. Ziefle, M.: The influence of user expertise and phone complexity on performance, ease of use and learnability of different mobile phones. Behaviour and Information Technology 21(5), 303–311 (2002)

26. Downing, R.W., Moore, J.L., Brown, S.W.: The effects and interaction of spatial visualization and domain expertise on information seeking. Computers in Human Behaviour 21, 195–209 (2005)
27. Czaja, S.J., Sharit, J.: Age differences in the Performance of Computer-based work. Psychology and Aging 8, 59–67 (1993)
28. Morrow, D., Miller, L.S., Ridolfo, H., Kokayeff, N., Chang, D., Fischer, U., Stine-Morrow, E.: Expertise and aging in a pilot decision making task. In: Proceedings of the Human Factors and Ergonomics Society 48th Annual meeting, pp. 228–232 (2004)
29. Ziefle, M., Schroeder, U., Strenk, J., Michel, T.: How young and older users master the use of hyperlinks in small screen devices. In: Proceedings of the SIGCHI conference on Human factors in computing systems 2007, pp. 307–316. ACM, New York (2007)
30. Davis, F.D.: Perceived usefulness, perceived ease of use, and user acceptance of information technology. MIS Quarterly 13, 319–340 (1989)
31. Adams, D.A., Nelson, R., Todd, P.A.: Perceived usefulness, ease of use, and usage of information technology: A replication. MIS Quarterly 16, 227–247 (1992)
32. Schajna, B.: Empirical evaluation of the revised technology acceptance model. Management Science 42, 85–92 (1996)
33. Schroeder, U., Spannagel, C.: The Role of Interaction Records in Active Learning Processes. In: Isaias, P., Nunes, M.B., dos Reis, A.P. (eds.) Proceedings of the IADIS Virtual Multi Conference on Computational Information Systems, pp. 99–104 (2005); Behaviour 21, 195–209 (2005)
34. Spannagel, C., Gläser-Zikuda, M., Schroeder, U.: Application of Qualitative Content Analysis in User-Program Interaction Research. Forum: Qualitative Social Research 6(2) (2006), http://www.qualitative-research.net/fqs-texte/2-05/05-2-29-e.htm
35. Jacareto Sourceforge Repository, http://jacareto.sourceforge.net/
36. Ziefle, M.: Spatial cues in small screen devices: Benefit or handicap? In: Proc. 12th IFIP TC13 Conference in Human-Computer Interaction, INTERACT (2009)
37. Ziefle, M., Bay, S.: How to overcome disorientation in mobile phone menus: A comparison of two different types of navigation aids. Human Computer Interaction 21(4), 393–432 (2006)

A Standalone Vision Impairments Simulator for Java Swing Applications

Theofanis Oikonomou[1], Konstantinos Votis[1,2], Peter Korn[3], Dimitrios Tzovaras[1], and Spriridon Likothanasis[2]

[1] Informatics and Telematics Institute, Centre for Research and Technology Hellas, 6th km Charilaou-Thermi Road, P.O. Box 60361, Thessaloniki, GR-57001 Greece
{thoikon,kvotis,tzovaras}@iti.gr
[2] Pattern Recognition Laboratory, Computer Engineering and Informatics, University of Patras, Rio Patras
{botis,likothan}@ceid.upatras.gr
[3] Sun Microsystems, Inc.,
17 Network Circle, MPK17-101, Menlo Park, CA 94025, USA
Peter.Korn@Sun.COM

Abstract. A lot of work has been done lately in an attempt to assess accessibility. For the case of web rich-client applications several tools exist that simulate how a vision impaired or colour-blind person would perceive this content. In this work we propose a simulation tool for non-web Java[TM] Swing applications. Developers and designers face a real challenge when creating software that has to cope with a lot of interaction situations, as well as specific directives for ensuring an accessible interaction. The proposed standalone tool will assist them to explore user-centered design and important accessibility issues for their Java[TM] Swing implementations.

Keywords: Human Computer Interaction, Web Accessibility, Simulation, software design, User-centered design.

1 Introduction

Despite the rapid evolution of Information and Communication Technologies (ICT) over the last years and the increasing acknowledgment of the importance of accessibility, the developers and designers of mainstream ICT-based products still act and struggle under total absence of structured guidance and support for adjusting their envisaged products and services with their user's real-time accessibility needs. As a result, a critical mass market of ICT based products, targeting older people and people with disabilities, remains highly locked.

Thus, the lack of non accessible software applications can cause large productivity losses, with many people being unable to fully participate at work, in education, or in a wide range of economic and social activities. The existing barriers on accessibility progress, reflects the current fragmented approaches to producing accessible products and services, which rather limit their economic potential and create a barrier to a thriving single market for them in Europe.

A. Holzinger and K. Miesenberger (Eds.): USAB 2009, LNCS 5889, pp. 387–398, 2009.

Moreover, there is mounting evidence that people with physical, cognitive and behavioural/physiological impairments such as visual, mobility, cognitive, hearing and speech inabilities, cannot access effectively ICT applications and services, especially due to the deficiencies in the ICT design and development process and the lack of accessibility support tools for developers.

So, many developers and designers are not fully equipped with evidence and knowledge related to the accessibility of their products or services [1]. Consequently, even the newest developments are not adequately accessible, missing the opportunity of tackling this issue at the development stage, when costs are compatible and solutions by design can be found, rather than making aftermarket adaptations. Moreover, they usually do not know how to specify accessibility requirements or how to design and test their product's compliance against the ones defined.

However, each user is different from the next. Monitoring the social situation in Europe with regard to the significant issue of inclusion, an estimate of >11% of Europe's population having some kind of disability, indicates that the spectrum of user diversity is enormous [2,3]. This becomes even more complex with the (un)availability of simulation and authoring tools for Java applications, since the power of Web 2.0 brings new sets of possibilities but also several challenges and difficulties on accessibility aspects [4].

Existing development tools and packaged solutions (e.g., several CAD tools or simulation environments) give little out-of-the-box assistance in most cases or, at worst, make it impossible to design and develop accessible ICT Java solutions for visual impaired users. It is important that the design and development of accessible ICT solutions can be supported in an automated fashion, as much as possible. Thus, although the existing simulation tools are considered to be a good reference for authoring tools, it is currently a work under progress. Thus, developers and designers need tools that provide process-integrated and constructive guidance to them in how to apply the accessibility principles.

This paper presents a Visual Impairment Simulation tool (VIStool) to achieve embedded accessibility design for the development of Java Swing applications.

2 Related Work

It is usually difficult for designers and developers to understand the problems users with disabilities face when accessing their software implementations that are not designed with their needs in mind. Thus, in order to have a better view of accessibility needs, in some cases developers use relevant simulation tools that can provide an opportunity for users to experience a software application (e.g. Web page) using simulated disabilities. It is obvious that simulation tools cannot simulate all kinds of disabilities and cannot provide the exact impact they have, but they provide certainly information and help designers make user interface content more accessible. These tools can enable, encourage, and assist users ("authors") in the creation of accessible applications.

On the visual impaired simulators side, work has already explored for Web applications accessibility as well as for assistive devices as the one that has been proposed by [5]. The aDesigner [6] is a disability simulator that helps Web designers to ensure that their pages are accessible and usable by the visually impaired. Web developers can use aDesigner in order to test the accessibility and usability of Web pages for low-vision and blind people. aDesigner is mostly oriented in testing the degree of colour contrast on the page, the ability of users to change the font size and the existence of alternate text for images. Color Doctor [7] is a simulator that can check colour accessibility. It converts any images displayed on the screen such as websites and other presentation contents into gray scale or colours that can be perceived by people with colour blindness. Color Doctor not only simulates website display, it is also possible to simulate real-time display of proposals, presentations, and moving images such as Flash by selecting the "Transparent" mode. Color Doctor shows the display content through four conversion filters: Grayscale, Protanopia, Deuteranopia and Tritanopia.

Furthermore, the Visual Impairment Simulator (VIS) for Microsoft Windows [8] is another tool that simulates everything displayed on users desktop. When the program runs, it manipulates the images on the user's screen so that it seems like the user has a visual impairment. Users can choose which impairment they wish to simulate from a drop down menu. The impairments that can be simulated are: Cataract, Color Blindness, Diabetic Retinopathy, Glaucoma, Hyperopia, Macular Degeneration, Magnifier and Retinitis Pigmetosa. The Vischeck [9] tool was created, in order to help web developers check their work for colour blind visibility. Also the WebAIM Low Vision Simulator [10] provides users with the opportunity to experience a web page as a user with visual disabilities. As it can be discerned, users can see the specified web page as if they suffer from Macular Degeneration, Cataract or Glaucoma. Finally Cambridge University has developed a vision impairment simulator which is included to the inclusive design toolkit [11]. The vision simulator modifies a digital image to show what the image might look like when viewed with a variety of different vision conditions. Each condition can be applied with different severity levels.

Even though most of visual impairment simulators are considered to be a good guide to the accessibility enhancement of Web sites and Microsoft applications, there are a number of major drawbacks regarding this effort. One major concern is that, they don't offer visual impaired simulation capabilities for other applications than Web such as Java Swing applications.

3 A Simulator for Embedded Accessibility Designs

3.1 Basic Concepts of the Simulator

The purpose of VIStool is to assist developers and designers to better empathise with those who have reduced vision capabilities, and to help understand how this loss affects the ability to interact with software applications and services. VIStool has been designed and developed with the objective to become a self learning software, which can be obtained as a standalone application, in order to present accessibility drawbacks and visual content problems of Java Swing applications to the developer/designer.

The philosophy behind the implementation presented here is to provide a complete free and open Source software application toolkit. It was considered that this kind of tool should be available as widely as possible and should be manipulated easily by experienced or not users. For that reason it was decided to be implemented with the Java programming language and its products that provide us an integrated machine-independent execution environment, simple GUI building facilities and so on. In our implementations we used the Sun Java™ Standard Edition Development Kit (JDK), the Java Accessibility Application Programming Interface (JAAPI) and the Netbeans IDE. A user-centered design method was applied in the implementation of the simulator in order to understand and extract user needs and system requirements as well as to produce appropriate design solutions that should be validated against the extracted requirements. For that reason two iterative phases have been decided to be followed. The first phase "Information Gathering" was conducted the first trimester of 2009, by performing a literature review survey. The user requirement collection started from the already assessed knowledge provided by the ACCESSIBLE project [12] software developers as well as representative organizations of people with disabilities. Identified users such as developers and designers have been contributing to the second phase, namely the interaction with users, which has been achieved via appropriate questionnaires and interviews. The results from the aforementioned phases were the foundation for the prototype design.

VIStool consists of the JAAPI that works as a bridge between the user's bundled Java Swing GUI and the simulator. The simulator has access to the impairments ontology that provides the information regarding all the implemented impairments and the appropriate controls over each of them. It then does the actual simulation which is presented back to the user through the user interface. A sketch of the VIStool architecture can be seen in Fig. 1.

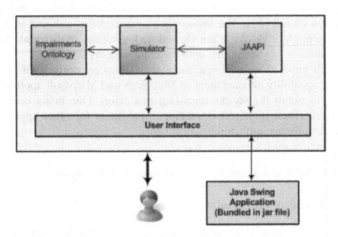

Fig. 1. VIStool architecture

3.2 Vision Impairment Capabilities

VIStool provides a reasonably accurate picture of some of the functional limitations and abilities that may be experienced with different types of visual impairments. Some of the most common causes of low vision in the developed world are cataracts, hyperopia, macular degeneration, glaucoma, etc. The International Classification of

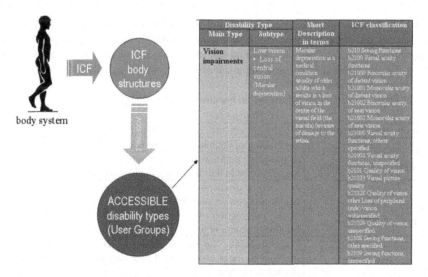

body system

Fig. 2. Using the ICF classification as a base for multiple user types

Functioning, Disability and Health (ICF) [13] provide a concrete classification of impairments of the body structures, which ensures no overlapping. In order to proceed in a structured manner, we worked on linking user types (e.g., disability types) to certain ICF body structures and their related impairments. The selection of the visual impairments that have been included to the simulator was based on the body functions from the ICF after translating them into relevant functional limitations. An example for the loss of central vision is depicted in Fig. 2.

The simulator has been developed in order to support colour blindness and various low vision impairments such as loss of central and peripheral vision, blurred vision, extreme light sensitivity and night blindness.

The loss of central vision creates a blur or blind spot, but side (peripheral) vision remains intact. This makes it difficult to read, recognize faces, and distinguish most details in the distance. Mobility, however, is usually unaffected because side vision remains intact. Typical examples of central vision loss are cataract and macular degeneration.

Loss of peripheral vision is characterized by an inability to distinguish anything to one side or both sides, or anything directly above and/or below eye level. However, central vision remains making it possible to see directly ahead. Typically, loss of peripheral vision may affect mobility and if severe, can slow reading speed as a result of seeing only a few words at a time. This is sometimes referred to as "tunnel vision". Typical examples of peripheral vision loss are glaucoma and retinitis pigmentosa.

Colour blindness is a lack of sensitivity to certain colours. Common forms of colour blindness include difficulty distinguishing between red and green, or between yellow and blue. Sometimes colour blindness results in the inability to perceive any colour. Colour blindness is problematic in driving vehicles, reading signs or maps, watching TV, working on a computer, understanding colourful graphics and charts etc. Within colour blindness capability the simulator supports Protanopia, Protanomaly, Deyteranopia, Deyteranomaly, Tritanopia, Tritanomaly, Achromatopsia and Achromatomaly.

All these impairments, especially central and peripheral vision loss, have a negative impact on computer use, since modern operating systems employ GUIs which require the use of eye-to-hand coordination to operate the mouse. A short description of the aforementioned low vision impairments can be found in Table 1.

Table 1. Low vision impairments short descriptions

Low Vision Impairment	Short Description
Cataract	A clouding of the lens in the eye that affects vision
Macular Degeneration	A medical condition usually of older adults which results in a loss of vision in the centre of the visual field
Glaucoma	A group of diseases that can damage the eye's optic nerve and result in vision loss and blindness
Retinitis Pigmentosa	In the progression of symptoms for retinitis pigmentosa, night blindness generally precedes tunnel vision
Hyperopia	Hypermetropia, far-sightedness or long-sightedness causes inability to focus on objects at near distance (or at any distance in extreme cases)
Night Blindness	Nyctalopia (Greek for "night blindness") is a condition making it difficult or impossible to see in relatively low light
Extreme Light Sensitivity	Hemeralopia (Latin for "sun blindness") is the inability to see clearly in bright light and is exactly opposite of Nyctalopia
Protanopia	A severe type of colour vision deficiency that is a form of di-chromatism in which red appears dark
Deyteranopia	A colour vision deficiency that moderately affects red-green hue discrimination
Tritanopia	An exceedingly rare colour vision disturbance in which there is a total absence of blue retinal receptors
Protanomaly	A mild colour vision defect which results in poor red-green hue discrimination
Deyteranomaly	Is by far the most common type of colour vision deficiency, mildly affecting red-green hue discrimination
Tritanomaly	A rare, hereditary colour vision deficiency affecting blue-yellow hue discrimination
Achromatopsia	Rod monochromacy is a rare, non-progressive inability to distinguish any colours
Achromatomaly	Blue cone monochromacy is a rare, total colour blindness that is accompanied by relatively normal vision, electoretinogram, and electrooculogram

3.3 Simulator Functionalities

The real-time interactions of developers with their Swing application forms are really important within the lifecycle design of their implementations. Thus, static and non interactive look and feel views of applications are fine when developers and designers developing independent forms, but this situation doesn't assist them concerning how form components should behave as the application is running in real time, where relevant modifications came about (e.g. modification of size, usage

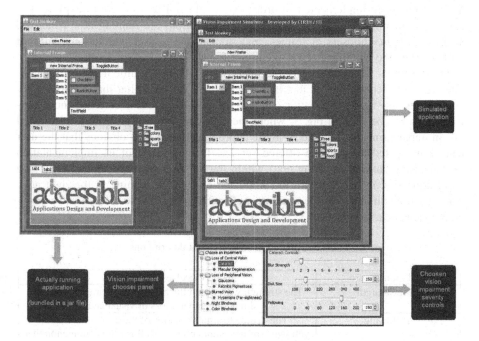

Fig. 3. VIStool initial state

Table 2. Comparative simulation controls usage

Simulation Controls Used	Cataract	Macular Degeneration	Glaucoma	Retinitis Pigmentosa	Hyperopia	Night Blindness	Extreme Light Sensitivity
Blur Strength	x	x	x		x		
Yellowing	x						
Disc Size	x	x					
Disc Count		x					
Disc Spread		x					
Relative Position to Mouse Cursor		x					
Severity Level			x				
Tunnel Size				x			
Whitening				x			
Transition Width				x			
Brightness						x	x

of combo boxes and buttons, change the ordering of tabs, etc). To overcome this, VIStool has been implemented in order to give the ability to users to explore, run and test their implementations. While their applications are running new windows, such as dialogs, choosers or frames, may appear due to user interactions. VIStool will simulate the window that has the user's focus.

On startup the user can specify the Java Swing GUI application he wants to simulate. The only requirement is that it is bundled in a jar file. After that VIStool takes control, runs the user's application and start the simulation. An overview of how VIStool looks can be seen in Fig. 3, where the user can select any of the implemented vision impairments to simulate from the appropriate panel. It is obvious that the user can be navigated through the offered services/functionalities of its implementation (e.g. pressing buttons, inserting text) within the left area where the actually running application lies, in parallel with the simulated application running in the right area. Thus, each modification to the running application is depicted to the simulated application view area.

Table 3. Simulation controls short descriptions

Simulation Controls	Short Description
Blur Strength	The strength with which the area in the cataract is blurred, simulating general loss of visual acuity
Yellowing	The degree to which the area of the cataract is made yellowish-brown, simulating the yellowing phenomenon that appears in some cases of cataracts
Disc Size	The size of the area affected
Disc Count	This controls the number of discs that are used to simulate the impairment. If this value is high, the disc will be more irregular, and if it is low, the impaired area will appear mostly or completely circular
Disc Spread	This controls how spread out the discs are that simulate macular degeneration. If the setting is high, the impairment will appear as a much wavier disc or even separated discs. If the setting is low, the impairment will appear mostly circular
Relative Position to Mouse Cursor	This setting was created to simulate the fact that many people with macular degeneration look out of the corner of their eye. So, the position of the centre of the impairment can be moved slightly, simulating this effect
Severity Level	This controls both the size of the unimpaired disc and the darkness of the impaired area. As the severity increases, the amount of unimpaired vision gets smaller and the impaired vision gets darker
Tunnel Size	The size of the area that is not yet completely black
Whitening	This simulates various degrees of a whitening effect where the entire inside of the visual field loses acuity
Transition Width	This setting changes how quickly the vision falls off to black. If it is set low, the transition will be a fairly sharp fade to black, if it is set to high, the transition will be gradual, starting at the centre of the visual field
Brightness	This controls how strongly the vision is illuminated

For each simulated impairment we can control various factors regarding the specific impairment from the appropriate control panel. This way we can simulate different degrees of severity for that particular impairment. The controls used by each impairment can be seen in Table 2, while a short description of the implemented impairment controls can be found in Table 3.

Consider the following case as an example. The user wants to simulate glaucoma. After selecting the impairment appropriate controls show up. As can be seen in Fig. 4 the potential patient that suffers from glaucoma may have some problems navigating through the application. This can be better understood when increasing the severity level of the impairment as seen in Fig. 5. This way the developer can better understand how a user with different degrees of vision impairments can perceive the application.

Finally, it is important to mention that the usage of a vision impairment simulator, like the proposed one, does not portray exactly how it is like to have a single or a combination of vision impairments. However, fully-sighted users who spend some time using the simulator's functionalities, throughout their design and development processes, can quickly acquire a sense of some of the design issues that should be taken into account in order to create accessible software applications.

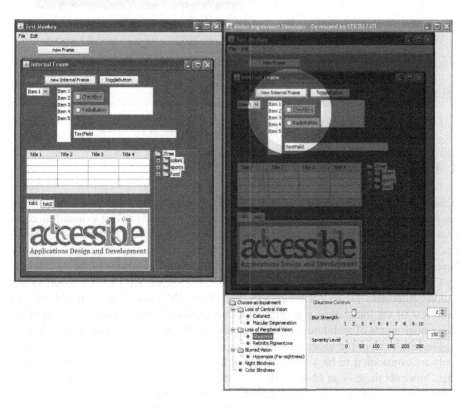

Fig. 4. VIStool simulating glaucoma

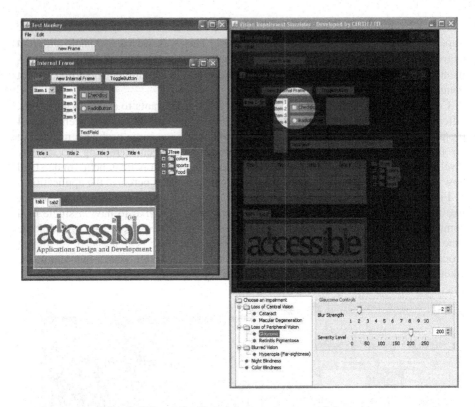

Fig. 5. VIStool simulating a more sever case of glaucoma

4 Evaluation Results

A first comparative evaluation analysis has been performed in order to verify design decisions and get input for modifications in future iterations. The evaluation comprised of a preliminary free exploration of the simulator's visual impairment capabilities of VIStool in comparison with existing vision impairment simulators. Thus, we have compared the functionality of VIStool with the functionalities of the Accessibility Colour Wheel [14], Inclusive Design Toolkit, aDesigner, ART [15], ColourDoctor, Colour Blindness [16], Vischeck, VIS, and WebAIM Low Vision simulators. An overview of the analysis is presented in Table 4, where we present the supported vision impairments of well known vision impairment simulators in addition to VIStool.

The results from the evaluation indicated that although most of existing simulation tools are considered to be a good reference for the simulation of Web pages and images, however there is an obvious shortage of simulators for Java Swing applications. Actually it should be considered that the support of these kinds of applications in contrast with Web and media content (e.g. images, presentations, etc.) is a work under progress.

Table 4. Comparative evaluation results

Vision Impairment \ Tools	VIStool	Accessibility Colour Wheel	Inclusive Design Toolkit	ADesigner	Art Simulator	Color Doctor	Color Blindness Simulator	Vischeck	VIS for Microsoft Windows	WebAIM for Low Vision Simulator
Deuteranope	x	x	x	x	x	x	x	x	x	
Tritanope	x	x	x	x	x	x	x	x	x	
Protanope	x	x	x	x	x	x	x	x	x	
Grayscale	x					x			x	
Cataract	x		x						x	x
Diabetic Retinopathy			x						x	x
Glaucoma	x		x						x	x
Hyperopia	x								x	x
Macular Degeneration	x		x						x	x
Retinitis Pigmetosa	x								x	
Protanomaly	x									
Deyteranomaly	x									
Tritanomaly	x									
Achromatopsia	x									
Achromatomaly	x									

5   Conclusion and Future Work

In this paper VIStool, a standalone tool for simulating various vision impairments, is presented. By making use of it developers would be assisted throughout the phases of the whole development process, while creating accessible Java™ Swing applications. With VIStool the developer has the ability to explore his application and test if the functionality he has implemented for each GUI component actually works and can be accessed by an impaired user. Furthermore, he can simulate not only various vision impairments but different severity levels for each impairment. Ongoing work is currently being done in several areas, including: improving VIStool capabilities in order to cover more vision or other impairment simulation situations and extending the functionalities of VIStool in order to apply the same simulation techniques to new and innovative JavaFX [17] applications that can be used for the development of Rich Internet applications.

Acknowledgments. This work was partially funded by the EC FP7 project ACCESSIBLE - Accessibility Assessment Simulation Environment for New Applications Design and Development, Grant Agreement No. 224145.

References

1. Harper, S., Khan, G., Stevens, R.: Design Checks for Java Accessibility. Accessible Design in the Digital World, UK (2005),
   http://www.simonharper.info/publications/Harper2005zr.pdf
   (accessed May 6, 2009)

2. Eurostat yearbook (2008), http://ec.europa.eu/eurostat (accessed May 6, 2009)
3. Report of the Inclusive Communications (INCOM) subgroup of the Communications Committee (COCOM), COCOM04-08,
   http://ec.europa.eu/information_society/activities/einclusion/docs/access (accessed June 22, 2009)
4. Kell, B., Sloan, D., Brown, S., Seale, J., Petrie, H., Lauke, P., Ball, S.: Accessibility 2.0: people, policies and processes. In: ACM International Conf. Proceeding Series, vol. 225, pp. 138–147 (2007), http://doi.acm.org/10.1145/1243441.1243471
5. Biswas, P.: Simulating HCI for special needs. ACM SIGACCESS Accessibility and Computing archive (89), 7–10 (2007) ISSN:1558-2337,
   http://doi.acm.org/10.1145/1328567.1328569
6. IBM Adesigner, http://www.alphaworks.ibm.com/tech/adesigner (accessed April 28, 2009)
7. Fujitsu Color Doctor 2.1,
   http://www.fujitsu.com/global/accessibility/assistance/cd/ (accessed April 28, 2009)
8. VIS simulator, http://vis.cita.uiuc.edu (accessed April 28, 2009)
9. Vischeck tool, http://www.vischeck.com (accessed April 28, 2009)
10. WebAIM low vision simulator,
    http://www.webaim.org/simulations/lowvision.php (accessed April 28, 2009)
11. Accessibility Inclusive Toolkit – visual impairment simulator, http://www-edc.eng.cam.ac.uk/betterdesign/downloads/impairmentsims/impairsim2.html (accessed April 28, 2009)
12. FP7 strep project ACCESSIBLE - Accessibility Assessment Simulation Environment for New Applications Design and Development, Grant Agreement No. 224145,
    http://www.accessible-project.eu/
13. ICF - International Classification of Functioning, Disability and Health. World Health Organization, http://www.who.int/classifications/icf (accessed March 10, 20009)
14. Accessibility Colour Wheel tool,
    http://gmazzocato.altervista.org/colorwheel/wheel.php (accessed June 28, 2009)
15. ART simulator, http://www.ubaccess.com/artsimulator.html (accessed May 28, 2009)
16. Colour Blindness Simulator –Etre,
    http://www.etre.com/tools/colourblindsimulator/ (accessed July 15, 2009)
17. JavaFX software applications, http://www.sun.com/software/javafx (accessed July 15, 2009)

AltText: A Showcase of User Centred Design in the Netherlands

Kathleen Asjes

Stichting Dedicon, Molenpad 2, 1016 GM Amsterdam, The Netherlands
kasjes@dedicon.nl

Abstract. In the information processing chain many documents are produced that are inaccessible to the reading impaired. The altText project aims to increase the accessibility of this content by: a) raising awareness among content providers about content adaption; b) allowing content providers to deliver content in a way that suits the needs of the information receiver; c) developing an online service that converts written text into several accessible formats (Braille, synthetic speech, large print or DaisyXML). The name of this service is the altText conversion portal. The paper argues that user centred innovation will be crucial to the success of this project.

Keywords: accessibility, altText project, hybrid content processing, accessible structures, usability research, conversion, user centred design, innovation.

1 Introduction

We are all familiar with the word 'accessibility', but what does it actually mean? When we talk about accessible content, for whom are we providing this content? Are we talking about a small percentage of users who are blind (about 1%) or do we include people with dyslexia (about 4%), or do we mean the 40% of users who use some kind of assistive technology on their computers?

In the current accessibility debate and activity, there is a strong focus on assistive technology and digital content. The accessibility of websites is assisted with worldwide known guidelines and closely monitored. The reasons for this focus are clear; digital media are rapidly developing and accessibility is mostly provided via add-on solutions to mainstream software and hardware. Although the recent developments in setting up e-government services and communication, official communication is still send in print in the Netherlands [1]. One example: you can fill in and submit your tax forms online, but the final outcome of the payment is send by post.

To facilitate the independence of anyone with reading disabilities, whether they are visually impaired, dyslexic or have trouble reading Dutch, the altText project aims to assist content providers in creating accessible material even when the chosen medium is analogue. The altText project integrates a number of findings and solutions from other projects (EUAIN [2], TeDUB [3], Lambda [4]) into one coherent framework. In this framework, solutions to the various problems of accessible text provision are implemented as views onto the content that therefore has to be provided in a semantically

A. Holzinger and K. Miesenberger (Eds.): USAB 2009, LNCS 5889, pp. 399–404, 2009.

enriched and structured way. The innovation within the altText project allows all content providers to produce accessible information in an efficient and cost-effective way. A content provider can upload documents to the portal where these are converted and made available in a collaborative web based editing environment. Content providers can review and correct the results of the conversion themselves, but also collaborate on difficult issues together with accessibility specialists. Lastly, the text is transformed into the preferred alternative format, for example Braille, synthetic speech, large print or DaisyXML (used for hybrid display of text synchronised with audio).

Interaction between the technical developers, experts from the accessibility organisation, end-users and content providers is crucial to the success of this project. This interaction has been facilitated all throughout the project, ensuring user centred innovation.

2 Accessible Structures

Increasingly more attention is being paid to accessibility in the traditional information processing chain. Accessibility is changing from being an afterthought that was considered at the end of the information provision process, to a catalyst for change at the beginning. Instead of allowing specialists to convert information into accessible formats after the content leaves the information chain, accessibility can be included in the core process. The technology is emerging which allows content providers to structure their information in such a way that it complies with existing accessibility legislation and guidelines. By integrating existing and emerging technologies within processing systems, it is possible to actively include the changing needs of end-users, and in so doing open new opportunities to provide information to everyone, in the format they prefer [5].

With a strong focus on creating awareness among content providers, the altText project aims to change the traditional information processing chain. The main focus in the project lies on applying 'accessible structures' to content. Structured information is the first big step towards high-quality accessible information. By structuring content more clearly, powerful new navigational possibilities emerge which are of benefit to all users, not only the visually impaired.

The structure of print material is mostly left to a range of visual cues, such as bold capital letters for the title of a chapter and bold italics for the heading of a subchapter. Even if adaptive technology allows the user to access a document, and read it following the 'visual structure' of the original, the adaptive device will flatten the visual structure, leaving a document with no structure at all. Without structure, navigation through the document is more difficult. Especially when the document is longer, finding information becomes more complex without structure detection. Providing documents with an "inner" structure makes it possible for adaptive devices to distinguish between a paragraph and a footnote, between a chapter and a subchapter. This enhances the level of accessibility of the whole document, allowing the user to move through it in the same way users without disabilities do when looking at the printed document, following the same "logic". In an ideal world, any document made available in electronic format should contain this inside structure which benefits everyone.

Highly structured documents are becoming more and more popular due to reasons that very seldom have to do with making them accessible to persons with disabilities. Some of the largest publishers are converting their old electronic texts into full XML documents so that it will allow them to look for certain portions of text that they can reuse in further editions, as well as to help them avoid double-production of the same text [6]. Whatever the reasons behind those decisions are, the use of highly-structured information is of great benefit to anybody accessing them, for whatever purpose. This then provides for:

- Consistency in the description of structural elements
- Understanding and predictability of structures
- Interaction with other standards
- Technical compliance with different devices
- Exchange of materials
- Flexibility and evolution

3 Hybrid Content Processing

Hybrid content is content that can be presented in different ways, suiting the preference of the content receiver. The altText project is one step towards the processing chain for hybrid content. It can inspire content providers in two ways; obtaining knowledge of accessible structures and creating output in several accessible formats. In the conversion portal workflow content providers enhance their content by adding structures. This workflow and online assistance also enables them to learn more about structured content and the problems involved in making content accessible. This awareness, and the learning curve of adding structure to content, can then be applied in their content creation phase. This is the first step towards total hybrid content processing by content providers. When they learn how to structure content, it will enable them to deliver content in different ways, suited to the needs of the information receiver.

The conversion portal is still an add-on accessibility layer, but has some major advantages over the current accessible content production methods. The portal assists the content provider to make their material accessible themselves. It is no longer the responsibility of the reading impaired receiver to ask for help when they receive inaccessible material, the content provider can take accessibility into account while producing material. Also, the content provider has a cost effective and flexible way of making their material accessible. They can do it themselves, on-demand, without asking help from a specialist organisation.

The conversion portal allows several input formats: word documents, open office text documents (.odt) and tagged .pdf. The main interchange format for content processing within the portal is XML. Accessible presentation imposes stricter requirements on the consistency of the structure and alternative structures in which the content is presented. Building on this level of strictness ensures a high level of consistency in the presentation. After investigation of several options, DaisyXML (www.daisy.org) promised to be the best interchange format for conversion into accessible output forms. DaisyXML is the format that provides the content in the portal with structural consistency that then can be modified according to taste. In order to convert the import formats into DaisyXML, the visual structure has to be included in the internal structure of the document. With the assistance of an analyser, the user learns if there are elements in the document that do not have a marked structure yet. The mark-up can be changed by the content provider, and analysed again until the validation process considers the document ready for conversion into DaisyXML. From the DaisyXML format, the portal can export the content as Braille print, Large Print or audio produced with synthetic speech. The audio can be presented with synchronised text online or plain audio (sent online or printed on cd). Depending on the type of information, the content provider and the receiver's preference, the output format can be different.

4   User Centred Innovation

The inclusion of all kinds of users is essential for solid system design in this project. Effort is invested to allow each participant in the chain of creation, (re)production, distribution and consumption processes to contribute to the development of the conversion portal. User and usability research are important throughout the development process, which is divided into several phases.

In the first phase of the project, content providers are requested to become involved in the project and provide documents they would normally send to out to the public, online as well as in print. The content providers in this case are civil servants from the communication department within a governmental organisation. This content is analysed to detect conversion issues in accessible content processing.

A first analysis of different input formats and material has revealed several issues with conversion into DaisyXML. The visual structure elements are very diverse and used in a different way each time. Test material has revealed that letter headings are often inserted into invisible tables, to allow a nice looking visual structure. This type of information is essential for the reader, and will likely be read out in the wrong order when converted into audio. Another problem in conversion is text hidden in pictures. The text in elements such as logo's and headers are often not recognised as text when they are embedded in a graphical picture. These types of elements need alternative text added, to allow including this text in the converted accessible format. From this phase we concluded the main issues in conversion are related to visual structure clues. See figure 1 for an example.

In the second phase of the project, the focus shifts from content providers to end-users, the receivers of accessible content. User requirements are determined for all output formats: Braille, synthetic speech, large print and DaisyXML. Most of these user requirements are known within specialist organisations, for example when it comes to Braille print according to National conventions, or large print. As synthetic speech is a rapidly developing technology, user requirement research was set up. A large group of students (n=1450) and adults (n=500) participated in rating several fragments in synthetic speech. This test group consisted of reading impaired and non-reading impaired respondents. Their appreciation varied widely, but generated a low average grade (4 out of 10). The additional feedback on the fragments has indicated that improvements have to be made to reading order, reading speed and pronunciation. This requirement has been taken on board in the system design, and in the implementation phase, trying to improve synthetic speech. In the last phase of the project, the improved speech will be tested with a similar group of end-users again.

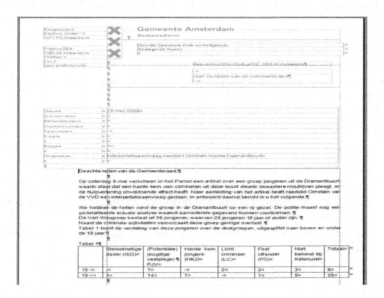

Fig. 1. Municipality letter. This is the first page of a letter to the municipality council members of Amsterdam. The (*grey elements*) are all part of the header. This includes information about the document (date, subject, sender, receiver) and contact information. While converting this document, the information placed in the *header on the first page* is not detected as text and disappears. The (*table at the bottom of the page*) is recognised as text, but once converted into audio, read out cell by cell, from left to right. This provides the reader with information about the categories and linear relations, but no insight into vertical relations within the category.

In the third phase, developers start building the altText portal framework. The information and issues gathered in the first two phases are addressed in the functional and technical design of the portal. In this development stage, the content providers are involved in building the prototype. After each development cycle, users of the portal (content providers) are requested to give feedback on its usability. Some first interviews among content providers has shown that the means for them to prepare their content have to be easy and straightforward, in order to convince them to make the effort. The project will therefore gather a list of suitable authoring tools for the annotation of different media types to allow the manual, semi-automatic or fully automatic conversion into accessible formats. Once the prototype has been developed, the output formats will be tested with end-users in the final phase of the project. This test will ensure if the gathered user requirements fit the expectations of a larger group of end-users.

5 Conclusion

The altText project will design and build a robust text processing framework. In the development of the framework prototype, interaction between the technical developers, accessibility experts, end-users and content providers plays an important role. Facilitating this interaction and including user- and usability research in the project, has ensured that the generated innovation is user centred. When the project finishes early 2010, the developed framework can be used to distribute content in suitable formats to end-users whilst maintaining the structural integrity of that content and ensuring the concerns of content providers are met.

The project will also provide some outcomes upon which further work can be based. In particular, the altText framework:

- provides a framework which can be integrated within different environments and organisations without the need for prior experience in this field
- allows interaction between users and content from a higher perspective
- identifies bottlenecks and optimal processes in the user to content communication path
- explores new user to content communication structures without disturbing existing ones

References

1. Van Dijk, J.A.G.M., Hanenburg, M.H.N., Pieterson, W.J.: Gebruik van Nederlandse Elektronische Overheidsdiensten in 2006. Universiteit Twente, Enschede (2006)
2. European Accessible Information Network, http://www.euain.org/
3. Technical Drawings Understanding for the Blind (TeDUB),
   http://projects.dedicon.nl/tedub/
4. Linear Access to Mathematics for Braille Devices and Audio-synthesis (LAMBDA),
   http://www.lambdaproject.org/
5. Franke, N., Keinz, P., Steger, C.: Testing the Value of Customization: When do customers really prefer products tailored to their preferences? Journal of Marketing 73, 5 (2009)
6. Müller, E., Andersson, S., et al.: Using XML for long-term preservation, Humboldt- Universität zu Berlin NDLTD (2008)

Usability Practice in Medical Imaging Application Development

Chufeng Chen[1], Jose Abdelnour-Nocera[1], Stephen Wells[2], and Nora Pan[2]

[1] School of Computing
Thames Valley University
St Mary's Road, Ealing – London UK, W5 5RF
[2] Siemens Molecular Imaging
23-38 Hythe Bridge Street
Oxford UK, OX1 2EP
chufeng.chen@tvu.ac.uk, jose.Abdelnour-Nocera@tvu.ac.uk,
stephen.wells@siemens.com, nora.pan@siemens.com

Abstract. Historically, development of medical imaging applications has focused on solving technical issues for small numbers of expert users. However, their use is now more mainstream and users are no longer willing to tolerate poor performance and usability. In this study we illustrate the application of user centred design methods in a medical imaging applications development company by using a usability comparative study of different regions of interest (ROI) tools. A use case analysis was used to judge usability efficiency and effectiveness of different ROI tools; and a user observation was also carried out which measured the accuracy achieved by these tools. We have found that useful results can be obtained by using these methods. We also generated some concrete suggestions that could be incorporated into future product development.

Keywords: User Centred Design, Medical Imaging, Siemens Molecular Imaging, Usability Comparative study, Region of Interest (ROI).

1 Introduction

Historically, development of medical imaging applications has focused on solving technical issues for small numbers of expert users. However their use is now more mainstream and users are no longer willing to tolerate poor performance and usability. Applying user centred design (UCD) methods for medical imaging applications should help to ensure applications are user friendly. In this study we illustrate the application of user centred design methods in a medical imaging applications development company (Siemens MI) by using a usability comparative study of different regions of interest (ROI) tools. Medical imaging applications often have a wide set of tools for drawing (ROIs) on medical images. These tools are used to delineate and quantify regions such as tumours. However, it is not clear which tools are better for end users in terms of effectiveness and efficiency. ROI tools need to be suitable for the particular needs of these users. A usability comparative study could be beneficial in improving the experience of users and also in avoiding the development costs of unnecessary features already present in existing tools.

A. Holzinger and K. Miesenberger (Eds.): USAB 2009, LNCS 5889, pp. 405–415, 2009.
© Springer-Verlag Berlin Heidelberg 2009

In section 2, this paper will review related studies for applying usability methods to this industry. Section 3 describes the development and practice of setting the ROI comparative study. Section 4 describes the methods used in the ROI comparative study. Results and findings are shown in section 5. Section 6 concludes the key challenges and findings of this study.

2 Background

People are living longer and longer and raising their life expectancy. However, diseases like cancer, diabetes and Alzheimer's etc. are becoming more frequent, and the number of chronically ill patients is also increasing. As a result, medical applications have become more and more important. These systems, however, are often not user friendly because of the complexity of medical applications. Furthermore, medical domain experts are no longer willing to tolerate poor performance and usability [1] & [6]. In order to improve usability of medical applications, many studies have focused on UCD process. For example, Zhang [2] developed a heuristic evaluation method which mainly focuses on medical devices' usability and safety issues. Palanque [3] also indicated that FDT (improvement of Formal Methods) can be applied in improving usability and safety of medical devices. Moreover, Bligard and Osvalder [4] developed an analytical approach for predicting and identifying use error (safety issues) and usability problems. However, these studies are analytical methods, and do not look at the user's experience.

In contrast, some studies have focused on the users' experience: Javahery & Seffah [5] considered a user study for improving medical device usability and safety. They evaluated a bioinformatics visualisation tool which was redesigned using a usability engineering framework called UX-P, which includes ongoing usability testing throughout the medical software design lifecycle. The UX-P framework provided guidance and structure during the early development phase of the product, and kept usability testing in the design lifecycle. Moreover, Ghulam [6] reviewed literature published from 1980 to 2005 in peer-reviewed journals of medical device technologies; they found that user involvement is a good method to improve usability of healthcare technologies. Furthermore, Silva [7] suggested using users' ideas for prototyping design of medical devices could improve usability of the user interfaces.

The above mentioned studies mainly revolve around the usability of medical devices rather than the software. However, some studies look at the usability of medical imaging interfaces. Mhiri and Despres [8] improved the medical imaging indexing efficiency by using the ontology method. They used the ontology technique to visualise the medical imaging reports through different semantic contents. Cannella [9] developed a new guideline to improve the usability of medical imaging applications' user interfaces. They created new abstract tags within medical imaging called the DICOM[1] format. These tags can be used by different medical imaging applications' interfaces, to automatically generate and standardise the visualisation and functionality of medical images.

---

[1] DICOM: Digital Imaging and Communications in Medicine (DICOM) is a standard for handling, storing, printing, and transmitting information in medical imaging.

These studies all concentrate on the visualisation of medical imaging user interfaces and there appears to be no prior usability research focussing on Region of Interest (ROI) tools used in medical imaging applications. Time is very important for these applications - an efficient, time-saving system results in higher patient throughput, which means both shorter waiting lists and, for private practices, more income. On the other hand, how good ROI tools are at doing what they are supposed to do is also important. An effective ROI tool results in accurate drawing and quantification.

These observations suggest that there is merit in conducting a usability assessment of ROI tools for improving efficiency and effectiveness. In doing this, it is also important to assess the benefits of considering UCD methods in the healthcare industry. By considering all the above issues, a usability comparative study of different ROI tools was conducted comparing different Siemens MI applications. As a result, it is possible to illustrate the benefits of using UCD methods for the future development of such products.

3   The Challenges of Applying Usability Methods to Medical Imaging Software

Introducing UCD to this kind of industry is a challenge because of the complexity of the medical imaging applications and the difficulties of getting large numbers of specialist clinical users for large usability studies. Furthermore, it can be hard to demonstrate to companies the value of adopting UCD in their development process as the benefits are not always easy to quantify. Relating sales to usability is complicated by the fact that these applications are high-value but sold in low-volume, and often bundled with other products.

In order to demonstrate the benefits of using UCD methods for medical imaging applications, we decided to study ROI tools as these are present in most applications, are implemented in a large variety of ways, and form a central and often time-consuming part of a doctor's workflow.

Most molecular imaging applications have a wide set of tools for drawing ROIs on medical images, e.g. drawing an ellipsoid around a specific area of interest such as a tumour. However, there appears to be no research to indicate which ROI tools are better for end users in terms of effectiveness and efficiency.

It is likely that some less user-friendly ROI tools may never be used at all. Some applications may include a range of tools which have almost identical functions (e.g. multiple tools that could be used to draw an ellipsoid). If the development of unnecessary or inefficient functions in these tools can be avoided this should both increase user satisfaction and reduce development costs.

It is also valuable to find out the best way of drawing ROIs in terms of optimising the usability efficiency of tools. Thus, the ROI comparative study compared the ROI tools of different applications to find evidence of useful features versus unnecessary ones.

We report our experience of doing the ROI comparison as a case study of implementing UCD methods in the development of medical imaging software. The ROI tools of each application were compared by a use case analysis to judge usability efficiency. To complement this, a user observation was also carried out which measured the accuracy achieved, the actual number of user actions and the time taken for each ROI tool when delineating a real tumour. The next section explains this in more detail.

4   Region of Interests Tools Comparison

We compared three different applications, which are listed as following:

Application **A** is a multi-modality oncology workstation application enabling advanced assessment of PET-CT[2]scans.

Application **B** is a client-server oncology platform that can review PET-CT scans.

Application **C** is an advanced workstation application for pre-clinical research that can analyze PET-CT scans.

Many of the tools can be regarded as falling under a small number of general types e.g. tools that create a 3D geometric shape as an ROI. This allows conclusions to be drawn about which general type of tools are most efficient.

Table 1. ROI tools in different applications

General Type	Specific Type of Tool	App A	App B	App C
2D geometric	Ellipse	YES	YES	YES
	Paintbrush shapes			YES
	Template shapes			YES
	Free draw shapes	YES	YES[3]	YES
2D iso-contour[4]	2D iso-contour	YES		YES
	Free draw 2D iso-contour	YES		YES
Convert 2D shapes to 3D	Convert 2D freeform shapes	YES		YES
	Convert 2D ellipses	YES		YES
3D geometric	Ellipsoid	YES	YES	YES
	Paintbrush 3D shapes (include Ellipsoid)			YES
	Template 3D shapes (include Ellipsoid)			YES
3D iso-contour	3D iso-contour (Threshold)	YES	YES	YES
Other special tools	Freeform Iso-contour	YES		
	Segmentation tools		YES	
	Interactive ROI threshold[5]			YES

---

[2] PET-CT: medical images include Positron Emission Tomography (PET) scans and Computed Tomography (CT) scans.

[3] Product B, Polyline is only really an annotation tool as quantification is not possible.

[4] Iso-contour tools allow users to automatically segment ROIs from a region.

[5] Interactive thresholding tools are similar to Iso-contour tools but using a different operating mechanism based on....

In addition, different applications often offer tools that can be regarded as being the same e.g. a tool to draw an ellipsoid, even if the exact sequence of mouse clicks is subtly different. This allows judgements to be made about which application has implemented a specific type of tool the best.

All available ROI tools in these applications were compared in terms of usability effectiveness and efficiency. ROI tools were broken down into use cases (the minimum user actions to create an ROI) for comparing usability efficiency.

Examples of an ROI tool are shown on figures 1 and 2.

All ROI tools of applications A, B and C are listed in table 1.

A use case analysis and user observation was carried out to compare the above ROI tools in terms of efficiency and effectiveness.

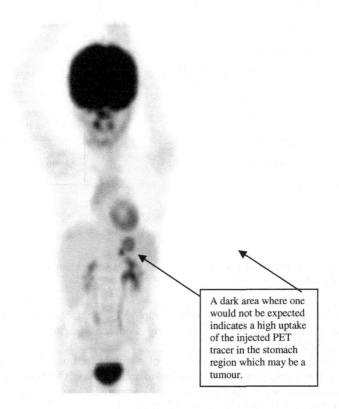

A dark area where one would not be expected indicates a high uptake of the injected PET tracer in the stomach region which may be a tumour.

Fig. 1. PET scan showing a tumour that needs to be measured

4.1 Comparison by Use Case Analysis

A use case describes what users can do in an application; it is represented as a sequence of simple steps. An example of a use case for creating an ellipsoid iso-contour is listed in table 2.

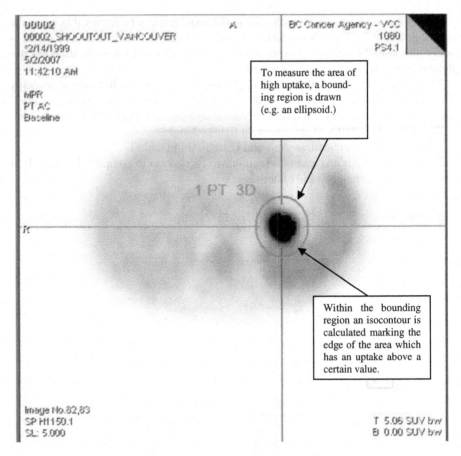

To measure the area of high uptake, a bounding region is drawn (e.g. an ellipsoid.)

Within the bounding region an isocontour is calculated marking the edge of the area which has an uptake above a certain value.

Fig. 2. Tumour segmentation by an ROI tool on an image slice through the volume of data at the level of the stomach

The standard actions needed to create a simple ROI using each tool were analysed. It could be argued that tools requiring a long sequence of actions are less efficient, and potentially less usable.

This analysis just looked at the creation of a simple ROI and did not include any fine tuning adjustments that could be applied to an ROI once it had been created.

Standard user actions in 2D ROI tools were compared. (Tools that allow the user to convert 2D shapes into 3D ROIs, and 3D ROI tools.)

Use case analysis allows the number of user actions to create ROIs to be compared in an objective manner. However, it is an abstract comparison of efficiency. In a real medical case the accuracy of the ROI is of great importance and so is the elapsed time taken to create it. An additional study with users was therefore carried out for measuring accuracy, the number of actual user actions, and the elapsed time taken to create an ROI on a real tumour when using each ROI tool.

Table 2. Example of a use case for isocountour tool

The Ellipsoid isocontour tool allows users to create an isocontour ellipsoid or sphere ROI covering multiple slices in the data series.

Standard user action	System response
1. Move the mouse cursor over the ruler icon and click on Ellipsoid isocontour (on the top right corner).	Display drop down list of different ROI tools.
2. Click and drag over the lesion area to draw the bounding ellipsoid shape.	Display bounding ellipsoid shape.
3. Adjust the SUV value in the input text dialog box to set the isocontour threshold that defines the ROI edge with the bounding shape.	Display isocontour SUV[6] edge.
4. Input label text for the ROI or just click OK.	A 3D ROI is created.

4.2 Comparison of User Observation

In order to complement the use case analysis, a user observation was arranged. Three experienced users were observed (one per application). Users were asked to follow a clinical scenario case and quantify the lesion as accurately and quickly as possible by using different ROI tools.

4.2.1 Scenario Case

A full body PET-CT DICOM dataset was selected as the scenario case. In this case there was a tumour in the stomach region. For this, they were asked to complete the following tasks:

1. Visualize the tumour and scroll through the slices to get a good visual impression of its size and shape. (Users were allowed to select different modalities of the dataset (i.e.Fused PET–CT or PET only) for the ROI quantification, and were allowed to select different zoom levels. Recording of the actual time and actual user actions to create the ROI started after this step).
2. Create a Region of Interest that covers the whole tumour.

---

[6] SUV Standard Uptake Value. A measure for the brightness of a voxel in PET image that is intended to be normalized and hence comparable between images.

3. Review the ROI and make any adjustments that are necessary to achieve an accurate delineation.
4. Measure the following values:
   a) Volume
   b) Max diameter
   c) Max SUV
   d) SUV mean

Users were asked to complete the above tasks by using each 3D ROI tool (2D ROI tools are not suitable for above scenario case). The time taken to use each tool was recorded. Approximately 20 minutes was taken for each user to complete the scenario for all the tools in one application.

4.2.2 Accuracy of Each ROI Tool

For the ROI comparative study, it was important to check if ROIs were drawn to an acceptable level of accuracy to avoid concluding that a tool is efficient if it draws fast but inaccurate ROIs. An assessment of the accuracy of a ROI requires a comparison to a 'gold standard' of some sort. This is difficult to achieve since the only definitive way to confirm the extent of a tumour is through surgical examination. It was decided that a reasonable approach would be to use an experienced nuclear medicine clinical doctor to delineate the tumour as accurately as possible, as if part of a diagnosis of the case without time constraints, and provide a report based on the scenario case dataset. He provided details on where he would place the ROI and what he thought the Max and Mean SUV should be.

These measurements could then be compared to the measurements of any future ROIs drawn on this tumour. ROIs with measurements that were close to this would be considered to be adequately accurate; those with a big deviation would be considered to be less accurate.

4.2.3 Limitation of the User Observation

A limitation of this user observation is that we only considered one user for each application rather than performing a large statistical survey. However, the purpose was simply to provide some confirmation from real examples for the conclusions drawn from the use case comparison.

The observation was performed on experienced users who work on the product definition and development of each application every day so were fully familiar with how all the tools functioned. It can therefore be assumed that there was no learning effect for these users in the order in which they used the tools. The purpose was to measure the speed and accuracy of a very experienced user using each tool on a real medical case. They were told to complete the scenario case as accurately and as quickly as possible. The learnability of each tool was not assessed in this study.

5 Discussion of Comparison

The use case analysis studied how many steps were required to create an ROI using each tool. We also conducted user observations to support the use case analysis and assess efficiency in terms of actual user actions, actual time and accuracy for completing the scenario. The discussions of our comparative findings are presented in the following sub sections.

5.1 Discussion of Use Case Analysis

The applications offer a wide variety of tools. We found that application **C** has the largest set of tools and **B** the smallest. However, this need not necessarily be a disadvantage as either application can contain the best tools available.

Looking at the standard user actions to create an ROI indicates that converting 2D shapes into a 3D ROI takes more user effort than the use of 3D iso-contour ROI tools and all ellipsoid tools. From this point of view, at least then these more sophisticated tools do indeed seem offer greater efficiency.

Use case analysis also indicates that equivalent tools in different applications require different numbers of user actions suggesting that some applications may have implemented tools in a more efficient and usable way. For example, applications **A** and **B** require two fewer actions than application **C** to create an ellipse, ellipsoid or 3D iso-contour.

5.2 Discussion of User Observation

The user observation of different types of tool showed that iso-contour tools (including an interactive threshold tool) have better accuracy and efficiency in terms of actual actions and timing. They required the least number of actions to adjust the initial ROI to make it accurate. This suggests that they are therefore suitable for a very busy environment (e.g. a medical doctor may need to complete up to 20 scan readings per day). The iso-contour tool of application **A** has the best timing and the iso-contour tool of application **B** has the best accuracy.

Tools to convert 2D shapes to a 3D ROI had the worst efficiency and the 3D geometric shape tools (without iso-contours) were in between.

Although most of ROI tools of application **C** required longer time and more actions, it provided almost all types of ROI tool which may suit users with different preferences. However, some of these tools have somewhat overlapping functionality which may be unnecessary (e.g. template and paintbrush, threshold and interactive threshold).

By considering use case analysis and user observation comparisons, we found that iso-contour tools (automatic contour) are the most efficient and among them, it was judged that iso-contour of application **A** has the best performance because it had a default pre-set threshold value for the isocontour edge. The choice of a sensible default meant that fine tuning was not required. It enables a user to complete an ROI drawing task in a short time.

5.3 Improvement Suggestions of the Comparative Study

The findings of the study were able to be fed back into the development process. For example:

1. Applying a pre-set isocontour threshold avoids the need for adjustment in most cases thus saving time.
2. An automatic calculation of ROI max diameter is efficient.
3. Some inefficient, inaccurate or overlapping ROI tools could be removed from future applications.
4. Manual drawing tools could be removed in favour of more sophisticated iso-contour tools.

The above suggestions could save development costs, improve the system efficiency, accuracy and increase the end-user satisfaction.

6 Conclusion

The complexity of medical imaging applications and the difficulties of getting large numbers of specialist clinical users for mass usability studies hinder the wide adoption of usability methods. However, we have found that useful results can be obtained by selecting suitable techniques, even if the scope of analysis and access to users are only limited. This is illustrated in this paper in the application of use case analysis (which does not require users) complemented by a small scale user observation to the topic of assessing the efficiency and accuracy of tools for drawing regions of interest. Possibly, the validity of our results was helped by the complexity of the specialist domain that the application is supporting and its small, relatively homogenous, well defined and known user base, which reduces the variability of findings. However, we also believe that the findings and benefits obtained with frequent direct access to end users cannot be replaced and are now working on suitable remote protocols to obtain usability and user experience data at different points in our lifecycle.

The study generated some concrete suggestions that could be incorporated into future product development. More importantly, it demonstrated that, despite the complexity of medical imaging and limited direct access to end users, the creative combination of relatively simple usability techniques yields tangible benefits, which pave the way for a broader adoption of UCD by development teams. Our future research will focus on methods and process integration and evaluation of the UCD process.

References

1. Timbleby, H.: User-centered methods are insufficient for safety critical systems. In: HCI and Usability for Medicine and Health Care, Austria, November 2007, pp. 1–20 (2007)
2. Zhang, J., Johnson, T.R., Patel, V.L., Paige, D.L., Kubose, T.: Using usability heuristics to evaluate patient safety of medical devices. Journal of Biomedical Informatics 36, 23–30 (2003)
3. Palanque, P., Basnyat, S., Navarre, D.: Improving interactive systems usability using formal description techniques: application to healthcare. In: HCI and Usability for Medicine and Health Care, Austria, November 2007, pp. 21–40 (2007)

4. Bligard, L.O., Osvalder, A.L.: An analytical approach for predicting and identifying use error and usability problem. In: HCI and Usability for Medicine and Health Care, Austria, November 2007, pp. 427–440 (2007)
5. Javahery, H., Seffah, A.: Refining the usability engineering toolbox: lessons learned form a user study on visualisation tool. In: HCI and Usability for Medicine and Health Care, Austria, November 2007, pp. 185–198 (2007)
6. Ghulam, S., Shah, S., Robinson, I.: User involvement in healthcare technology development and assessment, Structured literature review. International Journal of Health Care Quality Assurance 19(6), 500–515 (2006)
7. Silva, P.A., van Laerhoven, K.: Badideas for usability and design of medicine and healthcare sensors. In: HCI and Usability for Medicine and Health Care, Austria, November 2007, pp. 105–112 (2007)
8. Mhiri, S., Despres, S.: Ontology Usability Via a Visualization Tool for the Semantic Indexing of Medical Reports (DICOM SR). In: HCI and Usability for Medicine and Health Care, November 2007, pp. 409–414 (2007)
9. Cannella, V., Gambino, O., Pirrone, R., Vitabile, S., Legale, M.: GUI Usability in Medical Imaging. In: International Conference on Complex, Intelligent and Software Intensive Systems, pp. 778–782. IEEE, Los Alamitos (2009)

Current State of Agile User-Centered Design: A Survey*

Zahid Hussain[1], Wolfgang Slany[1], and Andreas Holzinger[2]

[1] Institute for Software Technology, Graz University of Technology, Austria
zhussain@ist.tugraz.at, slany@ist.tugraz.at
[2] Institute of Information Systems and Computer Media,
Graz University of Technology, Austria
a.holzinger@tugraz.at

Abstract. Agile software development methods are quite popular nowadays and are being adopted at an increasing rate in the industry every year. However, these methods are still lacking usability awareness in their development lifecycle, and the integration of usability/User-Centered Design (UCD) into agile methods is not adequately addressed. This paper presents the preliminary results of a recently conducted online survey regarding the current state of the integration of agile methods and usability/UCD. A world wide response of 92 practitioners was received. The results show that the majority of practitioners perceive that the integration of agile methods with usability/UCD has added value to their adopted processes and to their teams; has resulted in the improvement of usability and quality of the product developed; and has increased the satisfaction of the end-users of the product developed. The top most used HCI techniques are low-fidelity prototyping, conceptual designs, observational studies of users, usability expert evaluations, field studies, personas, rapid iterative testing, and laboratory usability testing.

Keywords: Agile Methods, Extreme Programming, Scrum, Usability, User-Centered Design, Survey.

1   Introduction

Due to their popularity, Agile software development methods are being adopted at an increasing rate in the industry. Recently, Dyba and Dingsoyr [1] presented a good review on the empirical studies of agile software development. However, agile methods are still lacking usability awareness in their development lifecycle, and the integration of usability/user-centered design into agile methods is not

---

* The research herein is partially conducted within the competence network Softnet Austria (www.soft-net.at) and funded by the Austrian Federal Ministry of Economics (bm:wa), the province of Styria, the Steirische Wirtschaftsförderungsgesellschaft mbH. (SFG), and the city of Vienna in terms of the center for innovation and technology (ZIT).

A. Holzinger and K. Miesenberger (Eds.): USAB 2009, LNCS 5889, pp. 416–427, 2009.

adequately addressed. Holzinger [2] points out the need for the awareness of various usability methods by software practitioners and their application according to the context of a project. Memmel et al. comment that "When usability engineering becomes part of agile software engineering; this helps to reduce the risk of running into wrong design decisions by asking real end users about their needs and activities" [3].

The efforts of integrating usability/HCI into software engineering have already been carried out for many years, e.g., IFIP WG 2.7/13.4[1] working group has been formed [4]. A recent work is compiled by Seffah et al. [5] in the form of a book containing chapters about various aspects of the integration of usability into the development process. However, since agile methods are a recent and emerging idea, there has not been much work carried out regarding the integration of usability/UCD into agile methods. The research carried out and presented in this paper aims at filling this gap and presents the preliminary results of a recently conducted online survey regarding the current state of the integration of agile methods and usability/UCD. The data was collected from 92 practitioners throughout the world. The results show that the majority of practitioners perceive that the integration of agile methods with usability/UCD has added value to their adopted processes and to their teams; has resulted in the improvement of usability and quality of the product developed; and has increased the satisfaction of the end-users of the product developed. The top most used HCI techniques are low-fidelity prototyping, followed by conceptual designs, observational studies of users, usability expert evaluations, field studies, personas, rapid iterative testing, and laboratory usability testing, respectively.

The next section thoroughly describes related literature studies. Section 3 describes details about the research method. Section 4 describes the results. Section 5 concludes the paper with future work.

2   Related Literature Studies

This section presents related work in two sub-sections: Related studies on agile usability/UCD in general and studies regarding surveys on agile methods and usability/UCD.

2.1   Related Studies on Agile Usability/UCD

In 2002, Kent Beck and Alan Cooper discussed the integration of XP, one of the popular agile methods, with interaction design and concluded that both approaches have strengths that can be integrated [6]. The focus of both methodologies on delivering value and on customers/users, as well as their iterative nature and continuous testing, make it possible to integrate them and reduce the shortcomings of each methodology, as agile methods need to know their true end-users and UCD benefits from a flexible and adaptive development methodology which runs throughout the project life-cycle [7]. Several studies exist that

---

[1] http://www.se-hci.org/

examine various aspects of the integration of agile methods and usability/UCD. Patton [8] gives details about the way of integrating interaction design into an agile process. Recently, Patton [9] describes the twelve best practices for adding user experience (UX) work to agile development. In their ethnographic field study, Chamberlain et al. [4] have described a framework for integrating UCD into agile methods. Armitage provides the guidelines for designers to work within agile methods [10]. Hodgetts [11] reports about his coaching experience for the integration of user experience design with agile methods. McInerney and Maurer [12] interviewed three specialists for integrating UCD within agile methods and were able to report the success of these methods. Miller [13] describes her experience of parallel tracks of interaction designers and developers that are highly connected and interleaved so that the interaction designers were always one iteration ahead. Blomkvist [14] describes the core principles of agile methods and UCD and outlines a model for bridging agile methods and UCD. Sy [15] describes her company's process of integrating agile methods with UCD in detail. Using Grounded Theory qualitative method, Ferreira et al. [16][17] have investigated several projects for the integration of UI design and agile methods. Fox et al. [18] also conducted a Grounded Theory qualitative study and describe the integration of agile methods and UCD in the industry.

Approaches to integrating agile methods and HCI practices vary. Constantine and Lockwood [19] focus on models in their agile usage-centered design. Kane [20] suggests integrating discount usability with agile methods. Beyer et al. [21] describe how Contextual Design, a UCD method, fits with agile methods. Holzinger et al. [22] [23] presented the idea of extreme usability by combining XP and usability engineering and embedded their ideas into software engineering education. Meszaros and Aston [24] report the introduction of usability testing based on paper prototypes into agile methods. Lee [25] describes combining scenario-based design, a usability engineering process, into agile methods. Obendorf and Finck [26] have described the integration of XP and scenario-based usability engineering. Brown et al. [27] report on using various artefacts, such as stories, sketches, and lists between interaction designers and agile developers. Ungar [28] describes the benefits of introducing Design Studio into the agile UCD process. Broschinsky and Baker [29] report on the successful use of personas in the XP process. Ambler [30] discusses strategies for tailoring user experience into agile methods using agile model-driven development. Wolkerstorfer et al. [31] and Hussain et al. [7], [32] have reported on the integration of various HCI techniques, e.g., field studies, personas, usability tests, paper prototypes, usability expert evaluations, etc., into their agile process. In the report of the special interest group regarding agile user experience, Miller and Sy [33] have referred to uncovering the best practices for agile UCD. Budwig et al. [34] report about the experience of UX teams working in Scrum, one of the popular agile methods, and describe the challenges, issues, and the solutions that they implemented to resolve those issues. Sy [35] describes "a framework for creating multi-sprint designs and getting them implemented without violating the Agile taboo against big design". Many of the studies mentioned above provide only anecdotal views and there is a need for quantitative as well as qualitative research in this area.

2.2   Related Studies Regarding Surveys on Agile Methods and Usability/UCD

There are few survey studies that exclusively regard agile methods and cover various aspects including their effectiveness and the potential problems [36][37][38][39][40]. Recently, two surveys were conducted among agile professionals for evaluating the success factors in agile software development projects and practices [41],[42]. None mentioned usability/UCD.

There are various survey studies regarding usability, usability professionals, and user-centered design dating back to 1993-94 [43],[44]. In the survey of Gunther et al. [45], the highest rated HCI techniques were usability testing followed by prototyping and heuristic evaluations. The survey results of Vredenburg et al. [46] show that UCD methods are gaining extensive acceptance in industry. Gulliksen et al. [47] conducted a survey of the usability profession in Sweden, showing that usability and user involvement has low priority in commercial projects. The highest rated HCI techniques were thinking aloud, lo-fi prototyping, interviews, field studies, and scenarios. In their survey study, Jerome and Kazman [48] point out the lack of coordination between developers and HCI practitioners. Surprisingly, heuristic evaluation was the least used technique. Ji and Yun [49] also conducted a survey in Korea among developers and usability practitioners, which not only showed differences between the type of output and customer requirements but also that practitioners were aware that usability/UCD methods have improved the usability of the developed product. In Switzerland, Vukelja et al. [50] conducted a survey among developers regarding the focus on design and development of user interfaces. Their results show that without the involvement of HCI practitioners, developers frequently develop user interfaces, and usability tests are rarely conducted. Zhou et al. [51] conducted their UCD survey in China showing that UCD methods can improve users' satisfaction and the competitiveness of the products developed. Recently in Norway, Bygstad et al. [52] conducted their survey regarding the integration of software development methods and usability. Their results show that usability testing is perceived to be less important than usability requirements, and companies believe that both software development methods and usability are integrated. Most companies use their own software development methods, followed by RUP, and Microsoft solution framework, while XP/agile methods were the least used methods. This study does not specifically focus on the integration of agile methods and usability. In a recent study, Dayton and Barnum [53] conducted two surveys regarding the impact of UCD within one company before and after moving to agile methods. Focusing mainly on usability testing, the results show that after transitioning to an agile process, the company becomes aware that the use of informal usability tests fits better with the agile process and that these are as effective as the formal usability tests conducted in a laboratory. This study mainly presents the results from a technical communicator's point of view, focuses on usability tests, presents views from just one company, and does not address other usability/HCI techniques. Nielsen Norman group has conducted a survey study regarding agile usability. They report that low-fi prototype are mostly used, usability professionals work in a parallel track, and faster usability methods work fine. This report is not publicly available though the summary is available at http://www.nngroup.com/reports/agile/.

To the best of our knowledge, no survey study except the Nielsen Norman group, has been conducted which specifically addresses the integration of agile methods and usability/UCD, focuses on both developers and usability professionals working in agile methods throughout the world, the HCI techniques used into agile methods, and their impact on the increased quality/usability of the products developed. Our research aimed at filling out this gap by conducting a survey and analyzing its results.

3   Method

This study used the online web-based survey methodology while covering both quantitative as well as qualitative research methods. A questionnaire was designed containing both close-ended multiple-choice questions and open-ended questions. A 5-point Likert scale was used for the close-ended multiple-choice questions; additionally don't know/no answer option was also provided. In total, there were 28 questions ranging from demographic questions to agile methods and practices, as well as HCI techniques and the impact of the integration of agile methods and usability/UCD. For the validity, usefulness, and readability of the survey content, feedback was received from two of the pioneers and experts in the field of agile usability/UCD.

The survey was targeted at practitioners (both usability professionals and developers) working in agile methods that integrate some HCI techniques, or where the role of a usability professional is practiced by someone in their agile team, or who have some usability/UCD awareness in their processes. The survey was posted and distributed to the agile-usability and XP Yahoo groups, the CHI mailing list, the Austrian HCI-UE group, the British HCI group, and through personal networks. The survey was implemented by using the open source survey tool "LimeSurvey". The survey was started in the second week of June 2009 and was closed after five weeks with 92 responses. Table 1 shows the various job titles of the respondents. The job title 'Other' includes a product manager, an analyst, a technical writer/usability, a business analyst, an academic researcher in HCI, and a researcher/programmer/student.

Table 1. The various job titles of the 92 respondents

Job title	Frequency	Percent
Executive / Director	14	15.22%
Project / Program Manager	12	13.04%
Developer / Software Engineer / Programmer	16	17.39%
Usability Engineer / UI/UX/Interaction Designer	33	35.87%
Consultant	11	11.96%
Other	6	6.52%

Table 2 shows the location of the respondents.

Table 2. Locations of the 92 respondents

Location	Frequency	Percent
Europe	42	45.65%
North America	35	38.04%
Australia & New Zealand	6	6.52%
South & Central America	4	4.35%
Asia	3	3.26%
Africa	2	2.17%

Table 3 shows the experience of the respondents in agile methods.

Table 3. Experience of the 92 respondents in agile methods

Experience	Frequency	Percent
1 Year	21	22.83%
2 - 5 Years	47	51.09%
6 - 10 Years	11	11.96%
11 - 20 Years	5	5.43%
No answer	8	8.70%

4   Results

This section presents the preliminary results.

Agile Software Development Methods. Scrum is highly used among various agile software development methods followed by Extreme Programming (XP), proving the consistency of their growing adoption in industry. Table 4 shows the various agile methods used. Note that multiple answers were possible to select. The 'Other' option in agile methods contains TSP/Agile Fusion, agile UCD, and home grown methods within the company.

HCI Techniques Used. As can be seen from Table 5, the top most used HCI techniques are low-fidelity prototyping, followed by conceptual designs, observational studies of users, usability expert evaluations, field studies, personas, rapid iterative testing, and laboratory usability testing, respectively. Note that multiple answers were possible. The 'Other' option in HCI techniques used contains contextual inquiry, non-formal usability tests (in person), participatory design, thorough UI specifications, high-fidelity prototyping, and model-driven inquiry. The use of low-fidelity prototyping, usability expert evaluations, and rapid iterative testing easily fit within the fast moving iterations of agile methods. The results are slightly different from those of [44][45][46][47][49][51].

Table 4. The various agile methods used (multiple answers possible)

Method	Frequency	Percent
Scrum	62	67.39%
Extreme Programming (XP)	44	47.83%
Lean Development	17	18.48%
Agile Unified Process/ Open UP	9	9.78%
Pragmatic Programming	7	7.61%
Crystal Methods	5	5.43%
Adaptive Software Development	3	3.26%
Other	11	11.96%

Table 5. The various HCI Techniques used (multiple answers possible)

HCI Techniques	Frequency	Percent
Low-Fidelity Prototyping	63	68.48%
Conceptual Designs	55	59.78%
Observational Studies of Users	52	56.52%
Usability Expert Evaluations	47	51.09%
Field Studies	43	46.74%
Personas	41	44.57%
Rapid Iterative Testing	37	40.22%
Laboratory Usability Testing	36	39.13%
Needs Analysis	33	35.87%
Goal-Directed Design	27	29.35%
Remote Usability Testing	24	26.09%
Conceptual Inquiry	24	26.09%
Ethnographic Research	21	22.83%
Automated Usability Evaluations	7	7.61%
Other	11	11.96%

The Impact of the Integration of Agile Methods and Usability/UCD.
The majority of the respondents consider that the integration of agile methods
with usability/user-centered design has added value to their adopted process and
to their teams, as most have selected 'Strongly Agree' or 'Agree' options. Table
6 shows the answers in frequency and percent. Only 4 respondents have selected
'Disagree' or 'Strongly Disagree'.

In Table 7, it can be seen that most respondents perceive that the adoption of the agile user-centered design process by their teams has resulted in the
improvement of usability and quality of the product developed.

In connection with the usability of the products, the majority of the respondents are also of the opinion that, due to the agile user-centered design process
adopted by their teams, the resulting product has increased the satisfaction of
its end-users (See Table 8).

Table 6. The integration of agile methods with usability/UCD has added value to the adopted process and to the teams

Answer	Frequency	Percent
Strongly Agree	27	29.35%
Agree	40	43.48%
Neutral	7	7.61%
Disagree	2	2.17%
Strongly Disagree	2	2.17%
Don't know / no answer	14	15.22%

Table 7. The adoption of an agile UCD process has resulted in the improvement of usability and quality of the product developed

Answer	Frequency	Percent
Strongly Agree	19	20.65%
Agree	41	44.57%
Neutral	10	10.47%
Disagree	6	6.52%
Strongly Disagree	2	2.17%
Don't know / no answer	14	15.22%

Table 8. The resulting product has increased the satisfaction of its end-users due to the adoption of an agile UCD process

Method	Frequency	Percent
Strongly Agree	20	21.74%
Agree	38	41.30%
Neutral	5	5.43%
Disagree	5	5.43%
Strongly Disagree	2	2.17%
Don't know / no answer	22	23.91%

5 Conclusion

Agile software development methods are flexible, iterative, and lightweight, making it easy to integrate usability/HCI techniques into them, while the focus of both methodologies on delivering value and on customers/users, as well as their iterative nature and continuous testing, further facilitate and enable this integration [7]. The survey results support this as the majority of respondents perceive that the integration of agile methods with usability/user-centered design has added value to their adopted process and to their teams. They also perceive that the adoption of an agile user-centered design process by their teams has resulted in the improvement of usability and quality of the product developed and has also increased the satisfaction of its end-users. The results are mostly consistent with [49][51].

The top most HCI techniques used are low-fidelity prototyping, followed by conceptual designs, observational studies of users, usability expert evaluations, field studies, personas, rapid iterative testing, and laboratory usability testing, respectively. The use of low-fidelity prototyping, usability expert evaluations, and rapid iterative testing easily fit into the fast pace of agile methods. The results are mostly consistent with Nielsen Norman report. Other techniques can be adapted using two parallel tracks of interaction designers and developers [15].

The preliminary results are presented in this paper. Detailed statistically analyzed results will be provided in future covering broader aspects of the integration of agile methods and usability/user-centered design. The results are promising and increase the hope that both communities of usability professionals and agile practitioners can work even closer to create successful products so that the use of those products can be brought to their full potential.

References

1. Dyba, T., Dingsoyr, T.: Empirical studies of agile software development: A systematic review. Information and Software Technology 50(9-10), 833–859 (2008)
2. Holzinger, A.: Usability Engineering for Software Developers. Communications of the ACM 48(1), 71–74 (2005)
3. Memmel, T., Reiterer, H., Holzinger, A.: Agile Methods and Visual Specification in Software Development: A Chance to Ensure Universal Access. In: Stephanidis, C. (ed.) HCI 2007. LNCS, vol. 4554, pp. 453–462. Springer, Heidelberg (2007)
4. Chamberlain, S., Sharp, H., Maiden, N.: Towards a framework for integrating agile development and user-centred design. In: Abrahamsson, P., Marchesi, M., Succi, G. (eds.) XP 2006. LNCS, vol. 4044, pp. 143–153. Springer, Heidelberg (2006)
5. Seffah, A., Gulliksen, J., Desmarais, M.C.: Human-Centered Software Engineering - Integrating Usability in the Development Process. Human-Computer Interaction Series. Springer, New York (2005)
6. Nelson, E.: Extreme programming vs. interaction design, FTP Online (2002)
7. Hussain, Z., Lechner, M., Milchrahm, H., Shahzad, S., Slany, W., Umgeher, M., Wolkerstorfer, P.: Agile User-Centered Design Applied to a Mobile Multimedia Streaming Application. In: Holzinger, A. (ed.) USAB 2008. LNCS, vol. 5298, pp. 313–330. Springer, Heidelberg (2008)
8. Patton, J.: Hitting the target: adding interaction design to agile software development. In: OOPSLA 2002 Practitioners Reports, Seattle, Washington. ACM, New York (2002)
9. Patton, J.: Twelve emerging best practices for adding UX work to agile development (June 2008), http://www.agileproductdesign.com/blog/emerging_best_agile_ux_practice.html
10. Armitage, J.: Are agile methods good for design? Interactions 11(1), 14–23 (2004)
11. Hodgetts, P.: Experiences integrating sophisticated user experience design practices into agile processes. In: Agile Conference, 2005, pp. 235–242 (2005)
12. McInerney, P., Maurer, F.: UCD in agile projects: dream team or odd couple? Interactions 12(6), 19–23 (2005)

13. Miller, L.: Case study of customer input for a successful product. In: Agile Conference, 2005, pp. 225–234 (2005)
14. Blomkvist, S.: Towards a Model for Bridging Agile Development and User-Centered Design. Springer, Netherlands (2005)
15. Sy, D.: Adapting usability investigations for agile user-centered design. Journal of Usability Studies 2(3), 112–132 (2007)
16. Ferreira, J., Noble, J., Biddle, R.: Agile development iterations and UI design. In: Agile 2007, pp. 50–58. IEEE Computer Society, Los Alamitos (2007)
17. Ferreira, J., Noble, J., Biddle, R.: Up-front interaction design in agile development. In: Concas, G., Damiani, E., Scotto, M., Succi, G. (eds.) XP 2007. LNCS, vol. 4536, pp. 9–16. Springer, Heidelberg (2007)
18. Fox, D., Sillito, J., Maurer, F.: Agile methods and User-Centered design: How these two methodologies are being successfully integrated in industry. In: AGILE 2008. Conference, pp. 63–72 (2008)
19. Constantine, L.L., Lockwood, L.A.D.: Usage-centered software engineering: an agile approach to integrating users, user interfaces, and usability into software engineering practice. In: ICSE 2003, pp. 746–747. IEEE Computer Society, Los Alamitos (2003)
20. Kane, D.: Finding a place for discount usability engineering in agile development: throwing down the gauntlet. In: Proceedings of the Agile Development Conference, ADC 2003, pp. 40–46 (2003)
21. Beyer, H., Holtzblatt, K., Baker, L.: An Agile Customer-Centered Method: Rapid Contextual Design. In: Zannier, C., Erdogmus, H., Lindstrom, L. (eds.) XP/Agile Universe 2004. LNCS, vol. 3134, pp. 50–59. Springer, Heidelberg (2004)
22. Holzinger, A., Errath, M., Searle, G., Thurnher, B., Slany, W.: From extreme programming and usability engineering to extreme usability in software engineering education (XP+UE→XU). In: COMPSAC 2005: Proceedings of the 29th Annual International Computer Software and Applications Conference (COMPSAC 2005), Washington, DC, USA, vol. 2, pp. 169–172. IEEE Computer Society, Los Alamitos (2005)
23. Holzinger, A., Slany, W.: (XP+UE→XU) praktische erfahrungen mit extreme usability. Informatik Spektrum 29(2), 91–97 (2006)
24. Meszaros, G., Aston, J.: Adding usability testing to an agile project. In: Agile Conference 2006 (2006)
25. Lee, J.C.: Embracing agile development of usable software systems. In: CHI 2006 extended abstracts on Human factors in computing systems, pp. 1767–1770. ACM, New York (2006)
26. Obendorf, H., Finck, M.: Scenario-based usability engineering techniques in agile development processes. In: CHI 2008, pp. 2159–2166. ACM, New York (2008)
27. Brown, J., Lindgaard, G., Biddle, R.: Stories, sketches, and lists: Developers and interaction designers interacting through artefacts. In: AGILE 2008. Conference, pp. 39–50 (2008)
28. Ungar, J.: The design studio: Interface design for agile teams. In: AGILE 2008. Conference, pp. 519–524 (2008)
29. Broschinsky, D., Baker, L.: Using persona with XP at LANDesk software, an avocent company. In: AGILE 2008. Conference, pp. 543–548 (2008)
30. Ambler, S.W.: Tailoring Usability into Agile Software Development Projects. Springer, London (2008)
31. Wolkerstorfer, P., Tscheligi, M., Sefelin, R., Milchrahm, H., Hussain, Z., Lechner, M., Shahzad, S.: Probing an agile usability process. In: CHI 2008: human factors in computing systems, pp. 2151–2158. ACM, New York (2008)

32. Hussain, Z., Milchrahm, H., Shahzad, S., Slany, W., Tscheligi, M., Wolkerstorfer, P.: Integration of extreme programming and user-centered design: Lessons learned. In: Abrahamsson, P., Marchesi, M., Maurer, F. (eds.) XP 2009. LNBIP, vol. 31, pp. 174–179. Springer, Heidelberg (2009)
33. Miller, L., Sy, D.: Agile user experience SIG. In: Proceedings of the 27th international conference extended abstracts on Human factors in computing systems CHI, Boston, MA, USA, pp. 2751–2754. ACM, New York (2009)
34. Budwig, M., Jeong, S., Kelkar, K.: When user experience met agile: a case study. In: Proceedings of the 27th international conference extended abstracts on Human factors in computing systems CHI, pp. 3075–3084. ACM, New York (2009)
35. Sy, D.: Coherent agile user-centered design. In: UPA 2009 International Conference, Usability Professional's Association (2009)
36. Ramachandran, V., Shukla, A.: Circle of life, spiral of death: Are xp teams following the essential practices? In: Extreme Programming and Agile Methods — XP/Agile Universe 2002. Springer, Heidelberg (2002)
37. Reifer, D.J.: How good are agile methods? IEEE Software 19(4), 16–18 (2002)
38. Rumpe, B., Schröder, A.: Quantitative survey on extreme programming projects. In: Extreme Programming and Agile Methods — XP/Agile Universe 2002 (2002)
39. Sillitti, A., Ceschi, M., Russo, B., Succi, G.: Managing uncertainty in requirements: a survey in documentation-driven and agile companies. In: 11th IEEE International Symposium on Software Metrics (2005)
40. Salo, O., Abrahamsson, P.: Agile methods in european embedded software development organisations: a survey on the actual use and usefulness of extreme programming and scrum. Software, IET 2 (2008)
41. Chow, T., Cao, D.B.: A survey study of critical success factors in agile software projects. Journal of Systems and Software 81(6) (2008)
42. Misra, S.C., Kumar, V., Kumar, U.: Identifying some important success factors in adopting agile software development practices. Journal of Systems and Software (in press, 2009) (Accepted Corrected Proof)
43. Rauch, T., Wilson, T.: UPA and CHI surveys on usability processes. SIGCHI Bulletin 27(3) (1995)
44. Rosenbaum, S., Rohn, J.A., Humburg, J.: A toolkit for strategic usability: results from workshops, panels, and surveys. In: CHI 2000: Proceedings of the SIGCHI conference on Human factors in computing systems. ACM, New York (2000)
45. Gunther, R., Janis, J., Butler, S.: The ucd decision matrix: How, when, and where to sell user-centered design into the development cycle, http://www.ovostudios.com/upa2001/ (accessed on June 10, 2009)
46. Vredenburg, K., Mao, J.Y., Smith, P.W., Carey, T.: A survey of user-centered design practice. In: CHI 2002: Proceedings of the SIGCHI conference on Human factors in computing systems. ACM, New York (2002)
47. Gulliksen, J., Boivie, I., Persson, J., Hektor, A., Herulf, L.: Making a difference: a survey of the usability profession in Sweden. In: NordiCHI 2004: Proceedings of the third Nordic conference on Human-computer interaction. ACM, New York (2004)
48. Jerome, B., Kazman, R.: Surveying the solitudes: An investigation into the relationships between human computer interaction and software engineering in practice. In: Human-Centered Software Engineering – Integrating Usability in the Software Development Lifecycle. Springer, Netherlands (2005)
49. Ji, Y.G., Yun, M.H.: Enhancing the minority discipline in the IT industry: A survey of usability and User-Centered design practice. International Journal of Human-Computer Interaction 20(2), 117–134 (2006)

50. Vukelja, L., Müller, L., Opwis, K.: Are engineers condemned to design? a survey on software engineering and ui design in Switzerland. In: Baranauskas, C., Palanque, P., Abascal, J., Barbosa, S.D.J. (eds.) INTERACT 2007. LNCS, vol. 4663, pp. 555–568. Springer, Heidelberg (2007)
51. Zhou, R., Huang, S., Qin, X., Huang, J.: A survey of user-centered design practice in China. In: IEEE International Conference on Systems, Man and Cybernetics, SMC 2008, pp. 1885–1889 (2008)
52. Bygstad, B., Ghinea, G., Brevik, E.: Software development methods and usability: Perspectives from a survey in the software industry in Norway. Interacting with Computers 20(3), 375–385 (2008)
53. Dayton, D., Barnum, C.: The impact of agile on user-centered design: Two surveys tell the story. Technical Communication 56(3) (August 2009)

Predicting Pointing Time from Hand Strength

Pradipta Biswas and Peter Robinson

University of Cambridge Computer Laboratory
15 JJ Thomson Avenue
Cambridge CB3 0FD, UK
{pb400,pr}@cl.cam.ac.uk

Abstract. Pointing tasks form a significant part of human-computer interaction in graphical user interfaces. We have developed a model to predict the task completion time for pointing tasks for people with motor-impairment. As part of the model, we have also developed a new scale of characterizing the extent of disability of users by measuring their grip strength. We have validated the model by conducting two trials involving people with motor-impairment and in both trials the model has predicted pointing time with statistically significant accuracy.

Keywords: Pointing tasks, interaction, performance, motor-impariment.

1 Introduction

Pointing tasks form a significant part of human-computer interaction in graphical user interfaces. Fitts' law [3] and its variations [12] are widely used to model pointing as a sequence of rapid aiming movements, especially for able-bodied users. Fitts' Law predicts the movement time as a function of the width and distance to the target. This law is found to be very robust and works in many different situations (even in space and under water). However the application of Fitts' Law for people with motor-impairment is debatable. They only conform to Fitts' Law when the task is very simple and thus requires less coordination between vision and motor-action [21] or there are other cues (e.g. auditory) besides vision [5].

We have developed a statistical model to predict the movement time of pointing tasks performed by people with motor-impairment. The model works by dividing the movement path in different phases. Prediction from our model is significantly (p<0.001) correlated with actual pointing time. As part of the model, we have also developed a new scale characterizing the extent of disability of users by measuring their grip strength.

2 Related Work

For disabled users, there is growing evidence that their interaction patterns are significantly different from those of their able-bodied counterparts [11, 17]. In

A. Holzinger and K. Miesenberger (Eds.): USAB 2009, LNCS 5889, pp. 428–447, 2009.

particular, the applicability of Fitts' law for motor-impaired users is debatable. Smits-Engelsman et. al. [21], Wobbrock and Gajos [5] found it to be applicable for children with congential spastic hemiplegia and motor-impaired people respectively, but Bravo et. al. [2] and Gump et. al. [7] obtained a different result. For real life pointing tasks, motor-impaired persons can not always control their movement following visual feedback. Their movements seem to be more ballistic (rapid and discrete movement without visual feedback, [7]). This may be a result of their poor coordination between perception and motor-action. This poor coordination causes more neuro-motor noise than the permissible limit of Fitts' law [14]. They obey Fitts' law when the task is very simple and thus requires less coordination between vision and motor-action [21] or there are other cues (e.g. auditory) besides vision [5].

There has been some work to develop an alternative to Fitts' law for motor-impaired people. Gump et. al. [7] found significant correlation between the movement time and the square root of movement amplitude (Ballistic Movement Factor [6]). Gajos, Wobbrock and Weld [5] estimated the movement time by selecting a set of features from a pool of seven functions of movement amplitude and target width, and then using the selected features in a linear regression model. This model shows interesting characteristics of movement patterns among different users but fails to develop a single model for all. Movement patterns of different users are found to be inclined to different functions of distance and width of targets.

3 Design of the Model

Able-bodied users move the mouse pointer towards a target by a single long sub-movement followed by some smaller sub-movements to home into the target. In the original formulation of Fitts' Law [3], it was assumed that a rapid aiming movement consists of two phases :

- An initial **ballistic phase**, which approaches the target.
- A **homing phase**, which is one or more precise sub-movements to home into the target.

However, this assumption does not hold for motor-impaired users because their movement is disturbed by many pauses and they rarely make a big movement towards the target. The main difference between the mouse movement of the motor-impaired and able-bodied users lie in the characteristics of the sub-movements [22]. The number of sub-movements for motor-impaired users is greater than that of able-bodied users and the main movement towards the target often consists of two or more sub-movements. The time spent between two sub-movements (described as pauses) also significantly affects the total task completion time. So our model estimates the total task completion time by calculating the average number of sub-movements in a single pointing task, their average duration, and the average duration of pauses. In the present study, we define a pause as the event when the mouse stops movement for more than 100 ms and a sub-movement is defined as a movement occurring between two pauses.

To reveal the characteristics of the sub-movements and the pauses, we clustered the points where the pauses occurred (i.e. a new sub-movement started) according to their positions. We evaluated the optimum number of clusters by using Classification Entropy [16] as a validation index. The optimum number of clusters was three. We found that about 90% of the sub-movements took place when the mouse pointer was very near the source (the pointer had not moved more than 20% of the total distance) or near the target (the pointer had moved more than 85% of the total distance). The sub-movements near the source and target are extremely variable and the remaining 10% of the sub-movements actually constituted the main movement. The positions of the cluster centres indicated three phases of movement

- **Starting Phase:** This phase consists of small sub -movements near the source, perhaps while the user gets control of the pointing device.
- **Middle Phase:** This consists of relatively large sub-movements and brings the pointer near the target.
- **Homing Phase:** This is similar to the homing phase in Fitts' Law, though the number of sub -movements is greater.

So our model divided the sub-movements and pauses during a pointing task into three classes based on their position with respect to the source and the target (Figure 1, the thick blue line depicts a sample cursor trace between a source and a target). The movement time is estimated as:

$$p_1(d_1 + s_1) + p_2 \cdot d_2 + f(Dist / v_2) + p_3(d_3 + s_3) - (s_1 + s_3)$$

Where,

$Dist$ Distance from source to target

p_1 Number of pauses near source

d_1 Average duration of a pause near source

s_1 Average duration of a sub-movement near source

p_2 Number of pauses in main movement

d_2 Average duration of a pause in main movement

v_2 Speed of movement in main movement

f Fraction of the total distance covered by the main movement

p_3 Number of pauses near target

d_3 Average duration of a pause near target

s_3 Average duration of a sub-movement near target

One difficulty in developing the model was to categorize users based on extent of their disabilities. Several clinical scales have been used to measure disability (e.g.

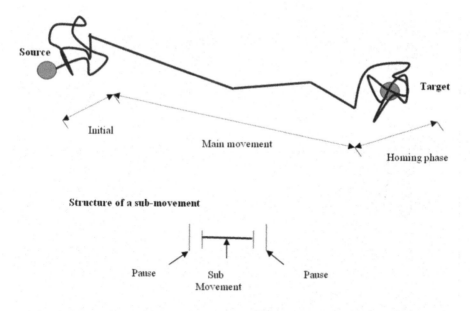

Fig. 1. Different phases of movement

Ashworth scale, the Weighted disability score, Tardieu Scale, Spasticity Grading [18] etc.), but they are not really applicable to modelling HCI. The clinical scales deal with a single disease and often are very subjective (e.g.: Ashworth scale for Spasticity) [18]. The descriptions of disease of the users are inadequate to calibrate a model numerically. So we have developed a new scale by evaluating the hand strength of motor-impaired users and then correlating this with their HCI performance such as task completion time, number of pauses etc. It has already been found that active ROM (range of motion) of wrist can be significantly correlated with the movement time of a Fitts' law task for children with spasticity [21]. Additionally, hand evaluation devices are cheap, easy to operate and have good test-retest reliability [13]. So these are reliable and useful tools for measuring physical strength making these results useful in practice. A pilot study of this model on a data set collected by a different researcher produced encouraging results [1]. In the next section, we present an experiment to collect pointing data from people with motor-impairment, and then use this to validate the model.

Figure 2 shows an example of use of the model. The thin purple line shows a sample trajectory of mouse movement of a motor-impaired user. It can be seen that the trajectory contains random movements near the source and the target. The thick red and black lines encircle the contour of these random movements. The area under the contour has a high probability of missed clicks as the movement lacks control and random there. A good interface should not have more than one target in this contour and the contour should help to decide the amount of separation between icons.

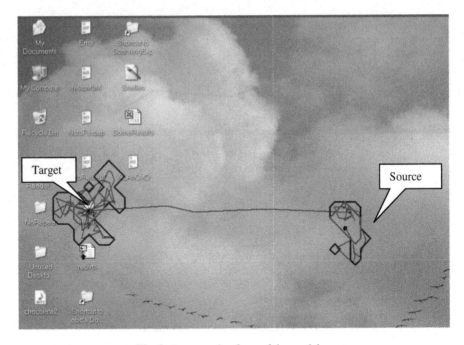

Fig. 2. An example of use of the model

4 Experiment

Our study consisted of pointing tasks. A sample screenshot of the task is shown in Figure 3. We followed the description of the multiple tapping tasks in ISO 9241 part 9.In this task the pointer initially located at the middle of the screen. The participants had to move it towards a target (one of the red dots, appearing a light grey in monochrome), and click on it. This process was repeated for all the targets. There

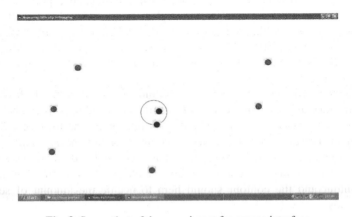

Fig. 3. Screenshot of the experiment for mouse interface

were eight targets on the screen and each participant performed the test twice (except participant P2, who retired after completing the first test). The distances to the targets ranged from 200 to 600 pixels while target widths were randomly selected as an integer between 16 and 48 pixels.

Material

We used a standard optical Mouse and an Acer Aspire 1640 Laptop with a 15.5" monitor having 1280×800 pixel resolution. We also used the same seating arrangement (same table height and distance from table) for all participants. We measured the following six variables for hand strength evaluation (Figure 4). Each variable was measured three times and we took the average. We evaluated only the dominant hand (the hand participants used to operate the mouse).

Grip Strength measures how much force a person can exert gripping with the hand. We measured it using a mechanical dynamometer.

Tip Pinch Strength measures the maximum force generated by a person squeezing something between the tips of his thumb and index finger. We measured it using a mechanical dynamometer.

Radial deviation is the motion that rotates the wrist away from the midline of the body when the person is standing in standard anatomical position. When the hand is placed over a table with palm facing down, this motion rotates the hand about the wrist towards the thumb. We measured the maximum radial deviation using a goniometer.

Ulnar deviation is the motion that rotates the wrist towards the midline of the body when the person is standing in standard anatomical position. When the hand is placed over a table with palm facing down, this motion rotates the hand about the wrist towards the little finger. We measured it with the goniometer.

Pronation is the rotation of the forearm so that the palm moves from a facing up position to a facing down position. We measured it using a wrist-inclinometer.

Supination is the opposite of pronation, the rotation of the forearm so that the palm moves from a facing down position to a facing up position. We measured it with the wrist-inclinometer.

Participants

We initially collected data from 10 motor-impaired and 6 able-bodied participants (Trial 1 in Table 1). The motor-impaired participants were recruited from a local centre, which works on treatment and rehabilitation of disabled people, and they volunteered for the study. To generalize the study, we selected participants with both hypokinetic (restricted movement, e.g. participants P1, P3, P4 etc.) and hyperkinetic (uncontrolled movement or tremor, e.g. participants P5, P6 etc.) movement disorders [4]. All motor-impaired participants used a computer at least once each week. Able-bodied participants were students of our university and expert computer users.

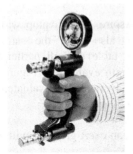

Measuring Grip Strength

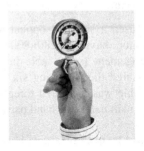

Measuring Tip-pinch Strength

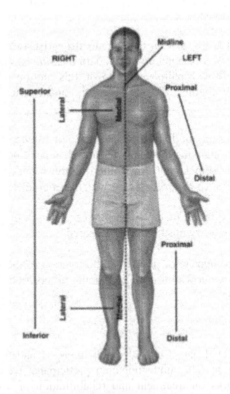

Standard anatomical position

Measuring ranges of motion

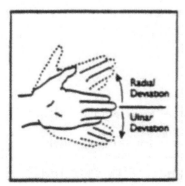

**Range of Motion of wrist
(Palm facing down)**

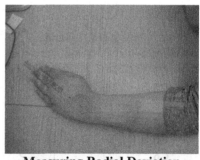

Measuring Radial Deviation

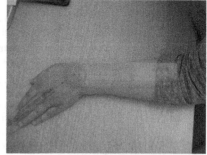

Measuring Ulnar Deviation

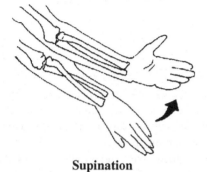

Pronation

Supination

Measuring Pronation

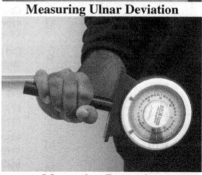

Measuring Supination

Fig. 4. Measurement of hand-strength

Table 1. List of Participants

	Age	Gender	Impairment	Trials Participated
C1	30	M		
C2	29	M		
C3	28	M	Able-bodied	Trial 1
C4	25	M		
C5	29	M		
C6	27	F		
P1	30	M	Cerebral Palsy reduced manual dexterity, wheel chair user.	Trial 1
P2	43	M	Cerebral Palsy reduced manual dexterity, also some tremor in hand, wheel chair user.	Trial 1
P3	25-45	F	One handed (dominant hand), the other hand is paralyzed.	Trial 1
P4	30	M	Dystonia, cannot speak, cannot move fingers, wheelchair user.	Trial 1
P5	62	M	Left side (non-dominant) paralysed after a stroke in 1973, also has tremor..	Trials 1 and 2
P6	44	M	Cerebral attack, significant tremor in whole upper body part, fingers always remain folded.	Trial 1
P7	46	F	Did not mention disease, difficulty in gripping things, no tremor.	Trial 1
P8	>45	F	Spina Bifida/ Hydrocephalus, wheelchair user.	Trials 1 and 2
P9	43	F	Did not mention disease, restricted hand movement, no tremor.	Trials 1 and 2
P10	>45	M	Cerebral Palsy from birth, restricted hand movement, no tremor.	Trials 1 and 2
P11	46	M	Multiple Sclerosis	Trial 2
P12	41	M	Cerebral Palsy, Hyper pressure, nocturnal epilepsy	Trial 2

Results

We found that the movement time significantly correlates ($\rho = 0.57$, $p<0.001$) with the number of pauses. We also correlated the average number of pauses per pointing task with the hand strength metrics. Figures 5 to 8 show the graphs of number of pauses with respect to Grip Strength, active ROM of Wrist (Ulnar + Radial Deviation) and active ROM of Forearm (Pronation + Supination) respectively. We found that some users did not have any range of motion in their wrist, though they managed to

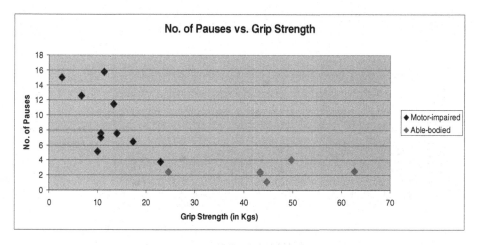

Fig. 5. Average number of Pauses per pointing task vs. Grip Strength

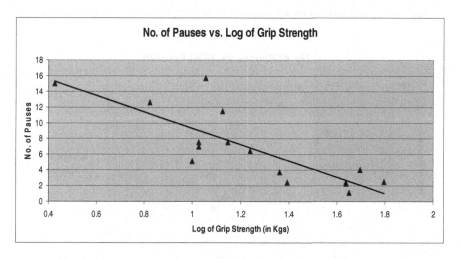

Fig. 6. Average number of Pauses per pointing task vs. Log of Grip Strength

move the mouse to perform the pointing tasks correctly. We also found that the natural logarithm of grip strength (Figure 6) significantly correlates with the mean ($\rho = -0.72$, $p<0.001$) and standard deviation ($\rho = -0.53$, $p<0.05$) of the number of pauses per pointing task. We did not find any correlation between that movement time and the distance, width or Fitts' Law index of difficulty (ID) [3] of the targets for motor-impaired users. This may be due to the presence of physical impairment and the number of pointing tasks (only 16) performed by the participants. We also did not find any significant correlations involving ranges of motion (Figures 7 and 8).

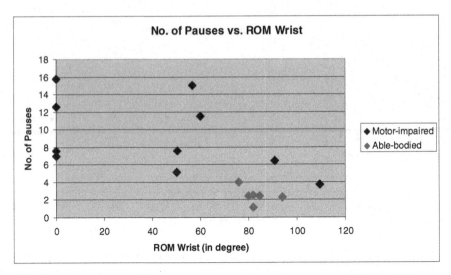

Fig. 7. Average number of Pauses per pointing task vs. Active range of ROM of Wrist

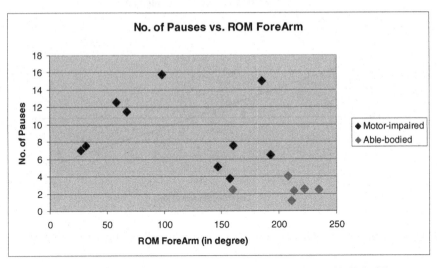

Fig. 8. Average number of Pauses per pointing task vs. Active range of ROM of Forearm

We divided the whole movement path into three phases and observed how the hand strength affects in the initial, main movement and homing phases. We found that grip strength significantly correlates with the average number of pauses near the source (Figure 9, $\rho = -0.61$, $p<0.01$) and near the target ($\rho = -0.78$, $p<0.001$). We also found that the mean and standard deviation of the velocity of movement were significantly correlated with grip strength (Figure 10, $\rho = 0.82$, $p<0.001$ for mean and $\rho = 0.81$, $p<0.001$ for standard deviation).

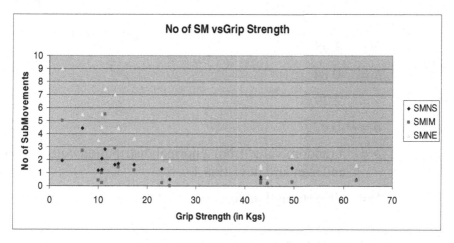

Fig. 9. Average number of Pauses per pointing task vs. Grip Strength (SMNS: Sub Movement Near Source, SMIM: Sub Movement in Middle SMNE: Sub Movement Near End)

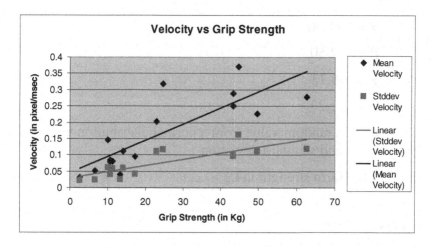

Fig. 10. Velocity of Movement vs. Grip Strength

5   The Model

We revised our model in the light of these results. Grip strength is used to predict the number of pauses near the source and destination, and also to predict the speed of movement. Probability distributions for the other factors were derived using the inverse transform method [17]. The model works based on following equations.

$$p_1 = \alpha + \beta \times \log(S) + 0.5 \times \rho \times \left(\chi \times e^{(\delta \times S)} \right)$$

Where

$$\alpha = \quad 3.95$$
$$\beta = \quad -0.84$$
$$\chi = \quad 2.29$$
$$\delta = \quad -0.02$$

$\rho =$ a random value from a normal distribution with mean 0 and standard deviation 1

$S =$ Grip strength in kg

$$p_3 = \alpha + \beta \times \log(S) + 0.5 \times \rho \times (\chi + \delta \times \log(S))$$

Where

$$\alpha = \quad 11.06$$
$$\beta = \quad -2.50$$
$$\chi = \quad 5.73$$
$$\delta = \quad -1.23$$

$\rho =$ a random value from a normal distribution with mean 0 and standard deviation 1

$S =$ Grip strength in kg

$$d_1 = \alpha \times e^{\beta \times (\chi + \delta \times \mu)}$$

Where

$$\alpha = \quad 3997279$$
$$\beta = \quad -0.16$$
$$\chi = \quad 140$$
$$\delta = \quad 100$$

$\mu =$ a random value from a uniform distribution between 0 and 1

$$d_2 = \alpha \times e^{\beta \times (\chi + \delta \times \mu)}$$

Where

$\alpha =$ 12956.60

$\beta =$ -0.11

$\chi =$ 140

$\delta =$ 100

$\mu =$ a random value from a uniform distribution between 0 and 1

$$d_3 = \alpha + \beta \times \log(S)$$

Where

$\alpha =$ 449.72

$\beta =$ -70.78

$S =$ Grip strength in kg

$$v_2 = \alpha + \beta \times \log(S) + 0.5 \times \rho \times (\chi + \delta \times \log(S))$$

Where

$\alpha =$ -0.12

$\beta =$ 0.14

$\chi =$ 0.007

$\delta =$ 0.03

$\rho =$ a random value from a normal distribution with mean 0 and standard deviation 1

$S =$ Grip strength in kg

$$MT = (p_1 - 1) \times d_1 + \alpha \times \frac{Dist}{v_2} + d_2 + (p_3 - 1) \times d_3$$

Where

$\alpha =$ 0.9

MT Movement Time

Dist Distance from source to target

p_1 Number of pauses near source

d_1 Average duration of a pause near source

d_2 Average duration of a pause in main movement

v_2 Speed of movement in main movement

p_3 Number of pauses near target

d_3 Average duration of a pause near target

We tested the performance of our model on 232 pointing tasks performed by 10 motor impaired and 6 able-bodied participants. The predictions were obtained by simulating each pointing task using Monte Carlo simulation. Figures 11 and 12 show the scatter plot and relative error in prediction. We calculated the relative error by using the following formula $\frac{(Predicted - Actual)}{Actual}$

In 10% of the cases the error was more than 80%, so the model has failed for those tasks. However, the predictions correlate significantly with actual values ($\rho = 0.65$, p<0.001) with error less than 40% in over half of the trials. The average relative error is -2% with a standard deviation of 57%.

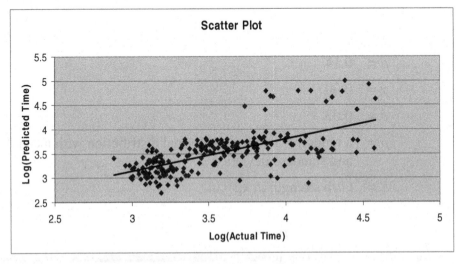

Fig. 11. Scatter plot of prediction

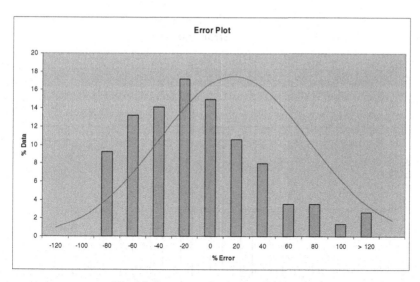

Fig. 12. Percentage error of prediction

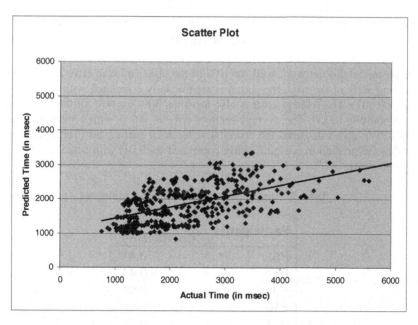

Fig. 13. Scatter plot between actual and predicted task completion times

We further validated the model by taking data from six participants (Trial 2). In this second trial (Trial 2 in Table 1), participants P5, P8, P9, P10 and two new participants took part. As most participants felt fatigue quickly, we ran the trial for six minutes for each participant. In total, they undertook 435 pointing tasks. Figures 13 and 14 show the scatter plot and relative error between actual and prediction. It can be

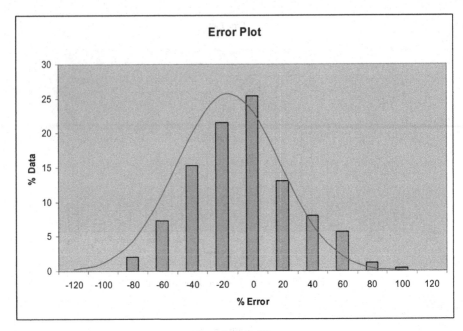

Fig. 14. Error Plot

seen the model did not work well for 10% of the tasks (relative error > 70%). For the remaining 90% of the trial, the actual is significantly correlated with prediction (ρ = 0.56, p<0.001). The relative error is also less than 30% for 60% of the trials (262 out of 435 pointing tasks). The average relative error is -16 % with a standard deviation of 34%. We also calculated the correlation for each participant (Table 2). It can be seen that the prediction is significantly correlated (p<0.01) with actual for five out of six participants.

Table 2. Correlation coefficients for each participant

Participants	Correlation Coefficients
P5	0.41*
P8	0.44*
P9	0.61*
P10	0.55*
P11	0.30
P12	0.46*

* p<0.01

6 Discussion

For able-bodied users, pointing performance is generally analysed in terms of Fitts' Law. However, Fitts' Law does not account for the users' physical abilities in predicting movement time [3, 15]. This seems reasonable for able-bodied users. However, our analysis indicates that people having higher hand strength also have greater control in hand movement and can perform pointing faster. The positive correlation between the velocity of movement and grip strength also supports this claim. As motor-impairment reduces the strength of hand, motor-impaired people loose control of hand movement. So the number of pauses near source and target are significantly affected by grip strength. The logarithmic relation between grip strength and number of pauses indicates that there is a minimum amount of grip strength (about 20 kg) required to move the mouse without pausing more than twice. This threshold of 20 kg can be used to determine the type of input device suitable for a user along with other factors like preference, expertise etc. Our analysis also showed that the flexibility of motion (as measured by range of measurement of wrist or forearm) is not as important as strength of hand (as measured by grip strength). Our model predicts pointing time by separately working on each individual phases and it also incorporates personal characteristics of users. In particular, we predicted the number of pauses near source and target and the velocity of movement based on the extent of disability of the user. The model has accurately predicted the task completion time for pointing tasks undertaken by motor-impaired users. The model can be used to predict task completion time for different interfaces and thus optimize interface layout based on minimum task completion time. It can also be used to generate design guidelines regarding minimum target separation, target size etc. for different degrees of motor-impairment.

The model did not work well for about 10% of pointing tasks. This 10% data deviated the average relative error from zero and also increased the standard deviation of relative errors. This failure can be attributed to various characteristics of users like effects of learning and fatigue, interest, expertise etc. In future we plan to incorporate more input parameters into the model. We also like to extend the scope of the model beyond pointing with a mouse. We would like to investigate different modalities of interaction like finger or stylus based input [8, 9, 10] and effects of situational impairments in interaction [19, 20], which will make the model useful for designing ubiquitous interfaces.

7 Conclusions

In this work, we have developed a model to predict movement time of pointing tasks for those motor-impaired people, who can use their hand to interact with a computer. The model works by dividing the movement path in three different phases. It has accurately predicted the pointing time undertaken by motor-impaired users. As part of the model, we have developed a new scale of characterizing the extent of disability of users by measuring their grip strength. Our study explains the effect of hand strength on pointing performance, which can be used to optimize interface layout (as done with Fitts' law for able-bodied people) and to choose proper input devices for motor-impaired users.

Acknowledgement

We would like to thank the Gates Cambridge Trust for funding this work. We are grateful to the participants at Papworth Trust and students of University of Cambridge for taking part in our experiments. We also would like to thank Adela Xu and Dr. Setor Knutsor of Papworth Trust for organizing the user trials and Prof. Jacob Wobbrock (Univ. of Washington), Dr. Neil Dodgson and Dr. Alan Blackwell (Univ. of Cambridge) for their useful suggestions.

References

1. Biswas, P., Robinson, P.: Automatic Evaluation of Assistive Interfaces. In: ACM International Conference on Intelligent User Interfaces (IUI) 2008, pp. 247–256 (2008)
2. Bravo, P.E., et al.: A study of the application of Fitts' Law to selected cerebral palsy adults. Perceptual and Motor Skills 77, 1107–1117 (1993)
3. Fitts, P.M.: The Information Capacity of The Human Motor System In Controlling The Amplitude of Movement. Journal of Experimental Psychology 47, 381–391 (1954)
4. Flowers, K.A.: Visual 'Closed-Loop' And 'Open-Loop' characteristics Of Voluntary Movement In Patients With Parkinsonism And Intention Tremor. Brain 99, 269–310 (1976)
5. Gajos, K.Z., Wobbrock, J.O., Weld, D.S.: Automatically generating user interfaces adapted to users' motor and vision capabilities. In: Proceedings of UIST (2007)
6. Gan, K.C., Hoffmann, E.R.: Geometrical conditions for ballistic and visually controlled movements. Ergonomics 31, 829–839 (1988)
7. Gump, A., et al.: Application of Fitts' Law to individuals with cerebral palsy. Perceptual and Motor Skills 94, 883–895 (2002)
8. Hoffmann, E.R., Sheikh, I.: Finger width corrections in Fitts' Law: Implications for speed-accuracy research. Journal of Motor Behavior 24, 259–262 (1991)
9. Holzinger, A.: Finger Instead of Mouse: Touch Screens as a means of enhancing Universal Access. In: Carbonell, N., Stephanidis, C. (eds.) UI4ALL 2002. LNCS, vol. 2615, pp. 387–397. Springer, Heidelberg (2003)
10. Holzinger, A., Höller, M., Schedlbauer, M., Urlesberger, B.: An Investigation of Finger versus Stylus Input in Medical Scenarios. In: Luzar-Stiffler, V., Dobric, V.H., Bekic, Z. (eds.) ITI 2008: 30th International Conference on Information Technology Interfaces, June 23-26, pp. 433–438. IEEE, Los Alamitos (2008)
11. Keates, S., Clarkson, J., Robinson, P.: Investigating The Applicability of User Models For Motion Impaired Users. In: Proceedings of ACM/SIGACCESS Conference On Computers And Accessibility, November 13-15 (2000)
12. Mackenzie, I.S.: Motor Behaviour Models For Human-Computer Interaction. In: Carroll, J.M. (ed.) HCI Models, Theories, And Frameworks: Toward A Multidisciplinary Science, pp. 27–54. Morgan Kaufmann, San Francisco (2003)
13. Mathiowetz, V., Weber, K., Volland, G., Kashman, N.: Reliability and validity of hand strength evaluation. Journal of Hand Surg (1984)
14. McCrea, P.H., Eng, J.J.: Consequences of increased neuro-motor noise for reaching movements in persons with stroke. Journal of Experimental Brain Research 162, 70–77 (2005)
15. Rosenbaum, D.A.: Human Motor Control. Academic Press Inc., California (1991)
16. Ross, T.J.: Fuzzy Logic with Engineering Application, International edn. McGraw-Hill Inc., New York (1997)
17. Ross, S.M.: Probability Models For Computer Science. Elsevier, Amsterdam (2002)

18. Scholtes, V.A.B., et al.: Clinical assessment of spasticity in children with cerebral palsy: a critical review of available instruments. Developmental Medicine and Child Neurology 48, 64–73 (2006)
19. Schedlbauer, M., Heines, J.: Selecting While Walking: An Investigation of Aiming Performance in a Mobile Work Context. In: AMCIS 2007 (2007)
20. Schedlbauer, M.J., Pastel, R.L., Heines, J.M.: Effect of Posture on Target Acquisition with a Trackball and Touch Screen. In: 28th International Conference on Information Technology Interfaces (ITI)
21. Smits-Engelsman, B.C.M., et al.: Children with congential spastic hemiplegia obey Fitts' Law in a visually guided tapping task. Journal of Experimental Brain Research 177, 431–439 (2007)
22. Trewin, S., Pain, H.: Keyboard And Mouse Errors Due To Motor Disabilities. International Journal of Human-Computer Studies 50(2), 109–144 (1999)

Analyzing Interaction Techniques Using Mouse and Keyboard for Preschool Children

Bettina Grünzweil and Michael Haller

Media Interaction Lab
Upper Austria University of Applied Sciences
Softwarepark 11, A-4232 Hagenberg (Austria/Europe)
{bettina.gruenzweil,michael.haller}@fh-hagenberg.at

Abstract. Nowadays, even very young children begin to use software applications – mostly playing games. Not surprisingly, both skills and abilities of preschool children differ not only from adults, but also from older children. In this paper, we analyzed preschool children in the kindergarten to show the most effective ways of interacting with an application. In contrast to related work, we mainly focus on how preschool children interact with applications using various interaction metaphors and devices.

Keywords: Preschool Children, Interaction, Mouse, Performance.

1 Introduction

In the past years, a lot of research has been done in the field of improving interfaces for children [11]. Growing up is a process of learning and during the first fifteen years the abilities and skills of children are changing rapidly [1]. Therefore, we cannot use software design guidelines designed for children ranging in age from about 10 to 12 for preschool kids.

As children today start using software in a very early age, the present study tests some of the most frequently used interaction techniques on preschool children, e.g. different dragging techniques (Drag-and-Drop vs. Sticky Drag-and-Drop [7]) using different devices such as keyboard and mouse. In the Sticky Drag-and-Drop interaction technique users click first on the object then move it without pressing the mouse button and finally they click again when the object reached the target (see Figure 1). Further results of our user test (e.g. detecting important regions of the screen, preferred colors etc.) can be found in [6]. Our key question during our test was to find out in which way desktop applications have to be designed so that preschool children can use them easily and efficiently.

A. Holzinger and K. Miesenberger (Eds.): USAB 2009, LNCS 5889, pp. 448–456, 2009.

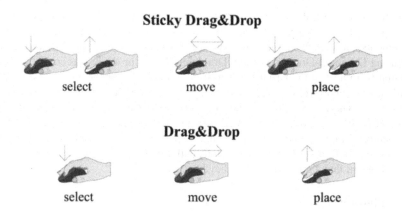

Fig. 1. Sticky Drag-and-Drop vs. Drag-and-Drop

2   Related Work

Several studies discuss the usage of input devices for children [2, 5, 8]. Inkpen conducted a study with children aged between 9 and 13 who already had experiences in using computers to compare Point-and-Click with Drag-and-Drop interfaces [11]. The Point-and-Click style to move an object was realized by Sticky Drag-and-Drop. The performance of children using Sticky Drag-and-Drop was significantly higher and the error rate was lower. In the same way, Hourcade tested kindergarten children [8, 9, 10]. In contrast to Inkpen and Hourcade, we wanted to test interaction techniques using mouse and keyboard *with children without any computer experience*.

A study of Donker and Reitsma compared mouse usage of preschool children, 7-year-old children and adults [3]. The results of this study showed that preschool children were able to aim and click with the same accuracy as adults, but they needed much more time. This result corresponds with the recommendations of the "Sesame Workshop" [13]. This non-profit education organization is developing media for education for more than 40 years. The experience-based guidelines indicate that the fine motor skills of preschool children are still developing.

Kail developed a formula for predicting the performance of children in these tasks depending on the performance time of adults [12]. According to Kail, the younger children are, the higher the difference between their time and the time, adults need for a certain task. The values decrease very rapidly between the first and the sixth year. After that, the negative slope of the curve gets less steep. This indicates that there is not only a difference between the performance of children and adults, but also a big difference between younger and older children.

3   User Study

In our user study, we wanted to test the performance between different devices (mouse vs. keyboard) and between two different interaction metaphors (Drag-and-Drop vs. Sticky Drag-and-Drop). We also evaluated the devices under two different setups, resulting in an overall of three different experiments. In the first experiment, the participants had to select objects, in the second, they had to choose horizontal movements, and finally, in the third experiment we measured the performance and error rate using Drag-and-Drop and Sticky Drag-and-Drop. The study was conducted with 42 children from a local kindergarten, who used a computer for their very first time. 55% of all participants were girls and 45% were boys, 96.34% were right-handed and 3.67% left-handed. The average age of the children was 4.53 years (SD=0.76). 14 children operated each experiment. A repeated measure within-subject design was used in our user study. Moreover, the order of the experiments was counterbalanced among participants. Before starting the user study, all children were able to try the device to make sure that they understood what they have to do.

3.1 Apparatus

For all three experiments, a 15.4" laptop with a resolution of 1440×900 pixels has been used. As depicted in Figure 2, the arrow keys and the space bar were the only keys that have been used in the experiments. For a quick identification, these keys were highlighted in color.

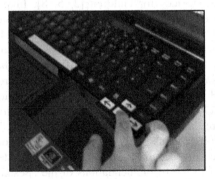
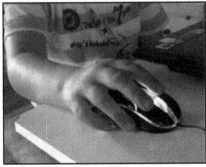

Fig. 2. *(left)* The keyboard and the mouse *(right)*, that have been used in the first two experiments

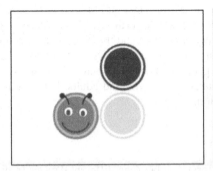
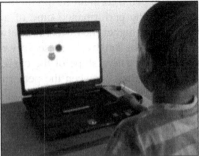

Fig. 3. Participants had to select the face of the object by using the key arrows and the space bar and the mouse

3.2 Experiment 1: Object selection

In the first experiment, children had to select one part of an object that consisted of three sub-objects (see Figure 3).

The sub-objects were linked together horizontally or vertically. One of the objects was the source object and another circle the target object (marked with a face). Using the keyboard, at the beginning of the experiment, the sub-object was active and highlighted by a colored ring. The participants had to move to the target object using the arrow keys and log in the target object by pressing the spacebar. Using the mouse, children had to move the mouse cursor to the target object and confirm the selection with a mouse-click. After a completed trial, all three objects were rearranged randomly.

3.3 Design and Procedure

All children were encouraged to move to and select as many target objects as possible. We tracked the number of correct and wrong selected target objects. While using the keyboard, the number of correct and wrong selected directions was stored. While using the mouse, the cursor movements were stored. The experiment stopped automatically after one minute.

3.4 Results

Using the mouse, averagely 14.77 objects were selected (SD=9.25) during the experiment, while the number of selected objects using the keyboard was 3.38 objects in average (SD=1.98). We also found a high significant difference using both devices ($F_{2,12}=18.84$, $p<0.001$).

81.36% of all target objects that were logged in correctly were selected by using the mouse, only 18.64% by using the keyboard. Altogether, 54.96% of all selected objects – right and wrong – were logged in by mouse, in contrast to 45.04% by keyboard.

An overall error rate of 36.73% occurred during the experiment. Errors are defined by selecting the wrong object or pressing the spacebar while the target object was still not activated. From these errors, 90.51% happened using the keyboard and only 9.49% occurred using the mouse. Again, we found a high significant difference ($F_{2,12}=23.79$, $p<0.001$).

3.5 Experiment 2: Horizontal Movement

In the second experiment, the object (a balloon or fish) had to be balanced (by moving to left and right). At the beginning the object was placed at the bottom of the screen. Using the keyboard, participants had to press the left and right arrow keys. In contrast, while using the mouse, the object was placed on the mouse cursor's position. During the experiment, vertically moving objects tried to collide with the balloon and the task was to not collide with those objects.

3.6 Design and Procedure

During the trials, the number of collisions, the duration of collisions and the path of the controlled object on the screen were tracked. The experiment was automatically stopped after passing ten collision objects.

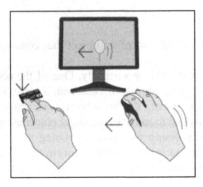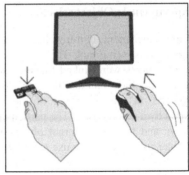

Fig. 4. Participants had to avoid collisions in the experiment 2. The balloon was controlled by using the key arrows and the mouse.

3.7 Results

The balloon collided on average with 4.62 objects (SD= 1.55) using the keyboard and with 3.15 objects using the mouse. We found a significant difference between the two devices ($F_{2,12}$=5.31, p<0.05).

3.8 Experiment 3: Object Movement

In this experiment, children had to pick up 26 objects and to put them into a basket (see Figure 5). The source objects had a size of 2 × 2cm on the used laptop screen, the target object measured a size of 6.5 × 5cm.

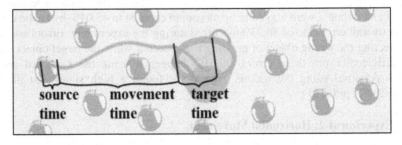

Fig. 5. Participants had to move the apples into the basket. The grey line shows a movement path.

The apples had a distance of 3 to 13 cm to the target object. Under the Drag-and-Drop condition, the selected objects moved back to their original position when the mouse-button was released before it reached the target object. To provide a visual feedback using Sticky Drag-and-Drop, the selected apple appeared transparent while moving the mouse. Notice that in this experiment, we only used the mouse device.

3.9 Design and Procedure

The task was to move as much apples as possible to the target object within 60 seconds. During this, we captured the mouse cursor as well as the number of source objects moved. An error occurred in the Drag-and-Drop scenario if the mouse button has been released *before* reaching the source object. An error occurred in the Sticky Drag-and-Drop scenario whenever children were clicking anywhere else than on the source objects to select and the target object to assign.

3.10 Results

On average 5.96 (SD=3.36) objects have been moved with the Sticky Drag-and-Drop interaction technique and 6.67 (SD=4.48) objects using the Drag-and-Drop technique. However, there was no significant difference between the mean of both methods, $F_{2,11}=0.38$, $p=0.54$.

A higher difference could be found comparing the error rates. On average 2.33 (SD=2.9) source objects selected by Drag-and-Drop did not reach the target, because the mouse button was released before the cursor reached the target object. This means that 28.57% of all objects selected with Drag-and-Drop did not reach their target. In contrast, using the Sticky Drag-and-Drop method, all children completed the task without any mistake. We measured a high significant difference between both methods ($F_{2,11}=7.59$, $p<0.01$).

To get a better understanding, we also tracked all mouse movements. Analyzing this data, we found out that the time children spent during the experiment can be classified in three categories: the source time, which is the time the cursor was placed on the source object, the movement time, which is the time between the source objects and the target object, and the target time, which is the time the cursor was placed on the target object (see Figure 6). Analyzing these traces, it becomes clear that by using Drag-and-Drop, the mouse cursor spent more time at the source and target objects than on the way between the objects; on average 41.83% of the time was spent for the movement from the source to the target and only 25.35% of the overall time was spent for the target time. In contrast, using the Sticky Drag-and-Drop method resulted in an overall of 37.82% total time spent for the movement and 19.77% of the overall time was spent for the target time. This results in a movement time of 42.36 %.

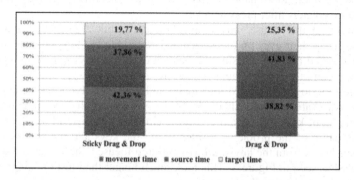

Fig. 6. Composition of time spent during the movement task

Although the children have to press and release the mouse button selecting and placing an object, it takes less time than by simply pressing and releasing the button as it is the case by using the Drag-and-Drop technique. Even children that were able to move more objects by using Drag-and-Drop achieved a higher percentage of source and target time than by using Sticky Drag-and-Drop (cf. Figure 7).

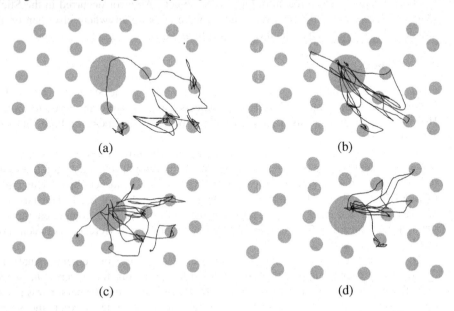

(a)   (b)

(c)   (d)

Fig. 7. These plots depict the movement of two different children using the Drag-and-Drop (a, c) and the Sticky Drag-and-Drop (b, d) metaphor

4 Discussion

The differences in performance and error rate between mouse and keyboard indicated that the mouse is preferred to the keyboard while designing applications for preschool children. The reason for this could be found in the steep learning curve of mouse usage. Children left their hand on the mouse all the time, but they release the keyboard immediately after pressing a key.

They watched the mouse only at the beginning, but after some minutes, they managed to keep their eyes on the screen and were able to click automatically when the cursor reached the target. Using the keyboard, they always put their fingers away from the keys shortly after clicking. Therefore, before they were able to press a key, they had to look to the keyboard. For many children, identifying the meaning of the used keys was hard as well, although the keys were highlighted and only a very limited amount of keys has been used. Some children just tried all the keys one after another. Because of the problems in identifying the keys and the fact that children release their hands from the keyboard, the children focused alternately the screen and the keyboard as seen in Figure 8. This took much longer than just clicking the mouse and was less intuitive as well.

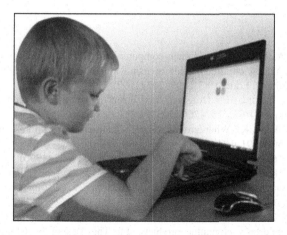

Fig. 8. Using the keyboard, the participants focused alternately the keyboard and the screen

Problems in using the mouse arose when children had to stop a movement precisely. This comes because the fine motor skills are still developing within preschool age. For the same reason, the standard deviations for the average selected or moved objects and collisions were relatively high; some children were already able to move their hands precisely and click accurately while others needed more time.

Unlike the assumption that preschool children would perform similarly to older children, significant differences in the amount of moved objects by Drag-and-Drop and Sticky Drag-and-Drop could not be found. Although children did not have any experience in using a mouse, they were able to move the objects with Drag-and-Drop. However, due to the error rate of Drag-and-Drop and the time children needed for selecting and placing the objects, Sticky Drag-and-Drop has more advantages than Drag-and-Drop – this was different with older children [11]. While all the objects selected with Sticky Drag-and-Drop reached their target, only 71.26% of the objects selected with Drag-and-Drop did. Additionally, even children that moved more objects using Sticky Drag-and-Drop needed more time for selecting and placing the objects with Drag-and-Drop than they did using Sticky Drag-and-Drop. This could be caused by the fact that keeping the mouse button pressed demands more concentration than simply moving the mouse.

5 Conclusions and Future Work

In this paper, we presented the results of three experiments that analyzed interaction techniques for preschool children. We showed that mouse interaction can be preferred to keyboard interaction, because of performance and error rate. Comparing mouse interaction styles, we found that Sticky Drag-and-Drop can be favored over Drag-and-Drop. Next, we want to analyze the behavior using interactive large surfaces (e.g. interactive tables) and develop design guidelines, which should help developers creating applications for preschool children.

References

1. Bruckman, A., Bandlow, A.: Human-computer interaction for kids, pp. 428–440 (2003)
2. Crook, C.: Young children's skill in using a mouse to control a graphical computer interface. Comput. Educ. 19(3), 199–207 (1992)
3. Donker, A., Reitsma, P.: Drag-and-drop errors in young children's use of the mouse. Interact. Comput. 19(2), 257–266 (2007)
4. Druin, A., Inkpen, K.: When are Personal Technologies for Children? Personal Ubiqutous Computing 5(3), 191–194 (2001)
5. Druin, A.: A place called childhood. Interactions 3(1), 17–22 (1996)
6. Grünzweil, B.: Richtlinien für die Erstellung von Applikationen für Kinder im Vorschulalter. Master Thesis, Digital Media, Upper Austria University of Applied Sciences (2008)
7. Hanna, L., Risden, K., Czerwinski, M., Alexander, K.J.: The role of usability research in designing children's computer products. In: The Design of Children's Technology. Morgan Kaufmann Series In Interactive Technologies, pp. 3–26. Morgan Kaufmann Publishers, San Francisco (1998)
8. Hourcade, J.P., Bederson, B.B., Druin, A.: Preschool children's use of mouse buttons. In: CHI 2004 extended abstracts on Human factors in computing systems, pp. 1411–1412 (2004)
9. Hourcade, J.P.: Learning from preschool children's pointing sub-movements. In: Proceedings of the 2006 Conference on interaction Design and Children, IDC 2006, Tampere, Finland, June 7-9, pp. 65–72. ACM, New York (2006)
10. Hourcade, J.P., Crowther, M., Hunt, L.: Does mouse size affect study and evaluation results?: a study comparing preschool children's performance with small and regular-sized mice. In: Proceedings of the 6th international Conference on interaction Design and Children, IDC 2007, Aalborg, Denmark, June 6-8, pp. 109–116. ACM, New York (2007)
11. Inkpen, K.: Drag-and-Drop versus Point-and-Click Mouse Interaction Styles for Children. ACM toChi 8, 1–33 (2001)
12. Kail, R.: Developmental Change in Speed of Processing During Childhood and Adolecense. Psychological Bulletin 109(3), 490–501 (1991)
13. Revelle, G.: Education via entertainment media: the Sesame Workshop approach. ACM Computers in Entertainment 1(1), 16 (2003)

The Use of ICT to Support Students with Dyslexia

Nadia Diraä, Jan Engelen, Pol Ghesquière, and Koen Neyens

K.U. Leuven - Belgium
{Nadia.Diraa,Jan.Engelen}@esat.kuleuven.be,
Pol.Ghesquiere@ped.kuleuven.be, Koen.Neyens@dsv.kuleuven.be

Abstract. The Katholieke Universiteit Leuven (K.U.Leuven) has a tradition of supporting students with a disability in order to guarantee equal opportunities to achieve their educational, personal and vocational goals. The K.U.Leuven policy is working towards inclusive education in the long term, by improving facilities and accommodation for certain target groups in the short term. Efforts have also been directed to make the learning environment more accessible for all kind of students, especially over the last few years. One of the target groups that has increasing numbers are students with learning disabilities (including dyslexia, dyscalculia, ...). To accommodate these students, the K.U.Leuven set off a project to evaluate the use of assistive technology (AT) for dyslexia. This small-scale study examined the experiences of two groups of students with dyslexia using 2 different software programs specifically developed to support this group of students. It was apparent that for students with dyslexia, reading and studying presents additional limitations which AT could facilitate to some extent.

Keywords: People with disabilities, Dyslexia, Assistive Technology, Accessibility.

1 Introduction

Dyslexia is a disorder in which a persistent problem arises with acquiring and applying reading and/or spelling at word level [1]. At this moment, there are growing numbers of students with dyslexia accessing higher education. At the K.U.Leuven, we have seen a yearly increase up to 20% of students with a learning disability since 2005-2006. Students with a learning disability like dyslexia now account for 41% of the students with a disability. In the Netherlands, about 14.000 out of 500.000 students have dyslexia; this is 3% of the total student population [2]. The same evolution is seen in the UK where the population of students with dyslexia has risen from 21.000 in 2004/2005 (2.4%) to 27.465 (3.1%) in 2007/2008 [3]. At the same time we see that evolutions in Internet and Communication Technologies (ICT) have created a lot of possibilities to prevent "handicap situations" (meaning a reduced accomplishment of life habits as a result of complex interactions between personal factors (personal characteristics such as impairments) and environmental factors) [4]. There are some studies demonstrating statistically significant impact of the use of a text reader on student text comprehension [5] [6].

In the period 2008-2009 knowledge and expertise in relation to accessibility of the digital learning environment and the use of ICT support within the K.U.Leuven has

A. Holzinger and K. Miesenberger (Eds.): USAB 2009, LNCS 5889, pp. 457–462, 2009.

been brought together and the support of several internal K.U.Leuven services has been started [7]. The digitalisation of the educational process that used to be an obstacle for students with impairments therefore now becomes a facilitating process and a real support for them. K.U.Leuven's Working Group on Digital Accessibility [8] has stimulated this project from an inclusive vision on the process of digital learning support. To address the needs of students with dyslexia, this project aimed to evaluate the effects of a campus wide introduction of AT for dyslexia.

2 Methodology

2.1 Special-Purpose Software

Students with special needs, especially dyslexia, are accommodated by the use of AT. For dyslexia, there are 2 software programs distributed in primary and secondary education in Flanders. These programs are also being used by students in higher education. At the start of this project, there were no numbers available about the number of students with dyslexia using AT. Since these programs became more and more popular among students, the Working Group on Digital Accessibility asked for funding to do some small-scale research on the application of ICT to facilitate students with dyslexia.

These AT consist of Kurzweil3000 and Sprint. **Kurzweil3000** [9] is a comprehensive reading, writing and learning software solution for students with special needs. The software can access documents in print (with the use of a scanner) or on the web, and electronic documents. Students can use it to read course material with increased speed; they can get visual and auditory feedback and use it for writing assignments.

Sprint [10] adds speech and language technology to a computer so that students can listen to documents, internet pages, email,... in fact to any available text on their computer, as Sprint reads them out loud. Sprint also can read aloud while text is being entered which helps in detecting mistakes.

This part describes how AT has been introduced to students with dyslexia at the K.U.Leuven. At the start of the academic year, the Disability Team of the K.U.Leuven organised an information session about assistive technology for students with dyslexia. This introduction was given by a remedial teacher. About 40 students with dyslexia were present. At the end of this session, the Disability Team made an appeal to participate in a small-scale research with two software programs for dyslexia: Kurzweil3000NL and Sprint. Kurzweil3000NL is a text reader with embedded study and writing skills localized for the Dutch language. It supports students with special needs by making it possible to access almost any document. Sprint is a comparable program that adds speech and language technology to a computer [10]. Both firms, Sensotec [11] and Jabbla [12], agreed to put the software at the disposal of the participating students for free in return for feedback.

There were about 40 students present at the information session, out of which 25 applied for participation in the study. Afterwards there were some more students who wanted to participate. They were also invited to the introductory sessions for each software program. Subsequently, introductory sessions were organised for the 2 different software programs. These introductions were given by trainers provided by the companies. At these sessions, the students were given the software program either on a usb stick (Sprint, 15 students) or on cd (Kurzweil3000, 17 students).

Table 1. Research Participants

Course	M/F	year of birth	Program	AT experience
Engineering	M	1981	Sprint	Yes
Engineering	F	1988	KW3000	N/A
Engineering	F	1990	KW3000	Yes
Computer Science	M	1987	KW3000	Yes
Geography	F	1988	KW3000	Yes
Geology	F	1986	SPRINT	No
Pharmaceutical Sciences	F	1988	SPRINT	No
Biology	F	N/A	SPRINT	N/A
Physiotherapy	M	1990	SPRINT	No
Rehabilitation Sciences	F	N/A	KW3000	N/A
Rehabilitation Sciences	F	N/A	KW3000	N/A
Political Sciences	F	1988	SPRINT	Yes
Law	F	1987	KW3000	N/A
Law	M	1986	SPRINT	Yes
Business Economics	F	1989	SPRINT	No
History	F	1990	KW3000	No
History	M	1988	KW3000	No
Anthropology	M	N/A	SPRINT	N/A
Educational Sciences	F	1985	KW3000	No
Educational Sciences	F	1987	KW3000	No
Educational Sciences	F	1978	SPRINT	No
Educational Sciences	F	1990	SPRINT	No
Educational Sciences	F	1989	KW3000	No
Educational Sciences	F	1986	SPRINT	No
Educational Sciences	M	1976	KW3000	No
Psychology	F	1987	KW3000	No
Psychology	F	1986	SPRINT	No
Psychology	F	1979	KW3000	N/A
Psychology	F	1989	KW3000	Yes
Psychology	F	1971	KW3000	No
Psychology	F	1990	SPRINT	No
Sexuality Studies	F	1987	SPRINT	No
Total:	F: 25		KW3000: 17	Yes: 7
32 participants	M: 7		SPRINT: 15	No: 18
				N/A: 7

2.2 Survey

All participants agreed to be interviewed 3 times during the academic year. The starting interview focused on their experience with ICT and their diagnosis of dyslexia. A second interview was held just after the first semester examinations and it focused on the possibilities of the AT, the problems and needs the students have faced, usability, and possible improvements. Finally, at the end of the academic year but before the June examinations, an evaluation of the project by the students was held.

2.2.1 First Survey

These semi-structured interviews were done by 2 master students in Educational Sciences. The first interviews consisted of 2 parts: one about the impact of dyslexia on their life, and one on the use and experience the participants have with ICT and AT in particular. On average, the students were satisfied by the, still growing, support from the Disability Team. The main problem is situated in the communication with teachers and teaching assistants especially during assessments. Many students find it difficult to disclose their disability to get digital course material. Another aspect is the lack of a generally accepted format for attesting dyslexia. At this moment, students with a disability are asked to provide (medical) documentation or attestation [13] for verification. The students also don't have a clear view on what to expect about reasonable adjustments and their rights. It seems that every faculty at the K.U.Leuven has some kind of support but there is not yet a single policy across the university. As a result of these interviews, additional training was provided for Kurzweil3000. The users of Sprint didn't indicate this need. Some students formulated reserves for using the software. They didn't want to become too dependent on it if they aren't sure they can continue to use the software for the full length of their education.

2.2.2 Second Survey
The second interview focused on the installation and use of ICT and the AT for dyslexia, on the accessibility of digital course material and on the drop outs. The installation of Kurzweil3000 proved to be rather difficult. The students started with demoversions which had to be removed from the computers before the final version could be installed. This resulted in the fact that after the demo-versions expired, only 6 out of 17 participants managed to install the new version without encountering any problems. However, not all these problems were due to the software. Some students had e.g. hardware that was not fit or had a broken cd-player. For Sprint, this was not an issue since the program was delivered on a usb stick which could be used on any computer with Windows installed. Most students used the AT to read course material on a higher speed than without. Some made mp3 files to listen to during other activities. Also the possibility to highlight in the electronic version of the text was found a plus. Negative aspects were the impossibility for the program to transpose mathematical and scientific formulae to speech, preparing files for text-to-speech could take some time, files needing to be divided in chapters no longer than 40 pages otherwise the program wouldn't load them. The availability of digital course material was another important issue. Some teachers have reservations towards putting to disposal digital versions of their course material. To counter this all students received a letter stating that they participated in a research project, with a signed agreement not to distribute any material given to them as part of this project. Some students felt uncomfortable to disclose their disability to get the digital course material. To meet further needs for electronic versions, the Disability Team set up a scan service for students with dyslexia. Here the students could scan the courses they wanted to study with the AT. Twice a week, this service was available for students during lunch hours. About 15 participants used the service to scan and prepare documents using the scanner and OCR. Also other students with dyslexia using AT, but not participating in the research project, made use of the scan service. At this phase of the study about 8 participants didn't use the program at all. Asked for the reasons, 4 still had problems installing Kurzweil3000. Others didn't want to invest too much time in acquiring the skills needed to make use of AT. Or they didn't want to participate in the interviews.

2.2.3 Final Survey

The final survey took place before the examinations in June 2009. Here we present only preliminary results since all the data haven't been studied in detail yet. This last interview focused on the use of the program, an evaluation and some remarks and feedback about the software programs. At that moment there were 10 participants out of 18 still using Kurzweil3000 and 11 out of 15 participants still using Sprint. Most participants only use the AT for text-to-speech assistance with reading. Some made efforts to improve their knowledge about the program but this is a minority. Furthermore, they didn't express interest in additional training to get a more profound knowledge of the AT. Negative aspects students expressed are: the time needed for scanning course material, problems acquiring digital material and the time needed to prepare this material for use with AT. They suggested filing digital course material in some kind of central repository for future use by other dyslexic students (which we plan for early 2010). Also they didn't find good use in the possibilities these software packages present for highlighting and structuring text, and creating outlines, word lists or study guides.

3 Conclusions

During the academic year 2008-2009, 32 students participated in a small-scale research on the use of AT for students with dyslexia. Both Kurzweil3000 and Sprint showed advantages and disadvantages. Students need to have some basic computer skills to be capable of using either software. There is a clear need for sufficient training to make fully use of all the possibilities this AT offers. Also other preconditions need to be in place to successfully implement this software. These preconditions consist of the availability of digital course material, the possibility/authorization to use ICT during courses and assessments, and sufficient computer skills for the students. As can be concluded from the survey, some participants dropped out of the research due to the lack of digital course material. They found that scanning all their readers and handbooks would take too much time since they are already limited in time due to their disability. The advantage of the AT, i.e. the possibility to read at higher speed didn't countervail the time they anticipated needing for scanning all material. With the further implementation of AT for dyslexia, K.U.Leuven needs to provide sufficient access to digital course material. Another precondition is the possibility to use ICT during courses and assessments. The use of ICT during courses didn't cause many conflicts. However, the use during assessments presented some problems. Some teachers didn't want students to use their own laptops or didn't want them to use any ICT at all. To counter the first problem, the Disability Team provided several clean laptops with the AT technology pre-installed. Another problem was the use of highlighted electronic documents. Some assessments allowed students to bring course material to examination but not all students with dyslexia were allowed to use their electronic documents. The possibility to use a function like "Find" in an electronic version would give them a remarkable speed advantage with regard to other students. The AT Kurzweil3000 has the facility to disable some functions and can keep a record of actions taken while using the program. Some faculties chose to prepare audio versions of the exams and mp3 players were put at disposal for students with reading impairments. A last but not at all the least precondition for success are the computer skills of the students. Most used a pc or laptop with Windows Vista or XP. Considering the amount of problems encountered while installing AT, most students needed assistance with this. There also needs to be sufficient training in the software programs to make sure the students understand the full capabilities of these AT.

References

1. van Dyslexie, D.: Brochure Stichting Dyslexie Nederland. Revised edn. (2003)
2. Broenink, N., et al.: Studeren met een handicap, p. 25. Verwey-Jonker Instituut (2001)
3. Higher Education Statistics Agency, Students and Qualifiers Data Tables, http://www.hesa.ac.uk/index.php/component/option, com_datatables/Itemid,121/task,show_category/catdex,3/#disab (accessed 10/07/09)
4. Fougeyrollas, P.: Québec: Cqcidih/Sscdih (1995b)
5. Dimmitt, S., Hodapp, J., Judas, C., Munn, C., Rachow, C.: Iowa Text Reader Project Impacts Student Achievement. Closing the Gap 24(6), 12–13 (2006)
6. Draffan, E.A., Evans, D.G., Blenkhorn, P.: Use of assistive technology by students with dyslexia in post-secondary education. Disability and Rehabilitation: Assistive Technology 2(2), 105–116 (2006)
7. OOP project, Verhoogde toegankelijkheid van onderwijsgerichte ICT toepassingen voor personen met een functiebeperking (K.U.Leuven funded project, 2006)
8. K.U.Leuven Working Group on Digital Accessibility, http://www.kuleuven.be/ digitaletoegankelijkheid/werkgroep.html
9. Kurzweil3000, http://www.kesi.com/kurz3000.aspx (accessed 10/07/09)
10. Sprint, http://www.jabbla.com/software/products.asp? Lid=4&pnav=;2;&item=11&lang=en (accessed 10/07/09)
11. Sensotec NV, http://www.sensotec.be/dyslexie/Producten/K3000/ Default.aspx
12. Jabbla, http://www.jabbla.com
13. K.U.Leuven Disability Team, http://www.kuleuven.be/studentservices/ disability.html (accessed 10/07/09)

Investigating of Memory – Colours of Intellectually Disabled Children and Virtual Game Addict Students

Cecília Sik Lányi

Virtual Environments and Imaging Technologies Laboratory,
University of Pannonia, Egyetem u. 10,
8200 Veszprém, Hungary
lanyi@almos.uni-pannon.hu

Abstract. We describe an investigation of memory colours. For this investigation Flash test software was developed. 75 observers used this test software in 4 groups: average elementary school children (aged: 8-9 years), intellectually disabled children (age: 9-15), virtual game addict university students (average age: 20) and university students who play with VR games rarely or never (average age: 20). In this pilot test we investigated the difference of memory colours of these 4 groups.

Keywords: Memory colour, intellectually disabled, virtual game addict.

1 Introduction

One of the most influential aspects on the quality of our lives is colour. Our use of memory colour occurs so often we usually don't even realize it is happening [1]. Another important impact colour has in our lives is on our learning processes. Disorders such as dyslexia are sometimes affected by colour. According to a web page on the testing of dyslexia the 'glare' of the white paper makes it hard for some dyslexic children and adults to read the page (Dyslexia, 2002) [2].

Many books and articles deal with the question of how colours influence the mood of people seeing them and how, e.g. in a picture the mood of a person can be expressed in colours. For artists, colour was always a vehicle to express moods [3]. Panton, as an artist, even gave the title of his booklet: "Choosing colours should not be a gamble. It should be a conscious decision. Colours have meaning and function" [4]. Hutchings discussed the use of colours during the ages, and pointed out that there are cultural differences that should be taken into consideration [5]. Robertson and his colleagues [6] found evidence of cultural and linguistic relativity, among others in colour categorization. Duncan and Nobbs [7] investigated the interrelationship between human emotions induced by colours and their psychophysical stimuli, and found differences between emotional colour scales established in Europe and the Far East.

Virtual Environment (VE): A synthetic, spatial (usually 3D) world seen from a first-person's point of view. The view in a VE is under the real-time control of the user. Virtual Reality (VR) and Virtual World are more or less synonymous with VE [8].

A. Holzinger and K. Miesenberger (Eds.): USAB 2009, LNCS 5889, pp. 463–475, 2009.

Multi-sensory VEs are closed-loop systems comprised of humans, computers, and the interfaces through which continuous streams of information flow. More specifically, VEs are distinguished from other simulator systems by their capacity to portray three-dimensional (3D) spatial information in a variety of modalities, their ability to exploit users' natural input behavior for human-computer interaction, and their potential to "immerse" the user in the virtual world [9].

Virtual reality games are popular among children and young people all over the world. According to Steinkuehler, the current global player populations of the three game titles (of dozens) that she has studied over the past few years (Lineage I, Lineage II and Word of Warcraft) totals over 9.5 million - a population which rivals, e.g. most US metropolises [10].

"The computer gaming industry has now surpassed the "Hollywood" film industry in total entertainment market share, and in the USA sales of computer games now outnumber the sale of books." (Doug Lowenstein, President, Interactive Digital Software Association) [11].

What is computer and video game addiction?

When time spent on the computer, playing video games or cruising the Internet reaches a point that it harms a child's or adult's family and social relationships, or disrupts school or work life, that person may be caught in a cycle of addiction. Like other addictions, the computer or video game has replaced friends and family as the source of a person's emotional life. Increasingly, to feel good, the addicted person spends more time playing video games or searching the Internet. Time away from the computer or game causes moodiness or withdrawal [12].

We are seeing more and more adults and adolescents struggling with real world relationships because of virtual world relationships they have created [13].

The Smith and Jones Wild Horses Center has the very first outpatient addiction treatment program for problem gamers in Europe. *"Computer and video games can be fun and innocent. Most people can play computer games without trouble. However, 20% of all gamers can develop a dependency on gaming. Many of these individuals have neglected family, romance, school, and jobs; not to mention their basic needs such as food and personal hygiene? All for a video or computer game"* [14].

Virtual reality games are popular among children and young people all over the world. There are a lot of 3D games nowadays. The properties of the heroes of these games are, however, very far from those of humans. Sometimes the surroundings are futuristic too. Children play with the computer games longer and longer every day, and thus the games have an influence on the aesthetic sense of the children. In this respect the question might be raised: are the memory colours of virtual game addict people influenced by VR games' colour, or not?

We know that the colour, shape and the name of objects are storing in different parts of the brain. Brain stores knowledge and colour separately [15]. Therefore the other question was to investigate in this pilot study whether a child with some intellectual disability or learning problems has other memory colours as the average children, or not?

2 Colourimetric Fundamentals

2.1 Colour

The electromagnetic radiation reaching our eye and producing there a sensation is called colour stimulus. The sensation produces the colour perception in our brain. In scientific literature three components of colour perception are distinguished: brightness, hue and colourfulness:

- Brightness: the sensation can be almost blending strong, medium or dim and dark.
- Hue is usually shown as a hue circle, where four distinguishable different areas are red, yellow, green and blue. A hue yellow hue can be reddish or greenish, but never bluish; a green hue can be yellowish or bluish, but never reddish, and so on (see: Figure 1) [16]. One can define the hues between two fundamental (or unique) hue, as e.g. green, bluish green, greenish blue, blue. Sometimes for the hues that are somewhere in the middle between two unique hues special names are used:

  o Yellow – red: orange
  o Green – yellow: lemon
  o Blue – green: cyan or turquoise
  o Red – blue: magenta or purple

- Colourfulness has been divided by MacDonald into a five value scale: Starting with gray (achromatic) up to the most brilliant colour. If no hue can be determined for a colour then it is gray (or white or black). Thus with increasing colourfulness one can speak about a gray, grayish, moderately vivid, vivid and very vivid colour perception.

The communication of the colour perception can thus be made in the following form: The complexion of the person who stands in front of me is medium bright, moderately vivid and reddish yellow [17].

The colour stimulus can be described in a definite way using a colour order system. The colour solid contains all the realizable surface colours. There are several colour systems in use, some of them are the RGB, CMYK, CIELAB, NCS. We performed our measurements using the CIELAB system, because this is – in contrary for example to the RGB or CMYK system a non-device dependent system, it is the system now recommended by international standards [18]. It can be used not only for surface colours, but also for defining colours produced on computer monitor screens. Figure 2. shows this colour system as a three dimensional body, with the lightness (the brightness of surface colours), chroma (representing colourfulness) axes and hue circle (or a^*, b^* axes to describe chroma and hue) where the hue is measured as a hue angle. In the CIELAB colour system one can describe the colour with the L^* lightness and the a^*, and b^* co-ordinates (in Figure 2 we show the a^*, b^* sections as two-dimensional planes). The a^*, b^* co-ordinates describe the amount of redness – greenness, and yellowness – blueness.

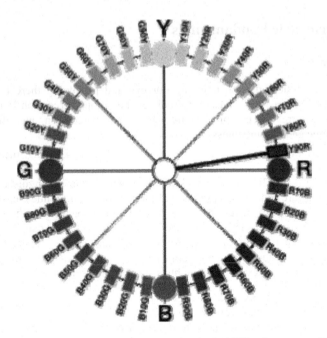

Fig. 1. Opponent colours and colour notation in the NCS colour system [16]

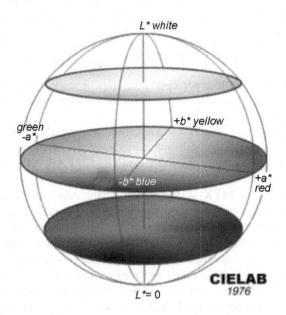

Fig.2. Three-dimensional graph of the real surface colours, in the system of lightness, chroma and hue

Visually the difference between two colours is described by saying: large, medium and small. In the CIELAB system, the colour difference can either be described as the Euclidian distance between the two points representing the colours in the three-dimensional space, or can be described by the lightness difference ($L*$), hue angle difference (h_{ab}), where

$$h_{ab} = \arctan(b*/a*), \text{ and } \Delta C*_{ab}: C* = (a* + b*)^{1/2}.$$

2.2 Memory Colours of Well Known Objects

The term memory colour is used for the colour of well-known, often seen object, as in our brain we attach a colour to the given object. One has to distinguish between memory colour and colour memory, the later is the colour we will reproduce after we have seen a coloured object. Memory colours are well stabilized products of our memory. They are colours we will pick from a high number of colour chips if one is asked to show the colour chip resembling the colour of human complexion, or sky blue, etc. Table 1 shows the $L*$, $a*$, $b*$ values of some memory colours.

Table 1. Memory colours for well-known objects according to different authors

Memory colour	$L*$	$h_{ab}*$	Reference
Caucasian skin	79.5	32.9	[19]
blue sky	54.0	238.8	[19]
green grass	50.0	138.5	[20]
oriental skin	63.9	49.0	[21]
deciduous foliage	33.6	145.3	[19]

3 Method

Flash test software was developed for the investigation of memory colours [22]. 75 observers used this test software in 4 groups: 20 average elementary school children (aged: 8-9 years), 10 intellectually disabled children (age: 9-15), 24 virtual game addict university students (average age: 20) and 21 university students who play with VR games rarely or never (average age: 20). The task was colouring pictures using the colour palettes introduced below and answering some questions. The experiment was made in a dark room using a laptop computer, the monitor of which was calibrated by an Eye-One apparatus. Every observer has good colour vision, we tested them with Colourlite Colour Test (see a shorter version of this test: http://www.colourvision.info/test_colour_vision_deficiency.htm)

3.1 The tests

The observers had to paint the grey pictures using different palettes.

The tests were based on 3 tasks:

i.   "Extended colour palette" (Figure 3),

ii.   "Given colour palette" (Figure 4), and

iii. "Answering questions" (Figure 5).

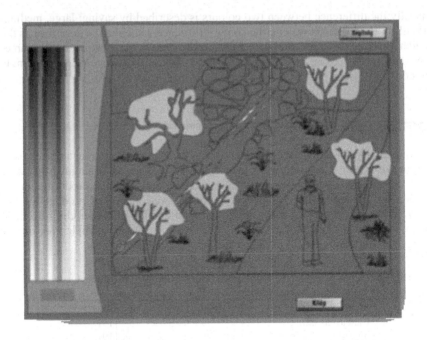

Fig. 3. Extended colour palette task: colouring the foliage

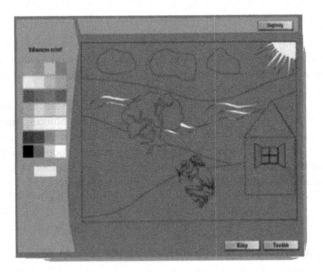

Fig. 4. Given colour palette task: colouring the sun

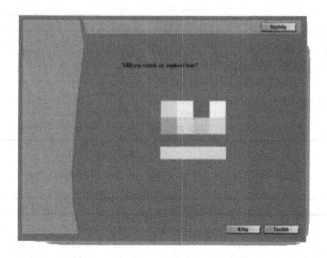

Fig. 5. Answering questions task: What kind of colour has the Caucasian skin?

The observers first solved the "Extended colour palette" tasks. Here the observer could choose from 576 colours. The second task: "Given colour palette" was made one week later. There were 7 colour groups, every colour group consisted of 4 colours. The last task: "Answering questions" was made one week later after solving the earlier task. At the 3rd task the test software asks some questions, for example: What kind of colour is the sky?, What kind of colour is the grass?

4 Results

The test software saved the chosen colours at the colouring tasks and the answers of the observers. So the software saved the L^*, a^* and b^* values of the Caucasian face skin, foliage, sky, tree trunk, cloud, grass, sun, stone, sand, flower, water: stream, sea.

Tables 2 and 5 show the average CIELAB L^*, a^*, b^* and the standard deviation. Based on the data of the pilot test, there was significant difference in the memory colours especially of grass and Caucasian face skin.

Table 2. Test results of the elementary school children

form	Mean			Standard deviation		
	L^*	a^*	b^*	L^*	a^*	b^*
sky	71.63	6.29	-35.08	9.63	8.91	14.89
tree trunk	44.66	10.69	24.85	5.74	6.44	2.79
cloud	69.75	7.81	-34.58	13.51	9.35	13.84
grass	76.85	-55.19	50.95	4.92	8.58	9.83
sand	83.59	-12.22	44.81	9.58	19.14	13.98

Table 2. (*Continued*)

	Mean			Standard deviation		
stone	51.02	0.05	0.83	13.67	4.20	5.89
foliage	70.85	-50.64	49.47	7.95	10.88	10.03
sun	94.90	-14.61	73.32	6.01	11.54	5.29
stream	67.95	-2.07	-24.75	9.27	15.50	20.51
Caucasian skin	86.07	4.17	31.90	5.92	11.50	13.24
sea	62.85	7.05	-37.54	7.37	10.92	14.01
flower	58.22	59.86	34.81	7.86	17.95	31.62

Table 3. Test results of the intellectually disabled children

	Mean			Standard deviation		
form	L^*	a^*	b^*	L^*	a^*	b^*
sky	65.42	5.26	-36.10	13.44	12.93	14.35
tree trunk	50.19	10.45	27.35	10.96	9.61	4.86
cloud	59.94	3.87	-31.87	15.22	12.51	16.83
grass	72.58	-49.13	45.84	13.07	12.15	9.62
sand	84.84	-10.58	44.65	19.23	16.02	18.40
stone	57.19	0.84	8.65	24.90	10.00	13.82
foliage	67.32	-44.77	44.45	17.03	20.89	11.48
sun	94.00	-12.87	68.52	10.58	18.52	7.73
stream	61.48	3.74	-35.32	14.78	11.75	13.22
Caucasian skin	71.58	8.71	40.39	20.60	15.56	14.89
sea	68.13	-0.71	-29.84	14.25	11.33	29.78
flower	60.84	50.94	46.87	15.34	30.71	23.93

Table 4. Test results of the virtual game addict university students

	Mean			Standard deviation		
form	L^*	a^*	b^*	L^*	a^*	b^*
sky	69.73	9.13	-36.20	7.39	7.43	12.75
tree trunk	40.87	39.13	26.47	7.67	3.49	1.98
cloud	87.93	-1.40	-14.87	6.87	6.56	9.52
grass	19.09	-41.20	14.03	6.84	5.89	5.31
sand	89.27	-14.07	48.87	16.53	15.86	13.76
stone	23.77	-3.07	-1.00	18.25	0.86	0.24
foliage	47.87	-38.60	37.93	2.32	0.68	4.02
sun	99.90	-24.20	71.13	0.45	2.95	14.73
stream	62.53	7.67	-35.27	9.65	7.80	9.58
Caucasian skin	81.47	0.73	28.93	17.51	7.92	8.68
sea	57.93	12.00	-40.53	8.67	7.49	10.16
flower	45.27	67.07	54.47	14.20	22.65	18.01

Table 5. Test results of the university students who play with VR games rarely or never

form	Mean			Standard deviation		
	L*	a*	b*	L*	a*	b*
sky	66.29	7.53	-34.71	9.07	11.40	11.75
tree trunk	41.35	16.82	31.18	6.31	0.81	7.80
cloud	80.71	0.53	-23.47	15.38	10.10	15.38
grass	64.65	-45.41	43.29	13.77	3.98	3.94
sand	93.00	-13.71	56.47	7.57	7.76	4.13
stone	64.59	-3.76	-0.53	13.37	0.98	0.57
foliage	68.00	-49.94	44.53	12.69	6.72	5.42
sun	99.82	-22.59	66.65	1.89	2.37	3.74
stream	65.18	-0.76	-26.24	9.05	7.29	2.85
Caucasian skin	94.88	-9.35	40.12	4.79	8.46	17.01
sea	66.94	1.94	-30.18	12.54	9.91	10.56
flower	49.12	72.59	38.12	7.29	5.79	30.35

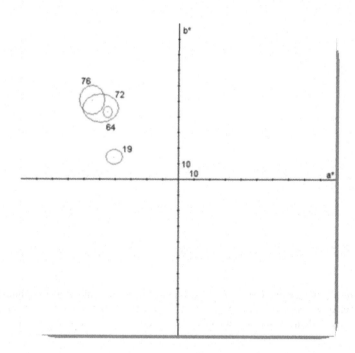

Fig. 6. The result of memory colour of grass, average elementary school children (red) *L*=76*, intellectually disabled children (green) *L*=72*, game addict university students (blue) *L*=19*, university students who play with VR games rarely or never (grey) *L*=64*

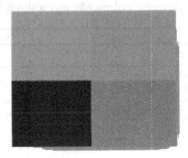

Fig. 7. Sample of the memory colour of grass, upper row: Average elementary school children, intellectually disabled children, lower row: game addict university students, university students who play with VR games rarely or never

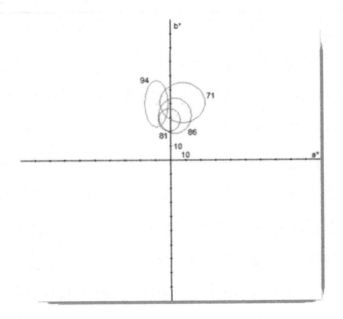

Fig. 8. The result of memory Caucasian face skin, average elementary school children (red) $L^*=86$,intellectually disabled children (green) $L^*=71$game addict university students (blue) $L^*=81$,university students who play with VR games rarely or never (grey) $L^*=94$

Figure 6 and Figure 7 show the „bad" influence on memory colour of VR games. There is no significant difference between the average elementary school children,intellectually disabled children and university students who play with VR games rarely or never, but the virtual game addict university students' results differ from the other 3 groups significantly. The grass' memory colour of the virtual game addict university students is darker. This result agrees with the results we had by

Fig. 9. Sample of the memory colour of Caucasian face skin, upper row: Average elementary school children, intellectually disabled childrenlower row: game addict university students, university students who play with VR games rarely or never

investigating the colours found in VR games, studied by game category: the colour of the grass of VR games was darker and browner, compared to the cartoon colours and the memory colours found in the literature [23], [24].

The results of Caucasian face skin are different too. The memory colour of game addict students is more grey.

The results show there was significant difference (p<0.5) in their memory colours between game addict university students and university students who play with VR games rarely or never. But there was no significant difference between the other three groups.

5 Summary

Answering the questions in the introduction:

Are the memory colours of virtual game addict people influenced by VR games' colour, or not?

Yes, there was a definite difference found between the game addict observers and the other 3 groups.

When a child has some kind of intellectual disability or learning problems are his/her memory colours modified, compared to the average children, or not?

We found difference only in case of the Caucasian face skin colour.

In our earlier research – where we measured the color use in virtual reality games – it was realized [23], that:

- in case of complexion colour : the colours are more yellowish than the memory colours.

- in case of grass colour: except for two categories (children and sport games) the colour of the grass was darker and browner, compared to the memory colours. So the colour of the grass in the virtual games is false too.

- in case of sky colour: it was found in most cases, that more types of blue colors are used, in some cases they were far from the natural sky colour, they were more grayish.

Unfortunately we observed that the designers of the virtual games did not take care of using natural colors [24]. These colors are very far from the memory colors too.

We would like to call the attention of the designers of virtual games to use more natural shades of colors that is to say, colors that are near to the natural ones. Otherwise these colours will influence the memory colours of people, especially of children who play with VR games frequently.

Acknowledgments. The author would like to thank Mrs. Andrea Kovács MSc student and Mr. Gábor Feitsher BSc. student developing the test software.

References

1. Denby, C.: Importance of Memory Color (2002),
   http://hubel.sfasu.edu/courseinfo/SL02/memory_color.htm
2. Dyslexia home page, http://www.dyslexia-test.com/color.html
3. Itten, V.: Kunst und Farbe, Otto Maier Verl. Ravensburg (1970)
4. Panton, V.: Choosing colours should not be a gamble. It should be a conscious decision. Colours have meaning and function as a title of his booklet, Danish Design Centre (1997)
5. Hutchings, J.B.: Color in anthropology and folklore. In: Nassau, K. (ed.) Color for science, art and technology. Elsevier, Amsterdam (1998)
6. Robertson, D., Davies, I., Davidoff, J.: Color categories are not universal: replications and new evidence from stone-age culture. J. of Exp. Psychology: General 129, 369–398 (2000)
7. Duncan, J., Nobbs, J.H.: Coloring our emotions: the measurement and application of our responses to color, Abstract. In: PICS 2004, Conference Glasgow (2004)
8. Bowman, D.A., Kruijff, E., Laviola Jr., J.J., Poupyrev, I.: 3D User Interfaces. Addison-Wesley, Reading (2004)
9. Stanney, K.M.: Handbook of virtual environments. In: Stanney, K.M. (ed.) Handbook of Virtual Environments: Design, Implementation and Applications. Lawrence Erlbaum Associates, Inc., Mahwah (2002)
10. Steinkuehler, C.: Massively Multiplayer Online Games – Based Learning. In: M3 – Interdisciplinary Aspects on Digital Media & Education, Workshop, Wien, Austria, November 23, pp. 15–16 (2006)
11. Lowenstein, D.: Essential facts about the video and computer game industry (2002), http://www.idsa.com/pressroom.html
12. Gameaddiction, http://www.mediafamily.org/facts/facts_gameaddiction.shtml
13. Molmann, S.: For online addicts, relationship float between real, virtual worlds (2008), http://edition.cnn.com/2008/BUSINESS/01/29/digital.addiction/index.html
14. Smith, Jones: (2006), http://www.smithandjones.nl/eng/index.html
15. Health24, http://www.health24.com/mind/Memory_and_cognition/1284-1297,12667.asp
16. Natural Color System - The International Language of Color Communication, Website found at, http://www.ncscolor.com/
17. MacDonald, L.: Color in Computer Graphics, 2nd edn. Lecture Notes. MacColor Ltd. (1998)

18. CIE Draft standard: Colorimetry – Part 4, CIE 1976 L*a*b* color space, CIE DS 014-4.1 (2006)
19. Bartleson, C.J.: Memory colors of familiar objects. J. OSA 50, 73–77 (1960)
20. Tarczali, T.: Investigation of color memory, PhD thesis, University of Pannonia (2007)
21. CIE TC 1-33 Color Rendering. Specifying Color Rendering Properties of Light Sources (1996)
22. Kovács, A.: Developing test software for investigation of memory color, MSc thesis work, University of Pannonia (2007)
23. Sik Lányi, C., Sik, A., Sik, G.: Virtual world – A brave new world – but what kind of colours are used in these virtual environments? Poster, 26th Session of the CIE, Beijing, China, July 4-11, vol. 1. D1, pp. 99–102 (2007)
24. Sik Lányi, C., Sik, A., Sik, G.: What Kinds of Colors are Used in the Virtual Games. In: 12th International Conference, HCI International 2007, Beijing, China, July 22-27. LNCS, vol. 4550-4566, poster, pp. 1285–1288. Springer, Heidelberg (2007)

A Sign Language Screen Reader for Deaf

Oussama El Ghoul and Mohamed Jemni

Research Unit of Technologies of Information and Communication UTIC[8]
Ecole Supérieure des Sciences et Techniques de Tunis,
5, Av. Taha Hussein, B.P. 56, Bab Mnara 1008, Tunis, Tunisia
oussama.elghoul@utic.rnu.tn, mohamed.jemni@fst.rnu.tn

Abstract. Screen reader technology has appeared first to allow blind and people with reading difficulties to use computer and to access to the digital information. Until now, this technology is exploited mainly to help blind community. During our work with deaf people, we noticed that a screen reader can facilitate the manipulation of computers and the reading of textual information. In this paper, we propose a novel screen reader dedicated to deaf. The output of the reader is a visual translation of the text to sign language. The screen reader is composed by two essential modules: the first one is designed to capture the activities of users (mouse and keyboard events). For this purpose, we adopted Microsoft MSAA application programming interfaces. The second module, which is in classical screen readers a text to speech engine (TTS), is replaced by a novel text to sign (TTSign) engine. This module converts text into sign language animation based on avatar technology.

Keywords: Screen reader, TTSing engine, Deaf, Avatar.

1 Introduction

Despite the technological advances in communication and information process, deaf people suffer from several difficulties to communicate and access to the information. Let know that visual information are visible, but not accessible for them if they are illustrated by textual representation. This is due to two main reasons: the illiteracy of the majority of deaf people and the non adapted information used by computers (like audible feedbacks). In this context, our project "Screen reader for deaf" aims to translate significant contents displayed in the screen after an event generated by user activities to sign language animation. The system represents a screen reader with an output different from those generated by classical screen readers.

The paper is organized as follows. Section 2 presents the motivation. Section 3 describes the survey of existing solutions for deaf accessibility. The technical architecture of classical screen readers is illustrated in section 4. The last section is devoted to describe our approach and to detail the technical architecture of the proposed system.

A. Holzinger and K. Miesenberger (Eds.): USAB 2009, LNCS 5889 pp. 476–483, 2009.
© Springer-Verlag Berlin Heidelberg 2009

2 Motivation

2.1 Literacy of Deaf

In 2003, the World Federation of Deaf confirmed that 80% of deaf people lack education or are undereducated, are illiterate or semi-literate [11]. Moreover Sign language is banned in many countries and programs. In addition, the average of deaf high school graduate is unable to exceed the fourth grade level. Deaf children have much trouble to read. Many of them still to have comprehension difficulties on reading into adulthood. Moreover, reading levels of hearing impaired is lower than the reading level of hearing students. In 1996, Marschark and Harris [8] have confirmed that their learning progress is extremely slow. In fact, the reading capability of the high-school graduate deaf is similar to the reading potential of 8 to 9 year old hearing child. Consequently, the gain of experience collected by deaf children in four years is equivalent to the gain of one year for hearing children [8].

2.2 Difficulty to Understand Menus and Textual Information

Because they can see visual information and use mouse and keyboard easily, we believe that visual computer contents are accessible for deaf. However, using computer and internet represents a big challenge for the majority of deaf people, due to their lack of education or their written language illiteracy. Understanding feedbacks or choosing menus is still difficult for hearing impaired because they are written in textual format. For this reason, their computer use is limited to the video chat or some deaf accessible websites. Furthermore, they have serious difficulties to use Hypertext links to navigate on the internet or to understand textual web contents. However, there exists few number of web contents on sign languages, mostly by embedding video files which contain sign language translations of the website's texts. These video translations are still limited to some administrative or deaf organization websites.

2.3 Many Audible Feedbacks

In general, computers are useable without having to listen to any sound. We can write text, navigate on the internet, or send mail without need for any hearing capacity. However, some sonorous feedbacks are generated by computers as alerts to certain events. An example is an error message or a sound to indicate that a new mail has arrived. These feedbacks require visual alternatives to be accessible by hearing impaired people. For example, when a new mail arrives, some applications show a message box or change the color of the mail client telling the user that there is a new message.

2.4 Deaf Have to Adapt Their Skills to Use Technology

Operating systems of different machines are available in a multitude of languages in the worlds except sign language and others spoken languages used by a minority of people. There are three reasons explaining this fact: the first is that the mainstream society chooses the mode of communication the most used (sign language is used by little number of people). The second reason is that there are hundreds of sign languages in the words. It's hard to make machines supporting this large number of visual languages. The last cause is due to the difficulties to implement an operating system using such languages because it requires the storage of many video sequences. Consequently, hearing impaired people have to adapt their communication need to the mode of communication chosen by mainstream society [9].

3 Survey of Existing Solutions

In order to improve the accessibility of hearing impaired people to the information and overcome the problems presented in last section many solutions and studies appeared during the last few years. In this section we illustrate three techniques offering to the deaf community a minimum of comfort to access to the information.

3.1 Websites Translation into Sign Languages

The most evident way to develop an accessible website to deaf person is to translate textual content into sign language. Many companies specialized on sign languages interpretation offer same services to translate websites' contents into sign language video sequences. However, the translation is a very hard task. It consumes times and money. The disadvantages of this solution can be summarized on the necessity of large bandwidth to be able to see video in streaming mode in the first hand, and in the second hand, textual links (Hypertexts) still inaccessible for reading disabled persons.

3.2 Hypertext in Sign Language or Pictograms

There exist very few websites in the World Wide Web based on sign language video interpretation. However, all these contents ignore Hypertext links despite their importance. Hypertext links are as significant as the information itself. In fact, they represent the most efficient and the most used navigation tool in the Web. If sign language contents exist, it would be hard to find by deaf users. Because, before to be able to see sign language content, a deaf should navigate several text-based web pages. As a solution, Andreas Kaibel and al. [6] have proposed a new technique which allows making Hypertext links in sign language format. All contents of pages are shown on video format accessible to deaf people[6]. In another hand, researchers have used pictograms as alternatives to the textual information in the Hypertext links[3].

3.3 Improving Deaf Users' Accessibility in Hypertext Structure

Due to its importance, some researchers have focused their studies to determine the impact of the hypertext structure on the accessibility (simplicity, content finding) of websites. It is argued that the structure of links between pages have an influence on the information finding [2]. The depth and breadth of website affect the speed of searching information. In fact, depth is the number of layers of nodes in the website structure and breadth is defined as the items number in the same node.

3.4 Synthesis

It is clear that many efforts are done to pick up the accessibility of deaf persons to the internet and digital information. However, these works are still insufficient to satisfy the need of deaf due to the cost and/or the difficulties to make. *Table1* illustrates the disadvantages and argues the unsatisfactory of each solution.

Table 1. Disadvantages of existing solutions

Solution	disadvantage
Websites translation into sign languages	- Cost (time and money); - Translation is limited to the content; - Navigation is difficult; - Need large bandwidth.
Hypertext in sign language or pictograms	- Cost (time and money); - Translation of hypertext links; - Easy navigation; - Hard to implement.
Improving deaf users' accessibility in hypertext structure	- Easier navigation; - Textual information; - Unusable for illiterates.

In this context, we propose a screen reader for deaf. The output is the translation of textual information, feedbacks, menus and message box into sign language. The proposed solution offers many advantages to deaf. The first one is the use of existing resources (such that, there is no need to develop operating systems or applications in sign languages). Furthermore, deaf can access to a wide range of web contents and not only to those presented in sign language. In particular, it becomes possible to read all existing textual web contents despite the medium quality of the translation. Moreover, the system is free and it is easy to use: the deaf has to put the mouse cursor over the text or the graphical content to be interpreted by a virtual character. The architecture of the proposed application is described in the next section.

4 Screen Reader Architecture

The most common definitions of a screen reader are in agreement that it is a software for visually impaired persons and that it serves to translate contents shown on the computer screen to vocal or/and Braille contents. Others definitions enlarge the set of persons who are able to use screen readers to illiterates or learning disabled persons because screen readers can read textual information. In this project, we have extended the set of screen reader users to cover persons who are learning disabled and hearing impaired.

In order to allow screen readers to access to the user interfaces, operating systems should have a specific architecture allowing screen readers manufactures to develop separate screen reader applications. In this context, Apple and Microsoft have developed their own architecture. For instance, in this work, we are using Microsoft design and our application has been developed on Microsoft Windows.

As shown on *figure1[1]*, the screen reader is a separate application but it communicates with the operating system and other applications via many interfaces. Thanks, to MSAA (Microsoft Active Accessibility) it becomes possible to communicate with the operating system in order to catch events, to get the focused GUI component and to read its textual properties and/or contents. In other words, MSAA represents an ideal interface to develop an application able to communicate and fetch textual information from the screen. However, some windows applications do not support or totally support the MSAA.

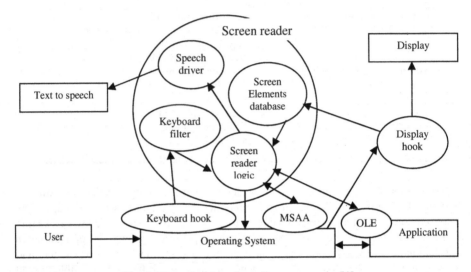

Fig. 1. General architecture of a screen reader [1]

To cover this gap screen readers use traditional techniques which consist on hooking keyboard and display. Captured keyboard events will be routed to the keyboard filter witch analyzes them and sends the result to be treated by the screen reader logic. At the same time, the display hook is responsible to monitor windows messages in order to determine screen updates and maintain an off-screen model (Screen Elements database). The off-screen model is a data structure with an associated API for screen information. It serves to specify to the screen reader information about the contents of the screen.

5   Our Approach

A screen reader for deaf is unlike any other screen reader not only because the output is in sign language but also for the reason that the input is based on the use of the mouse. For this reason, the classical screen reader architecture needs to be updated to satisfy new requirements (*figure2*). Firstly, the software should capture mouse events instead of keyboard events captured by screen readers for blind. Secondly, the application requires also an off-screen model to be used in the case of applications that do not support or support partially the MSAA technology. Concerning the output,

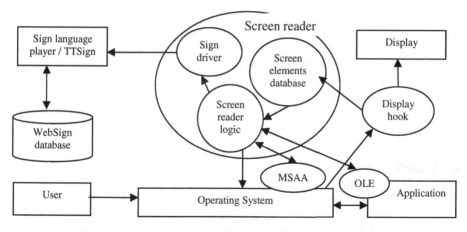

Fig. 2. Architecture of the proposed screen reader

we propose to integrate to the screen reader a new "text to sign language" engine. The system is controlled by a sign driver.

The difference between our tool and screen readers for blinds resides not only on the input/output modules but also on the screen reader logic. A screen reader for blind should read the focused object. However, a deaf needs to read the textual description of the mouse pointed objects. In another hand, unlike classical screen reader, our tool does not identify visual GUI objects. For example, when a new window is displayed on the screen of blind persons the system should indicate this information. Furthermore, if the user changes the focus to a button, the system should indicate that the focused object is a button and should also indicate the title of this button. However, this information is not essential for deaf because it is represented in visual way.

The Text to Sign player is an application developed in our research laboratory of technologies of information and communication UTIC [10]. It is based on the avatar

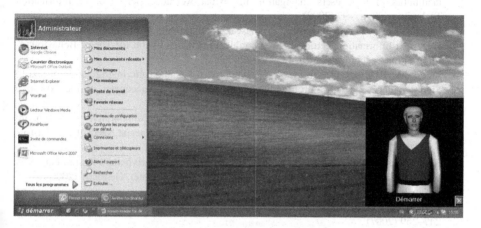

Fig. 3. Screenshot of the screen reader

technology. It can play directly signs by sending a movement request and it can interpret, in real time, textual sentences into Sign language. The player is described in previously published papers [4][5]. The two services are exploited as follow: most useful words and sentences (like open, close, save, shutdown ...) are stored locally and manipulated by the Sign driver. The movement requests are sent directly to the Sign player. If words or sentences are occasionally used (like texts in web pages or menus in newly installed applications), the system sends the entire sentence to the "text to sign" engine which contacts the server to get the translation using Websign database.

6 Conclusion

In this paper, we have presented a new screen reader dedicated to deaf using avatar technology and real time sign language machine translation. The system is tested locally with a small dictionary and we obtained promising results. In this step of the project, we have implemented only the part which uses the MSAA technology and we plan to start the development of message hooking solution soon.

As perspectives, we plan to ameliorate the websites interpretation, in the first step, by analyzing HTML tags. In a second step, we plan to run a set of experimentations with deaf persons.

Acknowledgments. We express our thanks to the anonymous reviewers of this paper and to Mr. Abdel Halim Chalbi, the Tunisian expert in sign language for his collaboration.

References

1. Blenkhorn, P., Evans, G.: Architecture and requirements for a Windows screen reader. In: Speech and Language Processing for Disabled and Elderly People (2000)
2. Fajardo, I., Cañas, J.J., Salmerón, L., Abascal, J.: Information structure and practice as facilitators of deaf users' navigation in textual websites. Behaviour & Information Technology 28, 87–97 (2009)
3. Fajardo, I., Canas, J., Salmeron, L., Abascal, J.: Improving Deaf Users' Accessibility in Hypertext Information Retrieval: Are Graphical Interfaces Useful for Them? Behaviour & Information Technology 25(6), 455–467 (2006)
4. Jemni, M., El ghoul, O.: An avatar based approach for automatic interpretation of text to Sign language. In: 9th European Conference for the Advancement of the Assistive Technologies in Europe, San Sebastián, Spain (2007)
5. Jemni, M., El ghoul, O.: A System to Make Signs Using Collaborative Approach. In: International Conference on Computers Helping People with Special Needs, Linz, Austria, pp. 670–677 (2008)
6. Kaibel, A., Grote, K., Knoerzer, K., Sieprath, H., Florian, K.: Hypertext in sign language. In: 9th ERCIM Workshop "User Interfaces For All". Königswinter, Germany (2006)
7. Lazar, J., Allen, A., Kleinman, J., Malarkey, C.: What frustrates screen reader users on the web: A study of 100 blind users. International Journal of Human-Computer Interaction 22, 247–269 (2007)

8. Marschark, M., Harris, M.: Success and failure in learning to read: The special case of deaf children. In: Reading comprehension difficulties: Processes and intervention, pp. 279–300. Lawrence Erlbaum, Mahwah (1996)
9. Rogers, T.: Access to information on computer networks by the deaf. The Communication Review 2, 497–521 (1998)
10. Research Laboratory of technologies of Information and Communication, http://www.utic.rnu.tn
11. World Federation of the Deaf (WFD), Position Paper regarding the United Nations Convention on the Rights of People with Disabilities, Ad Hoc Committee on a Comprehensive and Integral International Convention on the Protection and Promotion of the Rights and Dignity of Persons with Disabilities (June 24, 2003)

Spoken Dialogue Interfaces: Integrating Usability

Dimitris Spiliotopoulos, Pepi Stavropoulou, and Georgios Kouroupetroglou

Department of Informatics and Telecommunications
National and Kapodistrian University of Athens
Panepistimiopolis, Ilisia, GR-15784, Athens, Greece
{dspiliot,pepis,koupe}@di.uoa.gr

Abstract. Usability is a fundamental requirement for natural language interfaces. Usability evaluation reflects the impact of the interface and the acceptance from the users. This work examines the potential of usability evaluation in terms of issues and methodologies for spoken dialogue interfaces along with the appropriate designer-needs analysis. It unfolds the perspective to the usability integration in the spoken language interface design lifecycle and provides a framework description for creating and testing usable content and applications for conversational interfaces. Main concerns include the problem identification of design issues for usability design and evaluation, the use of customer experience for the design of voice interfaces and dialogue, and the problems that arise from real-life deployment. Moreover it presents a real-life paradigm of a hands-on approach for applying usability methodologies in a spoken dialogue application environment to compare against a DTMF approach. Finally, the scope and interpretation of results from both the designer and the user standpoint of usability evaluation are discussed.

Keywords: Speech, Spoken Dialog Interface, Usability, Usability Evaluation, Auditory User Interface, Human Computer Interaction, Accessibility, Computer Mediated Communication.

1 Introduction

The late years' research in communication, the world-wide-web and Human Computer Interaction (HCI) has led to significant advances in information access and revolutionized the way people exchange knowledge, learn and communicate. However, despite the newly designed approaches and technological advances, accessibility issues still constitute a barrier for a significant percentage of possible users, both mainstream as well as people with disability. People accessing the web or other educational material are usually presented with interfaces that, although make the information accessible; require either specific knowledge or expertise by the user. Moreover these are only designed as supplementary interfaces for use by special user groups in a specified modality or format as an alternative accessible means. Interfaces that are designed with only the accessibility as a solitary guide usually fail to present the real user with a usable means of communication.

A. Holzinger and K. Miesenberger (Eds.): USAB 2009, LNCS 5889, pp. 484–499, 2009.

Web technology is rapidly reaching maturity making it possible to practically use for most applications by the majority of potential users in the recent years. With high speed internet availability providing access to demanding multimodal services to all homes, most people can reap the benefits of real-time services ranging from voice banking to online socialising and beyond. Most high-level services are provided solely through web pages in the traditional point-and-click manner. In an effort to include the people with disability and boost *customer experience* most providers deploy spoken dialogue interfaces as a means for universal access as well as naturalness of information access.

The Web Accessibility Initiative (WAI) of the W3C and the emerging Web 2.0 [20] provide recommendations for creating, maintaining, extending and communicating accessible content. The creation of such content represents a harder task since it requires innovative design and multimodal implementation [28] according to the design-for-all directives while maintaining the scope of high-level user experience. The issues concerning universal accessibility in intelligent environments have been identified and deemed of utmost importance and benefit by the government bodies such as the European Union and the US Department of Education showing increased interest through appropriate accessibility initiatives, such as eInclusion of the eEurope [10].

Due to the complexity of natural language interaction, it is becoming very important to build spoken language interfaces as easily as possible using the enabling technologies. However, not all technologies involved in the process are of the same maturity, let alone standardisation. Furthermore, there is only a handful of platforms available for building such systems. Given the range, variability and complexity of the actual business cases it is obvious that the enabling technologies may produce working systems of variable usefulness due to design and/or implementation limitations.

As with all human-computer interfaces, speech-based interfaces are built with the target user in mind, based on the requirements analysis. However, they differ from traditional graphical user interfaces and web interfaces. The use of speech as the main input and output mode necessitates the use of *dialogue* for the human-machine communication and information flow. Information is received by the speech interface and presented to the user in chunks, much alike a dialogue between two humans. The input is recognised, interpreted, managed, and the response is constructed and uttered using speech. The naturalness is indeed far more enhanced than using forms and buttons on a traditional web interface. Apart from that, the use of Dual-Tone Multi-Frequency (DTMF) navigation over telephony is also a very common approach. However, such approach is seldom tailored for all users, is static and very unnatural. As a result, the performance of the resulting application does not always meet satisfactory levels in usability. It is, therefore, imperative that usability is ensured by design and verified by evaluation in a spoken dialogue interface when that is either deployed from the start or replaces a DTMF menu-driven approach.

The rest of this paper discusses the background of speech-based Human-Computer Interaction and elaborates on the spoken dialog interfaces. It explores what usability is and how it is ensured for natural language interaction interface design and implementation, both from the designer and the application deployment (business use) points of view. Hands-on experience on business-oriented spoken dialogue interfaces has shown that the designer can benefit from summative evaluation in the pre-deployment phase. The benefit from the transition to a spoken dialogue interface from a DTMF interface that provides a relatively large amount of services to a wide range of users is of utmost importance. This work presents the results of usability testing performed over a pre-deployed natural language dialogue system and a DTMF approach for the same real-life application domain, showing how usability engineering is applied for the design and implementation of a state-of-the-art voice user interface and evaluated by the target users.

2 Natural Language Interaction

People acquire communicative skills over time through the experience of using and operating the user interfaces. As the level of user adeptness rises, the speed and accuracy of the operation increases. The user adapts to the system and interacts more efficiently. The level of absolute efficiency corresponds to the actual system design, and can be assessed either as a full system or as a breakdown of its fundamental design modules or processes. In order to evaluate usability of such interfaces it is important to understand their design requirements and their architecture.

The use of speech as input/output for interaction requires a spoken language oriented framework that adequately describes the system processes. W3C has defined the Speech Interface Framework to represent the typical components of a speech-enabled web application [19].

Speech interaction is context-dependent. The context of the user input is analysed by the system in an attempt to understand the *meaning* and *semantics* within the application domain. The interaction itself is called a *dialogue*. The spoken dialogue interfaces handle human-machine dialogue using natural language as the main input and output. A general depiction of a Spoken Dialogue Interface is shown in Figure 1.

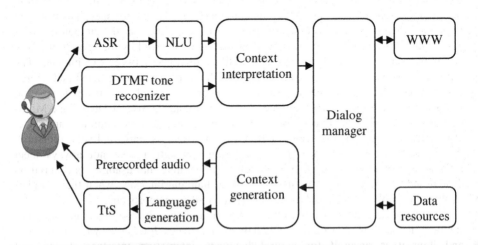

Fig. 1. Spoken dialog interface framework

Broadly speaking, a generic dialogue system comprises of three modules:

- Input – commonly includes automatic speech recognition (ASR) and natural language understanding (NLU). The ASR converts the acoustic user input into text while the NLU parses the text in order to semantically interpret it. Additionally, a DTMF tone recognizer may be included in order to allow for such input.
- Dialogue Management – is the core of the dialogue system. It handles a unique and complete conversation with the user, evaluating the input and creating the output. In order to do that, it activates and coordinates a series of processes that evaluate the user prompt. The dialog manager (DM) identifies the communicative act, interprets and disambiguates the NLU output and creates a specific dialogue strategy in order to respond. It maintains the state of the dialog (or belief state), formulates a dialog plan and employs the necessary dialog actions in order to fulfil the plan. The DM is also connected to all external resources, back-end database and world knowledge.
- Output – usually in includes a natural language generator (NLG) coupled with a text-to-speech synthesizer (TtS). The NLG renders the dialog manager output from communicative acts to proper written language while the TtS engine converts the text to speech and/or audio. A lot of applications, for the sake of customer satisfaction, use prerecorded audio queues instead of synthetic speech for output. In that case, the dialogue manager forms the output by registering all text prompts and correlating them with prerecorded audio files.

When building a speech-based human-computer interaction system, certain basic modules must be present [23]. The Dialogue Manager is responsible for the system behavior, control and strategy. In general, a dialogue with a machine is a sequential process and contains multiple turns that can be initiated by the machine (system initiative), the user (user initiative), or both (mixed initiative). The ASR and NLU recognize the spoken input and identify semantic values. The language generator and TtS or the prerecorded audio generator provides the system response. The dialogue is usually restricted within the thematic domain of the particular application. The performance of the particular modules is an indication of usability issues. The ASR accuracy and the lack of language understanding due to out-of-grammar utterances or ambiguity hinder the spoken dialogue. Moreover, the lack of pragmatic competence of the dialogue manager (compared to the human brain) and the response generation modules sometimes overcomplicate the dialogue and frustrate the user.

3 Usability

The term usability has been used for many years to denote that an application or interface is *user friendly*, *easy-to-use*. These general terms apply to most interfaces, including web interfaces and more importantly speech-based web interfaces. Usability is measured according to the attributes that describe it, as explained below [25]:

- Usefulness – measures the level of *task enablement* of the application. As a side results it determines the *will* of the user to actually use it for the purpose it was designed for.

- Efficiency – assesses the *speed, accuracy* and *completeness* of the tasks or a user's goal. This is particularly useful for evaluating an interface sub-system since the tasks may be broken down in order to evaluate each module separately.
- Effectiveness – quantifies the system *behaviour*. It is a user-centric measure that calculates whether the system behaves the way the users expect it to. It also rates the system according to the level of *effort* required by the user to achieve certain goals and respective *difficulty*.
- Learnability – it extends the effectiveness of the system or application by evaluating the user's effort required to do specific tasks over several repetitions or time for training and expertise. It is a key measure of user experience since most users expect to be able to use an interface effortlessly after a period of use.
- Satisfaction – it is a subjective set of parameters that the user's are asked to estimate and rank. It summises the user overall *opinion* about an application based on whether the product meets their *needs* and performs *adequately*.
- Accessibility – is a very important and broad discipline with many design and implementation parameters. For spoken dialogue interfaces, it can be through of as an extension of the aforementioned usability attributes to the universal user. Speech and audio interfaces are suitable for improved accessibility [11, 5, 12].

3.1 Interaction Design Lifecycle (Interfaces) and Usability

The basic interaction design process is epitomized by the main activities that are followed for almost every product. There are four stages in the lifecycle of an interface:

- Requirements specification and initial planning
- Design
- Implementation, testing and deployment
- Evaluation

In terms of usability there are three key characteristics pertaining to user involvement in the interaction design process [26]:

- User involvement should take place throughout all four stages.
- The usability requirements, goals and evaluation parameters should be set at the start of the development
- Iteration through the four stages is inevitable and, therefore, should be included in the initial planning.

Figure 2 shows how usability generally integrates with the development of an interface.

3.2 Speech Interfaces and Usability

Spoken dialogue interfaces may be of three types depending on their design:

a. DTMF replacement
b. Simple system or user-directed question-answering
c. Open-ended natural language mixed-initiative conversational system

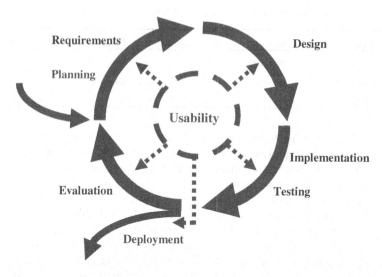

Fig. 2. Typical interface lifecycle and usability

Type (a) systems are the very basic menu-driven interfaces where a static tree-based layout is presented to the user. The user may respond with yes/no and navigate through the menu through options. Such systems are not user-friendly, typically used for very limited domain services, and require patience and time from the user in order to complete a task. The main advantage is that they are very robust, since the user is presented with only a few options at any time, and can only go forward or backwards in the tree-structured menu.

Type (b) systems use more advanced techniques in order to accommodate a more natural interaction with the user. The menus may be dynamic, have confirmation and disambiguation prompts as well as more elaborate vocabulary. Still, the system or the users have to use voice responses within the grammar. Such systems have reusable dialogue scripts for dialogue repair. The small grammars keep the system relatively robust. Such systems are used for most applications at the moment, providing a trade off between efficiency and robustness.

Type (c) systems are used for large scale applications. These systems are targeted for user satisfaction and naturalness. The users may respond to natural "how may I help you" system prompts with equally natural replies. The utterances may be long, complex and exhibit great variety. The dialogue is dynamic and the demand for successful ASR is high, as is the use of statistical or machine learning methods for interpretation. The dialogue management is task-based, the system creating tasks and plans of actions to fulfil. The users expect high-level natural interaction, a very important element to factorise in usability parameterisation.

It is obvious now that each type of design entails particular usability expectations. Each type is expected to excel in certain aspects.

Table 1. Usability impact on spoken dialogue interface development lifecycle

Type	Requirements	Design	Implementation	Evaluation	Deployment
DTMF	low	medium	low	low	low
Q&A	medium	medium	low	medium	low
Open	high	high	medium	high	medium

Table 1 shows how usability is taken into account in each stage of the product lifecycle, based on the experience from the development and testing of nationwide-size spoken dialogue business applications. The development of such applications is an iterative process, as mentioned before. Practitioners in industrial settings agree that usability parameters as well as testing is also part of the iterative process. Open systems possess the highest potential for usability integration. In that respect, the remainder of this chapter refers mostly to open systems and less to the other two types. These days, such systems are the centre of the attention by researchers, developers and customers alike, focusing on advanced voice interaction and high user satisfaction. The use of natural voice response (both acoustic and syntactic) and the natural dialogue flow constitute the state-of-the-art in spoken dialogue interfaces.

4   Usability Evaluation

Usability evaluation is usually performed either during or at the end (or near the end) of the development cycle. The methodologies that can be used for that differ in their scope, their main difference being that, when a product is finished (or nearly finished), *usability testing* serves for fine-tuning certain parameters and adjusting others to fit the target user better. During the design phase, usability evaluation methods can be used to probe the basic design choices, the general scope and respective task analysis of a web interface. Some of the most common factors to think about when designing a usability study are:

- Simulate environment conditions closely similar to real world application use.
- Make sure the usability evaluation participants belong to the target user group
- Make sure the user testers test all parameters you want to measure
- Consider onsite or remote evaluation

4.1   Methodologies

Usability evaluation for speech-based web interfaces is carried upon certain usability evaluation methods and approaches on the specific modules and processes that comprise each application. Each approach measures different parameters and goals. They all have the same goal, to evaluate usability for a system, sub-system or module. However, each approach targets specific parameters for evaluation. Depending on whether they are deployed during the design or production phase, and whether they focus on the user interaction or a sub-system performance parameter, there are two distinct classes of methodology – evaluative usability testing and Wizard-of-Oz (WOZ) testing [14].

4.1.1 Wizard-of-Oz (Formative Evaluation)

It is a common approach that is used not only for speech-based dialogue systems but for most web applications. It enables usability testing during the early stages by using a human to simulate a fully working system. In the case of speech-based dialog systems, the human "wizard" performs the speech recognition, natural language understanding, dialog managements and context generation. Cohen et al. [4] list the main advantages of the WOZ approach:

- Early testing – it can be performed in the early stages in order to test and formulate the design parameters as early in the product lifecycle as possible.
- Use of prototype or early design – eliminates problems arising later in the development such as integration.
- Language resources - Grammar coverage for the speech recognition (ASR) and respective machine learning approaches for interpretation (NLU) are always low when testing a non-finalised product. Low scoring for ASR-NLU may hinder the usability evaluation, however, the use of the human usability expert eliminates such handicap.
- System updates – the system, being a mock-up, can be updated effortlessly to accommodate for changes imposed from the input from the test subjects, making it easier to re-test the updated system in the next usability evaluation session.

The WOZ approach is primarily used during the initial design phase to test the proposed dialogue flow design and the user response to information presentation parameterisation. Since errors from speech recognition and language interpretation are not taken into account, the resulting evaluation lacks the realistic aspect. Expert developers usually know what to expect from the speech recognition and interpretation accuracy because these are domain dependent.

There are two requirements for successful usability testing, the design of the tasks and the selection of participants. The participants are required to complete a number of tasks that are carefully selected to test the system. In a dialogue system the primary concern to evaluate is the dialogue flow. Other tasks consist of testing the natural language interface of such aspects as linguistic clarity, simplicity, predictability, accuracy, suitable tempo, consistency, precision, forgiveness, and responsiveness, which make the interface easy and transparent to use.

4.1.2   Usability Testing Using Working Systems (Summative Evaluation)

As mentioned before, usability testing can take place during the design phase, the implementation or after the deployment of a speech-based dialogue interface. At the end of the implementation, pre-final versions of the system should be tested by potential users in order to evaluate the usability. For spoken dialogue interfaces, a set of 15 objective (quantitative or qualitative) and subjective usability evaluation criteria have been proposed [7], including modality appropriateness, input recognition adequacy, naturalness, output voice quality, output phrasing adequacy, feedback adequacy, adequacy of dialogue initiative relative to the task(s), naturalness of the dialogue structure relative to the task(s), sufficiency of task and domain coverage, sufficiency of the system's reasoning capabilities, sufficiency of interaction guidance, error handling adequacy, sufficiency of adaptation to user differences, number of interaction problems [1] and overall user satisfaction.

Moreover, Bernsen & Dybkjær [2] have used evaluation templates for their DISC evaluation model as best practice guides while, later, they formed a set of guidelines for up-to-date spoken dialogue design, implementation and testing, covering seven major aspects [3]. These aspects can be used as the basis for usability evaluation strategies. Many frameworks and methodologies have been developed and used for evaluation of spoken dialogue systems in recent works [8, 9, 13, 15, 17, 18, 21, 24, 30].

5   Usability Evaluation of a Spoken Dialogue System: Case Study

There are two requirements for successful usability testing, the design of the tasks and the selection of participants. The participants are required to complete a number of tasks that are carefully selected to test the system. In a dialogue system the primary concern to evaluate is the dialogue flow.

A comparison between a DTMF system and a spoken language interface is expected to reveal no major differences accessibility wise. Both modalities are for example equally appropriate for a blind person trying to access a service by phone. Significant differences are however expected with respect to usability issues. In particular, DTMF systems are exclusively menu driven using a strictly hierarchical and static navigation process. This essentially means that the customer needs to navigate through various levels of menus listening to every option to finally be transferred to a human agent and be asked the general "how may I help you" question. This is especially true for complex domains taking into account that the options list should be kept short for cognitive reasons. Natural Language Interfaces, on the other hand, allow for a more dynamic and shorter dialog flow. Hence they allow for greater efficiency, flexibility and naturalness.

Furthermore, it is often the case that there is no exact mapping between the user's request and the menu options presented to him and hence the user is left confused with no option that suits his needs (which in turn leads to hang-ups or mis-interpretations). On one hand, the large number of possible options is prohibitive resulting in a dysfunctional, over-complicated menu structure, on the other hand DTMF system design is most often developer rather that user centered. In contrast spoken dialogue interfaces utilize machine learning techniques in order to model user behaviour. The system is thus better adapted to the user's mental model allowing for a more natural interaction.

With respect to learnability considerations, the intrinsically arbitrary nature of the mapping between concepts and DTMF tones makes options difficult to remember, especially in the case of complex menu trees and users that rarely call the system. Speech, of course, is for most users the most natural way to interact and the mode they are most experienced with.

Finally, DTMF systems are by definition restricted in choice of wording, which can sometimes be confusing when it comes to use of jargon, especially for elderly people who are not very technologically aware. For example, an elder who wants to make use of video calling capability on his mobile phone may not be aware that he needs to choose the 3G services option in the DTMF menu. In the case of a spoken language system, he could – in theory at least – express his request in his own words.

On the other hand, recognition technology in the case of spoken language systems is still error prone, and it has been shown that speech recognition accuracy greatly affects the user's experience. Furthermore, spoken language systems – especially mixed-initiative ones – are more difficult, time-consuming and costly to develop, ultimately posing the question whether there should be a trade-off between user satisfaction and engineering considerations. It should also be noted that the general population is not very familiar and experienced with such systems. Performance usually goes down first, before it goes up again, once the users are trained. DTMF systems are in contrast more familiar to users, easier to develop, simpler and thus almost error free. In addition, DTMF systems are constantly directing the user through the interaction, so most of the times the user knows what to do.

All issues mentioned above affect key usability criteria such as efficiency, effectiveness, user-satisfaction and ease of learning. Since these usability criteria apply to both types of systems, the two modalities can be compared based on metrics defined for each criterion, irrespectively whether the exact metric per se can apply to both types of systems. Such metrics can be hang-ups, no-input rates, no-match events (or pressing a non available DTMF key for DTMF systems respectively), interaction duration, number of dialog steps/turns (whereas the user input may be an utterance or a sequence of DTMF keys), successful task completion, use of barge-in capability, subjective evaluation questionnaires.

In the following section we will present a case study whereas a DTMF system of moderate complexity is compared to a spoken dialog interface. Both systems serve the same services for a Customer Care call centre of a Mobile Telephony company. Thus, they give users distant access to services by phone. We will first present the two systems in light of the usability criteria analyzed throughout this paper, and then we will present the usability evaluation of each system.

5.1 System Description

Figure 4 shows the basic architecture of both systems. The DTMF system has a three level menu with a number of options at each level ranging from 3 to 4. As is, the user needs to go through three steps to choose the deepest embedded in the tree option. The same can be accomplished within a single dialog turn in the case of the Spoken Dialogue system leading to more efficient interaction. Also worth noting that while both systems have barge-in functionality, DTMF users will still need to listen to all options if what they want is presented last. Furthermore, in the DTMF system the user is presented with 9 options – corresponding to user requests – while the Spoken Dialogue system at this point handles approximately 30 high-level request categories (that basically means that 21 categories are subsumed under the "other" option in the DTMF menu). Categorization of requests was based on the analysis of the domain and callers' utterances. As a result the speech based system is bound to achieve greater coverage and be more useful and effective.

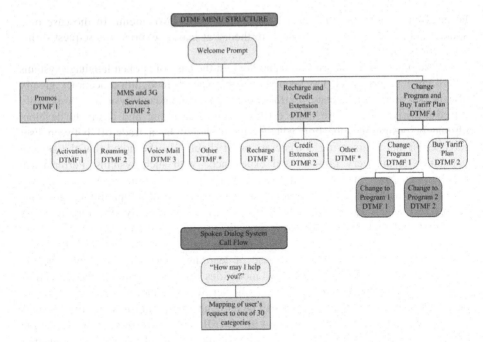

Fig. 3. DTMF and Speech-based dialogue systems basic architecture. Optimal tree traversal is faster for the former. Error handling, universals, help sub-dialogs in the Spoken Dialog system and some sub-menus in the DTMF system are excluded for ease of presentation.

5.2 Usability Evaluation: Procedure, Results and Discussion

During usability testing seven participants were asked to perform five tasks each, using the DTMF and the spoken language functionality. None of the participants had used the particular systems before, all but one had used DTMF systems before, and only two had used natural language systems before. Choice of tasks was based on stats from real usage, so that the most common tasks were chosen. Also tasks were chosen so that they correspond to options found high and leftward in the tree structure, as well as more deeply embedded. Finally, one task corresponded to a request not represented in the DTMF menu. For each task, successful completion, call duration and dialogue steps, number of barge-ins and no-inputs were monitored. In addition, at the end of the testing session, each participant was asked to fill in a relevant questionnaire. Table 2 shows example questions (based on [6, 16, 22, 29], among others) used as subjective evaluation criteria and the usability aspect they correspond to. Participants were asked to assess the two systems on a Likert scale from 1 to 5. Finally, as a control parameter, participants were asked to compare the systems (e.g "Which system is more useful?") and state which system/modality they preferred.

Figures 5 and 6 present the results for the objective criteria. While task completion ratio is almost the same for the two systems, calls to the speech based system required fewer steps and were almost two times shorter compared to calls to the DTMF system. Barge-in functionality was most often used during the interaction with the DTMF system. This was expected, since users are more familiar with DTMF systems

Table 2. Example questions from the usability questionnaire. Each question is mapped to the usability parameter it assesses.

Example Question / Statement	Usability Parameter
The system is useful	Usefulness
The interaction was boring	User satisfaction-Engagement
The interaction was frustrating	User satisfaction-Engagement
The interaction with the system is fast and efficient	Efficiency
There were many repetitions in the interaction	Efficiency
The interaction with the system is natural	Naturalness
I always knew what to do/say	User expertise-Expected behaviour
High concentration was required while using the system	Ease of use-Task ease
I could recover from errors quickly	Error handling / error tolerance
I felt I had control during my interaction with the system	Interaction control-dialog initiative

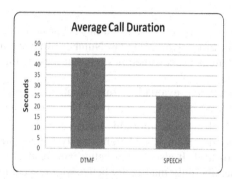
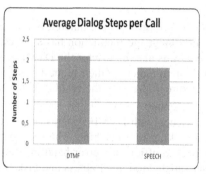

Fig. 4. Average call duration in seconds. Calls made to the Spoken Dialog System were significantly shorter. Number of Dialog Steps/Turns. A caller's utterance corresponds to a sequence of one or more DTMF tones. As within an utterance the user may provide more than one piece of information, similarly in a DTMF system an expert user may press more than one keys within a single turn.

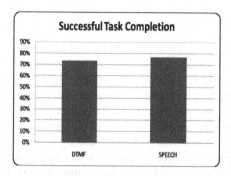
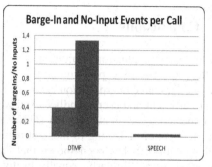

Fig. 5. Percentage of tasks completed successfully and average number of barge-ins and no-input events per call

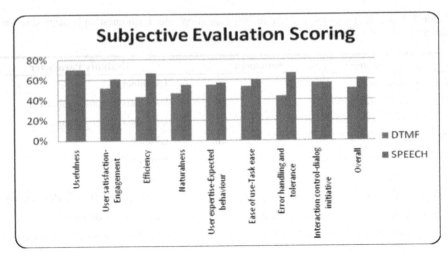

Fig. 6. Subjective Evaluation Scoring. Scores are presented as percentages of the highest score possible.

and DTMF prompts are inherently longer, as all options are listed there. Furthermore, natural language interaction has a different turn taking protocol. Number of no input events was also higher for the DTMF system as users sometimes felt that they had no menu item matching their request.

Figure 7 presents the results of the subjective evaluation. In general, the speech based system ranked higher and was preferred by all users but two. These users had experience with DTMF systems only, and felt more comfortable using such a system than talking to a machine. The speech based system scored significantly better with respect to efficiency, error handling and overall. It also scored better with respect to user satisfaction, naturalness and task ease, and only marginally better with respect to expected behavior and user expertise. The latter can be accounted for, considering that most participants had greater experience with DTMF. As far as error handling and dialog repair are concerned, natural dialog systems are more flexible and robust, whilst DTMF systems usually just force the user to start over again from the root of the menu. Finally, both systems were considered equally useful.

6   Conclusions

A usability evaluation paradigm was described that compared two systems of different modalities performing the same task. Despite recognition errors (25% natural language interpretation error rate) the speech based system proved to be faster, more efficient and user friendlier. And while the increase in speed of task completion is expected to be greater for the DTMF system, as users become more familiar with the application (adapting to menu structures, memorizing choices, using the barge-in functionality), it has been shown that expert, familiarized users are not necessarily satisfied users. Similarly, equally useful, effective (note that task completion rates were similar) and accessible interfaces, can differ vastly with regards to the end-user experience and satisfaction. Especially in the case of disabled users, who often have limited options for use of an alternative modality or a multi-modal interface, it is thus critical that the system is not only accessible but as usable as possible. Appropriate modalities are not necessarily usable modalities.

Finally, the following should be noted: Firstly, it has been shown in the literature [27] that there are differences between usability testing results and real use results. Our data from the first days of the speech-based system's launch corroborate this claim. In particular, there is a high ratio of no-input events and hang-ups (18,8% and 13,5% respectively). We do expect, however, that this percentage will decrease as users become more experienced with the interface. Lack of familiarity on behalf of the end user is a drawback for current open-ended speech interfaces.

Secondly, as mentioned above, speech interfaces can be costly and cumbersome to develop. Nevertheless, they can prove easier to manage and cheaper to upgrade. For example, due to the in-depth analysis of caller requests, future services may be broken down or reassigned to other sub- or top-level categories and new service queues effortlessly. New services can be added without any need to change the structure of the spoken dialogue application, as no menus or list options are actually presented to the user. Thus, since there is really no need to redesign, smooth transition is assured during major updates and the user experience is retained. The latter is considered to be a key parameter for user satisfaction. However, there are still issues to be considered with respect to system's need for re-training and change in content.

Finally, in this case study, a speech interface is compared to a DTMF system of moderate complexity. It might as well be the case that when compared to a simple DTMF system, there is no gain in user satisfaction. Our experience from such a simple call services application indicates that there is no difference in subjective evaluation. As an objective criterion, however, a 1.5% decrease in inner transfers (resulting from errors in routing) was monitored from the moment the speech-based system was launched. Similarly, we would expect a significant gain in user satisfaction for complex domains. In any case, early usability testing can facilitate the choice of the appropriate for each application modality, but more importantly help create an interface that it both functional as well as familiarly usable since the user feedback can be used right from the design phase.

Acknowledgements

The work described in this paper has been funded by the KAPODISTRIAS Programme of the Special Account for Research Grants, University of Athens.

References

1. Bernsen, N.O., Dybkjaer, H., Dybkjaer, L.: Designing Interactive Speech Systems: From First Ideas to User Testing. Springer, London (1998)
2. Bernsen, N.O., Dybkjær, L.: A Methodology for Evaluating Spoken Language Dialogue Systems and Their Components. In: International Conference on Language Resources and Evaluation, pp. 183–188. ERLA, Athens (2000)

3. Bernsen, N.O., Dybkjær, L.: Building Usable Spoken Dialogue Systems. Some Approaches. Int. J. Lang. Data Proc. 28(2), 111–131 (2004)
4. Cohen, M., Giancola, J.P., Balogh, J.: Voice User Interface Design. Addison-Wesley, Boston (2004)
5. Duarte, C., Carriço, L.: Audio Interfaces for Improved Accessibility. In: Pinder, S. (ed.) Advances in Human Computer Interaction, pp. 121–142. I-Tech Education and Publishing KG, Vienna (2008)
6. Dutton, R.T., Foster, J.C., Jack, M.A., Stentiford, F.W.M.: Identifying usability attributes of automated telephone services. In: European Conference on Speech Communication and Technology, pp. 1335–1338. ISCA, Berlin (1993)
7. Dybkjær, L., Bernsen, N.O.: Usability Issues in Spoken Language Dialogue Systems. Nat. Lang. Eng. 6(3-4), 243–272 (2000)
8. Dybkjær, L., Bernsen, N.O.: Usability Evaluation in Spoken Language Dialogue Systems. In: ACL Workshop on Evaluation Methodologies for Language and Dialogue Systems, pp. 9–18 (2001)
9. Dybkjær, L., Bernsen, N.O., Minker, W.: Evaluation and Usability of Multimodal Spoken Language Dialogue Systems. Speech Communication 43(1-2), 33–54 (2004)
10. eEurope 2005: An Information Society for All. Online Project Web Site (2005), http://europa.eu.int/information_society/eeurope/2005/index_en.htm
11. Fellbaum, K., Kouroupetroglou, G.: Principles of Electronic Speech Processing with Applications for People with Disabilities. Technology and Disability 20(2), 55–85 (2008)
12. Freitas, D., Kouroupetroglou, G.: Speech Technologies for Blind and Low Vision Persons. Technology and Disability 20(2), 135–156 (2008)
13. Hajdinjak, M., Mihelic, F.: The PARADISE evaluation framework: Issues and findings. Comp. Ling. 32(2), 263–272 (2006)
14. Harris, R.A.: Voice Interaction Design: Crafting the New Conversational Speech Systems. Elsevier, Amsterdam (2005)
15. Hartikainen, M., Salonen, E.-P., Turunen, M.: Subjective Evaluation of Spoken Dialogue Systems Using SERVQUAL Method. In: International Conference on Spoken Language Processing, pp. 2273–2276. ISCA, Jeju (2004)
16. Kamm, C.A., Litman, D., Walker, M.A.: From novice to expert: The effect of tutorials on user expertise with spoken dialogue systems. In: International Conference on Spoken Language Processing, pp. 1211–1214. ISCA, Sydney (1998)
17. Kamm, C.A., Walker, M.A., Litman, D.: Evaluating spoken language systems. In: American Voice Input/Output Society Conference, AVIOS, San Jose, pp. 187–197 (1999)
18. Larsen, L.B.: Issues in the Evaluation of Spoken Dialogue Systems using Objective and Subjective Measures. In: 8th IEEE Workshop on Automatic Speech Recognition and Understanding, pp. 209–214. IEEE Press, New York (2003)
19. Larson, J.A., Raman, T.V., Raggett, D.: W3C Multimodal Interaction Framework, http://www.w3.org/TR/mmi-framework/
20. Larson, J.A.: W3C Speech Interface Framework, http://www.w3.org/TR/voice-intro/
21. Litman, D.J., Pan, S.: Designing and evaluating an adaptive spoken dialogue system. User Modeling and User-Adapted Interaction 12(2-3), 111–137 (2002)
22. Love, S., Dutton, R.T., Foster, J.C., Jack, M.A., Stentiford, F.W.M.: Identifying salient usability attributes for automated telephone services. In: International Conference on Spoken Language Processing, pp. 1307–1310 (1994)
23. McTear, M.F.: Towards the Conversational User Interface. Springer, London (2004)

24. Moller, S., Englert, R., Engelbrecht, K., Hafner, V., Jameson, A., Oulasvirta, A., Raake, A., Reithinger, N.: MeMo: Towards Automatic Usability Evaluation of Spoken Dialogue Services by User Error Simulations. In: 9th International Conference on Spoken Language Processing, pp. 1786–1789 (2006)
25. Rubin, J., Chisnell, D.: Handbook of Usability Testing, Second Edition: How to Plan, Design, and Conduct Effective Tests. Wiley Publishing, Inc., Indianapolis (2008)
26. Sharp, H., Rogers, Y., Preece, J.: Interaction Design: Beyond Human-Computer Interaction. John Wiley & Sons, Inc., New York (2002)
27. Turunen, M., Hakulinen, J., Kainulainen, A.: Evaluation of a Spoken Dialogue System with Usability Tests and Long-term Pilot Studies: Similarities and Differences. In: 9th International Conference on Spoken Language Processing, pp. 1057–1060 (2006)
28. van Kuppevelt, J., Dybkjær, L., Bernsen, N.O. (eds.): Advances in natural multimodal dialogue. Springer, The Netherlands (2005)
29. Walker, M.A., Litman, D.J., Kamm, C.A., Abella, A.: Evaluating spoken dialogue agents with PARADISE: Two case studies. Comp. Speech Lang. 12(3), 317–347 (1998)
30. Walker, M.A., Kamm, C.A., Litman, D.J.: Towards developing general models of usability with PARADISE. Nat. Lang. Eng. 6(3-4), 363–377 (2000)

Usability and Accessibility of eBay by Screen Reader

Maria Claudia Buzzi[1], Marina Buzzi[1], Barbara Leporini[2], and Fahim Akhter[3]

[1] CNR-IIT, Pisa, Italy
[2] CNR-ISTI, Pisa, Italy
[3] Zayed University, Dubai, U.A.E
{Claudia,Marina}.Buzzi@iit.cnr.it,
Barbara.Leporini@isti.cnr.it, Fahim.Akhter@zu.ac.ae

Abstract. The evolution of Information and Communication Technology and the rapid growth of the Internet have fuelled a great diffusion of eCommerce websites. Usually these sites have complex layouts crowded with active elements, and thus are difficult to navigate via screen reader. Interactive environments should be properly designed and delivered to everyone, including the blind, who usually use screen readers to interact with their computers. In this paper we investigate the interaction of blind users with eBay, a popular eCommerce website, and discuss how using the W3C Accessible Rich Internet Applications (WAI-ARIA) suite could improve the user experience when navigating via screen reader.

Keywords: eCommerce, accessibility, usability, blind, ARIA.

1 Introduction

Ever since the late 1990s, a burgeoning number of electronic commerce (eCommerce) websites have attracted countless visitors and consumers.

Usability is a key factor in the success of these eCommerce systems. The term "usability" is precisely defined by the International Organization for Standardization in the ISO 9241, a multi-part standard covering a number of aspects for people working with computers: "the extent to which a product or website can be used by specified users to achieve specified goals with effectiveness, efficiency and satisfaction in a specified context of use" [9]. Many factors can impact user experience, such as rapidity of finding the desired information, efficiency and security when carrying out the transaction, reliability of the delivery service behind the website, etc.

The Web is an important new information resource for people with special needs, since they can retrieve various kinds of information by themselves through the Web.

Blind people can easily access the Web using a screen reader (a software application that interprets and announces what is being displayed on the screen) or non-visual browsers such as voice browsers (the latter possibility does not eliminate the use of screen readers for interacting with the OS and other applications).

A. Holzinger and K. Miesenberger (Eds.): USAB 2009, LNCS 5889, pp. 500–510, 2009.

However, the Web is becoming more difficult for blind users as more visual content, such as image links, is being used in Web sites. Blind users' problems can range from mere annoyance at wasted time and effort, to having to abandon a task, or ask for sighted help.

Special-needs persons are a rapidly growing segment of consumers in Europe, mainly due to the increasing median age of the population to be considered when designing eCommerce services.

According to the American Foundation for the Blind, more than twenty million Americans, age 40 and older, are experiencing significant vision loss [1]. And when they attempt to acquire information in the cyber-world, they must overcome a number of barriers that cannot be overcome through training the blind, but only through the intentional development of accessible pages.

In particular, blind people who have mobility problems may successfully utilize on-line eCommerce services. Unfortunately these websites have complex layouts, crowded with active elements that are often difficult to navigate via screen reader. Indeed, it has been acknowledged that blind people face the serious problem that reading certain Web pages is quite difficult [7, 14, 17, 18].

The challenge to web designers is to create a website that is not only visually attractive and informative, but is also accessible and friendly to visually-impaired people.

When designing for blind users, it is necessary to consider the three main interacting subsystems of the Human Processor Model: the perceptual, motor and cognitive systems [4].

Sightless persons perceive page content aurally and navigate via keyboard. This makes the "reading process" time-consuming and sometimes difficult and frustrating, if the contents are not designed with special attention to their needs. Thus, various obstacles make it too hard for blind people to fully understand the structure of a Web page. However, if the Web page is well structured with the help of headings or intra-page links, such as a "skip to main content" link, blind users can easily understand the table of contents or arrive at the main content quickly [14].

The cognition aspect of the interaction is important, since many learning techniques are only relevant to people with good vision and may not apply to someone with a visual impairment. Thus, alternative ways to deliver the identical content should be provided. Furthermore, a blind person may develop a different mental model of both the interaction and the learning processes, so it is crucial to provide an easy overview of the system and contents.

Non-visual perception can lead to:

1. Content serialization.
   A screen reader reads the contents sequentially, as they appear in the HTML code. This process is time-consuming and annoying when part of the interface (such as the menu and navigation bar) is repeated in every page. As a consequence, blind users often stop the screen reading at the beginning, and prefer to navigate by Tab Keys, from link to link, or explore the content row by row, via arrow keys.
2. Content and structure mixing.
   The screen reader announces the most important interface elements such as links, images, and window objects as they appear in the code. For the blind user, these elements are important for figuring out the page structure, but require additional cognitive effort to be interpreted.

3. Table.

If the table's content is organized in columns, the screen reader (which reads by rows) announces the page contents out of order; consequently the information might be confusing or misleading for the user.

4. Lack of context.

When navigating by screen reader the user can access only small portions of text and may lose the overall context of the page; thus it may be necessary to reiterate the reading process.

5. Lack of interface overview.

Blind persons do not perceive the overall structure of the interface, so they can navigate for a long time without finding the most relevant contents.

6. Difficulty understanding UI elements.

Links, content, and button labels should be context-independent and self-explanatory.

7. Difficulty working with form control elements.

For example, the new JAWS (an acronym for Job Access With Speech, a popular screen reader) version (v. 10) simplifies the interaction with forms since it can automatically activate the editing modality (for text input) when the virtual focus arrives at the text box (for instance when the user presses the Tab key). However, with previous screen reader versions the user may experience great difficulty, since switching between exploration and editing modalities is required (i.e. form mode on/off).

8. A blind person is unable to access multimedia content such as video streaming, video conferencing, and captioning.

If an alternative description is not present, the user may lose important content.

In this paper we analyze the accessibility and usability of eBay, a popular eCommerce website. Specifically, we show the interaction with the home and result pages. Then we discuss how WAI-ARIA [19], the suite developed by the Web Accessibility Initiative (WAI) group of W3C, might facilitate interaction for the blind. Section 2 presents related works, Section 3 describes the exploration of eBay via screen reader, highlighting potential problems and Section 4 introduces the WAI-ARIA suite, discussing the advantages of structuring the content in landmarks/regions.

2 Related Works

It is essential to implement both usability and accessibility principles when designing a user interface (UI). Accessibility is a basic pre-requisite for allowing users to have access to the web page content, while usability provides online users with simple, efficient, rapid and satisfying navigation and interaction.

Navigation is vital for special-needs persons, and especially for the blind, since it is crucial for them to be aware of their current location on the webpage and how to return to the beginning, or how to reach a certain point in the material [5].

ECommerce systems pose new challenges with respect to classic user-centered product design, where the target is a set of homogeneous users.

Various studies investigate the usability of eCommerce systems and include a general discussion on accessibility, but to our knowledge only a few focus on totally blind persons [16, 2, 15, 8].

Petrie et al. [16] presented the results of accessibility testing of 100 websites with users with various (visual, motor and perceptual) disabilities, showing that websites that are accessible for differently-abled users can also be visually pleasing.

Concurrently, they addressed different aspects of accessibility that do affect visual design, such as visual structure, color contrast, and text size, aspects of design that can affect all users, not only the disabled. Specifically the study tested 100 websites spread out over five sectors (including eCommerce) with automated verification and user testing involving 51 differently-abled users, including 10 totally blind users.

Of the eCommerce websites analyzed, eBay.co.uk was chosen as a case study. Although pages were cluttered, authors registered a 100% task success rate among users, including the totally blind, observing that a complex layout is possible without necessarily compromising accessibility. However, since details of the user test are not specified it is difficult to evaluate the potential difficulties of each task: where the target is located in the site, the number of steps needed to complete the task, ease of use and performance. This affects user satisfaction. Concerning this last point the authors recorded that the blind encountered more difficulties than did other differently-abled users.

Organizing a page in logical sections enhances the experience of the blind user when navigating a page in two ways: it provides a page overview and offers the possibility of jumping from section to section. Specifically, heading levels may improve navigation since screen readers have special commands for moving from one heading to another.

Brudvik et al. [2] present an interesting study on how sighted users associate headings with a web page, observing very different results depending on factors such as whether the page has a hierarchic structure, how users identify sections, etc. Furthermore authors applied techniques of information retrieval (i.e. training data and a classifier), developing a system for automatically inferring from the context (font, size, color, surrounding text, etc.) if a phrase "works semantically" (and may function) as a heading, and dynamically adds the heading level using Javascript. The system called HeadingHunter was evaluated using human-labeled headings gathered from the study and showed high precision (0.92 with 1 the max).

Most common website usability factors involve meeting business objectives while providing a satisfying user experience. Therefore, accessibility should be seen as a challenge to designers and implementers rather than as a constraint.

Parmanto et al. showed that simplification and summarization may enhance usability of crowded web sites for the visually impaired [15]. To simplify user interaction via screen reader, irrelevant content is removed according a strategy that also takes into account the genre of the website (eCommerce, News, etc.). Furthermore, summarization provides users with a page overview that facilitates user orientation.

A pilot usability study conducted by authors with two visually impaired subjects on the original and the transformed Yahoo!News website, offered promising results.

In general, different approaches may be applied to transform on-fly web pages, in order to improve interface usability and content accessibility, such as using an intermediary proxy server or specific client-side solutions (e.g. modified browser, plug-in, etc.). However, the automatic simplification or on-fly transformation, applied to any website, might lead to the accidental removal of content interesting for the user.

We suggest the use of WAI-ARIA to reach a similar result (page overview, easy orientation, access to main contents, etc.) while maintaining the website content unaltered.

Last, an interesting study by Gladstone et al., investigates the use of a natural language interface for simplifying interaction for the blind [8]. Specifically, the Online Shop of the Royal National Institute of Blind People was redesigned, creating fully accessible and usable interfaces while guaranteeing that they were visually attractive. The use of natural language in association with a user profile allows the system to respond to a greater range of phrases, improving its effectiveness and efficiency.

3   Exploring eBay via Screen Reader

For this study, eBay.com was selected to evaluate accessibility and usability of eCommerce websites via screen reader. We chose eBay.com as a case study due to the simplicity and clarity of its graphical user interface and because it is one of the most reputable websites in the online auction business. The richness of a UI is the strength of an eCommerce service, but the environment's complexity can create difficulties when interacting via screen reader.

3.1   Evaluation Methodology

The eBay home and result pages were analyzed with a usability inspection, carried out independently by three of this paper's authors, who are also accessibility experts.

The pages were navigated using the screen reader JAWS for Windows (http://www.freedomscientific.com) v. 9.0 and 10. We used both the MS IE version 7.0 and the Mozilla Firefox version 3.0.5 browsers.

The test was carried out by the authors independently and observations were annotated by everyone. Afterwards, outcomes were compared, discussed and integrated in a face-to-face meeting.

One author has been totally blind since childhood and uses the JAWS screen reader every day; thus she knows this tool's functions very well and is able to use advanced commands. By analyzing the test results we noticed that in spite of her great expertise using JAWS, she was unable to perceive the exact structure of the layout.

The sighted authors carried out the same test mainly using JAWS basic commands (carried out with PC screen turned off).

Therefore, integrating both these outcomes led to a more accurate analysis. The different experiences of the authors when using JAWS allowed us to cover a variety of interaction modalities: i.e. basic commands, simulating the level of novice users, and advanced screen reader functions for experienced users.

3.2   Interacting with the eBay Homepage

In order to evaluate eBay navigation aspect, we accessed the content of the home page to monitor the accessibility and usability aspects via the JAWS screen reader. In our evaluation, we referred to the usability criteria reported in [13], [14].

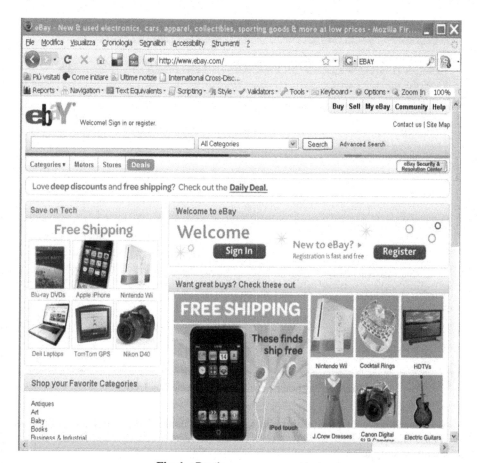

Fig. 1. eBay home page screenshot

By accessing the eBay home page (Fig. 1), we observed the following features:

- Number of links

  Over 100 links are detected by JAWS when loading the Web page. There are far too many links to be navigated, and it is hard for a blind user to orientate him/herself among the links or find the interesting ones (Fig. 2). The exploration could be simplified by reducing the number of links, or by grouping them according to the interest.

- Headings

  No heading level is detected by JAWS. Headings can help blind users understand the main structure of the page content. Headings could give a blind user an overview of the content by executing a specific screen reader command to list all headings within the page – i.e. all main areas in which the content can be structured. For instance, that effect can be obtained with the JAWS screen reader by pressing Insert+F6. Moreover, a more appropriate effect can be provided via ARIA landmarks [19] (see Section 4 for details). For instance, in [3] the authors

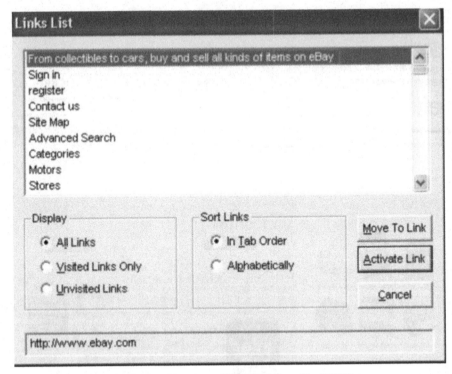

Fig. 2. eBay home page links list detected by JAWS

used landmarks for partitioning the page content using Wikipedia Editing Page as a case study.

- Search functions

  By navigating content in a sequential way or by using advanced interacting JAWS commands -- e.g., letter "e" to move onto edit fields, or "f" to navigate among the form elements -- the blind user encounters an edit field. By exploring around that edit field, he/she can guess that the field is used to search for something within categories; in fact, below the edit box there are a combobox for categories and a "search" button. A specific label for the edit field should be added to make the UI clearer.

- Graphical map

  The page contains some links recognized as a map, in which alternative descriptions are not provided. After the sentence "Welcome to eBay", the JAWS screen reader detects three graphic map links: image map link "ws/eBayISAPI.dll?SignIn&ru=http%3A%2F%2Fwww.ebay" (corresponding to the "Sign In" Button), image map link "ws/eBayISAPI.dll?RegisterEnterInfo" (corresponding to the "Register" Button) and Image map link "246". For a blind user those links are useless. Fortunately these links are also duplicated close to the logo (upper left side), thus the screen reader is able to intercept and communicate them to the user.

- Navigation links and shortcuts
  Neither local navigation links (e.g. "skip to content") nor shortcuts to activate main links are used in the home page. The user has to read the page in a sequential way by using the arrow keys or the Tab key, wasting time.

3.3 Exploring a Search Result

Let us now consider the result page when looking for a specific product. Suppose one is interested in buying audio books. A blind user accesses the home page, moves onto the Edit field, and writes the word "audiobooks". After the user presses the Enter key, the result page is loaded. In this case a heading associated with the desired word is used. Thus, as soon as the page is loaded, by typing the letter "h" the JAWS virtual focus moves towards the result main section. From this point, the user can explore the items found in a sequential way.

Fig. 3 shows the result page; the search query is "audiobooks". Fig. 4 reports a segment of page content read by JAWS.

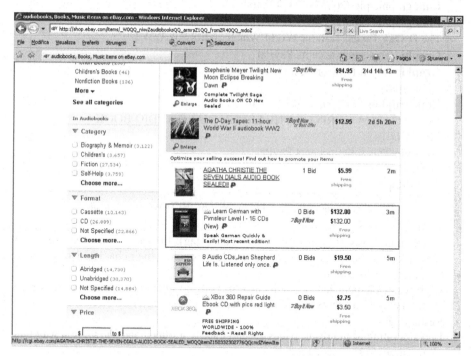

Fig. 3. eBay result page screenshot obtained with the search string "audiobooks"

The main features observed for the result page can summarized as follows:

- No rendering structure
  All the found items or a subset of them are rendered in a sequential way without any structure (e.g. an item list, a heading for each product, and so on). Indeed, the default rendering customization is settled on "List", but the list is not implemented

Heading level 1 audiobooks
Link [Save this search]
View as List
Link [Customize view]
Sort by Best Match
Price
Link Time Left
Featured Items
Link graphic pict/2603757004156464_2
Link graphic Enlarge
Link Stephenie Meyer Twilight New Moon Eclipse Breaking Dawn
Graphic This seller accepts PayPal
Complete Twilight Saga Audio Books ON CD New Sealed
Graphic Buy It Now $94.95
Free shipping 24d 14h 12m
Link graphic pict/2603744737436464_1
Link graphic Enlarge
The D-Day Tapes: 11-hour World War II audiobook WW2
Graphic This seller accepts PayPal
Graphic Buy It Now or Best Offer $12.95
2d 5h 20m
Link graphic pict/1503323027766464_1
Link AGATHA CHRISTIE THE SEVEN DIALS AUDIO BOOK
SEALED!!
Graphic This seller accepts PayPal
1 Bid $5.99
Free shipping 2m

Fig. 4. Segment of the result items read by the JAWS screen reader

in a standard way (i.e. with the <ul> HTML tag). In other words, the user must read all elements by the arrow keys, in order to explore their characteristics.

- Graphical functional links
  Each result element has a graphical link with no alternative descriptions, which should be used to access a specific product.
- Result pages
  Links pointing to the result pages are not clearly grouped and shown in a way that allows them to be reached quickly.

4   Discussion

Using ARIA would enhance eBay's usability in many ways, as explained and exhaustively illustrated by the ARIA best practices document [19].

First of all, structuring the web page in logical sections can provide blind users with a page overview. An important guideline for simplifying user navigation is related to the logical partitioning of content. As mentioned in the previous section, no heading has been used to partition the page into different areas.

In this perspective, landmarks could guide the user to the main areas in which the page can be split. In particular, the eBay home page could be partitioned into areas such as "Login", "Search", "Actions" (e.g. "buy", "sell", "my ebay", etc.), "Great buys", "From our Sellers", "Shop favorite categories", and "Choose language". In this way, the user could quickly refer to the desired page section.

Analogously, the result page could be split into logical sections.

ARIA offers the following default landmarks: application, banner, main, navigation, search, complementary, contentinfo, log and status. If the logical section does not fit one of these landmarks, it is possible to use the role region and specify a title:

<div role="main"> ... <div role="region" title="Great buys">...

The "flow to" property may be used to force the screen reader to navigate these sections in an order (established by the web designer) that should reflect how the user navigates the page (e.g. <flow to="Great buys">).

Having common standard navigation landmarks with the same meaning would provide a blind user with a consistent navigation experience on every website. Furthermore, cognitive- and learning- disabled users could take advantage of collapsed/expanded regions to manage the amount of information processed at any one time [19].

These basic considerations for improving interaction via screen reader should be integrated according to the observations reported below.

Making eCommerce websites suitable for the abilities and skill levels of all users is a great challenge. Obviously, the needs of sighted users as well as the blind must still be considered when defining the graphical interface.

Information should be provided through both visual and auditory channels, the design should be optimized for reading via screen reader, the interface must be easy to use via keyboard, and no additional cognitive effort should be required of the blind user.

In this study we investigated the interaction of blind users with eBay, via screen reader. We analyzed the eBay home page and one result pages to verify the usability.

The results have shown that both pages contain some features that could be improved. Specifically, we suggested ways in which ARIA would enhance usability in these two important pages.

In conclusion, we believe that our suggestions could have general applications, and that applying ARIA would enhance usability via screen reader in any eCommerce environment.

References

1. American Foundation for the Blind, http://www.afb.org/Section.asp?SectionID=15
2. Brudvik, J.T., Bigham, J.P., Cavander, A.C., Ladner, R.E.: Hunting for headings: sighted labeling vs. automatic classification of headings. In: 10th international ACM SIGACCESS conference on Computers and accessibility, pp. 201–208 (2008)
3. Buzzi, M., Buzzi, M.C., Leporini, B., Senette, C.: Improving Interaction via Screen Reader Using ARIA: An Example. In: 18th International World Wide Web Conference (WWW 2009) Developers Track (2009), http://www2009.org/pdf/www09dev_proceedings.pdf

4. Card, S.K., Moran, A., Newell, T.P.: The Psychology of Human-Computer Interaction. Lawrence Erlbaum Associates Inc., New Jersey (1983)
5. Debevc, M., Verlic, M., Kosec, P., Stjepanovic, Z.: How Can HCI Factors Improve Accessibility of m-Learning for Persons with Special Needs? In: Stephanidis, C. (ed.) HCI 2007. LNCS, vol. 4556, pp. 539–548. Springer, Heidelberg (2007)
6. Disability Rights Commission: The web access and inclusion for disabled people. Technical report, Disability Rights Commission (DRC), UK (2004)
7. Fukuda, K., Saito, S., Takagi, H., Asakawa, C.: Proposing new metrics to evaluate web usability for the blind. In: CHI 2005 on Human factors in computing systems, pp. 1387–1390. ACM, New York (2005)
8. Gladstone, K., Rundle, C., Alexander, T.: Accessibility and Usability of eCommerce Systems. In: Miesenberger, K., Klaus, J., Zagler, W.L. (eds.) ICCHP 2002. LNCS, vol. 2398, pp. 11–18. Springer, Heidelberg (2002)
9. International Standard Organization (ISO), ISO 9241-11: Ergonomic Requirements for Office Work with Visual Display Terminals (VDTs), Part 11: Guidance on Usability, 1st ed., International Organization for Standardization, Geneva, CH, 1998-03-15 (1998)
10. Harrison, C., Petrie, H.: Severity of usability and accessibility problems in eCommerce and eGovernment websites. In: People and Computers XX. Engage, pp. 255–262. Springer, Heidelberg (2005)
11. Huang, A.W., Sundaresan, N.: A semantic transcoding system to adapt Web services for users with disabilities. In: Fourth international ACM conference on Assistive technologies, pp. 156–163 (2000)
12. International Standards Organization (1992 - 2000). Standard 9241: Ergonomic requirements for office work with visual display terminals, http://www.iso.org
13. Leporini, B., Andronico, P., Buzzi, M., Castello, C.: Evaluating a modified Google user interface via screen reader. Universal Access in the Information Society 7(1-2) (2008)
14. Leporini, B., Paternò, F.: Applying web usability criteria for vision-impaired users: does it really improve task performance? International Journal of Human-Computer Interaction (IJHCI) 24(1), 17–47 (2008)
15. Parmanto, B., Ferrydiansyah, R., Saptono, A., Song, L.: AcceSS: accessibility through simplification & summarization. In: 2005 International Cross-Disciplinary Workshop on Web Accessibility (W4A), pp. 18–25. ACM Press, New York (2005)
16. Petrie, H., Hamilton, F., King, N.: Tension, what tension?: Website accessibility and visual design. In: 2004 international cross-disciplinary workshop on Web accessibility (W4A), pp. 13–18 (2004)
17. Takagi, H., Asakawa, C., Fukuda, K., Maeda, J.: Accessibility designer: visualizing usability for the blind. In: 6th international ACM SIGACCESS conference on Computers and accessibility, pp. 177–184 (2004)
18. Theofanos, M.F., Redish, G.: Bridging the gap: between accessibility and usability. Interaction 10(6), 36–51 (2003)
19. W3C. WAI-ARIA Best Practices. W3C Working Draft (February 4, 2008), http://www.w3.org/TR/wai-aria-practices/

Video Relay Service for Signing Deaf - Lessons Learnt from a Pilot Study

Christophe Ponsard[1], Joelle Sutera[2], and Michael Henin[3]

[1] CETIC Research Centre, Charleroi (Belgium)
cp@cetic.be
[2] SISW, Walloon Interpretation Centre for Deaf People
joelle.sisw@swing.be
[3] SISB, Brussels Interpretation Centre for Deaf People
michaelhenin73@hotmail.com

Abstract. The generalization of high speed Internet, efficient compression techniques and low cost hardware have resulted in low cost video communication since the year 2000. For the Deaf community, this enables native communication in sign language and a better communication with hearing people over the phone. This implies that Video Relay Service can take over the old Text Relay Service which is less natural and requires mastering written language. A number of such services have developed throughout the world. The objectives of this paper are to present the experience gained in the Walloon Region of Belgium, to share a number of lessons learnt, and to provide recommendations at the technical, user adoption and political levels. A survey of video relay services around the world is presented together with the feedback from users both before and after using the pilot service.

1   Introduction

Hearing impairment is an invisible disability that is omnipresent in the society. It is estimated that 8% of the population suffer from hearing loss to some degree. Deaf people have very specific communication needs which are crucial for their personal development and their successful integration, especially for those using sign language as their native language.

For a signing deaf, establishing a clear communication with a hearing people requires the help of a third party that will carry out oral-to-sign interpretation. This can be a relative. However in a number of circumstances where neutrality, autonomy or confidentiality is necessary, the services of a professional interpreter are sought. The significant difference of demand and supply in the number of available interpreters requires advance booking (days or even weeks) and the chances are slim to find one for short term or for urgent matters. Moreover, most of the working time of these interpreters is spent in travelling to the location of their clients.

Good quality video communications have become affordable with the generalization of high-speed Internet, advances in the web-cam technology, and the

A. Holzinger and K. Miesenberger (Eds.): USAB 2009, LNCS 5889, pp. 511–522, 2009.
© Springer-Verlag Berlin Heidelberg 2009

high performance video codec. This enables signing deaf to communicate with each other in their native languages at a distance otherwise they were restricted to textual form of communication (FAX, SMS, email, chat) in the past. Video communication enables new forms of interpretation to communicate with hearing people. They include:

- *Video Remote Interpretation (VRI)*: provides interpreting services for in-person situations, using video communication. The hearing and deaf participants are together, in the same location, but the interpreter is located remotely.
- *Video Relay Service (VRS)*: provides telephone access via video communication, instead of traditional text-based systems (TTY) and the associate text relay service (TRS). They are intended for use across telecommunication equipment where a phone call is being placed. The three parties (Deaf, Hearing, and Interpreter) are in different locations.

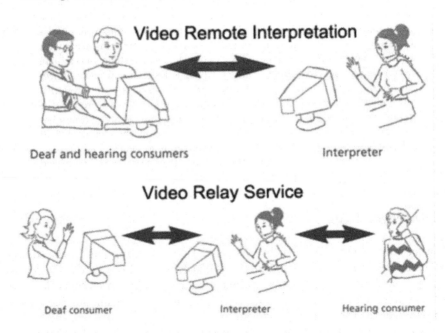

Fig. 1. VRI vs VRS (taken from [15])

Although a number of VRS running across the world (US, UK, Sweden, Denmark, Germany, etc.), there exist very few documentation to describe their return of experience related to the various dimensions of the deployment of such a service. The aim of this paper is to present our experience of deploying a VRS in Belgium and analyse those in the light of the existing VRS following the above dimensions. Our pilot project has been running since January 2008 with the pace of one to two half days a week. It involves mainly 4 professional sign language interpreters (in turn) and deaf people scattered on about 8 different locations (deaf associations, city house, private house, places hiring deaf people). We have only considered routine usage and not emergency calls that require a more specific and advanced organisation.

This paper is structured as follows. Section 2 gives an extensive overview of the state of the art of VRS around the world. A synthesis of the main expectations and fears collected from potential and actual users of the pilot project are reported in the section 3. This synthesis enables to check the extent these expectations and fears are important and how to overcome them. The section 4 summarizes a number of lessons learned and recommendations from our pilot project. Section 5 presents a series of related work. Finally, we draw a set of conclusions of our work in the pilot project and highlight our future directions on deployment.

Note that it the context of this paper, we will only consider normal usage, not emergency calls which requires a more specific and advanced organisation.

2 An Overview of Video Relay Centre around the World

We give here an overview of a number of VRS, our purpose is not to be exhaustive but representative of various ways VRS have developed and are organized.

2.1 United States

The US were the pioneer in text relay service (TRS) with system running already in the 70's allowing deaf people to use the phone although not through American sign language (ASL). There is a very wide network covering all the US with more than 15 different operators [22]. This development was pushed by "American With Disabilities Act " (A.D.A, 1990). Since 2000, with the technological maturation of video communication, video relay have developed allowing deaf to use ASL.

Due to their maturity, US relay centres are a model to follow. They are regulated by the Federal Communications Commission (FCC) which issued a number of rules such as the need to run 24/7 (since 2006), to answer 80% of the calls in less than 2 minutes (since 2008). The calls must be either originate or terminate within the US.

VRS is funded through the Interstate Telecommunications Relay Fund. This fund was created by the FCC, originally to fund TRS services. The money comes from a tax on the revenue from all telecommunications companies operating in the US. The tax on revenue is set by the FCC yearly and has been steadily increasing as the number of VRS minutes continues to climb. In 2009, some fraud was detected about unjustified minutes calling for more control and ethics.

2.2 United Kingdom

UK has a strong tradition of TRS back to the 80's. It was first called TypeTalk [17]. Nowadays this service runs 24/7. It is funded by British Telecom on behalf of the UK communications industry.

The first VRS was set up by a deaf and sign language led social enterprise called Significan't, their service is called SignVideo [16] and employs only fully qualified and registered sign language interpreters. Service is accessible during office hours with a few minutes waiting time. On the average the cost is 60% of the cost of a face-to-face interpretation. For deaf users, this cost can be supported by Access to Work and the National Health Services.

Another VRS available in the UK is organized by the British Deaf Association (BDA) in partnership with a VBS operator, CSD Inc, originating from the US. A VRS experiment was also organized by the RNID (Royal National Institute for Deaf) had to close in 2007 due to lack of funding.

2.3 Sweden

Sweden was a quick to organize VRS, already in 1997 based on ISDN technology. Today there are 5 VRS running in Sweden, during week days from 8AM to 8PM. The service is subsidised by the government and is totally free for the users both for local and international calls. The hardware is also supported by the government. The technical solution often relies on the MMX platform which is widely used in Nordic countries [13]. It is a total communication platform (audio/video/chat) and supporting both wired and mobile calls.

Sweden is quite advanced in the use of video on 3G mobile phones. Although the resolution is quite low, the mobility is a key advantage and specific use and "short sign language" (roughly equivalent to SMS) has developed. A specific project studied how to adapt the VRS to this use and ended in 2006. As a result users can now call the video relay service using their 3G telephone, IP based video telephone or web client as well as their traditional ISDN video telephone, so in complete independence of the technology [3].

2.4 Denmark

The national Danish video relay service is provided by The Labourmarket Centre North, an organisation managed by the municipality of Aarhus. It targets mainly deaf and hard of hearing employees in Denmark. Development has started in 2005 and the full deployment is planned for 2009. It is funded by the Ministry of Employment. 19 job centres from 19 municipalities located in the central Jutland Region have showed there interest in the service, in order to support deaf and hard of hearing people getting a job. The technical solution is quite complete and is based on the MMX platform [12].

2.5 France

TRS have been organized in France from 1982 to 1996, run by France Telecom and relying on the "minitel" (a general public text terminal very widespread in this period). It was ended due to the evolution of technology (Internet) and cost reasons.

Video Relay Services are only starting to emerge in France under the pressure of deaf associations led by UNISDA [19]. Two VRS are developing

- *Visio08* organized by Websourd, an association run by deaf people. It is primary located in the Toulouse area [21]. The current interface is on a PC equipped with a high quality webcam and a specific software combining a communication window and textual information.
- *Viable France* primary located in Paris [20]. It is based on the solution of an US provider which also sells a specific very usable terminal (VPAD) including a touch screen, flash and WiFi connectivity. This device is also used by the interpreters.

There is still no clear funding scheme identified although an anti-discrimination law was voted in 2005 requiring the set up of relay centres. So far the above VRS are running in pilot phase with end users or with specific contracts with users in companies.

3   User Survey Related to Video Relay Services

In complement with the previous wide scale overview, we give in this section a survey reflecting the feedback collected from users about the specific technical interface and more generally about their expectations and fears w.r.t. VRS. Some of them were collected among potential users and other among pilot users. This allowed us to check how those were confirmed or not by the experience.

3.1   Perception of Video Terminals

As stated before, there are four different kinds of user interface for interacting in video mode: three wired and one mobile. Those are illustrated in figure 2.

- *videophone:* it provides a simple and familiar phone interface with only some extra buttons. A frequent concern here is the size of the screen.
- *TV with video set-top box:* boxes that can be connected to a television are developed by some manufacturers like Leadtek and D-Link. They are much appreciated as they enable a very convivial use on the TV set in the living room and are simple to use. A potential drawback is privacy.
- *computer with webcam:* any recent computer can be turned into a videophone device using a webcam (often integrated in laptop screens nowadays) and an adequate client software, preferably compliant with videophony standards to interoperate: generally SIP in Europe, older H.323 standard in US.
- *mobile:* 3G phones now support video at lower resolution than wired videophony but with the fantastic advantage of mobility.

It appears that each device has a potential benefit for some kind of users: older deaf users may prefer a telephone like interface or the fact that it can more easily cope with incoming calls, younger users may prefer to use their laptop. For sign language interpreters image size is not so an issue: trial on 8 inch videophones where successful and even on PC full screen image is not used as other client related data are useful to display.

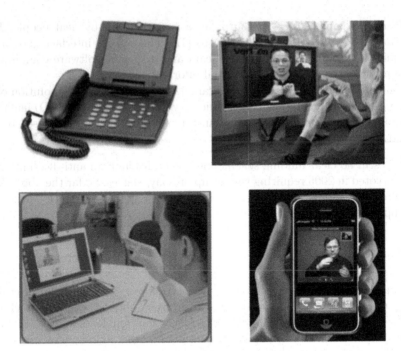

Fig. 2. Different kinds of video communication interfaces

3.2   Expectations and Fears of Deaf Users

The deaf users surveyed were composed of a sample of 10 active deaf people of various backgrounds: employee, teacher, psychotherapist auxiliary, social assistant. The main expectations stated were the following

- rapid, direct and pleasant communication to speed up decisions and improve organisation
- being able to call for services such as plumber, doctor, banker, tour operator, etc. Those are usually not reachable by FAX, email or SMS.
- reduce the need to move for processing requests.
- more autonomy, especially w.r.t. relatives and friends.
- ability to use sign language rather written language for distant communication.
- large availability.

and the main fears:

- it won't work because I tried with some webcam and it was jerky (or someone told me).
- it won't work because there were previous experimentations and nothing came out of it.
- communication through a screen is more difficult, I prefer to be in physical presence with the interpreter.

- the videophone will not be comfortable enough to use because of the screen size.
- it will cost too much as hardware or communication.

The above feedback can be summarized in a few requirements which very similar to those stated by UNISDA: accessibility for all, all the time, free, simple to use and meeting quality standards [18].

3.3   Expectations and Fears of Sign Language Interpreters

The interpreters surveyed where composed of a sample of 5 professional interpreters working across Wallonia and Brussels. The main expectations stated were the following:

- reduction in travel time and of the associated stress and costs, currently more than 50% of the time is spend in travels.
- more time for the actual interpretation work.
- the service could trigger more demands because it is currently only partly being answered.
- possibility to work from home.

and the main fears:

- I don't want to work all the day on a screen but I could agree to try part of my time.
- it won't work in some context: if the call is too technical, too long, etc.
- how to use the communication device ?
- what if... person not present, does not understand, second call, etc.

Those resulted in a number of recommendations about the scope of the VRS, deontological aspects, organisation of training. These are detailed in the next section.

3.4   Point of View of Hearing Users

Hearing users interacting with deaf people see the following potential benefits of the system:

- greater autonomy of the deaf employee at work.
- ability to get in touch with deaf employee for example if absent from work.
- ability to get in touch with deaf client to discuss some limited issue or to plan a meeting with physical interpretation.
- more personal contact.
- better reactivity and better understanding the using written language over fax or email.

4 Lessons Learnt and Recommendations

4.1 About the System Configuration

There is no single unique terminal solution either for the deaf user and the sign language interpreters. For deaf people, a videophone can be recommended for older or less computer literate people but also for its ability to stay on all the time to get incoming calls and for the greater privacy it provides despite its smaller screen size. In case the primary use of communication is not VRS but other deaf friends, a more comfortable situation could be a set-top-box connected to the television in the living room. Finally if a PC is already available, converting it to a video device is a cheap solution. If this is a laptop, it is also very mobile. Using Mobile 3G strongly depends on the country.

For the sign language interpreter, trials were successful both with video devices and computer. A computer is probably necessary in both cases for accessing the client profile and history or for keeping track of the accounting and billing. Having a PC solution enables more integration such as the automatic opening of the client file from the incoming call identification and the monitoring of the call duration. The interpreters should be trained to the use of the system.

In case all the interpreters are busy, the deaf user should be placed in waiting queue and a wait video should be designed to be played in this context to provide a short explanation.

4.2 About the Interpretation Room

Sign language interpreters should be installed in separated individual quiet room, with enough space and very good lightning conditions which is important for the image quality. The background is also important as well as the clothing which should follow usual contrast rules for easing the identification of the hands and the facial expressions.

The seat should be fully adjustable in order to have a comfortable interpreting position. A mirror is also useful to control its appearance (the videophone/software can also act as a mirror).

For the call with the hearing person, a phone should be available preferably with a headset rather than using hand free mode.

4.3 About the Interpreter Behaviour

The sign language interpreter should have a number of reflexes on the way to react on an incoming call and when facing a number of special events such as absence, answer machine, etc.

When picking up a deaf call, the sign language interpreter should have a standard way to present herself, possibly using an impersonal identification number (for anonymity and traceability purposes). It should then go through the process of the request.

Most phone calls are generally quite simple and short requests, taking typically 5-10 minutes once the right person is reached. However the interpreter should be able to identify potentially problematic requests such as:

- the deaf user does not know who to call: the interpreter should not help in identifying a person or look after a number in a directory.
- complex technical explanations should not be handled in VRS but an appointment for a physical interpretation can be made.
- strong emotional context, such as health problems, law suit: an appointment for a physical interpretation is also recommended.
- the deaf user just wants to chat with the interpreter.

When trying to contacting a hearing people, a number of special cases can also occur such as: nobody answers, a wrong person answers (possibly at the correct number or because of a wrong number), there is an answer machine or an automatic call dispatcher (typically in help desks of big administrations/corporations). The interpreters should report those problems and ideally let the deaf sort them out.

When a hearing person is reached, the interpreter should introduce the interpretation context clearly and make sure the persons has understood it. Then he can switch to interpretation using the first person to impersonate the deaf user. This can be somewhat disturbing if the voice does not match, e.g. female interpreter for a male deaf client.

5   Related Work

An e-practice study reports on the TEGNKOM deployment in Denmark which was presented in section 2 [9]. The main lessons learned in this experience highlighted:

1. the importance of cross-sector partnership including the end user.
2. the need of professional support to help in the adaptation to new ways of working, especially to adapt to new ICT solutions.
3. the confirmation of the high impact VRS can have on the target groups. By supporting every day communication, it helps them avoiding marginalisation at the labour market.

The e-practice study also proposes an interesting classification of various impact dimensions of VRS:

- *the user dimension* which the way such a service is perceived by the various users: deaf people, hearing people (deaf relatives, deaf co-workers, people in administration facing deaf citizens), sign language interpreters;
- *the technical dimension* which is about the communication infrastructure, both hardware (terminals such as visiophone, set-top-box or PC with webcam) and software (softphones and IT management services for call management, billing...);
- *political dimension* which is about convincing deaf associations, interpreter associations and public authorities that the service is worth being adopted and funded. We will refer to this classification in the next part of this related work.

About the *user dimension*, a sociological survey was reported by [4]. It highlights interesting issues in the context of a private use. Some of them for the deaf users are: the realisation of autonomy w.r.t. travels and relatives, to be able not only to place calls to but also to get calls from hearing people (hence the need to communicate its number and to have a technical solution to notice incoming calls), the discovery of the fact that the callee can be absent, the use of a phone directory, the projection and perception of its own image.

The *technical dimension* has been covered more extensively in the literature, typically about the minimal acceptable resolution, video frame rate, bandwidth requirements [1,2,6,8]. Those requirements are now well known. Efficient, interoperable and affordable solutions are available, based on standards such as SIP (signalling), h.264 (video codec).

About *political dimension*, a success factor in the organisation of a VRS is the involvement of the Deaf community itself. This is the experience reported by Websourd and Significan't [11]. Our own experience confirms this and will also drive the way it will evolve in the future. As highlighted in our survey, the way it should be supported by the public authorities is variable depending on the country context. A study in France reports about the main possibilities such as by the state, by the user, as universal service [18]. The universal service, as currently deployed in the US, is identified as the most appropriate solution for preserving the equality of rights.

More general work are also available related to the use of ICT by the Deaf community. [7] gives a general overview of the use of ICT for deaf people using current as well as future technologies. The focus is on communication, e-learning and barrier-free access to information. It is illustrated by various projects of the Austrian Center for Sign Language. A similar work was done in Belgium [14]. [10] investigates the impact of using video communication in a web-based learning context. In particular it focuses on usability issues by deaf users. It reports on the way such users react when faced to a video-based technology and details some particular requirements which can be usefully transposed to VRS such as the use of explanatory video in sign language.

6   Conclusions and Perspectives

In this paper, we presented a number of lessons learned and some recommendations from the deployment of a video relay service in the Walloon Region of Belgium. Although they only reflect a partial experience, still we discussed them in the light of other existing similar services and of the expectations and fears of a number of users, especially from the point of view of the interface they have with the hardware and with the hearing person through the sign language interpreters. Although they may not be fully generalised, they can still be a set of useful guidelines to be further consolidated.

A video relay service can help achieving many expectations improving the daily lives of several people but the path to achieve this milestone is quite difficult. Our experience is that it requires a substantial effort both at technical and organisational level. It should be supported by a critical mass of people. The current pilot in the Walloon region proved too small for this quest. Currently there are on-going discussions with interpreters of the Brussels Region so as to broaden the scope of our pilot set-up. It is also important to have the full support of the deaf communities especially through the deaf federations (i.e. FFSB [5] and Fevlado fevlado, respectively for the North and South parts of Belgium) who can then lobby the public authorities.

Acknowledgement

This project was financially supported by the Walloon Region (Ministry of Health and Social Affairs). We also thank the Belgian French Federation of Deaf People, the deaf users, associations and sign language interpreters who have contributed to this work.

References

1. Blades, F., Collins, J.: Remote Sign Language Interpreting, D223, SignWorks Project (June 1998)
2. Blades, F., Collins, J.: Transmission and Reception of BSL by Videophone, D221, SignWorks Project (June 1998)
3. Bystedt, P.: Access to video relay services through the Pocket Interpreter (3G) and Internet (IP). Towards an inclusive future Impact and wider potential of information and communication technologies (2007)
4. Dalle-Nazbi, S.: Technologies visuelles et e-inclusion. initiatives de sourds. Innovation: The European Journal of Social Science Research 21(4) (2008)
5. FFSB, Fédération Francophone des Sourds de Belgique, http://www.ffsb.be
6. Hellstrom, G.: Quality Measurement on Video Communication for Sign Language. In: Proc. of the 16th Int. Symp. on Human Factors in Telecom. (May 1997)
7. Hilzensauer, M.: Information technology for deaf people, In: Ferreira, C. (ed.) Intelligent Paradigms for Assistive and Preventive Healthcare. Studies in Computational Intelligence, vol. 19, pp. 183–206. Springer, Heidelberg (2006)
8. ITU, Supplement 1 (05/99) to Series H – Application profile – Sign language and lip-reading real-time conversation using low bit-rate video communication (1999)
9. Johnston, A.B.: Video relay service for deaf and hard of hearing. European e-practice use case (2007), http://www.epractice.eu/en/cases/tegnkom
10. Kosec, P., Debevc, M., Holzinger, A.: Towards Equal Opportunities in Computer Engineering Education: Design, Development and Evaluation of Videobased e-Lectures. International Journal of Engineering Education 25(4), 763–771 (2009)
11. Lorant, C., Corréa, J., Sangla, J., Lombard, I.: Video Relay Service: Definition, Objectives and Deployment (in French). In: Online proceedings of the UNISDA conference (January 2009), http://www.unisda.org/spip.php?article282
12. Netwise, MMX Multimedia
13. Netwise, MMX Multimedia, MMX Call Center for Interpreter Services – helping the deaf community (2006), http://www.netwisecorp.com/upload/news/netwise_news/netwise_news_200%6_winter.pdf
14. Ponsard, C., Molderez, J.-F.: How can NTIC help Deaf People (in French). Wallon Region, Ministry of Social Matters (2003)

15. SignOnVRI, http://www.signonvri.com
16. SignVideo, http://www.signvideo.co.uk
17. Text Relay UK, http://www.textrelay.org
18. UNISDA, 2006 Report - part 2 - french relay centers (in French), http://www.unisda.org/spip.php?article58
19. UNISDA, http://www.unisda.org
20. Viable France, http://www.viable.fr
21. Visio08, http://www.visio08.com
22. Wikipedia, Video Relay Service, http://en.wikipedia.org/wiki/Video_Relay_Service

Using a Log Analyser to Assist Research into Haptic Technology

Fannar Freyr Jónsson and Ebba Þóra Hvannberg

University of Iceland, School of Engineering and Natural Sciences,
Hjardarhaga 2-6, 107 Reykjavik, Iceland
{ffj,ebba}@hi.is
http://www.hi.is/

Abstract. Usability evaluations collect subjective and objective measures. Examples of the latter are time to complete a task. The paper describes use cases of a log analyser for haptic feedback. The log analyser reads a log file and extracts information such as time of each practice and assessment session, analyses whether the user goes off curve and measures the force applied. A study case using the analyser is performed using a PHANToM haptic learning environment application that is used to teach young visually impaired students the subject of polynomials. The paper answers six questions to illustrate further use cases of the log analyser.

Keywords: Log analyser, logging tool, multimodal, haptic, voice, audio, visually impaired, blind.

1 Introduction

Qualitative data on problems and design improvement proposals are useful for a usability evaluation. A number of quantitative measures are also used for usability evaluation such as time to complete a task, completion of a task and frequently navigated areas of an application. Such measures are often performed by observing the user during interaction, but can also be gathered automatically [2]. In particular, eye gazing is becoming more popular since it can reveal where exactly the user is looking. Evaluation tools which analyse modern user interactions such as gestures have also been developed [4]. Haptic and tactile interaction has been developed for several years, in particular, as a viable technology for visually impaired users [3,5,7,8,9].

The vast number of research studies performed to learn more about the usability and usefulness of haptic technologies in learning environments has motivated us to develop a tool to aid the evaluator in gathering and analysing objective measures. Examples include studies on how to map visual properties to haptic properties, to help the understanding of these properties by visually impaired users [6,10], or how to use audio feedback to indicate the position of the PHANToM [2,9]. Another motivation for our work is that a think-aloud protocol is not

A. Holzinger and K. Miesenberger (Eds.): USAB 2009, LNCS 5889, pp. 523–531, 2009.
© Springer-Verlag Berlin Heidelberg 2009

realistic when an audio is added to an interface since it may increase a user's burden during interaction. Hence the need for objective measures increases.

In this paper we describe a log analyser which we have developed to help researchers with post-analyses on log files. The main purpose of the log analyser is to decrease the time it takes to analyse the log files and to provide additional functionalities to research studies. We describe some use cases of the log analyser. Then we give an example of using it on a research study which we have carried out to compare the advantages of haptic, audio and voice cues on four types of exercises, which are meant to teach young blind students about polynomials.

2   Description of the Log Analyser

Before we describe some of the use cases of the log analyser, we will briefly describe the reference application, a learning environment which we have developed to aid a student in learning about polynomials [1]. A teacher can enter any polynomial of xy into the learning environment's user interface and the PHANToM haptic device will allow the student to feel the two dimensional curve through force feedback. The user interface is displayed in Fig. 1. After entering a formula in an input box, the polynomial is drawn and the student can start following the curve.

Currently, the software is implemented with a magnetic effect of a specific force to help the user stay on the curve. As the student traverses the curve, he or she

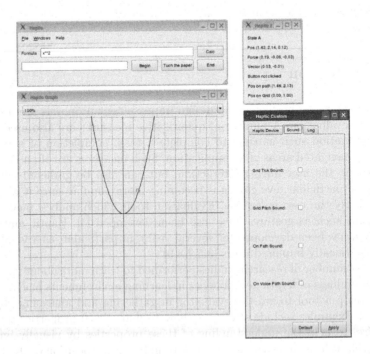

Fig. 1. The user interface of the reference application, the learning environment

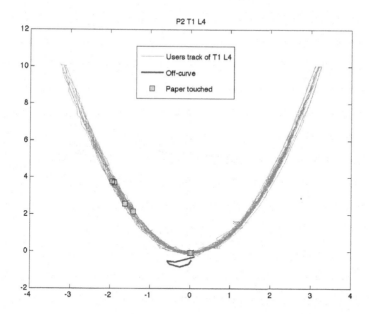

Fig. 2. Visualisation of the trajectory along the xy axis for $y = x^2$. (*Best viewed in colour*)

will also feel a grid to enable orientation and distance travelled. The software can be configured to play audio as the curve is traversed, talk out loud when the user goes off curve and to talk out loud the x, y co-ordinates on demand when the user presses a button on the pen. The stiffness of the pen can be configured.

When the user is learning about the shape of the mathematical polynomial, the software logs every movement and other data, such as when the user is off curve and when the user presses the button on the pen. Each line in the log file is marked with the current time. Through the software's user interface, the evaluator is able to note the beginning and end of a task and the software then marks these times to the log file and annotates it with "Begin task #" or "End task #". When the student is doing auxiliary tasks, such as comparing the felt curve to reference polynomials on tactile paper or other models, the evaluator can note these actions through the interface of the software, which then logs it to the log file and annotates it accordingly.

This log file which the learning environment creates contains a lot of information and will be very difficult to read. Therefore our focus is creating a prototype of a research tool for making it easier to analyse and work with these kinds of log files. The log analyser is a research tool and its purpose is to help the researcher with post-analyses. The data from the log file is read into the log analyser which then extracts information from it. After a session, the log analyser can describe the trajectory of a movement, both in two dimensions or in time as is shown in Fig. 2 and Fig. 3. Other main use cases of the log analyser will now be described.

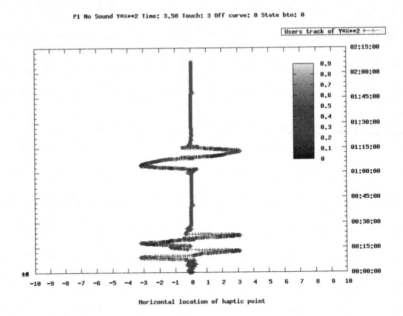

Fig. 3. Visualisation of the trajectory along the time/xy axis. (*Best viewed in colour*)

2.1   UC1: Practice or Session Time

The evaluator can get the beginning and end time of a practice or the session time of the student.

2.2   UC2: Tracking of a Trajectory

The trajectory is displayed in two ways, both on xy axis, or as an xy-time axis. See Fig. 2 and Fig. 3.

2.3   UC3: Duration and Number of Times Off Curve

The log analyser shows when the user is on the curve and when he is off the curve. It will also show how long the student spends off the curve and how often he or she goes off the curve. Visual display of when the user is off curve as seen on Fig. 2 (red line).

2.4   UC4: Passing a Reference Point

In order to understand better how the user examines the curve, it is possible to enter a reference point and ask the log analyser to count the number of times the reference point is passed. This information can also be visually displayed as seen on Fig. 4. In this example the markings s1 to s8 are the predefined areas we want to find out how often the users enters.

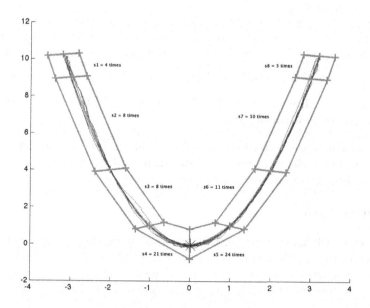

Fig. 4. Visualisation of the trajectory splitted into eight areas

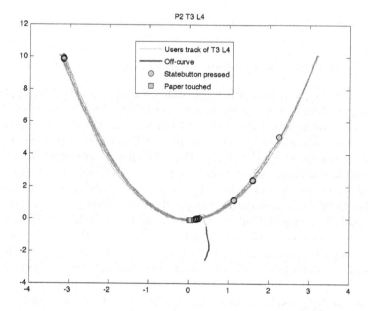

Fig. 5. Visualisation of the trajectory along the xy axis for $y = x^2$. (*Best viewed in colour*)

2.5   UC5: Number of Times an Auxiliary Task, Such as Comparing to a Reference

To learn how often the student compares to a reference, such as a tactile paper with a polynomial. Visual display of when an auxiliary task is performed is marked as a green circle as seen on Fig. 5.

2.6   UC6: Number of Times the User Asks to Listen to Co-ordinates or Other Additional Aid

This use case is to get better knowledge how often the user asks for further aids, such as reading of the co-ordinates. Visual display of when a button is pressed, as seen on Fig. 2, is marked with a green box on the curve.

2.7   UC7: Force

The force the PHANToM peripheral outputs as the user is following the curve is written to the log file. Using this number the tool calculates in a post-session analysis the length of the force, the highest given force, the lowest given force, the average force and then calculates the median and standard deviation for the session.

3   Case Study Using the Log Analyser

In order to validate the functionality of the log analyser we set out the following question:

Can the log analyser give realistic results by using the proposed use cases?

We tested the log analyser with a research study of the reference application, a learning environment for polynomials, to evaluate the outcomes of different haptic, audio and speech cues provided to visually impaired, young people. Altogether nine students, six of them seeing but blind folded and three visually impaired, participated in the study. The participants are asked to solve four tasks with three different effects: no sound effect (T1), continuous stereo sound (T2), and using speech synthesiser (T3) to give xy co-ordinates. The four tasks entail identifying the co-ordinates $x = y = 0$ on the curve $y = x$, and identifying polynomials of varying difficulties: $y = x$ (medium), $y = 2x + 2$ (difficult), and $y = x^2$ (easy). In each of these three tasks the user got three different polynomials to compare to on tactile paper, where one of them was correct. Below are excerpts of research questions based on the use cases in previous section:

3.1   Research Questions Associated with Use Case 1, Session Time

Question 1. Is there a difference in how long users take to solve each task depending on the effects (T1,T2,T3) or polynomials?

There is not a significant difference between effects. Examining the means, we notice that with the speech synthesiser users took longer to finish the task than using the other effects on average. T1, no sound, took M=2.61 minutes on average, N=32, while T3, speech, took M=3.17 minutes on average. There is a significant difference between the polynomials, with the difficult polynomial taking the longest.

3.2 Research Questions Associated with Use Case 3, Off Curve

Question 2. Is there a difference in how often users go off curve depending on the effects (T1,T2,T3) or polynomials?

There is not a significat difference between effects. However, there is a significant difference between polynomials, with $y = x^2$ going most frequently off the curve, most likely because of the steepness of the trajectory. Otherwise, users seem to follow the trajectories nicely. Looking only at those who are going off the curve, we note that T3, speech, are going off the curve on average M=1.22, N=9, average for T2, continuous sound, is M=1.75, N=4 and T1, no sound, the average is M=1.0, N=7.

3.3 Research Questions Associated with Use Case 5, Comparing to a Reference

Question 3. Is there a difference between each effect how often users compare to an object?

There is not significant difference between each effect. Still it seems that users are a little more confident using speech than using no effect. Average comparisons using T1, no sound, is 3.38 times, T2, continuous sound, is 3.12, and for T3, speech, users compare to the reference on average 2.79 times during a session.

3.4 Research Questions Associated with Use Case 6, Additional Aid (Speech Synthesiser)

Question 4. Do users, who ask for speech, take longer to solve the task than other users?

A regression analysis shows that there is a significant relationship between the number of times users asked for speech and the time it took to finish the task ($p < 0.05$, Beta=0.390).

Question 5. Do users ask for speech aid more often for the more difficult tasks?

From the data we see that users ask for speech more often in the difficult task, y=2x+2 than in the other tasks, or M=10.62 compared with the task where users asked for speech aid most seldom $y = x$, find $x = y = 0$, M=2.89.

3.5   Research Questions Associated with Use Case 7, Force

Question 6. Does the device need to use more force on users depending on the task being solved?

There is a significant difference between tasks (p=0, partial eta squared=0.488) meaning that there is a considerable effect, with the highest average force being applied with $y = x^2$.

The conclusion of these research questions is that there is not a significant difference in the objective measures between effects. As expected there is a significant difference between tasks.

The evaluator can observe the user and use the interface of the learning environment to record the user's behaviour in research questions 1 and 3 and work out the results. We term such use cases as integrated observation. Such collection and analysis are more reliable than a manual one and prevents human mistakes. In questions 2, 4, 5 and 6 above there is no easy way for an evaluator to observe and analyse them, i.e. automatically from the tool.

To emphasise the need for an integrated or automatic observation we found an inconsistency in research question 1 where the evaluator had forgotten to record when the user finished and/or started a new task which lead to misleading information, hence the need to be automatically collected and analysed. Therefore the log analyser is highly connected to the learning environment.

4   Conclusions

A log analyser has been developed for the purpose of aiding researchers in working with log files and doing post-analyses on them. This study has shown that such a tool can be very useful and that the log analyser can find new, previously uknown results. For example, earlier research on the learning environment did not look into the reference points.

To answer the question *"Can the log analyser give realistic results by using the proposed use cases?"* we used the log analyser on log files from our reference application, a learning environment, by posing some questions. We conclude from this experiment that the implemented use cases of the log analyser are useful for post-analyses on the data.

In this paper, we have only given a few examples of the analyser's utilities but plan to explore its usefulness further and particularly the qualities of force and the path traversed. In particular, future work will include the following research question:

Can the log analyser be leveraged by other applications than the reference application, the learning environment, described in this paper?

References

1. Birgisson, M.T.: Staerdfraedistafur. In: Tolvunarfraediskor, Verkfraedideild. Reykjavik, Haskoli Islands (2008)
2. Crossan, A., Brewster, S.: Multimodal Trajectory Playback for Teaching Shape Information and Trajectories to Visually Impaired Computer Users. ACM Trans. Access. Comput. 1(2), 1–34 (2008)

3. Fritz, J.P., Barner, K.E.: Design of a haptic data visualization system for people with visual impairments. IEEE Transactions on Rehabilitation Engineering 7(3), 372–384 (1999)
4. Gouy-Pailler, C., et al.: A Haptic Based Interface to Ease Visually Impaired Pupils' Inclusion in Geometry Lessons. In: Universal Access in Human-Computer Interaction. Applications and Services, pp. 598–606 (2007)
5. Lee, J.C., et al.: Haptic pen: a tactile feedback stylus for touch screens. In: Proceedings of the 17th annual ACM symposium on User interface software and technology. ACM, Santa Fe (2004)
6. Ramloll, R., et al.: Constructing sonified haptic line graphs for the blind student: first steps. In: Proceedings of the fourth international ACM conference on Assistive technologies. ACM, Arlington (2000)
7. Wall, S., Brewster, S.: Feeling what you hear: tactile feedback for navigation of audio graphs. In: Proceedings of the SIGCHI conference on Human Factors in computing systems. ACM, Montreal (2006)
8. Wall, S.A., Brewster, S.A.: Tac-tiles: multimodal pie charts for visually impaired users. In: Proceedings of the 4th Nordic conference on Human-computer interaction: changing roles. ACM, Oslo (2006)
9. Yu, W., Brewster, S.: Evaluation of multimodal graphs for blind people. Universal Access in the Information Society 2(2), 105–124 (2003)
10. Yu, W., Ramloll, R., Brewster, S.A.: Haptic Graphs for Blind Computer Users. In: Brewster, S., Murray-Smith, R. (eds.) Haptic HCI 2000. LNCS, vol. 2058, p. 41. Springer, Heidelberg (2001)

Usability in Public Services and Border Control

New Technologies and Challenges for People with Disability

Giuliano Pirelli

European Commission Joint Research Centre
Via E. Fermi 2749, I-21027 Ispra (VA) Italy
giuliano.pirelli@jrc.ec.europa.eu

Abstract. The paper starts with a brief overview of the scale of disability and associated challenges and puts them in the context of the public policy on disability. It then analyses the usability challenges in public services and border control, including the issues of accessibility, safety and communication. These need to be addressed in future policy proposals, to provide the best assistance by new technologies to elderly people and people with disabilities, avoiding creating new barriers due to incorrect or incomplete initial conception. With increasing flux of novel security technology in mass transportation systems, and particularly the use of biometric identification in airports, the challenge of usability is recognized. This paper analyses these issues in the context of users with disability in an idealized process of Simplifying Passenger Travel (SPT).

Keywords: disability, usability, accessibility, security, safety, biometrics, assistive technologies, airport, border control, mass transportation, transportation systems, policy.

1 Introduction

As new security technologies are introduced in public services, such as border control and mass transportation systems, their accessibility for the disabled needs to be evaluated. A large part of the population is directly or indirectly concerned with disability of permanent or temporary nature.

The problems encountered by people with disabilities in every day life highlight problems encountered by many other people. The elderly, or even any person, has to spend some time to get used to new systems, regardless if they directly use new technologies, or the new technologies influence their operating schemas.

While the use of new home equipment lets time to get acquainted, unfamiliar locations with frequently changing procedures may generate stress. This is for instance the case in an airport, with complex check-in procedures and security controls, requiring the user to follow new rules and interact with new equipment.

The new technologies should help the system's designers in facilitating the users' tasks. Nevertheless, quite often the users are confronted with significant difficulties. *A new set of invisible barriers* limit an easy access to new challenging solutions. Therefore, great attention has to be paid to usability issues. Care to the specific

A. Holzinger and K. Miesenberger (Eds.): USAB 2009, LNCS 5889, pp. 532–552, 2009.

difficulties encountered by people with disabilities is a way to help them and - at the same time - to find solutions useful for all other citizens.

1.1 Current Trends

Recent studies have highlighted a number of demographics trends in Europe, which must be born in mind when considering the introduction of new technologies in large scale public applications.

Taking into account the needs of people with disability, not only is an obligation, but adds different ways of perceiving problems and *finding solutions for all users*: ramps for people with physical impairment are used for luggage, simplified web pages for people with visual impairment are used for small screens of mobile phones, the small dot on button 5 for the blind is used in darkness or when touch typing, TV captioning and screens in bus or metro with stations' names for people with hearing impairment are used in noisy situations and by foreign users.

The specific needs of the elderly and of people with disability have to be considered in order to allow a *design for all* approach in the aspects related to the data's' privacy and to the travel documents' identity controls, checked by manual or automatic readers.

With increased levels of threats to public transportation system in recent years, there is now heightened emphasis on risk mitigation by deploying new security technologies for identification, detection and surveillance. Airports are a good example where the goal of security enhancement is being pursued aggressively by the deployment of mass spectrometry and biometric technologies.

It is often the case that when security is the main focus, ethical and social concerns are often forgotten in the false belief that the latter are an impediment to the security objectives. Nevertheless, new technologies may be used in defining a smarter process design rather than just automating existing tasks. Thus may ensure greater acceptability by the end users while satisfying the functional and security objectives.

1.2 The Challenges for Disability

The average age of the population is continuing to increase. The group of *elderly people* is often characterized by good experience of life and availability of money, which they wish to spend and *fully participate in the social life*: traveling, using the Internet, taking the best advantage of the new available technologies, of course if all of them will be of easy access.

Due to an average *longer expectation of life*, in some cases also a larger number of elderly people will be affected by some form of disability. On the other side, the progresses in the medical field allow people to survive to severe accidents or difficult birth, in some cases with different limitations or disabilities.

The so called *Silver Economy* concept recognizes the importance of designing systems usable by the elderly [1]. It requires long term development and sustainability of social and care services, assistive technologies and accessibility of these services, with encouragement in order to improve the quality of services. It seems like that even if older people do not view themselves as disabled, they increasingly come together with this group in order to reinforce the lobby pressure.

1.3 Nature of Disability

For such reasons, the distinction between people with or without disabilities is becoming less sharp. Moreover, a large number of people without a *permanent disability* might suffer, at some point in life, from *temporary disabilities,* e.g. due to temporary impairments: broken legs, plastering, crutches, wheelchair, broken or wet or lost glasses, less concentration and longer reaction time due to lack of prescribed drugs, reduced vision or reduced hearing or increased reaction time due to fatigue, jet lag or illnesses, pregnant ladies, parents traveling with many children, language or communication problems, etc. In this paper, the concept of disability is used in a large comprehensive sense, including permanent disability and temporary disability or temporary impairment.

1.4 The Scale of Disability

It is quite difficult to use a unique common definition of disability and a common reference schema, since each country has collected slightly *different statistical data, which can hardly be compared* and used in a single table. Nevertheless, we have to be aware that a very large part of the population in directly or indirectly concerned by disability.

According to the European Disability Forum, disabled people represent *50 millions of persons in the European Union* (10% of the population). One in four Europeans has a family member with a disability. People with reduced mobility represent more than 40% of the population [2].

A similar information is provided also by Eurostat: *44.6 millions* persons aged 16-64 living in private households in *25 European countries* (15.7% of the population) stated that they had a long-standing health problem or disability (LSHPD) [3].

Figures of the same order are available *also for the USA*: 54.4 millions people, about one in five residents of the USA (19%) report some level of disability. Among those with a disability, *35 millions* (12%) are classified as having a *severe disability.* Among those with disabilities, 31% with severe disabilities and 75% with non-severe disabilities are employed, compared with 84% of people in this age group without a disability. A portion of people with disabilities - 11 millions aged 6 and older - need personal assistance with everyday activities [4].

These data are presented in Table 1 and Fig. 1.

Table 1. Population and people with disability in USA and EU (millions)

	population	number of people with disability	% of people with disability in the population	number of people with severe disability (USA) or reduced mobility (EU)	% of people with severe disabilty in the population	number of people with severe disability needing personal assistance	number of people within 16-64 years with disability
USA	300	54	19 %	35	12 %	11	
EU	500	50	10 %	45			16

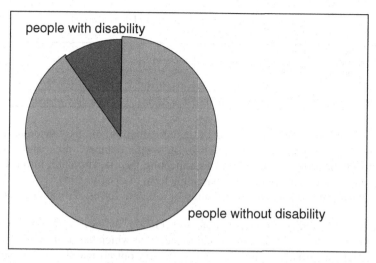

Fig. 1. Population and people with disability in EU

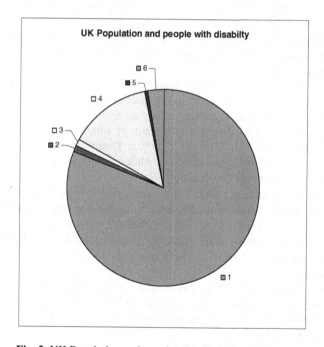

Fig. 2. UK Population and people with disability (millions)

- 1: Population without disability (50).
- 2: Wheelchairs users (0.7).
- 3: Deaf people (0.7).
- 4: Hearing impaired people (8.3).
- 5: Blind or partially sighted people (0.3).
- 6: Hidden disabilities: diabetics (1.8).

Table 2. People with disability in UK (millions)

	people with disability	wheel-chair users	deaf people	hearing impaired people	blind or partially sighted people	diabetics people (hidden disability)	parking badges for people with disability
UK	10.100	0.750	0.700	8.300	0.300	1.800	2.300

In order to have a rough idea of the distribution on the different forms of disabilities, it is preferable to refer to a single country, thus allowing easier comparisons of different approaches in collecting the statistic data. In the UK alone an estimated 14% of the population has some form of disability [5].

Fig. 2 and Table 2 show the distribution of different forms of disability in the UK:

- The UK Disability Discrimination Act (1995) defines a disabled person as someone with "a physical or mental impairment which has a substantial and long-term adverse effect on his (sic) ability to carry out normal day-to-day activities". Disabilities are diverse and range in severity. They may be either visible or invisible, or both. The key types of disability relate to problems with mobility, sensory mechanisms, learning and communication difficulties, mental health issues and hidden disabilities like diabetes, epilepsy and heart disease. Many of these forms of disability are treatable or may be alleviated by broader changes in social perceptions [6].

- The term *disabled person* covers people with a wide range of disabilities and health conditions - from a visual impairment to arthritis, cancer, multiple sclerosis, heart disease, depression, Downs Syndrome and diabetes. There are over 10 millions disabled people in Britain; of which, 4.6 millions are over State Pension Age and 0.7 millions are children. Disability increases with age: only 10% of adults aged 16-24 are disabled, while one third of people between the age of 50 and retirement age are disabled [7].

- It is estimated that there are about 9.8 millions people in the UK with some form of disability - one in seven of the population. At the last count, in 1996, there were 750,000 wheelchair users in the UK. In 2002-03, 19% of men and 13% of women reported having hearing difficulties. In terms of hidden disabilities, there are about 1.8 millions diabetics in the UK and over 350,000 people with epilepsy, for example [8].

- According with the Royal National Institute of the Blind (RNIB), about 152,000 people are on the register of blind people, and 155,000 on the register of partially sighted people. 24 % of all registered blind people who have an additional disability are also deaf [9].

- According with the Royal National Institute of the Deaf (RNID), 9 millions adults are deaf or hard of hearing, of which: 8.3 millions with mild to moderate deafness and 700,000 with severe to profound deafness; 2.5 millions aged 16 to 60 and 6.5 millions aged over 60 [10].

When considering the problem from the point of view of the *difficulties encountered in traveling*, the available statistics often indicate the number of people who do -

within some limits - travel, but can hardly consider the larger majority who cannot travel, due to the existing barriers. Therefore, when considering share of the disabled in public transport, it is fair to assume that a larger majority of the disabled are unable to travel due to the existing barriers [11].

The following data in UK are provided by the Disabled Persons Transport Advisory Committee (DPTAC) [12]:

- Disabled people are unable to use 70% of buses and 40% of the rail network. Almost 50% of disabled people list transport as their main local concern and feel their employment opportunities have been reduced because of poor public transport. 60% of disabled people have no car in the household, compared with just 27% of the general population who have no car. Compared with the general public as a whole, disabled people travel a third less often. 60% of the rail network is inaccessible to disabled people according to the Strategic Rail Authority [13].
- The number of *parking badges* for disabled people (Blue Badges) on issue in England stands at *2.3 millions* [14].

2 Public Policy on Disability

2.1 The EU Transport Regulation on the Disabled Air Passengers' Rights

The European Union has extensive laws for mobility rights and equal treatment of the disabled passengers. This includes right to boarding, assistance, mobility equipment and accessible information.

On 5 July 2006, the European Union adopted a new Regulation concerning the rights of disabled persons and persons with reduced mobility when traveling by air [15]. The regulation entered into force on 26 July 2008 [16].

The Regulation provides for compulsory assistance to persons with reduced mobility; no reservation can be refused on the ground of disability; some exceptions are possible though; operators and airport managers must ensure that the staff has appropriate assistance training.

The overall principle and aim of the Regulation is to protect any passenger with reduced mobility or sensory impairment, intellectual disability or any other cause of disability, age or psychological problems, and whose situation needs appropriate attention and the adaptation to his or her particular needs of the service made available to all passengers. The following aspects of the Disabled Air passengers' Rights are particularly defined:

- *Boarding:* An airline shall not refuse, on the ground of reduced mobility or disability, to accept the reservation of a person or to embark a person, except for safety reasons established by national, Community or International law (which should be publicly available in accessible formats) or if the size of the aircraft or its doors makes the embarkation or carriage of a disabled person physically impossible. If boarding is denied, the disabled passenger has the right to be informed about the reasons thereof, and to receive re-imbursement or re-routing.
- *Assistance:* A disabled passenger has the right to receive assistance, which must be adapted to his/her specific needs. 48 hours before departure prior notification is

nevertheless required. If the passenger does not notify his or her needs, the airline shall however do all efforts to assist the person anyway in order to allow the person for traveling.

- *Mobility equipment and assistive devices:* Thanks to the new Regulation, the disabled has the right to bring mobility equipment and assistive devices and/or to travel with his or her assistance dog in the cabin.
- *Accessible information:* Essential information provided at airports and on board the aircraft, should be provided in accessible formats for disabled air passengers, according to their needs.
- *Complaints:* In case of discrimination, the disabled passenger can contact the managing body of the airport, or the airline concerned. In case of no satisfaction, the person can address the enforcement bodies that will be set in each Member State.

2.2   The International Convention on the Rights of Persons with Disabilities

The Convention was agreed by an Ad Hoc Committee of the UN General Assembly in New York on 25 August 2006. On 30 March 2007, the Convention has been opened for signature. The European Community has signed the Convention as a State Party. Following ratification by the 20th party, it came into force on 3 May 2008. To date, 50 countries are parties to the convention, while a further 93 have signed but have not yet ratified.

The Convention aims to promote, protect and ensure the full and equal enjoyment of all human rights and fundamental freedoms by all persons with disabilities, and to promote respect for their dignity. The Convention will cover 650 millions people in the world, including 50 millions in the EU alone [17].

The adoption of the Convention embodies the paradigm *shift from charity to rights, from a medical model to a social / Human Rights model.* Disabled people are no longer considered as victims or patients, they are *persons with rights and a full role to play in society.*

This achievement is a success for the EU. In May 2004, the Council mandated the Commission to negotiate on behalf of the Community on matters falling under Community competence. Community competence mainly stems from legislation adopted on the basis of Article 13 of the EC Treaty, which enables the Community to take action to combat discrimination based, *inter alia*, on disability. The successful conclusion of these negotiations constitutes a landmark for the *European Community* in that it will, for the first time ever, become party to a comprehensive UN human rights convention.

3   Role of Assistive Technologies

Research in Assistive Technologies may contribute improving the quality of life of all citizens and their access to the Information Society. The work will aim at fostering the inclusion and at empowering from the security standpoint a portion of the population that is currently, at least partially, excluded and that might be exposed to gratuitous security risks. There is the potential for a significant activity of harmonisation of national initiatives, identification of best practices, assessment and demonstration of technologies, and awareness raising, in a complex and multilingual field, which exactly corresponds to the role of the EC Joint Research Centre (JRC).

JRC contributed to disability aspects in several areas. Particularly, the VOICE and SESAMONET Projects, described hereafter, achieved excellent results and demonstrated the feasibility of applications of low-cost and high-performance new technologies for all citizens, in a *design for all* approach.

3.1 The VOICE Project

The VOICE Project aimed at the promotion of automatic recognition of speech in conversation, conferences, television broadcasts and telephone calls [18]. It started in 1996 at JRC and developed prototypes of user friendly interfaces allowing an easier use of commercial products in translating the spoken voice into PC screen messages and subtitles. The Project achieved significant results in years 1996-97 and provided a better definition of the requirements of people with special needs. It was then sponsored and funded by the DG-XIII-TIDE (previous to Directorate General Information Society) in years 1998-2000. Through the project, more than one hundred workshops were organized in order to develop an awareness raising process on the potentialities of voice-to-text recognition systems. Approximately 6,000 participants attended the workshops, in which a prototype of automatic subtitling, developed for this aim, was presented and used for live subtitling of speeches, as demonstration of feasibility and validation on the field.

In years 2001 and 2002 the activities addressed the harmonisation of television subtitling, in collaboration with the European Broadcasting Union and the CENELEC Normalisation Committee, with the support of Directorate General Enterprise. The Conference "eAccessibility by Voice", held at Ispra (Varese), Italy, was one of the closing events of the European Year of People with Disabilities 2003. The Conference brought together representatives of European countries, television broadcasters, Associations of people with disabilities and many experts from all over Europe.

Collaboration has been established with the Department of Interdisciplinary Studies in Translation, Languages and Cultures (SITLeC) of the University of Bologna at Forlì, for a few conferences for raising the broadcasters and professional subtitlers' awareness of the potential of speech-to-text technology in the production of real time subtitles. As result of that, interpreters of the University of Forlì achieved a good level of performance in the use of speech to text technology to produce - for the first time in Italy - real time subtitles of several conferences and debates.

3.2 The SESAMONET Project

The SESAMONET Project (SEcure and SAfe MObility NET) is a RFID and GPS based guidance system for visually impaired people. The Project's objective was the development of an integrated electronic system to increase mobility of people with visual disabilities and their personal safety and security.

The system is based on an electronic path made of RFID tags, a custom-designed walking cane, and a smart phone or PDA (Personal Digital Assistant). Each RFID tag provides position signals via a dedicated walking stick to a smart phone containing information about the location, and a recorded voice - via a Bluetooth headset - guides the visually impaired person along the route. The prototype system uses RFID micro-chips embedded in the ground. The microchips can be recycled from the electronic tracking of cattle. The technical aspects have been patented by the EC [19].

In collaboration with the municipal authorities of Laveno (Varese), Italy, on the Major Lake, a full scale pilot project of about two kilometers along the lakeshore has been equipped with microchips. An other path has been equipped at the Parco Prealpi Giulie and the system has been demonstrated at the eInclusion Conference held in Vienna on November 2008. Other new paths are being set up.

3.3 Motivation in Public Services and Border Control

On the following years, the activities moved from the area of people with hearing or visual impairment to address a larger spectrum of problems. The field of applications was further extended considering the difficulties encountered by people with other disabilities, as well as by elderly and disadvantaged people, in view or their Inclusion / Exclusion in the social life. This deals with situations in which a citizen cannot effectively interact with an ICT-mediated environment, and more generally with all citizens, who can some time in their lives have a temporary or a permanent disability.

New initiatives have taken into account aspects of safety and security related to disability in the new JRC's Actions, as BORSEC (Border Security) and SCNI (Security of Critical Networked Infrastructures).

4 Usability Issues in Border Control

4.1 Usability Challenges in Biometric Access Control

Usability of biometrics has received attention in recent years with their increasing use in commercial and government applications. Early lead was taken by NIST in the area of biometric usability standards, user interaction models and sample quality / usability relationship [20].

User acceptance requires that the users perceive the real need and the system's utility e.g. convenience for them. Reliability of recognition and data security can establish trust in a biometric system. Conversely, problems with usability will diminish the confidence. The system's acceptance also depends on personal attitudes and minorities may be particularly sensitive in this field [21]. Context also matters in the acceptance of biometrics: using biometrics in passports is considered to be more useful than using them for monitoring work hours [22].

Nadel has highlighted procedural considerations in biometric usability; these include factors such as information, guidance and ergonomics [23]. Fondeur stresses features like autonomy, fault tolerance, minimum habituation adaptability and performance [24]. Lack of commonly accepted methods and metrics or for biometric usability was also recognized. Proceedings of a recent usability workshop provide an excellent overview of this topic [25]. Holzinger has analysed and presented several aspects of usability engineering for software developers [26].

4.2 System's Convenience

4.2.1 Accessibility

Physical accessibility for people with reduced mobility is now becoming a norm; however access to information systems by the disabled is not fully explored. Nevertheless, the latter aspect is particularly important to ensure a regular flow of passengers in the airport, since a good communication and information system may speed up all the activities: check-in, identity controls, hand luggage checks, reaching the gates, boarding the plane. Biometrics in access control combines the physical and information domains, e.g. when biometric identification is used in the end-to-end air travel process [27].

4.2.2 Safety in Emergency Situations

A person with sensory or cognitive impairment or under linguistic barriers *may react in an unexpected way or just not react at all.* A deaf person might continue his way since he cannot hear a normal appeal, or will not open a bag or will not take out an un-allowed object (for instance a pair of scissors) or do so in a too quick or dangerous way, being frightened by the unforeseen situation. This may give rise to a security or safety issue or exacerbate an emergency situation, such as during evacuation. A practical challenge is therefore how to *communicate effectively to all users in an emergency* as well as in normal situations?

Someone will consider the presence of people with disabilities as an *ethic problem* and will feel the need to provide them with *additional help*, in order to save an individual life, even before that of other users.

Someone else will consider their presence as a *pragmatic problem* and try avoiding that they may in some way be an *obstacle for others* and delay the main flow in an escape lane, confusing other people with requests of information and help. There is a concrete risk that a wheelchair follows down and blocks an emergency exit, or that a blind person looses his way or that a deaf person follows his own *visual logic* since he or she cannot listen to messages from the loudspeakers.

4.2.3 Awareness and Training

Three layers may be considered: awareness, information and training. They would be beneficial for all involved personnel.

- *Awareness:* to think that there are people with disabilities and that there may exist specific problems in applying standard security controls on them, as well as problems for their safety, particularly in emergency situations.
- *Information:* on different kinds of disabilities and different kinds of technical aids wered or used by them, e. g. risk of warming up a metal prosthesis or deregulating or destroying a electronic prosthesis by intense magnetic field and of possible interferences in the other sense (the assistive device may disturb the control equipments).
- *Training:* on how to select people to submit to a special control and on how to perform such control, considering that the large majority of the passengers declaring themselves as people with disability will really have such a disability, while some of them may be, in exceptional circumstances, kamikaze wearing explosives inside the technical aids or prosthesis.

4.2.4 Accessible Communication: Redundant Information Systems

Information systems are not perfect nor are the people using them. Therefore information provision to users in a process needs to be designed on the basis of cognitive limitations as well as expectations of the end users. Design factors to consider are:

- *What* would the different users *wish* to know (content).
- What they *need* to *know* (relevance).
- *When* people need such *information* (timeliness).
- *How they* will best *understand* it (communication channel).
- How *they* will *remember* it (retention for later use).
- What information needs to be *repeated* (re-enforce).

With respect to the disabled, the above factors need to be considered for the specific modes of disability. Therefore the communication channels in a public service context need to be adapted to diverse disability profiles.

Redundancy is often one of the solutions that may help in providing more complete and more efficient information. This is valid also in supporting people with disability in their traveling process and in the identity controls.

In order to help overcoming usability needs in access control, different supports should be made easily available: a general pamphlet, a short video-clip, information via loudspeakers, information on a screen, via radio or television. Often people miss a part of each channel of information: redundancy may provide the missing pieces of information in a different format as well as on a different moment. In stations or airports, in noisy situations, in different languages, it is difficult to understand the full information from loudspeakers. The information on the screens is more detailed and available for longer time.

People with some limitations do not get the full information. Blind people or people with visual impairment have to relay only on audio information, while deaf people or people with hearing impairment have to relay only on visual information. For them, as well as for people with communication problems (just only with limited knowledge of a foreign language) this *re-ensuring redundancy* is lost and the partially got pieces of information generate uncertainty, insecurity, typically in unfamiliar situation. *This uncertainty affects of course the directly concerned person, but also all the other users* as well as the services' providers and the whole system: a lost passenger may delay the entire queue and, in some cases, the departure of a flight.

It often happens that a form has to be filled in rather quickly: terms used in it may appear more difficult, due to specific vocabulary or specific syntax and may require more time or receive a wrong answer. For many people there is an *obvious* association of deafness and the use of *sign language*. On the contrary, while a considerable number of deaf people use sign language, an even more considerable number of them *do not use it* and the large majority of people with (medium) hearing impairment do not know it at all. Subtitling or just simple written messages may ensure a better comprehension. In many cases, lips reading may be sufficient, but this is easier in the user's mother tongue.

4.3 Certification for the Users of Assistive Devices

Dealing with disability related problems is difficult due to the lack of a common rule in defining and trusting certificates of disability status and of wearing technical aids. On which basis, for instance, the security staff in an airport may select the people who should avoid electronic controls since they wear a pace maker or a cochlear implant or a metallic prosthesis? Which categories of aids should be considered in order to perform the appropriate security checks? Which kind of documents should demonstrate their status and certify the use of prosthesis or medical devices?

An aspect to be considered is that of trusting the oral declarations of the users, about their disabilities and their need of technical aids. Even a written document provided by them will generate a similar problem of trust. Even if delivered and stamped by hospitals or disability associations or national authorities, it is difficult to verify the source in a quick way. The formats and languages of the documents certifying a disability are quite different in different countries. A harmonisation in this field is necessary in order to give them a more official value and make them more comparable and easier understandable in a shorter time.

A *European Disability Card* or a *European Medical Aids Card* would help the users to get an appropriate assistance, and the controllers to perform the appropriate checks. If this international card will be equipped with RFID, it could send information to the checking equipment, which will in turn send back a warning to avoid the gate (or switch off the control, if the RFID is well trusted).

4.4 Technical Certification of Assistive Devices

People needing special medical care or people with disabilities use a wide range of new equipments. Many border security controllers are not familiar with them and cannot judge the ways of use of them, as well as of risks of damaging or destroying the visible external equipment or even generate serious consequences on the invisible internal coupled equipment and possibly on some vital functions (pace-makers, cochlear implants).

As a complement to the previously proposed information about the need of using an Assistive Device (related to the person), technical information on the device itself should be made available on the same card or on a different one (related to the device).

The border controllers should know whether the control equipment may interfere, deregulate or destroy such device: therefore they should know which users should avoid the normal line and how to perform a special check. If the medical equipment can be detached from the holder, as in the case of hearing aids or the external part of a cochlear implant, should such equipment pass through the x-ray or magnetic field checks? Who should write down a set of specifications and operational limits?

4.5 Usability of Biometrics in Identity Documents - Open Questions

The proposals presented in this Section 4 are part of the results of the research Adaptive Multimodal Biometrics for Advanced Trusted Traveler Paradigm, described with more details in Section 5. The study has brought up new questions on the challenges of usability and security in the context of the passengers with disability. We highlight a few of them here:

- *Electromagnetic interference:* Risk to assistive medical implants such as pacemakers and cochlear implants due to EM interference of the detection devices at security checkpoints.
- *Explosives*: Risk of hiding explosives or other items of security threat in wheel chairs and other belongings; risk of explosion due to personal oxygen container prescribed on medical grounds.
- *Certification:* Who should certify / prescribe the use of medical devices on-board for a passenger and what is an acceptable form of certification / prescription in all EU countries? Who should certify the quality of medical equipment - what are the requirements for such certification? International Forms with medical information, as MEDIF / FREMEC (Frequent Traveler's Medical Card) are provided by the airlines companies to manage some practical information and probably to defend themselves in case of problems with the passengers, more them defending the latter, who in principle need more help.
- *Automated control:* What are the design criteria for the accessibility of eGates for a range of passengers with disability as well as the elderly? What are the procedures for emergency evacuation and how they are built into the design of eGates?
- *Data protection and privacy:* May the users with disability be known a priori (in the booking procedure or in airports)? Should this information be included in the electronic passport, in order to speed up the controls? The information stored on the ePassport may be completed by additional information, preferably stored on a personal data card, creating in such a way multi-function identity documents (e.g. identity + disability / medical needs).

5 Biometrics in Airport

In 2008, the Institute for the Protection and Security of the Citizen (JRC-IPSC) performed a project that analysed the usability of security technologies in an airport departure process. [28]. The study's objectives were:

- To develop formal concept of a secure airport and define an Advanced Trusted Traveler (ATT) paradigm based on adaptive multimodal biometrics.
- To investigate the requirements of a cross-border technical infrastructure for multimodal biometrics for air travel process.
- To identify usability issues, including those of the disabled, regarding biometrics based ePassport and trusted traveler cards.

The main achievement of the project in its first year was the definition of a *Secure Airport Concept:* development of a probabilistic model for the security of airport passenger departure process based on SPT (Simplifying Passenger Travel) Ideal Process Flow [29].

The Project examined the Usability Issues, developing a study of usability requirements through workshops and meetings with airport operators and users: definition of a framework for the assessment of passenger departure process; process metrics of security and (in)convenience for a number of disable user profiles.

5.1 A Framework for Usability and Security Assessment

Initial scoping of the study of the usability issues in air travel process has been carried out in the light of the previous work on general biometric usability already carried out by NIST in the USA.

We illustrate our methodology for a novel model for usability assessment on a case study of passenger departure process at airports for which we have chosen IATA / SPT ideal process as the formal process definition.

In the present research, the scope of the usability study was to examine the accessibility of the disabled and elderly passengers to the passenger departure process, with or without biometric identification. The study concentrated on the impact of border security measures on disabled people, particularly in the phase of the identity controls. On one side, the use of biometrics is expected to speed up checks and provide more reliability, on the other side, the risk of non acceptance of the system by the users might limit its general use.

5.2 The Analytical Framework

Referring to the definition: "Usability is the effectiveness, efficiency and satisfaction with which a *specified set of users* can achieve a *specified set of tasks* in a particular environment", in the present research the specified *set of users* consisted of the different types of disable passengers as well as the elderly, while the specified *set of tasks* were the main passenger tasks involved in the airport passengers' process. The specific usability context was set by the Simplified Passenger Travel process for seamless airport journey. Fig. 3 shows a high level abstraction of the SPT process model.

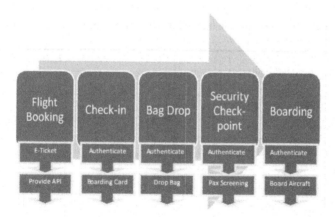

Fig. 3. High-level abstraction of the Ideal Process Flow Departures Process (Passenger's view)

On the other hand, security is defined in terms of the risk posed to the assets by the threats that may be natural or man-made. When developing a framework for common security and usability analysis, we need to take into account the primary stakeholders: the citizen on one hand and authorities on the other. This is shown in Table 3.

Table 3. A framework for concurrently analyzing usability and security for persons with disability

Citizen with disability	*Usability*	The citizen may face specific *inconvenience* due to the choice of technologies or the design of the process in which they are deployed.	*What is the relationship between risks and inconvenience in a system?*
	Assistive Needs	Authorities are responsible for offering assistance as per the needs of a person with disability	Authorities may perceive specific security *risks* from a person with specific profile
		Obligations	*Security*
		Authorities responsible for a Service	

An analytical framework was developed for a joint usability-security assessment along the process dimension. A table, in the form of a spreadsheet, considered the inconvenience encountered by users with different abilities all along the typical situations encountered by them in the airport passenger process. Table 4 shows the task / user profile matrix used in the analysis.

The *rows* in Table 4 represent the *tasks* in the normal progression order encountered by the passengers, from the initial stage of scheduling and booking a flight online, by telephone or at a travel agency, to the practical problems eventually

Table 4. Scope of usability study in the SPT process with respect to a range of user profiles

	Sensorial disability: blind	Sensorial disability: deaf	Mental disability: psychological	Physical disability: motor	Elderly	Temporary disability
Scheduling a flight						
Booking a flight						
Approaching the airport						
Check in						
Communications						
Passport control						
Emergency escape						
Reaching the plain						
Flight						
Luggage control						
Leaving the airport						

encountered in reaching the airport, parking and starting the check-in procedures and baggage drop. Particular attention was then paid to the next steps of identity controls, by human personnel or by automatic e-gates as well as hand luggage controls. Then the next steps: reaching the security gate, passing the final boarding controls, going onto the plane, flight, disembarkation, arrivals controls, baggage collection and exit from the airport.

The *columns* in Table 4 represent different *types* of disability: from visual or hearing or mental disability, to motor disability, as well as the problems related to the elderly or passengers with temporary impairment, such as being pregnant or using crutches or traveling with several children.

5.3 Analysis of the SPT Process - Results

By filling in the matrix presented in Table 4, it started becoming a tool for collecting information, organizing ideas and suggesting possible solutions. Each intersection in the table, i.e. each cell, represented a particular context of user / task pair in the SPT process. For a selected set of cells, usability problems were identified from the passengers' point of view as well as potential security problems from the operators' point of view. After a first iteration, the matrix was then refined, extending the numbers of rows and columns in order to consider more different cases.

The spreadsheet was first populated with analytical information in a qualitative form. A quantitative evaluation was then carried out to identify various factors contributing to passenger inconvenience as well as the security risk to the departure process. This method was repeated for selected user profiles. A partial snapshot of the resulting analysis is shown in Table 5; more details are provided in Table 6. The inconvenience and risk factors were quantified on a scale of 1-5 and aggregated on a *per-profile* and *per-process* stage basis. (1 indicates a least inconvenience or security risk, while 5 indicates a most inconvenience or security risk).

Care was concentrated on the usability aspects related to biometrics and disability and particularly to communication problems, often underestimated in many situations. The difficulties that have been highlighted should contribute at fostering the inclusion and at empowering from the security standpoint a portion of the population that is currently, at least partially, excluded and might be exposed to gratuitous security risks.

The user needs in mass transport - at airports and railways stations - and the security aspects have been discussed with a few members of associations of people with disabilities and in meetings and workshops at the airports of Malpensa and Berlin Schoenfeld (April, June 2008), at the international congress *A global world of communication* in Vancouver, organised by the Canadian and the International association of people with hearing impairment (July 2008), and at the EDIS conference *Management of transport networks and management of security in ports, airports and railways* in Genoa (September 2008).

Results for a set of the most significant cases were plotted in a graphical form, thus helping in redefining with more precision the previous data and any correlations between different sets. Fig. 4 shows a specific user profile evaluation set of the departure process for inconvenience and security risk. The situation that has been analysed considers a conventional passport control. Further analysis will concentrate on the biometrics passport controls at eGates.

Table 5. Quantification method for security risk and passenger inconvenience for a passenger profile (partial set)

	Sensorial Disability: Hearing (permanent)			
	deaf **with internal equipment** (cochlear implant		deaf or hard of hearing **with external equipment** (hearing aids)	
	Inconv.	*sec.risk*	*inconv.*	*sec.risk*
body control: frontal clear communication or unpredictable reactions; electromagnetic interference	5	3	3	2
bags control: frontal clear communication or unpredictable reactions; electromagnetic interference	3	3	3	3
identity control: no voice recognition systems; no voice-guided semi-automatic systems	1	1	1	1

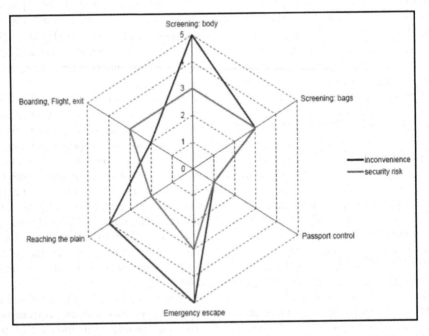

Fig. 4. Security risk and inconvenience profile of the SPT process for passengers with cochlear implant

These data underlined a significant difference between the passengers' feelings of inconvenience and the security risks. Users with assistive aids, as pace makers or cochlear implants, of course attach the greatest importance to their equipment, both the implanted part and the external one. From the point of view of security, the risk is rather limited, mainly related to possible magnetic interference or hidden explosives.

This situation is unbalanced, since it may bring to a superficial control, sufficient to reduce the security risk, but dangerous for the user: for instance only a passenger with pace maker may avoid the electromagnetic controls, while a passenger with cochlear implant has to insist in order to avoid such controls that might deregulate the implant; sometimes the external part of the assistive devise may be passed through X-rays control with a similar risk; also hygienic aspects should be more considered in manipulating personal medical devices. For this reason, the figures previously indicated were normalized, increasing the level of the security risk in order to indicate not a real greater risk but a need for greater attention.

For the above reasons, the matrix was expanded by further information, separating the responsibility of the security controllers and that of the airport's handlers. This allowed a more precise interpretation of different situations form the point of view of the passenger and his feelings of inconveniences, in such a clearer way as to better define the same situations from the point of view of what the airport's authorities should do. Nevertheless, this also doubled the number of columns. In order to limit its proliferation, further distinction within the data registered into the latter two columns - i.e. security risk or need of special care for accessibility - was presented only by using a set of colors for the different concerned actors, as indicated in Table 6:

Table 6. Quantification method for security risk and passenger inconvenience

not applicable	marks from 5 (max) to 1 (min): no strict correspondence between passenger's inconvenience and security risks					0: no additional problem
	passenger's equipment, with risk of damage, and requiring additional security control					
	passenger's inconvenience (worried about personal risks)					
	5: passenger has an internal equipment	4: external equipm linked to the internal	3: external equipm	2:	1:	
	security risk (metal, explosives, electromagnetic interference)					
	5: passenger's equipm explosives / interference	4:	3:	2:	1: risk reduction in control's level	
	passenger requiring help to overcome physical barriers					
	passenger's inconvenience (difficulties in overcoming physical barriers)					
	5: physical or visual impairment	4: hearing impairment	3:	2: access web site or telephone call center	1: limited additional difficulties	
	security risk (limited risk, but special help needed)					
	5: equipment or staff to help overcoming	4: written info and staff to help	3:	2: accessible web site and call center	1: risk reduction in control's level	

- either the passengers' feelings of inconvenience (blue for values 5-4-3 / azure for values 2-1) with respect to the security risks (pink for values 5-4-3 / rose for values 2-1);
- or the passengers' need for help in order to overcome barriers or the passengers' need for help in order to overcome barriers (dark green for values 5-4-3 / light green for values 2-1) with respect to the obligation of providing some additional help (brown for values 5-4-3 / beige for values 2-1).

On the other side, examining more steps in the passenger process added a considerable number of rows and the dispersion on too many situations created difficulties in comparing the numeric values attributed to different but similar cases. In order to limit the data to analyse in the rows, some simplification had to be made: concentrating on situations in the departure process and making the hypothesis that a similar situation in the arrival or transfer passenger control could be defined by the same numeric value (e.g. hand luggage security checks for the first or the second flight; same difficulties in reaching the airport as well as leaving from it, etc.).

Finally, all the numeric values in Table 6 have been re-attributed in a more standardized way, easier to be presented to the airport's authorities: for instance, level 5 for each passenger with an implanted assistive device or with a physical or visual impairment. Applying this approach to the *tasks* and *types* (rows and columns) of the table, a large matrix was generated. These values have then been applied to the final tables on the user (in)convenience and security risk. Unfortunately these data cannot fit in the format of this publication. They are available for further discussion in view of validation tests, which actually are the next step, in collaboration with a few associations of people with disabilities.

6 Conclusions

As new security technologies are introduced in public services, such as border control and mass transportation systems, their accessibility for the disabled needs to be evaluated, since a large part of the population is directly or indirectly concerned with disability. This paper highlights the importance of the topic and the dimension of the problem. It proposes an awareness raising process and analysis of possible ways for helping elderly people and people with disabilities to obtain the best assistance from new technologies, avoiding creating new barriers due to difficulties of use or incorrect or incomplete initial conception.

There are policy challenges in promoting equal access for all to mainstream products and services. These challenges require accessibility norms or standards for services of general interest, promoting social inclusion and equality of opportunities, by using the potential of new technologies and spreading examples of good practice. Use of many new systems requires some form of technical awareness. As a result, such systems may inadvertently create new classes of *disabled people*, i.e. users that are unable to use new equipment properly. Therefore, information technologies may generate new cases of *technical disability*. This is particularly true when the users need to use new technologies infrequently or in unusual complex situations, such as traveling in an unknown context, under stress and fatigue.

With increasing flux of novel security technology in mass transportation systems, and air transport processes in particular, the challenge of usability is recognized. This paper has analysed these issues in the context of users with disability in an idealized process of Simplifying Passenger Travel (SPT). The paper presented a common framework for analyzing security risks and inconvenience for the disabled in the SPT process and showed that it allows examining the two aspects in a balanced way. The framework can be used to devise risk-managed inspection policies for the disabled passengers with assistive devices.

Acknowledgement. The work described in this paper has been carried out in collaboration with several JRC colleagues, with whom the author jointly participated in various projects and benefited from constructive discussions while developing these concepts. VOICE project was initiated under the JRC Exploratory Research grant in 1996-1997 and continued under the funding of Directorate General Information Society in 1998-2000. SESAMONET was carried out under the JRC-IPSC Exploratory Research grant in 2005-2006. Part the work related to Usability in Airport Security was carried out under the JRC-IPSC Exploratory Research grant in 2008.

References

1. Silver Economy Network of European Regions,
   http://www.silverlife-institute.com/uploaded_files/docs/bulletin_en_070924_1190989084.pdf
2. European Disability Forum (EDF),
   http://www.edf-feph.org/Page_Generale.asp?DocID=12534
3. Eurostat - Statistics in focus - Population and social conditions, 26/2003 - Employment of disabled people in Europe in 2002 - Preliminary estimates for year 2002 of the survey for the European Year of People with Disabilities (2003)
4. Report on 2005, issued by the United States Census Bureau (December 2008),
   http://www.cjwalsh.ie/2009/02/us-disability-statistics-practical-application-in-europe/
5. The Social Firms UK Website - Disability Facts and Stats,
   http://www.socialfirms.co.uk/document/format_uploaded/download.php/doc690.html
6. Disability Facts and Stats,
   http://www.socialfirms.co.uk/document/format_uploaded/download.php/doc690.html
7. Family Resources Survey 2003-2004, http://83.137.212.42/sitearchive/DRC/Newsroom/key_drc_facts_and_glossary/number_of_disabled_people_in.htm
8. http://www.socialfirms.co.uk/document/format_uploaded/download.php/doc690.html
9. Data at 31 March (2006),
   http://www.ic.nhs.uk/statistics-and-data-collections/social-care/adult-social-care-information/people-registered-as-blind-and-partially-sighted-triennial-2006-england
10. http://www.rnid.org.uk/information_resources/aboutdeafness/statistics/statistics.htm#deaf

11. The UK Department for Transport, Parking badges for disabled people, data for 2007, `http://www.dft.gov.uk/pgr/statistics/datatablespublications/public/parkingbadges/parkingbadgesdisabled07.pdf`
12. `http://www.dptac.gov.uk/consult/03.htm`
13. `http://83.137.212.42/sitearchive/DRC/Newsroom/key_drc_facts_and_glossary/transport.html`
14. Data on March 2007, `http://www.dft.gov.uk/pgr/statistics/datatablespublications/public/parkingbadges/parkingbadgesdisabled07.pdf`
15. Official Journal of the European Communities, `http://eur-lex.europa.eu/LexUriServ/site/en/oj/2006/l_204/l_20420060726en00010009.pdf`
16. Civil Aviation Authority - Consumer Protection Group, `http://www.caa.co.uk/docs/33/CAA_CPG_PRM_Update.pdf`
17. Final report of the Ad Hoc Committee on a Comprehensive and Integral International Convention on the Protection and Promotion of the Rights and Dignity of Persons with Disabilities, `http://www.un.org/esa/socdev/enable/rights/ahcfinalrepe.htm`
18. The VOICE Project, `http://voice.jrc.it`
19. The SESAMONET Project, `http://silab.jrc.it/SESAMONET.php`
20. Biometric Usability, NIST, `http://zing.ncsl.nist.gov/biousa/`
21. Sasse, A.: User Perception of the Technology and Acceptance, `http://zing.ncsl.nist.gov/biousa/docs/workshop08/day1/6Sasse/sassebiomdc_june08.pps`
22. Patrick, A.: Acceptance of Biometrics, `http://zing.ncsl.nist.gov/biousa/docs/workshop08/day1/7Patrick/Andrew-Patrick-Acceptance-of-Biometrics.pdf`
23. Nadel, L.D.: Usability Considerations for Face Image Capture at US-VISIT Ports of Entry, `http://zing.ncsl.nist.gov/biousa/docs/workshop08/day2/2Nadel/Usability_Face_Image_Capture_at_US_VISIT_POE.pps`
24. Fondeur, J.-C.: Usability of Biometrics for Border Crossing, `http://zing.ncsl.nist.gov/biousa/docs/workshop08/day2/5Fondeur/Usability%20of%20Biometrics%20for%20Border%20Crossing%201.1.pdf`
25. The International Workshop on Usability and Biometrics, June 23-24 (2008), `http://zing.ncsl.nist.gov/biousa/html/workshop08.html`
26. Holzinger, A.: Usability Engineering for Software Developers. Communications of the ACM 48(1), 71–74 (2005)
27. BAA, miSense - the Connected Journey, `http://www.baa.com/portal/site/baa/menuitem.6a4740fe62e293a4b03f78109328c1a0/`
28. Secure Airport, Advanced Trusted Traveler Paradigm using Adaptive Multi-modal Biometrics, `http://serac.jrc.it/index.php?option=com_content&task=view&id=137&Itemid=238`
29. SPT: Ideal Process Flow V 2.0 (December 1, 2006), `http://www.iata.org/NR/rdonlyres/31BD66A2-4446-4514-A911-3EA9DDAC7CAA/0/IPF_V20_FINAL.pdf`

Author Index